Female Urinary Incontinence

Anne P. Cameron

Editor

Female Urinary Incontinence

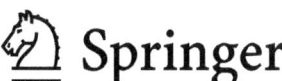 Springer

Editor
Anne P. Cameron
Urology
University of Michigan
Ann Arbor, MI, USA

ISBN 978-3-030-84351-9   ISBN 978-3-030-84352-6   (eBook)
https://doi.org/10.1007/978-3-030-84352-6

This Springer imprint is published by the registered company Springer Nature Switzerland AG
The registered company address is: Gewerbestrasse 11, 6330 Cham, Switzerland

Contents

Part I   Diagnosis and Etiology of Incontinence in Women

1   **Epidemiology, Definitions, and Cost of Incontinence in Women**   3
Cynthia S. Fok, Rachael Gotlieb, and Nissrine Nakib

2   **Anatomy and Physiology of Female Urinary Incontinence**   19
Felicity Reeves and Tamsin Greenwell

3   **Diagnosis of Urinary Incontinence in Women**   51
Elizabeth Dray and Haritha Pavuluri

4   **Urodynamic Testing of Female Incontinence**   61
Anne P. Cameron

5   **Historical Treatment of SUI and UUI in Women**   85
Justina Tam and Una J. Lee

Part II   Conservative Treatment

6   **Behavioral Therapy and Lifestyle Modifications
for the Management of Urinary Incontinence in Women**   107
Kimberly Kenne and Catherine S. Bradley

7   **Physical Therapy and Continence Inserts**   127
Paige De Rosa, Ilana Bergelson, and Elizabeth Takacs

Part III   Medical and Surgical Treatment of UUI

8   **Medical Therapy with Antimuscarinics and ß3-Agonists**   147
Sophia Delpe Goodridge and Leslie M. Rickey

9   **Posterior Tibial Nerve Stimulation for Female Urge
Urinary Incontinence**   165
Giulia Lane

10 Sacral and Pudendal Neuromodulation (SNM) 177
    Priyanka Gupta

11 Botulinum Toxin for Overactive Bladder 193
    Sophia Janes, Sara M. Lenherr, and Anne P. Cameron

12 Augmentation Cystoplasty in the Non-neurogenic
    Bladder Patient 207
    Aisha L. Siebert, Elizabeth Rourke, and Stephanie J. Kielb

13 Advanced Options for Treatment of Refractory Urgency
    Urinary Incontinence 221
    Elizabeth Rourke, Alice Wang, and Melissa Kaufman

Part IV Surgical Treatment for SUI

14 Urethral Bulking Agents. 235
    Alexandra L. Tabakin and Siobhan M. Hartigan

15 Burch Colposuspension 257
    Ali Luck and Samantha Raffee

16 The Innovation of Midurethral Slings: Where We've
    Been and Where We Are Today 273
    Suzette E. Sutherland and Ellen C. Thompson

17 Autologous Fascial Sling. 295
    Annah Vollstedt and Priya Padmanabhan

18 Managing Complications After Surgical Treatment
    of Stress Urinary Incontinence 317
    Alyssa K. Gracely

19 Failure of Treatment of Stress Urinary Incontinence 343
    Caroline Dowling and Sandra Elmer

Part V Other Contributors and Causes of Incontinence

20 Prolapse as a Contributing Factor to Stress and Urgency
    Urinary Incontinence 371
    Whitney Horner and Carolyn W. Swenson

21 Incontinence After Complex Urinary Reconstruction:
    Orthotopic Neobladder and Gender-Affirming Surgery 387
    Amanda C. Chi, Nancy Ye, Virginia Li, Krystal DePorto,
    and Polina Reyblat

22 Rare Conditions Causing Incontinence and Their Treatment 407
    Ariana L. Smith and Andrea C. Yeguez

Part VI   Incontinence in Special Populations

23   Incontinence in Older Girls and Adolescents 429
Esther K. Liu and Kristina D. Suson

24   Female Neurogenic Incontinence 453
Jenny N. Nguyen and Doreen E. Chung

25   Urinary Incontinence in the Elderly 465
Casey G. Kowalik and Lara S. MacLachlan

**26   Maximizing Intraoperative Performance and Safety
During Incontinence Surgery** 477
Kristin Chrouser and Keow Mei Goh

**27   Experimental Therapies and Research Needs for Urinary
Incontinence in Women** 497
Casey G. Kowalik and Rena D. Malik

Index 519

Summary

Female urinary incontinence has a significant impact on a woman's quality of life and her overall health. Incontinence puts women at risk for urinary tract infections and limits their activities of daily living such as work, exercise, and intimacy. This problem also has substantial economic impact for a woman, with expensive pads or other protective devices and contributes significantly to healthcare expenditures.

Unfortunately, incontinence in women is infrequently discussed in medical visits despite most women wanting to address their leakage. There have been substantial shifts in the diagnosis and treatment of women with incontinence in the past 5 years. There are new medical therapies (beta three agonists), new minimally invasive therapies such as PTNS, dramatic shifts in the utilization of mesh products, and countless new therapies in human trials.

This book will be a comprehensive review of the: etiology, anatomy, diagnosis (including an in depth review of urodynamics), treatments from conservative to the most complex surgery, and future directions of care of female incontinence. There are several guidelines on female incontinence such as the AUA/SUFU guidelines on stress incontinence and overactive bladder that will be references in treatment algorithms. In this book, we will also focus on incontinence in poorly understood populations such as older children, the elderly, women post-reconstruction, and trans women. For completeness, we will include parts on non-standard causes of incontinence that are often neglected in these reviews such as fistulas and urethral diverticulum.

The book will be structured as follows. It will begin with an in depth review of the etiology and diagnosis of incontinence. This will include a review of the cost of incontinence, a detailed chapter on diagnosis, and a separate chapter on urodynamics given the paucity of good references on this topic. This chapter will include detailed visual examples for the reader. Along with a chapter covering anatomy of the bladder and urethra/pelvic floor, a historical review of treatments of the past will be included since so many women have undergone these therapies and have altered anatomy.

Conservative treatments will be discussed in detail in Part II, including patient and provider handouts on behavioral modification and how to perform pelvic floor exercises.

Part III will cover medical therapy, minimally invasive treatments all the way through radical surgical approaches with a chapter focusing on the little-known subject of management of treatment failures. Part IV will be centered on the treatment of stress incontinence with chapters progressing from least invasive to most invasive therapies and a chapter on mesh complications and treatment failures which is a controversial topic.

Many other pelvic floor disorders can result in incontinence although they are not typically discussed in works focusing on female incontinence. Given the importance of other pelvic floor anomalies in the differential diagnosis of incontinence, I have included chapters in Part V on the intersection of prolapse with female incontinence, incontinence diagnosis and management following major reconstruction such as neobladder or penile inversion vaginoplasty, and incontinence due to more rare conditions such as fistulas.

Part VI will focus on special populations with incontinence who have different treatment paradigms and cautions such as pediatric patients, the elderly, and women with neurogenic lower urinary tract dysfunction. I have included a chapter on fecal incontinence and its intersection with urinary incontinence since so few practitioners address both problems simultaneously, but should. The concluding chapter will focus on research needs and the ever expanding horizon of new developments in the field of incontinence in women.

This book will serve as a comprehensive text directed towards primary care providers, gynecologists, urologists, learners, and those trained in female pelvic medicine and reconstructive surgery (FPMRS). It will, when appropriate, contain patient or provider handouts and treatment flow charts which are excellent reference tools for clinical care.

Given the topic of incontinence specifically in women and the burgeoning rise of women in the field of FPMRS, I propose an all-female author list to provide the opportunity for these women to showcase their knowledge. I am a board member of the Society of Women in Urology and SUFU with many superb contacts and have many of these gifted women, all experts in the field in mind for chapter authors (see outline below). They are comprised of an international group of female urologists and urogynecologist who were each picked for chapters based on their particular expertise.

Audience Primary care providers, urologists, gynecologists, female urologists, pediatric urologists, urogynecologist, functional gastroenterologist, basic and translational scientists, medical students entering any of these fields, urology and gynecology residents, and fellows.

Contributors

Ilana Bergelson Department of Urology, University of Iowa, Iowa City, IA, USA

Catherine S. Bradley Obstetrics and Gynecology: Female Pelvic Medicine and Reconstructive Surgery, University of Iowa, Iowa City, IA, USA

Anne P. Cameron Urology, University of Michigan, Ann Arbor, MI, USA

Amanda C. Chi Department of Urology, Kaiser Permanente Southern California, Los Angeles, CA, USA

Kristin Chrouser University of Michigan Department of Urology, VA Ann Arbor Healthcare System, Ann Arbor, MI, USA

Doreen E. Chung Department of Urology, Columbia University Irving Medical Center, New York, NY, USA

Krystal DePorto Department of Urology, Kaiser Permanente Southern California, Los Angeles, CA, USA

Paige De Rosa Department of Urology, University of Iowa, Iowa City, IA, USA

Caroline Dowling Eastern Health, Department of Urology, Box Hill, VIC, Australia

Monash University, Eastern Health Clinical School, Level 2, Box Hill, VIC, Australia

Epworth Healthcare, Richmond, VIC, Australia

Elizabeth Dray University of South Carolina School of Medicine Greenville, Greenville, SC, USA

Sandra Elmer Epworth Healthcare, Richmond, VIC, Australia

Department of Urology, Royal Melbourne Hospital, Parkville, VIC, Australia

Department of Urology, Austin Health, Heidelberg, VIC, Australia

Cynthia S. Fok Department of Urology, University of Minnesota, Minneapolis, MN, USA

Keow Mei Goh University of Michigan Department of Urology, VA Ann Arbor Healthcare System, Ann Arbor, MI, USA

Sophia Delpe Goodridge Wellstar Urology, Roswell, GA, USA

Rachael Gotlieb Medical School, University of Minnesota, Minneapolis, MN, USA

Alyssa K. Gracely Chesapeake Urology Associates, Salisbury, MD, USA

Tamsin Greenwell Department of Urology, University College London Hospitals (UCLH) and University College London (UCL), London, UK

Priyanka Gupta University of Michigan, Ann Arbor, MI, USA

Siobhan M. Hartigan Hunterdon Urological Associates, Flemington, NJ, USA

Whitney Horner Female Pelvic Medicine & Reconstructive Surgery, Department of Obstetrics & Gynecology, University of Michigan, Ann Arbor, MI, USA

Sophia Janes Division of Urology, Department of Surgery, University of Utah Health, Salt Lake City, UT, USA

Melissa Kaufman Vanderbilt University Medical Center, Urology, Nashville, TN, USA

Kimberly Kenne Obstetrics and Gynecology: Female Pelvic Medicine and Reconstructive Surgery, University of Iowa, Iowa City, IA, USA

Stephanie J. Kielb Department of Urology, Northwestern University Feinberg School of medicine, Chicago, IL, USA

Casey G. Kowalik Department of Urology, University of Kansas Health System, Kansas City, KS, USA

Giulia Lane Department of Urology, University of Michigan, Ann Arbor, MI, USA

Una J. Lee Section of Urology and Renal Transplantation, Virginia Mason Medical Center, Seattle, WA, USA

Sara M. Lenherr Division of Urology, Department of Surgery, University of Utah Health, Salt Lake City, UT, USA

Virginia Li Department of Urology, Kaiser Permanente Southern California, Los Angeles, CA, USA

Esther K. Liu Detroit Medical Center Urology, Detroit, MI, USA

Ali Luck Department of Women's Health, Obstetrics & Gynecology, Female Pelvic Medicine Reconstructive Surgery, Henry Ford Health Systems, Detroit, MI, USA

Lara S. MacLachlan Institute of Urology, Lahey Hospital & Medical Center, Burlington, MA, USA

Rena D. Malik Department of Surgery, Division of Urology, University of Maryland School of Medicine, Baltimore, MD, USA

Nissrine Nakib Department of Urology, University of Minnesota, Minneapolis, MN, USA

Jenny N. Nguyen Department of Urology, Columbia University Irving Medical Center, New York, NY, USA

Priya Padmanabhan Beaumont Hospital, Department of Urology, Royal Oak, MI, USA

Haritha Pavuluri University of South Carolina School of Medicine Greenville, Greenville, SC, USA

Samantha Raffee Department of Urology, Female Pelvic Medicine Reconstructive Surgery, Henry Ford Health Systems, Detroit, MI, USA

Felicity Reeves Department of Urology, University College London Hospitals (UCLH), London, UK

Polina Reyblat Department of Urology, Kaiser Permanente Southern California, Los Angeles, CA, USA

Leslie M. Rickey Departments of Urology and Obstetrics, Gynecology & Reproductive Sciences, Yale School of Medicine, New Haven, CT, USA

Elizabeth Rourke Department of Urology, Vanderbilt University, Nashville, TN, USA
Vanderbilt University Medical Center, Urology, Nashville, TN, USA

Aisha L. Siebert Department of Urology, Northwestern University Feinberg School of medicine, Chicago, IL, USA

Ariana L. Smith Division of Urology, Department of Surgery, University of Pennsylvania Health System, Philadelphia, PA, USA

Kristina D. Suson Children's Hospital of Michigan, Pediatric Urology, Detroit, MI, USA

Suzette E. Sutherland Female Urology/Urogynecology, UW Medicine Pelvic Health Center, Seattle, WA, USA
Department of Urology, University of Washington School of Medicine, Seattle, WA, USA

Carolyn W. Swenson Female Pelvic Medicine & Reconstructive Surgery, Department of Obstetrics & Gynecology, University of Michigan, Ann Arbor, MI, USA

Alexandra L. Tabakin Division of Urology, Rutgers Robert Wood Johnson Medical School, New Brunswick, NJ, USA

Elizabeth Takacs Department of Urology, University of Iowa, Iowa City, IA, USA

Justina Tam Section of Urology and Renal Transplantation, Virginia Mason Medical Center, Seattle, WA, USA

Ellen C. Thompson Department of Urology, University of Minnesota School of Medicine, Minneapolis, MN, USA

Annah Vollstedt Beaumont Hospital, Department of Urology, Royal Oak, MI, USA

Alice Wang Vanderbilt University Medical Center, Urology, Nashville, TN, USA

Nancy Ye Department of Urology, Kaiser Permanente Southern California, Los Angeles, CA, USA

Andrea C. Yeguez Division of Urology, Department of Surgery, University of Pennsylvania Health System, Philadelphia, PA, USA

Part I
Diagnosis and Etiology of Incontinence in Women

Chapter 1
Epidemiology, Definitions, and Cost of Incontinence in Women

Cynthia S. Fok, Rachael Gotlieb, and Nissrine Nakib

Introduction

Pelvic floor disorders in women are common. Pelvic floor disorders include pelvic organ prolapse, urinary incontinence, and anal incontinence. This chapter focuses specifically on the epidemiology of urinary incontinence (UI). In this chapter, we discuss (1) definitions of urinary incontinence, (2) rates of urinary incontinence, (3) risk factors for urinary incontinence, (4) costs of urinary incontinence, and (5) social disparities in female urinary incontinence.

Definitions of Urinary Incontinence in Women

In women, urinary incontinence, defined as involuntary loss of urine, is a common bothersome complaint [1]. Urinary incontinence can manifest in many ways and can come from many etiologies. Characterizing and defining the symptom of urinary incontinence can help in a woman's evaluation and treatment.

In 2010, the International Urogynecological Association (IUGA) and the International Continence Society (ICS) convened a joint task force to report on the terminology of female pelvic floor dysfunction. This document has provided much of the terminology on female urinary incontinence [1]. Please see the summary of the definitions listed in Table 1.1.

C. S. Fok (✉) · N. Nakib
Department of Urology, University of Minnesota, Minneapolis, MN, USA
e-mail: csfok@umn.edu; naki0003@umn.edu

R. Gotlieb
Medical School, University of Minnesota, Minneapolis, MN, USA

© The Author(s), under exclusive license to Springer Nature Switzerland AG 2022
A. P. Cameron (ed.), *Female Urinary Incontinence*,
https://doi.org/10.1007/978-3-030-84352-6_1

Table 1.1 Definitions of urinary incontinence

Type of urinary incontinence	Definition
Stress incontinence	Complaint of involuntary loss of urine on the effort of physical exertion, or on sneezing or coughing
Urgency incontinence	Complaint of involuntary loss of urine associated with urgency
Postural incontinence	Complaint of involuntary loss of urine associated with the change of body position
Nocturnal enuresis	Complaint of involuntary urinary loss of urine which occurs during sleep
Mixed incontinence	Complaint of involuntary loss of urine associated with urgency and also with effort or physical exertion or on sneezing or coughing
Continuous incontinence	Complaint of continuous involuntary loss of urine
Insensible incontinence	Complaint of urinary incontinence where the woman has been unaware of how it occurs
Coital incontinence	Complaint of involuntary loss of urine with coitus
Functional incontinence	Complaint of involuntary loss of urine that is associated with a separate physiologic or pathologic process

Functional incontinence is urinary incontinence that is associated with a separate physiologic or pathologic process. This is important as these causes may be reversible. Common causes of functional incontinence can be remembered by the mnemonic *DIAPPERS* [2]

- *D*rugs (e.g., bethanechol)
- *I*nfection (e.g., urinary tract infection)
- *A*trophy (e.g., menopause)
- *P*sychological disorders (e.g., delirium, depression, dementia)
- *P*harmacological (e.g., diuretics, narcotics, sedatives)
- *E*ndocrine (e.g., hyperglycemia, hypercalcemia)
- *R*estricted mobility
- *S*tool impaction

Overactive bladder, although not a disease itself, is a condition that is often included in the discussions of urinary incontinence. Overactive bladder syndrome is "urinary urgency, usually accompanied by frequency and nocturia, with or without urgency urinary incontinence, in the absence of urinary tract infection or other obvious pathology [1]."

Rates of Urinary Incontinence

In discussing rates of urinary incontinence, we first must define prevalence and incidence. *Prevalence* is defined as *all* cases in a given population at a specific time divided by the number of individuals at risk for disease in that population. *Incidence* is the number of *new* cases in a population over a period of time divided by the total number of individuals followed in that time period.

Urinary incontinence in women is common. For the subsequent data described, we will be focusing primarily on prevalence rates of urinary incontinence in the United States. The reported prevalence of urinary incontinence in the literature is a variable based on how the question was asked and in what population. The reported prevalence of any type of urinary incontinence ranges from 5% to 64% in large epidemiological studies. Please see a summary of the large epidemiological studies in female urinary incontinence listed in Table 1.2.

Table 1.2 Summary of large epidemiological studies in female urinary incontinence

Study	Prevalence urinary incontinence by type	Total incontinence
Women's Health Initiative n = 23,296 postmenopausal women 50–79 years old	SUI: 51% UUI: 49% MUI: 14%	Highest reported prevalence with 64% of women reported having any experience of an episode of UI [3]
National Health and Nutrition Examination Survey (NHANES) (2005–2016) Cross-sectional survey of US women 20 years and older 2001–2004 cohort n = 4229 2005–2016 cohort n = 15,003	SUI: 26% UUI: 10% MUI: 16%	49.6% reported any UI [4] 53% reported any UI [5] 30% reported moderate to severe urinary incontinence in the 2005–2016 cohort which is an increase from the 17.1% in the 2005–2010 cohort [5, 6]
Group Health Cooperative n = 3536 women 30–90 years old	SUI: 14% UUI: 5% MUI: 21%	45% of reported urinary incontinence defined as "leakage of any amount that occurred at least monthly" [7]
Nurses' Health Study Female registered nurses 30–55 years enrolled in 1976. UI questions were first asked in 1996 Incidence of new UI in this cohort was assessed from 2000 to 2002 [9]	Incidence of: SUI: 2% UUI 0.7% MUI 0.9%	34.1% at least one episode of urine leakage monthly during the previous 12 months [8] 9.2% reported at least monthly episodes of UI during the prior 12 months 27.6% reported new UI during the prior 12 months [9]
Epidemiology of Lower Urinary Tract Symptoms (EpiLUTS) [10] Adults 40 years and older n = 15,861 women	SUI: 31.8% UUI: 24.4%	
Kaiser Permanente Continence Associated Risks Epidemiologic Study (KP CARES) [11] 25–84 years old women	SUI: 15%	
Reproductive Risks for Incontinence Study at Kaiser (RRISK) [12] Women between 40 and 69 years		28.6% reported at least one episode of urinary incontinence weekly

Rates of Urinary Incontinence by Age

The prevalence of urinary incontinence has been found to increase with age. The Group Health Cooperative found 28% of women 30–39 years old reported urinary incontinence, whereas 55% of women 80–90 years old reported urinary incontinence. In women 30–39 years of age, 45% reported stress incontinence, 10% reported urgency incontinence, 41% reported mixed incontinence, and 8% reported severe urinary incontinence. This is in contrast to women 80-90 years of age where only 16% reported stress incontinence, 20% reported urgency incontinence, 53% reported mixed incontinence, and 33% reported severe urinary incontinence [7]. The Nurse's Health Study showed that as age increases the incidence of stress incontinence decreases, while the incidence of urgency incontinence increases with age [9]. Although the EPIC study is not a population-based study of US adults, this is a study of adults 18 years and older from Canada, Germany, Italy, Sweden, and the United Kingdom. This study also demonstrates a strong relationship between urinary incontinence and age in women. The prevalence rates were 7.3% for women 39 years and younger, 13.7% for women 40–59 years, and 19.3% for women over 60 years [13].

The NHANES cohort showed the stress incontinence is most common in women 40–59 years (32%) but urgency incontinence and mixed incontinence were higher in those over 60 years (19% and 25%, respectively). Furthermore, women less than 40 years were less likely to be bothered by their symptoms, and older women were more likely to report moderate or severe/very severe symptoms [5]. The Health, Aging, and Body Composition Study shows that 21% of women 70–79 years old report at least weekly urinary incontinence. In this cohort, the rates of predominantly urgency incontinence were similar stress incontinence (42% urgency incontinence, 40% stress incontinence) [14].

Rates of Urinary Incontinence by Race or Ethnicity

NHANES data from 2001 to 2004 showed that the odds of stress urinary incontinence were approximately 2.5 times higher in white and Mexican-American women than African American women when controlling for age, parity, BMI, and activity level with different prevalence of urinary incontinence based on race/ethnicity [4]. Updated NHANES 2005–2016 again reported that non-Hispanic Black women had the highest prevalence of urgency incontinence at 18% compared to 9% for other groups. This group also had the lowest prevalence of stress incontinence at 16% compared to 28% for other groups [5].

Reproductive Risks for Incontinence Study at Kaiser also reported that African American and Asian American women were less likely than Caucasian women to report urinary incontinence [10]. Studies also show that Caucasian women (41%) are more likely to report urinary incontinence than African American (31%) or

Latina women (30%) but Latina women (9%) are less likely to report mixed incontinence than African American (14%) or Caucasian (15%) women [15]. This difference in incontinence rates continues as women age with the Health, Aging, and Body Composition Study showing that in women 70–79 years old Caucasian women are twice as likely to report weekly incontinence than African American women (27% versus 14%) [14].

The Establishing the Prevalence of Incontinence (EPI) study from 2002 to 2004 showed the overall prevalence of urinary incontinence in women in southeastern Michigan was 14.6% for African American women and 33.1% for Caucasian women. Although the number of leakage episodes did not differ between the groups, the quantity of urine loss was significantly higher in African American women. Half of the Caucasian women (50.1%) reporting incontinence reported losing a few drops, whereas half of African American women (50.6%) reporting incontinence reported losing urine to the point of wetting their underwear or pad. There was furthermore a difference seen in the rates of stress incontinence and urgency incontinence between the two groups but no difference in mixed urinary incontinence. Approximately 39.2% of Caucasian women reported stress incontinence compared to 25% of African American Women; in contrast, 23.8% of African American women reported urgency incontinence compared to 11% of Caucasian women [16].

The Hispanic Established Populations for the Epidemiologic Study of the Elderly (Hispanic EPESE) showed that 15% of Mexican American Women reported any symptoms of urinary incontinence within the last month. Those with incontinence did tend to be older, completed less formal education, and had higher acculturation rates. The women experiencing incontinence also tended to have more impact on their daily lives, prior use of estrogen, prior pregnancies, and more deliveries. In this population experiencing urinary incontinence, mixed urinary incontinence was most common (41.8%), followed by urgency incontinence (33.1%), and then stress incontinence (10%) [17].

Huang et al. reported that 70% of Asian American Women reported any urinary incontinence symptoms in the past 12 months. Approximately 27% report daily symptoms and 38% report weekly symptoms. Of those that report urinary incontinence, there is an even number that report stress (27%) and urgency (25%) incontinence [18].

Risk Factors for Urinary Incontinence

There are multiple risk factors that may predispose a woman to urinary incontinence. Risks factors such as age, race/ethnicity, pregnancy/delivery, family history, physical activity, smoking, and obesity are commonly implicated. Urinary incontinence is also associated with pelvic floor disorders including prolapse, irritable bowel syndrome, prior pelvic surgery including hysterectomy, neurological illnesses including multiple sclerosis, Parkinson's illness, dementia, and other illnesses such as diabetes and urinary tract infections.

Age

As noted above in the prevalence section, increasing age is a well-established and unfortunately non-modifiable risk factor for urinary incontinence. Age is associated with a higher prevalence of any urinary incontinence. Older women are also more likely to report more bothersome urinary incontinence, more severe urinary incontinence, and urgency or mixed urinary incontinence symptoms [5, 7].

Parity and Mode of Delivery

Blomquist et al. derived data from the Mother's Outcome after Delivery (MOAD) study, a longitudinal cohort study of parous women, from October 2008 to December 2013. Participants were recruited from a community hospital 5–10 years after their first delivery (index birth) and followed up annually for up to 9 years. Follow-up ended in April 2017. Among 1528 women (778 in the cesarean birth group, 565 in the spontaneous vaginal birth group, and 185 in the operative vaginal birth group), the median age at first delivery was 30.6 years, 1092 women (72%) were multiparous at enrollment (2887 total deliveries), and the median age at enrollment was 38.3 years. For spontaneous vaginal delivery, the 15-year cumulative incidences of SUI were 34.3% (95% CI, 29.9–38.6%) and OAB 21.8% (95% CI, 17.8–25.7%). Compared with spontaneous vaginal delivery, cesarean delivery was associated with a significantly lower hazard of SUI and OAB [19].

Family History

Women with UI, including stress, urgency, and mixed UI, show familial aggregation. Studies of twins using a Danish population-based twin registry suggest that urgency and mixed UI have a significant genetic component [20]. Furthermore, a Swedish twin registry revealed the presence of a strong genetic risk for stress UI [21]. Genetic loci have been suggested for both urgency UI [22] and stress UI [23].

The Pelvic Floor Disorders Network published a genome-wide association study (GWAS) of 2241 cases of urgency UI and 776 controls from the Women's Health Initiative that identified six loci associated with urgency UI [24]. Penney et al. performed a GWAS using the Nurses' Health Study (NHS) to identify genetic variants associated with the risk of UI [25]. They identified eight single nucleotide polymorphisms (SNPs) located on two loci, chromosome 8q23.3 and 1p32.2, that were significantly associated with UI. For the UI subtypes, no SNP reached genome-wide significance. This GWAS provides initial evidence of genetic associations for UI and merits further research.

Physical Activity

High-impact exercising is associated with an increased risk of urinary incontinence. This association is seen even in younger nulliparous women. The prevalence of urinary incontinence in nulliparous women who participate in high-impact exercising is 38.6% compared to women who do not, 19.9%, but is likely due to the increase in activity rather than causative and women should not be advised to avoid physical activity [26].

Smoking

In the Nurses' Health II Study (NHS II), current smoking appeared to increase frequent or severe leaking urine by 20% and 34%, respectively [27]. Other studies have shown similar results. The SWAN study reported a 38% increased risk of moderate/severe incontinence among current smokers relative to never smokers [28]. According to the Norwegian Epidemiology of Incontinence (EPINCONT) study, there was a 40% increased risk of severe incontinence in current smokers relative to never smokers among 27,936 women aged 20–64 years [29]. There are several reasons why this might be the case. One may be the decrease in collagen production associated with smoking which in turn may weaken supporting structures and ligaments in the pelvic floor. Another may be the direct effects of a smoker's cough which may damage the urethral sphincter. There are also other direct and indirect effects on the bladder and urethral function from other smoking-related comorbidities, including vascular disease, asthma, and COPD [30]. All women who smoke should be advised to quit given the negative impact on continence and multiple other health risks.

Pelvic Surgery

Pelvic surgery impacts the pelvic floor in many different ways. Most epidemiologic studies use prior hysterectomy as proxy for prior pelvic surgery. There is not a clear relationship between urinary incontinence and prior hysterectomy. The Group Health Cooperative found that history of hysterectomy was associated with increased odds of not only having urinary incontinence (odds ratio 1.33, $p = 0.004$) but also having severe urinary incontinence (odds ratio 1.55, $p = 0.002$) [7]. This is contrasted to the Nurse's Health study which did not find any relationship between the history of hysterectomy and urinary incontinence [9].

Comorbid Conditions

There are many comorbid conditions that may be associated with an increased risk of urinary incontinence.

Obesity

It is well-established that obesity confers an increased risk of urinary incontinence [31]. Obesity is defined as ≥ 30 kg/m2, and the World Health Organization (WHO) estimates that 1.9 billion and 600 million adults >18 years of age are overweight and obese, respectively, throughout the world [32]. Etiologically, four factors associated with obesity are hypothesized to increase the risk of UI: increased abdominal fat, which increases intravesical pressure; urethral hypermobility and increased abdominal pressure, which cause detrusor instability; and intervertebral disk herniation, which affects innervation of the bladder [33]. Urodynamic studies support the existence of these processes, having found that weight loss leads to a decrease of intravesical pressure and an increase of cystometric capacity. In a study by Bulbuller et al., 120 obese females undergoing laparoscopic sleeve gastrectomy (LSG) were asked to complete the International Consultation on Incontinence Questionnaire-Urinary Incontinence-Short Form (ICIQ-UI-SF) and Incontinence Impact Questionnaire (IIQ-7) prior to surgery and 6 months after the surgery [34]. They found that of the 120 patients, 72 (60%) complained of UI preoperatively. Among these 72 patients, 23 (31.95%) described urge incontinence, 18 (25%) stress incontinence, and 31 (43.05%) mixed-type incontinence. At 6 months postoperatively, the percentage of excess weight loss was 70.33% (SD =14.84%). For all three UI subtypes, the 6-month postoperative ICIQ-UI-SF and IIQ-7 scores decreased significantly compared to the preoperative scores ($P < 0.05$). Scores for the preoperative and postoperative ICIQ-UI-SF questionnaire are as follows: For UI, it was 8.76 and 2.64; SI 8.77 and 2.57; and MI 10.58 and 3.74. Scores for the IIQ-7 questionnaire showed the following: For UI, it was 6.73 and 2.53; SI 7.10 and 2.27; and MI 7.68 and 3.16. Hence, women who are overweight or obese can be counselled that weight loss will improve their UUI or SUI and should be encouraged to make this effort.

Constipation

According to a meta-analysis of 16 observational studies with 35,629 participants and 6054 urinary incontinence patients, constipation is significantly associated with urinary incontinence risk in women, OR 2.46 (95% CI 1.79–3.38). However, further prospective studies are needed to clarify the causality [35]. Since constipation is a bothersome problem in and of itself providing women with advice to regulate their stool consistency will be of benefit.

Pelvic Pain

Based on our clinical impression, one may expect to see a significant correlation between pelvic floor muscle pain (PFMP) and "irritative" voiding symptoms. However, in a study by Meister et al. which is an analysis of association between PFMP and urinary frequency as well urgency *incontinence*, there did not seem to be a correlation after controlling for postmenopausal status [36]. They hypothesized that further study with a longer urinary distress index questionnaire, which includes additional irritative symptoms, may be necessary to better address a correlation.

Chronic Respiratory Disease

The presence of chronic lung disease (CLD) in women has been shown to be associated with urinary incontinence. This is even more pronounced in older women and is associated with more distress than their age-matched peers without CLD. A study by Button et al. prospectively observed women with cystic fibrosis (CF, $n = 38$), chronic obstructive pulmonary disease (COPD, $n = 27$), and 69 healthy women without CLD [37]. The majority of women in all three groups reported episodes of incontinence (CF 71%; COPD 70%; healthy women 55%). Compared to age-matched healthy controls, women with CF reported more episodes of incontinence, more commonly stress incontinence. Furthermore, women with CLD were twice as likely to develop incontinence than healthy women.

Diabetes Mellitus (DM)

The Group Health Cooperative found that DM is not a risk factor for urinary incontinence but is a risk factor for having severe urinary incontinence (odds ratio 1.83, $p = 0.01$) [7].

The pathophysiology of how DM is related to urinary incontinence is that DM may increase the risk of UI as a result of detrusor overactivity [38].

The Cost of Urinary Incontinence

Urinary incontinence can be costly to both an individual woman and society. There are direct costs and indirect costs. Direct costs are the costs directly related to management or treatment of a condition, such as in self-care products (e.g., incontinence pads), medical care (e.g., diagnosis, treatment, testing, physical therapy), medication costs, and treatment of urinary incontinence associated complications (e.g., skin breakdown, falls). Indirect costs are the lost productivity and wages associated with seeking care and treatment. In addition to the economic costs, many women also may experience pain, suffering, and decreased quality of life secondary to their urinary incontinence.

Any Urinary Incontinence

Urinary incontinence is a common and expensive condition. The annual costs of urinary incontinence in the United States have been quoted as high as $19.5 billion a year. Of that cost, $4.2 billion a year for community-dwelling adults and $5.3 billion for institutionalized elderly [39]. United States' expenditures for female urinary incontinence in 2004 were estimated to be over $206 million and increased to $246 million in 2013 [40]. At one point, the national costs of urinary urgency incontinence in the United States were estimated to be $65.9 in 2007 and were predicted to rise to $82.6 billion in 2020 [41]. The fact that the US adult incontinence market was estimated to be a $7.2 billion industry in 2015 has prompted the development and sales of many newer and reusable incontinence products [42].

The Diagnostic Aspects of Incontinence Study (DAISy) group reported in 2006 that women with severe urinary incontinence may pay $900 annually for routine care. Costs include things such as incontinence products, toilet paper, paper towels, and laundry. This mean annual care for all women with incontinence of $494.12 a year is particularly significant as the reported annual income for most women in this survey was less than $100,000, with 53% under $40,000 [43].

Reproductive Risks for Incontinence Study at Kaiser found women were paying on average over $250 annually in out-of-pocket costs for urinary incontinence. Weekly costs ranged from $0.93 per week to $7.82 per week as the severity of incontinence went from moderate to severe. Costs increased for women who experienced mixed urinary incontinence, had more severe urinary incontinence, had higher body mass index, and were African-American [44].

Stress Incontinence

Looking at nonsurgical treatments for stress incontinence, there was a cost-effectiveness analysis comparing pelvic floor therapy, a disposable incontinence tampon, a self-fitting pessary, or a provider-fitted incontinence pessary. This study found the most cost-effective nonsurgical treatment to be pelvic floor therapy [45].

The Stress Incontinence Surgical Efficacy (SISTEr) Trial from the Urinary Incontinence Treatment Network (UITN) looked at the cost of self-management strategies for women with stress incontinence and found women spent nearly $750 annually in out-of-pocket costs for stress incontinence management. They also found that women were willing to pay $118 +/− $132 per month for complete resolution of symptoms. Women with higher household incomes or more episodes of urinary incontinence were willing to spend more [46]. Furthermore, the SISTEr Trial showed that on average the costs of self-management decrease by 72% ($625 per woman per year) at 2 years after stress incontinence surgery [47].

Urgency Incontinence

After behavioral modification and pelvic floor therapy, anticholinergic and beta-agonists are the next line in the treatment of urinary urgency incontinence. There are multiple medications available including generic medications. One study looking at the costs of medications to Medicare beneficiaries showed that from 2000 to 2015, women spent on average $168 a year on medications [48].

Urgency incontinence medication costs were compared to costs for percutaneous tibial nerve stimulation (PTNS), intravesical botulinum toxin injection, and sacral neuromodulation over a 24-month period. During this time frame, costs for patients that were started on medications and stayed on the medications were on average $1787. The mean costs rose to $6626 for those treated to PTNS, $7032 for those who went to combination mirabegron/antimuscarinics, $10,183 for onabotulinum-toxinA, and $39, 952 for those who underwent sacral neuromodulation [49].

ROSETTA showed that for sacral neuromodulation the cumulative per person cost during the 2-year study period was $35,680 as compared to $7460 for intravesical botulinum toxin injection [50].

Social Disparities in Female Pelvic Floor Disorders

When reading the existing literature on female pelvic floor disorders, one must be mindful of the social disparities that exist. There are differences in knowledge, health care access, and health care-seeking behaviors based on factors such as age, race/ethnicity, socioeconomic status, and location of residence. These disparities may impact the generalizability of some of the existing literature on female pelvic floor disorders.

The current literature shows that there are disparities in the knowledge, care-seeking behaviors, and treatment of women with pelvic floor disorders including urinary incontinence.

Several studies have shown that there are racial disparities that exist in women's knowledge regarding risk factors and treatment options for urinary incontinence. One analysis of responses of community-dwelling adult women in Connecticut to the Prolapse and Incontinence Knowledge Questionnaire show that African American women were significantly less likely to recognize childbirth as a risk factor for urinary incontinence. Women of color were also significantly less likely to know about risk factors, preventative strategies, and curative treatment options for urinary incontinence [51].

Study of Women's Health Across the Nation (SWAN) study did not find racial or ethnic, socioeconomic, and education status as factors preventing midlife women from seeking treatment of urinary incontinence. In this study, the duration of symptoms and having regular medical care were the factors that were more significantly associated with seeking treatment [52].

Analysis of the NHANES data from 2005 to 2016 showed that the odds of self-reported urgency incontinence symptoms increased with lower socioeconomic status [53].

A retrospective study examining pelvic floor therapy attendance rates at an urban tertiary care center showed that Latina women tended to be less likely to initiate or complete pelvic floor therapy than those who did not identify as Latina [54].

One study looked at the use of sacral neuromodulation among Medicare beneficiaries from 2001 through 2010 and found that during this period those that underwent implantation were more likely female, White, under the age of 65, and lived outside the western United States [55].

Anger et al. found that in female Medicare beneficiaries, there are differences in the diagnosis of stress incontinence, likelihood of undergoing sling surgery, and postoperative complications of sling surgery based on race. From 1999 to 2001, Caucasian women were more likely to be given a diagnosis of stress incontinence than non-Caucasian women. During this time, Caucasian and Latina women were much more likely to undergo sling surgery than African American or Asian American women; however, non-Caucasian women were twice as likely to have postoperative complications after sling surgery. Non-Caucasian women were statistically more likely to have non-urologic complications, pelvic organ prolapse, and urinary obstruction than Caucasian women during the first year after sling surgery. This trend was also seen in the diagnosis of urgency incontinence or repeat incontinence procedure but did not reach statistical significance [56]. Stanford University looked at complication rates of women who underwent outpatient urethral sling placement from 2005 to 2011. This study found that women who had at least one unplanned hospital visit during the first 30 days after surgery were more likely to be African American and have Medicaid insurance [57].

Conclusion

Urinary incontinence is a common problem that many women experience. The prevalence of urinary incontinence is influenced by many factors including age, race/ethnicity, family history, and other comorbidities. The costs of urinary incontinence for each individual woman may be variable, but there is a significantly high overall societal cost. Health disparities influence the treatment and care of women who suffer from urinary incontinence.

References

1. Haylen BT, de Ridder D, Freeman RM, Swift SE, Berghmans B, Lee J, et al. An International Urogynecological Association (IUGA)/International Continence Society (ICS) joint report on the terminology for female pelvic floor dysfunction. Neurourol Urodyn. 2010;29(1):4–20.
2. Demaagd GA, Davenport TC. Management of urinary incontinence. P T. 2012;37(6):345–61H.
3. Hendrix SL, Cochrane BB, Nygaard IE, Handa VL, Barnabei VM, Iglesia C, et al. Effects of estrogen with and without progestin on urinary incontinence. JAMA. 2005;293(8):935–48.
4. Dooley Y, Kenton K, Cao G, Luke A, Durazo-Arvizu R, Kramer H, et al. Urinary incontinence prevalence: results from the National Health and Nutrition Examination Survey. J Urol. 2008;179(2):656–61.
5. Lee UJ, Feinstein L, Ward JB, Kirkali Z, Martinez-Miller EE, Matlaga BR, et al. Prevalence of urinary incontinence among a nationally representative sample of women, 2005–2016: findings from the urologic diseases in America Project. J Urol. 2021;205(6):1718–24.
6. Wu JM, Vaughan CP, Goode PS, Redden DT, Burgio KL, Richter HE, et al. Prevalence and trends of symptomatic pelvic floor disorders in U.S. women. Obstet Gynecol. 2014;123(1):141–8.
7. Melville JL, Katon W, Delaney K, Newton K. Urinary incontinence in US women: a population-based study. Arch Intern Med. 2005;165(5):537–42.
8. Grodstein F, Fretts R, Lifford K, Resnick N, Curhan G. Association of age, race, and obstetric history with urinary symptoms among women in the Nurses' Health Study. Am J Obstet Gynecol. 2003;189(2):428–34.
9. Lifford KL, Townsend MK, Curhan GC, Resnick NM, Grodstein F. The epidemiology of urinary incontinence in older women: incidence, progression, and remission. J Am Geriatr Soc. 2008;56(7):1191–8.
10. Coyne KS, Sexton CC, Thompson CL, Milsom I, Irwin D, Kopp ZS, et al. The prevalence of lower urinary tract symptoms (LUTS) in the USA, the UK and Sweden: results from the Epidemiology of LUTS (EpiLUTS) study. BJU Int. 2009;104(3):352–60.
11. Lukacz ES, Lawrence JM, Contreras R, Nager CW, Luber KM. Parity, mode of delivery, and pelvic floor disorders. Obstet Gynecol. 2006;107(6):1253–60.
12. Rortveit G, Subak LL, Thom DH, Creasman JM, Vittinghoff E, Van Den Eeden SK, et al. Urinary incontinence, fecal incontinence and pelvic organ prolapse in a population-based, racially diverse cohort: prevalence and risk factors. Female Pelvic Med Reconstr Surg. 2010;16(5):278–83.
13. Irwin D, Milson I, Hunskaar S, Reilly K, Kopp Z, Herschorn S, Coyne K, Kelleher C, Hampel C, Artibani W, Abrams P. Population-based survey of urinary incontinence, overactive bladder, and other lower urinary tract symptoms in five countries: results of the EPIC Study. Eur Urol. 2006;50:1306–15.
14. Jackson RA, Vittinghoff E, Kanaya AM, Miles TP, Resnick HE, Kritchevsky SB, et al. Urinary incontinence in elderly women: findings from the Health, Aging, and Body Composition Study. Obstet Gynecol. 2004;104(2):301–7.
15. Sze EH, Jones WP, Ferguson JL, Barker CD, Dolezal JM. Prevalence of urinary incontinence symptoms among black, white, and Hispanic women. Obstet Gynecol. 2002;99(4):572–5.
16. Fenner DE, Trowbridge ER, Patel DA, Patel DL, Fultz NH, Miller JM, et al. Establishing the prevalence of incontinence study: racial differences in women's patterns of urinary incontinence. J Urol. 2008;179(4):1455–60.
17. Espino DV, Palmer RF, Miles TP, Mouton CP, Lichtenstein MJ, Markides KP. Prevalence and severity of urinary incontinence in elderly Mexican-American women. J Am Geriatr Soc. 2003;51(11):1580–6.
18. Huang AJ, Thom DH, Kanaya AM, Wassel-Fyr CL, Van den Eeden SK, Ragins AI, et al. Urinary incontinence and pelvic floor dysfunction in Asian-American women. Am J Obstet Gynecol. 2006;195(5):1331–7.
19. Blomquist JL, Muñoz A, Carroll M, Handa VL. Association of delivery mode with pelvic floor disorders after childbirth. JAMA. 2018;320(23):2438–47.

20. Rohr G, Kragstrup J, Gaist D, Christensen K. Genetic and environmental influences on urinary incontinence: a Danish population-based twin study of middle-aged and elderly women. Acta Obstet Gynecol Scand. 2004;83(10):978–82.
21. Wennberg AL, Altman D, Lundholm C, Klint A, Iliadou A, Peeker R, et al. Genetic influences are important for most but not all lower urinary tract symptoms: a population-based survey in a cohort of adult Swedish twins. Eur Urol. 2011;59(6):1032–8.
22. Norton P, Milsom I. Genetics and the lower urinary tract. Neurourol Urodyn. 2010;29(4):609–11.
23. McKenzie P, Rohozinski J, Badlani G. Genetic influences on stress urinary incontinence. Curr Opin Urol. 2010;20(4):291–5.
24. Richter HE, Whitehead N, Arya L, Ridgeway B, Allen-Brady K, Norton P, et al. Genetic contributions to urgency urinary incontinence in women. J Urol. 2015;193(6):2020–7.
25. Penney KL, Townsend MK, Turman C, Glass K, Staller K, Kraft P, et al. Genome-wide association study for urinary and fecal incontinence in women. J Urol. 2020;203(5):978–83.
26. Almousa S, Bandin van Loon A. The prevalence of urinary incontinence in nulliparous adolescent and middle-aged women and the associated risk factors: a systematic review. Maturitas. 2018;107:78–83.
27. Danforth KN, Townsend MK, Lifford K, Curhan GC, Resnick NM, Grodstein F. Risk factors for urinary incontinence among middle-aged women. Am J Obstet Gynecol. 2006;194(2):339–45.
28. Sampselle CM, Harlow SD, Skurnick J, Brubaker L, Bondarenko I. Urinary incontinence predictors and life impact in ethnically diverse perimenopausal women. Obstet Gynecol. 2002;100(6):1230–8.
29. Hannestad YS, Rortveit G, Daltveit AK, Hunskaar S. Are smoking and other lifestyle factors associated with female urinary incontinence? The Norwegian EPINCONT Study. BJOG. 2003;110(3):247–54.
30. Bump RC, McClish DK. Cigarette smoking and urinary incontinence in women. Am J Obstet Gynecol. 1992;167(5):1213–8.
31. Dumoulin C, Hunter KF, Moore K, Bradley CS, Burgio KL, Hagen S, et al. Conservative management for female urinary incontinence and pelvic organ prolapse review 2013: summary of the 5th International Consultation on Incontinence. Neurourol Urodyn. 2016;35(1):15–20.
32. Subak LL, Richter HE, Hunskaar S. Obesity and urinary incontinence: epidemiology and clinical research update. J Urol. 2009;182(6 Suppl):S2–7.
33. Cummings JM, Rodning CB. Urinary stress incontinence among obese women: review of pathophysiology therapy. Int Urogynecol J Pelvic Floor Dysfunct. 2000;11(1):41–4.
34. Bulbuller N, Habibi M, Yuksel M, Ozener O, Oruc MT, Oner OZ, et al. Effects of bariatric surgery on urinary incontinence. Ther Clin Risk Manag. 2017;13:95–100.
35. Lian WQ, Li FJ, Huang HX, Zheng YQ, Chen LH. Constipation and risk of urinary incontinence in women: a meta-analysis. Int Urogynecol J. 2019;30(10):1629–34.
36. Meister MR, Sutcliffe S, Badu A, Ghetti C, Lowder JL. Pelvic floor myofascial pain severity and pelvic floor disorder symptom bother: is there a correlation? Am J Obstet Gynecol. 2019;221(3):235.e1–e15.
37. Button BM, Holland AE, Sherburn MS, Chase J, Wilson JW, Burge AT. Prevalence, impact and specialised treatment of urinary incontinence in women with chronic lung disease. Physiotherapy. 2019;105(1):114–9.
38. Mokdad AH, Bowman BA, Ford ES, Vinicor F, Marks JS, Koplan JP. The continuing epidemics of obesity and diabetes in the United States. JAMA. 2001;286(10):1195–200.
39. Hu TW, Wagner TH, Bentkover JD, Leblanc K, Zhou SZ, Hunt T. Costs of urinary incontinence and overactive bladder in the United States: a comparative study. Urology. 2004;63(3):461–5.
40. Feinstein L, Matlaga B. In: Services UDoHaH, editor. Urologic diseases in America. National Institutes of Health: US Government Printing Office; 2018. p. 14.
41. Coyne KS, Wein A, Nicholson S, Kvasz M, Chen CI, Milsom I. Economic burden of urgency urinary incontinence in the United States: a systematic review. J Manag Care Pharm. 2014;20(2):130–40.

42. Alam PA, Huang JC, Clark BA, Burkett LS, Richter LA. A cost analysis of icon reusable underwear versus disposable pads for mild to moderate urinary incontinence. Female Pelvic Med Reconstr Surg. 2020;26(9):575–9.
43. Subak LL, Brown JS, Kraus SR, Brubaker L, Lin F, Richter HE, et al. The "costs" of urinary incontinence for women. Obstet Gynecol. 2006;107(4):908–16.
44. Subak L, Van Den Eeden S, Thom D, Creasman JM, Brown JS, for the Reproductive Risks for Incontinence Study at Kaiser (RRISK) Research Group. Urinary incontinence in women: direct costs of routine care. Am J Obstet Gynecol. 2007;197(6):596.e1–9.
45. Simpson AN, Garbens A, Dossa F, Coyte PC, Baxter NN, McDermott CD. A cost-utility analysis of nonsurgical treatments for stress urinary incontinence in women. Female Pelvic Med Reconstr Surg. 2019;25(1):49–55.
46. Subak LL, Brubaker L, Chai TC, Creasman JM, Diokno AC, Goode PS, et al. High costs of urinary incontinence among women electing surgery to treat stress incontinence. Obstet Gynecol. 2008;111(4):899–907.
47. Subak LL, Goode PS, Brubaker L, Kusek JW, Schembri M, Lukacz ES, et al. Urinary incontinence management costs are reduced following Burch or sling surgery for stress incontinence. Am J Obstet Gynecol. 2014;211(2):171.e1–7.
48. Kinlaw AC, Jonsson Funk M, Conover MM, Pate V, Markland AD, Wu JM. Impact of new medications and $4 generic programs on overactive bladder treatment among older adults in the United States, 2000–2015. Med Care. 2018;56(2):162–70.
49. Kraus SR, Shiozawa A, Szabo SM, Qian C, Rogula B, Hairston J. Treatment patterns and costs among patients with OAB treated with combination oral therapy, sacral nerve stimulation, percutaneous tibial nerve stimulation, or onabotulinumtoxinA in the United States. Neurourol Urodyn. 2020;39(8):2206–22.
50. Harvie HS, Amundsen CL, Neuwahl SJ, Honeycutt AA, Lukacz ES, Sung VW, et al. Cost-effectiveness of sacral neuromodulation versus onabotulinumtoxinA for refractory urgency urinary incontinence: results of the ROSETTA randomized trial. J Urol. 2020;203(5):969–77.
51. Mandimika CL, Murk W, Mcpencow AM, Lake AG, Miller D, Connell KA, et al. Racial disparities in knowledge of pelvic floor disorders among community-dwelling women. Female Pelvic Med Reconstr Surg. 2015;21(5):287–92.
52. Waetjen LE, Xing G, Johnson WO, Melnikow J, Gold EB, (SWAN) SoWsHAtN. Factors associated with seeking treatment for urinary incontinence during the menopausal transition. Obstet Gynecol. 2015;125(5):1071–9.
53. Lee JA, Johns TS, Melamed ML, Tellechea L, Laudano M, Stern JM, et al. Associations between socioeconomic status and urge urinary incontinence: an analysis of NHANES 2005 to 2016. J Urol. 2020;203(2):379–84.
54. Shannon MB, Genereux M, Brincat C, Adams W, Brubaker L, Mueller ER, et al. Attendance at prescribed pelvic floor physical therapy in a diverse, urban urogynecology population. PM R. 2018;10(6):601–6.
55. Laudano MA, Seklehner S, Sandhu J, Reynolds WS, Garrett KA, Milsom JW, et al. Disparities in the use of sacral neuromodulation among Medicare beneficiaries. J Urol. 2015;194(2):449–53.
56. Anger JT, Rodríguez LV, Wang Q, Chen E, Pashos CL, Litwin MS. Racial disparities in the surgical management of stress incontinence among female Medicare beneficiaries. J Urol. 2007;177(5):1846–50.
57. Dallas KB, Sohlberg EM, Elliott CS, Rogo-Gupta L, Enemchukwu E. Racial and socioeconomic disparities in short-term urethral sling surgical outcomes. Urology. 2017;110:70–5.

Chapter 2
Anatomy and Physiology of Female Urinary Incontinence

Felicity Reeves and Tamsin Greenwell

Abbreviations

POD   Pouch of Douglas
POP   Pelvic organ prolapse
PUJ   Pelvi-ureteric junction
SUI   Stress urinary incontinence
TVT   Tension free vaginal tape
VUJ   Vesico-ureteric junction

Learning Objectives
- To describe the normal anatomy of the female pelvis and perineum
- To describe the normal physiology of micturition and be aware of related pathology and effects
- To describe the relation of the pelvic organs to each other
- To list the blood and nerve supply to the female pelvis and lymphatic drainage
- To understand the clinical relevance of anatomy with regard to causes of urinary incontinence in women
- To apply this knowledge to clinical practice when assessing and managing a female patient with urinary incontinence

F. Reeves
Department of Urology, University College London Hospitals (UCLH), London, UK
e-mail: felicity.reeves@nhs.net

T. Greenwell (✉)
Department of Urology, University College London Hospitals (UCLH) and University College London (UCL), London, UK
e-mail: tamsin.greenwell2@nhs.net

A. P. Cameron (ed.), *Female Urinary Incontinence*,
https://doi.org/10.1007/978-3-030-84352-6_2

Introduction

It is essential to have accurate working knowledge and understanding of the normal anatomy and physiology of the lower urogenital tract and female pelvis. This supports the diagnosis, differential diagnosis, formulation of a management plan, and understanding of conditions affecting the female genitourinary tract and pelvic floor that contribute to urinary incontinence. McGuire recognised that not all stress urinary incontinence was related to problems with urethral support (hypermobility incontinence) and described the Valsalva leak point pressure in urodynamic evaluation to aid differentiation between hypermobility and intrinsic sphincter deficiency [1]. His work surrounding the loss of the urethro-vesical angle in women with hypermobility stress incontinence also aided this differentiation. Measurement of intraurethral pressure and abdominal pressure during coughing helped to understand that one of the mechanisms of hypermobility stress urinary incontinence was urinary leakage when raised intraabdominal pressure was transferred to the urethra as well as the bladder due to this loss of normal urethro-vesical angle [2]. Incontinence in women can be stress and/or urgency or continuous from fistula, congenital ectopic ureters, or overflow. Causes can be divided into anatomical causes, neurological causes, idiopathic, iatrogenic (post-surgery and/or post-radiotherapy) and obstetric. The integral theory of Petros encompasses the hammock theory from Delancey and others to explain the multifactorial causes for urinary incontinence in women [3]. The integral theory states that '*prolapse and most pelvic floor symptoms such as urinary stress leakage, urge leakage, abnormal bowel, and bladder emptying mainly arise from laxity in the vagina and its supporting ligaments*' [3]. Ligamentous strength is reliant on oestrogen and postmenopausal women may suffer from ligamentous laxity that responds to hormone replacement therapy. Hormonal changes during pregnancy are also important. From 3 months gestation, hormonal changes affect the type and amount of collagen produced with a resultant increase in ligament laxity and weakness. Although the hormonal changes of pregnancy resolve post-partum, the ligamentous weakness and laxity remain. Because the pelvic floor muscles are interlinked with the ligaments of the pelvis, laxity in the pelvic ligaments also adversely affects muscular strength and coaptation and can result in reduced urinary or faecal continence [3]. The importance of the uterus as a central anchoring point must also not be underestimated, and loss of this central support following hysterectomy often leads to pelvic floor weakness with subsequent development of urinary incontinence or pelvic organ prolapse. The perineal body, despite measuring only 4 cm, provides strength and central support between the posterior vagina and rectum. It is often stretched and weakened during vaginal delivery. Whilst Caesarean section eliminates the physical musculoskeletal stretching and trauma of vaginal childbirth on the pelvic floor, the hormonal changes that lead to connective tissue weakness during pregnancy and after birth remain and will still influence continence and pelvic floor support. Maximal urethral closure pressure has been found to be 42% lower in women with stress incontinence compared to those without [4].

This chapter is presented in sections: the physiology of voiding, the bony pelvis and ligaments, the pelvic sidewall, the perineum, the pelvic floor, the lower urinary tract and reproductive organs, the levels of uterine support, and the blood supply, lymphatics, and nerve supply of the female pelvis. Urinary continence relies on intact and co-ordinated interrelationships between all the above. Where possible, the clinical relevance of anatomical and/or physiological pathology leading to urinary incontinence has been emphasised to aid understanding of both the pathophysiology and management.

Definitions

1. The perineum is the diamond-shaped area below the pelvis. The urethra, the vagina, the rectum, and the anus in women pass through it to their sites of termination.
2. The pelvis is a basin-shaped bony structure below the abdomen and above the perineum and lower limbs that connects the spine to the lower limbs. The pelvic organs, muscles, nerves, lymphatics, and vasculature are contained within it.
3. The pelvic floor is a funnel-like sheet of muscle made up of four main muscles that aids directly with pelvic organ support and indirectly with abdominal organ support. It is pierced by, and aids in the control of the rectum, vagina, and urethra. It separates the pelvic cavity from the perineum.
4. The superficial perineal pouch is the space inferior to the perineal membrane and superior to the superficial perineal fascia (of Colles). It contains the ischiocavernosus, bulbospongiosus and superficial transverse perineal muscles.
5. The deep perineal pouch is the space inferior to the deep pelvic floor fascia and superior to the perineal membrane. It contains the deep transverse perineal muscles and the compressor urethrae.
6. A modified Martius labial fat pad flap (MMLFPF) is an interposition flap loosely based upon the bulbospongiosus flap described by Martius. It is harvested on a vascular pedicle from the fatty tissue within the labia majora and used to augment healing and improve local tissue quality following vaginal and urethral surgery.
7. The fistula is an abnormal connection between two epithelial surfaces most commonly between the vagina and the bladder, i.e. a vesico-vaginal fistula.
8. The stress urinary incontinence (SUI) classification (as defined by Blaivas and Olsson) is based on videourodynamic (VUDS) findings and assesses the position of the bladder neck at rest and with cough relative to the inferior margin of the pubic symphysis (IMPS).

    Type 0 – a history of SUI but no SUI demonstrated on VUDS

    Type I – less than 2 cm descent of bladder neck on cough or strain with SUI. Well supported bladder neck at rest

    Type IIa – >2 cm descent of the bladder neck on cough or strain with SUI Well supported bladder neck at rest

    Type IIb – abnormally low resting position of the bladder neck (below the level of the IMPS) with SUI demonstrated on cough or strain

    Type III – normal resting position of the bladder neck with an open bladder neck and SUI at rest (intrinsic sphincter deficiency) [5]

Physiology of Voiding

Normal voiding is defined as a 'voluntary continuous detrusor contraction that leads to complete bladder emptying within a normal time span, in the absence of obstruction' [6]. During voiding, it has been demonstrated that there is a fall in urethral pressure through active relaxation of the urethra prior to any rise in detrusor pressure, which allows for a coordinated void.

The normal bladder stores urine at low pressure and empties volitionally when socially acceptable. This involves a complex and delicate interplay between the autonomic nervous system and higher control centres.

During the storage phase, sympathetic stimulation from the thoracolumbar spine causes relaxation of the detrusor muscle via B3 receptor mediation and co-ordinated bladder neck contraction via alpha-1 receptors mediation, with noradrenaline as the neurotransmitter.

During the voiding phase, preganglionic parasympathetic nerves originating from the S2-S4 segments of the spinal cord cause contraction of the detrusor muscle consequent to release of acetylcholine from postganglionic parasympathetic neurons via the activation of M3 muscarinic channels (which are G-coupled receptors resulting in increased calcium, calmodulin interaction, and consequent increases in myosin light chain kinase). Parasympathetic stimulation additionally reduces urethral sphincter tone via nitric oxide release.

Somatic innervation, via Onuf's nucleus (located in the anterior horn of the sacral spinal cord), from the pudendal nerve stimulates contraction of the external urethral sphincter via nicotinic receptors with acetylcholine as the neurotransmitter.

At a higher level, the pontine micturition centre is responsible for the coordination of micturition, receiving signals when the bladder is full via stretch receptors in the bladder and sending stimulatory signals via the parasympathetic system to the bladder and inhibitory signals via the somatic system to the external urethral sphincter to stimulate a coordinated void. The pontine micturition centre also receives signals from the prefrontal cortex, the thalamus, the pons, and the medulla.

In neurological conditions, such as following a cerebrovascular accident (CVA or stroke), affecting the frontal cortex, social incontinence may occur due to disinhibition and inability to override the need to void and defer until a socially convenient time. In spinal cord lesions, depending on the level, reflex voiding can occur if the distal autonomous spinal cord remains intact. In a complete spinal injury, this can lead to discoordination of voiding with resultant detrusor sphincter dyssynergia such that the bladder contracts against a closed urethral sphincter leading to high bladder pressure and a risk of renal failure consequent to impaired ureteric drainage and transmission of the high bladder pressures to the kidneys. Other neurological conditions such as multiple sclerosis and Parkinson's disease can present with a spectrum of bladder and bowel dysfunction, but most commonly present with neurogenic detrusor overactivity associated urgency incontinence. Detrusor overactivity is the urodynamic finding of contraction of the detrusor during the bladder filling phase in association with symptoms of urgency and /or urgency incontinence. Where the generated detrusor pressure is greater than the urethral sphincter tone and pressure, there will be urinary leakage.

Bony Pelvis and Pelvic Ligaments

Loss of urethral and bladder neck support was first hypothesised as a cause for stress urinary incontinence in 1922 by Bonney [7]. There is a need for physical support of the pelvic organs, and the importance of the uterus to provide an anchoring point for ligaments has been highlighted. The hormonal changes of pregnancy and following menopause adversely affect collagen composition and strength of ligaments, which in turn reduces the effectiveness of muscular contraction against the ligaments. Bony pelvis dimensions may also impact continence, with women with stress incontinence reported having sub-pubic angles 2.3–3 degrees wider than age-matched continent women [8].

The Pelvic Bones

The bones of the female pelvis are lighter and thinner than those of the male pelvis (Figs. 2.1 and 2.2). The fused innominate bones: the ischium, the ilium, and the pubis form the acetabulum and the anterolateral bony pelvis, whilst the sacrum and coccyx bones form the posterior aspect of the bony pelvis (Figs. 2.1 and 2.2). In the female pelvis, there is a wider angle of the pubic arch and a shallower sacral curve than in the male pelvis, which produce a larger pelvic inlet and outlet to facilitate vaginal childbirth. It is possible to palpate the iliac crest, pubic tubercle, and ischial tuberosity during clinical examination of the vagina and perineum (Fig. 2.4).

When standing, the pelvic inlet is tilted anteriorly and is bounded by the superior border of the pubic symphysis, the posterior border of the pubic crest, the arcuate line of the ilium, the anterior border of the ala of the sacrum, and the sacral promontory (Fig. 2.1). The pelvic outlet boundaries are the tip of the coccyx, the ischial tuberosity and the sacrotuberous ligaments, the inferior ramus of the pubis, and the inferior margin of the pubic symphysis. (Figs. 2.1, 2.2, and 2.4). Five fused vertebrae form the sacrum which contains eight foramina (four on each side) for the paired sacral nerves (S1, 2, 3, and 4) (Fig. 2.9).

The pubic symphysis is a cartilaginous joint cranial to the external genitalia and is the site of articulation of the two pubic bones. The superior ramus of each pubic bone forms the superior aspect of the obturator foramen. The inferior aspect of the obturator foramen is formed by the union of the inferior ramus of the pubic bone and ischial bone to form the ischiopubic ramus.

The bony pelvis is divided into the greater pelvis (or 'false pelvis' so termed as it is part of abdominal cavity) and the lesser pelvis (or true pelvis). The greater pelvis is incomplete anteriorly, bounded laterally by the ilium and posteriorly by the

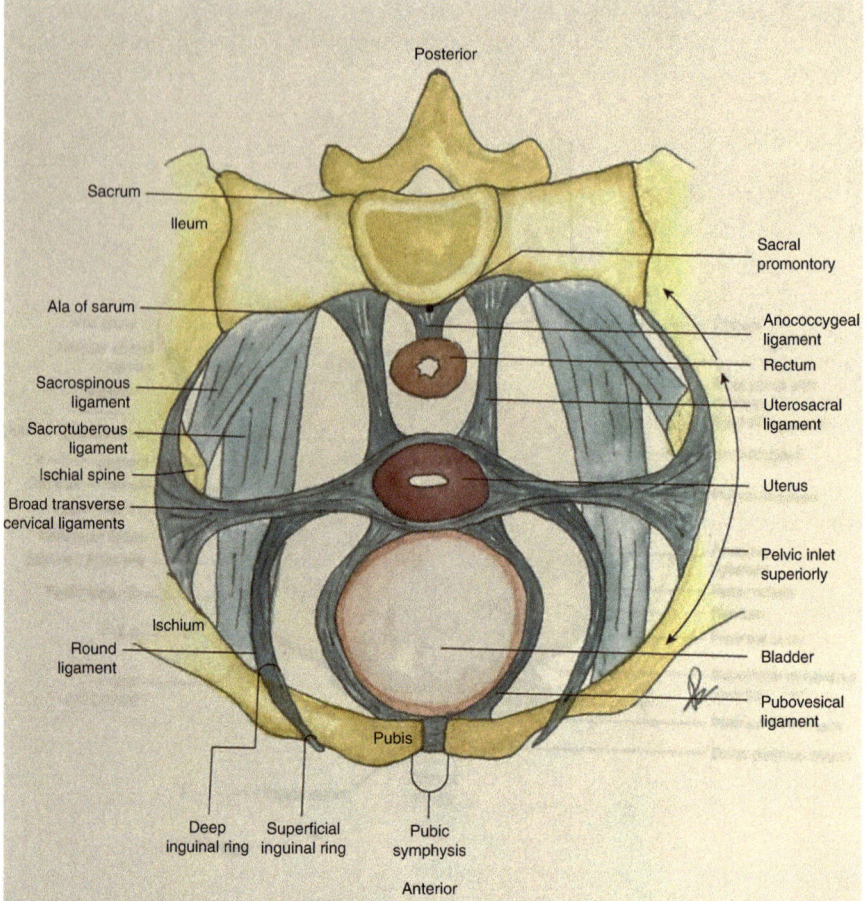

Fig. 2.1 Bony pelvis and ligaments in transverse plane

base of the sacrum. The lesser (true) pelvis contains the pelvic inlet and sits behind the pelvic brim. It is bounded by the sacrum and coccyx posteriorly, the inner surfaces of the ilium and the ischium anterolaterally, and the pubic symphysis anteriorly (Figs. 2.1, 2.2, and 2.4).

Pelvic Ligaments Figs. 2.1 and 2.4

Ligaments are bands of connective tissue that hold bones together to allow joint articulation or support internal organs. The ligaments of the pelvis include:

1. The Sacrospinous ligaments which attach the sacrum to the ischial spine bilaterally.
2. The Sacrotuberous ligaments which attach the sacrum to the ischial tuberosity bilaterally.

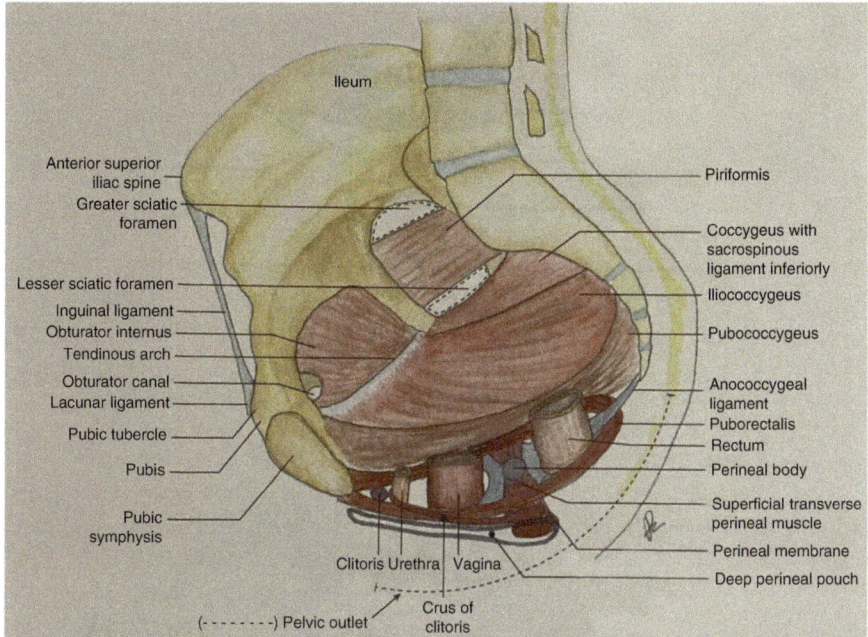

Fig. 2.2 Saggital view of pelvis from medical aspect with left hemipelvis removed. Levator ani and pelvis organs transected to demonstrate relation

3. The Inguinal ligaments (Poupart's ligaments) which extend from the anterior superior iliac spine to the pubic tubercle bilaterally and mark the transition from the pelvis into the lower limb.
4. The Lacunar ligaments which are moon shaped and extend from the medial inguinal ligament to the pubic tubercle on each side.
5. The Sacroiliac ligaments which have an anterior and posterior part and extend from the sacrum to the iliac bone across the sacroiliac joints on each side.
6. The Obturator ligaments which cross superior to the obturator membrane bilaterally.

The collagen-based connective tissue of these ligaments responds to changes in oestrogen and progesterone. Oestrogen maintains the strength of ligamentous collagen, and hence, ligamentous weakness can be seen in postmenopausal women. Ligamentous weakness can also be seen (although less commonly) in nulliparous women due to congenital connective tissue weakness and collagen disorders [3]. Hysterectomy as well as causing loss of central physical support may also reduce the blood supply to the cardinal and uterosacral ligaments, causing additional ligamentous weakness consequent to ischaemic change.

The greater and lesser sciatic notches are on the posterior aspect of the ischium separated by the ischial spine. The sacrotuberous and sacrospinous ligaments traverse these notches to create the greater and lesser sciatic foramina. The sacrospinous ligament can be palpated vaginally, and in sacrospinous fixation operations for the treatment of vaginal prolapse, the vaginal wall is sutured to this ligament to provide support (Fig. 2.4).

The arcus tendinous fascia pelvis is a strong band of connective tissue attaching the ischium above the ischial spine to the lower part of the pubic bone.

Pelvic Foramina

The greater sciatic notch is a notch in the posterior aspect of the bony pelvis inferior to the posterior superior iliac spine and the superior to the ischial spine. The notch is converted to the greater sciatic foramen by the crossing sacrospinous and sacro-tuberous ligaments. All neurovascular structures travelling into and out of the pelvis must pass through it. It contains the piriformis muscle. The superior gluteal nerve (from L4-S1 nerve roots of the sacral plexus) and vessels exit the pelvis into the gluteal region above the piriformis muscle through the greater sciatic foramen. The inferior gluteal nerve (from L5-S2 nerve roots of the sacral plexus) and vessels, the sciatic nerve (from nerve roots L4-S3), the posterior femoral cutaneous nerve (from nerve roots S1-3), and the nerve to quadratus femoris (from nerve roots L4-S1) exit the pelvis into the gluteal region or the lower limb, below the piriformis muscle, through the greater sciatic foramen (Fig. 2.2). The nerve to obturator internus (from nerve roots L5-S2) and the pudendal nerve (from nerve roots S2-4) and internal pudendal vessels also exit the pelvis through the greater sciatic foramen to curl around the sacrospinous ligament at the level of the ischial spine and enter the perineum via the lesser sciatic foramen.

The lesser sciatic notch is a small notch inferior to the ischial spine on the posterior aspect of the bony pelvis (Fig. 2.2). It is converted into the lesser sciatic foramen by the crossed paths of the sacrospinous and sacrotuberous ligaments. It contains the tendon of the obturator internus muscle and is the entry and exit point to the perineum. The nerve to the obturator internus muscle (from nerve roots L5 to S2) along with the internal pudendal vessels and the pudendal nerve (from the nerve roots S2-S4) enter the perineum via the lesser sciatic foramen.

The pudendal nerve passes between the piriformis and coccygeus muscles (Figs. 2.2, 2.4, and 2.9) into the pelvis via the greater sciatic foramen and then crosses around the sacrospinous ligament to enter the perineum via the lesser sciatic foramen. It travels in Alcock's (pudendal) canal anteriorly along the lateral wall of the ischiorectal fossa alongside the internal pudendal artery and vein. Alcock's canal is a sheath of thickened obturator internus fascia. Immediately before entering or on entering Alcock's canal, the pudendal nerve branches to give off the inferior rectal nerve (from nerve roots S2-4) (Fig. 2.4). It then branches at the posterior border of the perineal membrane into the perineal nerve and the dorsal nerve of the clitoris. The perineal nerve branches to form a superficial (cutaneous) and a deep (muscular) perineal nerve which innervate the striated muscles of the superficial and deep perineal pouches, the lower vagina, and the labia. The dorsal nerve of the clitoris provides sensory innervation and is essential for normal sexual function (Fig. 2.4).

The pudendal nerve and the internal pudendal vessels are the main perineal neurovascular supply (described further in the section on the female perineum). The pudendal nerve innervates the external striated (voluntary) urethral sphincter, and pudendal nerve damage can lead to sensory loss in the labia and clitoris as well as faecal and urinary incontinence. The pudendal nerve is particularly at-risk during vaginal childbirth and, less commonly, in professional cycling. It is possible to perform a pudendal nerve block with transvaginal local anaesthetic injection into the region of the ischial spine during labour if needed for pain relief.

The obturator nerve (from nerve roots L2-4) and vessels exit the pelvis into the medial compartment of the thigh via the obturator canal which is situated in the superomedial aspect of the obturator foramen. An accessory obturator nerve (nerve roots L3 and L4) exits the pelvis via the mid-lateral aspect of the obturator foramen in 25% of people. The obturator foramen is the site of trocar passage when performing a transobturator mid-urethral sling for SUI. Care should be taken to puncture the obturator membrane as medial as possible to avoid the obturator nerve and vessels and the accessory obturator nerve. The obturator nerve is also at risk of inadvertent stimulation during endoscopic bladder tumour resection, especially with lateral wall tumours. Stimulation can cause an unexpected powerful thigh adduction (the obturator kick) which risks inadvertent bladder perforation (Fig. 2.8).

Pelvic Side Walls

The Muscles of the Pelvic Side Wall (Table 2.1)

The body and rami of the pubic bones along with the pubic symphysis form the anterior pelvic wall. The obturator internus muscle and the lesser sciatic foramen form the lateral pelvic wall. The sacrum, the ilium, and the sacroiliac joints form the posterior pelvic wall. The piriformis muscle lies posterolaterally and exits the pelvis via the greater sciatic foramen to insert into the femur. The sacral plexus and the internal iliac vessels pass medial to the piriformis muscle. The piriformis muscle originates on the anterior surface of the sacrum and the gluteal surface of the ilium and inserts into the greater trochanter of the femur. It acts as a lateral (external) rotator of the extended hip and an abductor of the flexed hip. Its innervation is by the nerve to piriformis (sacral plexus roots S1-2). The obturator internus muscle originates on the inner (pelvic) aspect of the obturator membrane and the adjacent inferior margin of the superior pubic ramus and inserts into the greater trochanter of the femur. Its tendon exits the perineum into the thigh via the lesser sciatic foramen. It acts as a lateral rotator of the extended hip and abductor of the flexed hip. Its innervation is from the nerve to the obturator internus (nerve roots L5, S1, and S2). The coccygeus muscle originates on the ischial spine and inserts into the inferior sacrum and the coccyx. It acts to support the pelvic organs and flex the coccyx. Its innervation is from the anterior roots of the S4 and S5.

Table 2.1 Muscles of the pelvic floor and walls

Muscle	Origin	Insertion	Action	Nerve supply	Blood supply
Obturator internus	Obturator membrane and ipsilateral inferior ramus of the pubis and the ischium	Medial surface of greater trochanter of femur	Lateral femoral rotation at the hip	Nerve to obturator internus, L5, S1	Superior gluteal artery
Piriformis	Anterior sacrum	Medial superior border greater trochanter of femur	Lateral femoral rotation at the hip	L5, S1, S2	Superior and inferior gluteal and internal pudendal arteries with corresponding veins.
Levator ani	Ischial spine Body of pubis Obturator internus fascia – tendineus arch	Perineal body, perineal membrane Anococcygeal body Walls of vagina, rectum and anal canal	Pelvic organ support, sphincter to anorectal junction and vagina Counteracts increased abdominal pressure	Pudendal nerve (S2-4) 4th sacral nerve	Inferior gluteal artery, inferior vesical artery, pudendal artery. Corresponding veins and lymphatics
Coccygeus	Ischial spine Sacrospinous ligament	Inferior sacrum and coccyx	Pelvic organ support Coccygeal flexion	4th and 5th sacral nerves	Inferior vesical, inferior gluteal and pudendal arteries with corresponding veins and lymphatics

The endopelvic fascia covers the internal aspect of the pelvic side wall. It forms a strong fascial sheet that blankets both the piriformis and obturator internus muscles. Internal to this fascia are the pelvis vessels, and external to it are the spinal nerves. The sacral plexus overlies the piriformis muscle (and is discussed in more detail in the section on nerve supply).

The Pelvic Floor

The pelvic floor (also known as the pelvic diaphragm) is the funnel-shaped muscular floor of the pelvic cavity. It is composed of the levator ani muscles (nerve supply anterior root of S4 and branches from the pudendal nerve S2, 3, and 4), the coccygeus muscles (nerve supply from the anterior roots of S3 and S4), the perineal membrane, and deep transverse perineal muscles within the deep perineal pouch.

The Pelvic Diaphragm Muscles (Figs. 2.2 and 2.4)

The pelvic diaphragm forms the floor of the pelvic cavity and the roof of the perineum. It is composed of the levator ani muscles anteriorly and the coccygeus muscle posteriorly. Levator ani has three parts: (1) puborectalis, which is a U-shaped sling of muscle originating and inserting into the pubic bones that passes around the anorectal junction; (2) pubococcygeus, which originates from the inner aspect of the pubic bones and inserts into the coccyx; and (3) iliococcygeus, which arises from the arcus tendineus of the obturator fascia and inserts into the coccyx.

The pelvic diaphragm is attached proximally to the body of the pubic bone, the arcus tendineus of the obturator fascia, and the ischial spine. Distally, it is attached to the perineal body (a midline fibromuscular raphe), the anococcygeal body, the coccyx, the anococcygeal ligament, the walls of the vagina, the walls of the rectum, and the walls of the anal canal. The levator ani mainly acts to support and stabilises the pelvic (and by default the abdominal) organs. It does have a secondary sphincteric action by maintaining the angle of the anorectal junction and of the angulation of the proximal vagina and urethra relative to the mid and distal vagina and urethra. This action is particularly important at times of increased abdominal pressure or straining such as during vaginal childbirth or defecation.

The perineal body is a pyramidal midline fibromuscular structure sited at the junction between the posterior anorectal perineal triangle and the anterior urogenital perineal triangle (Refer to the section on the Perineum). It provides a central attachment for the muscles and supports of the pelvic floor and perineum. Damage to the perineal body, particularly a risk during vaginal childbirth, may contribute to pelvic organ prolapse (POP), urinary, and faecal incontinence. The pelvic ligaments are only able to provide unaided pelvic organ support for short periods. Long-term pelvic organ support is dependent upon the interaction between the pelvic musculature and the ligamentous attachments.

The levator ani is covered by a tough sheet of fascia – the endopelvic fascia which is composed of a mesh-like group of collagen fibres interlaced with elastin, smooth muscle cells, and blood vessels. This is contiguous with the transversalis fascia of the abdominal wall. The endopelvic fascia lies immediately above the levator ani and attaches to the ischial spine, the arcus tendineus, the ileopectineal (Cooper's) ligament, and the arcuate line (from the sacral promontory to the pectineal line on the pubic bone).

The area of the endopelvic fascia that attaches the uterus to the pelvic side wall is the parametrium. The intermediate layer of the parametrium is condensed at the level of the cervix to form the cardinal and uterosacral ligaments. The endopelvic fascia continues down to form a sheet attaching the proximal vagina to the pelvic sidewalls – the paracolpium [9]. Delancey described three levels of utero-vaginal support [1].

Level I is the support from the parametrium, the cardinal ligaments, the uterosacral ligaments, the pubocervical ligaments, and the paracolpium, which suspend the cervix and superior vagina to the pelvic walls.

Level II is the support from the paracolpium, which suspends and fixes the mid vagina directly to pelvic side walls laterally and to the levator ani muscles posteriorly. The pubocervical fascia supports the bladder and merges with the endopelvic fascia and the anterior vaginal wall. The posterior vaginal wall merges with the endopelvic fascia to support the rectum and aids in the prevention of posterior vaginal wall prolapse.

Level III support is from the attachment of the distal vagina laterally to the levator ani, anteriorly to the urethra and posteriorly to the perineal body. The perineal body, in turn, is connected to the perineal membrane laterally on both sides of the pelvis and aids in support and stabilisation of the distal vagina [9].

The fascia of the pelvis is in continuity with the retroperitoneal fascia and has three layers referred to as strata; the endopelvic fascia represents the outer strata. The intermediate strata contain neurovascular elements within a fatty layer and require definitive mobilisation to access the pelvic organs. The intermediate strata of the fascia of the pelvis condense to form stronger ligamentous attachments to support the pelvic organs. These include the posterior and lateral vesical, the uterosacral, and the cardinal ligaments. The inner stratum of the pelvic fascia lies deep to the peritoneum and covers the bladder dome and anterior rectum. The urethra and vagina pass through the levator ani at the urogenital hiatus, which is the weakest area of the anterior pelvic diaphragm, and then pass through the deep perineal pouch before exiting into the perineum (Figs. 2.2, 2.4, and 2.5). The urogenital hiatus is supported anteriorly by the levator ani and the pubic bones and posteriorly by the external anal sphincter and perineal body [9]. The resting levator ani muscle tone in normal situations maintains closure of the urogenital hiatus by pulling the urethra, vagina, and rectum towards the pubic bone. If levator muscle damage and weakness occur (such as after vaginal childbirth), it is no longer possible to close the urogenital hiatus in this manner, and the connective tissue of the supportive fascia eventually fails and prolapses, and/or urinary or faecal incontinence develops [9].

Uterine Support (Figs. 2.1 and 2.3)

Uterine supports not only need to be strong to maintain the position of the uterus but also require the ability to expand during pregnancy. There are several levels of uterine support, and it follows that after a hysterectomy and disruption of this support, there is a risk of vaginal vault prolapse. Connective tissue surrounds all the pelvic organs, and in some areas, this has increased in density to form additional fibromuscular ligaments for support. This connective tissue is continuous with the extraperitoneal components of the abdominal wall but is separated from the ischiorectal fossa below by the levator ani muscles and pelvic fascia.

The broad ligament is a double layer of the peritoneum and folds as a sheet over the body of the uterus running laterally to attach the uterus to the pelvic sidewall.

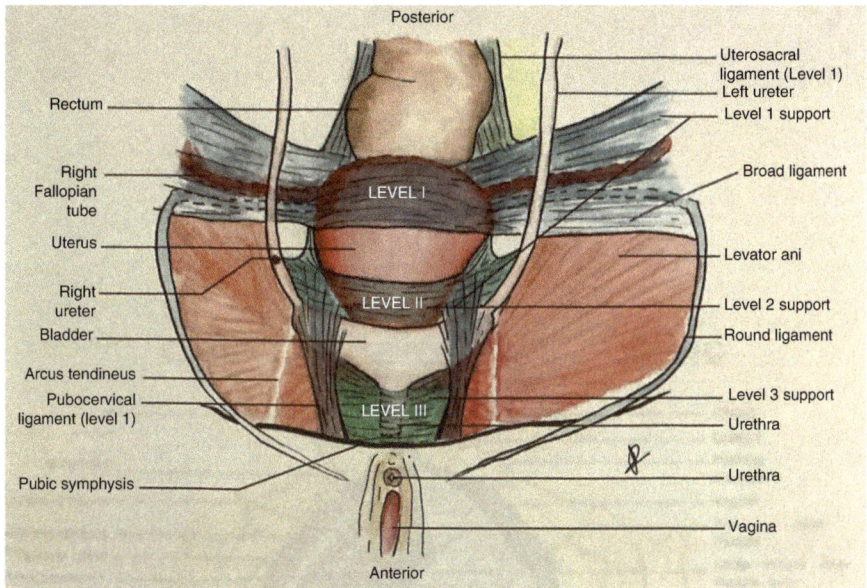

Fig. 2.3 Cross section a pelvis demonstrating three levels of vaginal and uterine support

The fallopian tubes run in the upper border of the fold of the broad ligament. The broad ligament is a protective layer for the female pelvic organs. Between the layers of the broad ligament (the parametrium) lie the suspensory ligaments of the ovaries, the round ligament of the uterus, uterine and ovarian vessels, and lymphatics. The suspensory ligament of the ovary attaches the medial aspect of the ovary to the uterus at the junction between the uterus and the fallopian tube. It contains the ovarian vessels and lymphatics.

The round ligament of the uterus is a continuation of the ovarian ligament. It runs from the ovary and uterus to the pelvic brim, enters the deep inguinal ring at the midpoint of the inguinal ligament, travels through the inguinal canal, and terminates in the subcutaneous tissues of the labia majora. It is the gubernacular remnant.

Most of the support for the uterus comes from three sets of ligaments, the cardinal, the pubocervical, and the uterosacral ligaments. The *cardinal (or transverse cervical) ligaments* are fan-shaped fibro-muscular ligaments that run from the cervix and vaginal vault to the lateral walls of the pelvis. They are found within the inferior section of the broad ligament providing lateral support to the cervix. The *uterosacral ligaments* pass posteriorly from the sides of the cervix to the middle of the sacrum and the fascia overlying piriformis. They provide posterior tension and are palpable on rectal examination as they run either side of the rectum. When standing erect they are vertical in position. The *pubocervical ligaments* are attached between the pubic symphysis to the cervix and bladder anteriorly. Laterally, the bladder is supported by the visceral pelvic fascia.

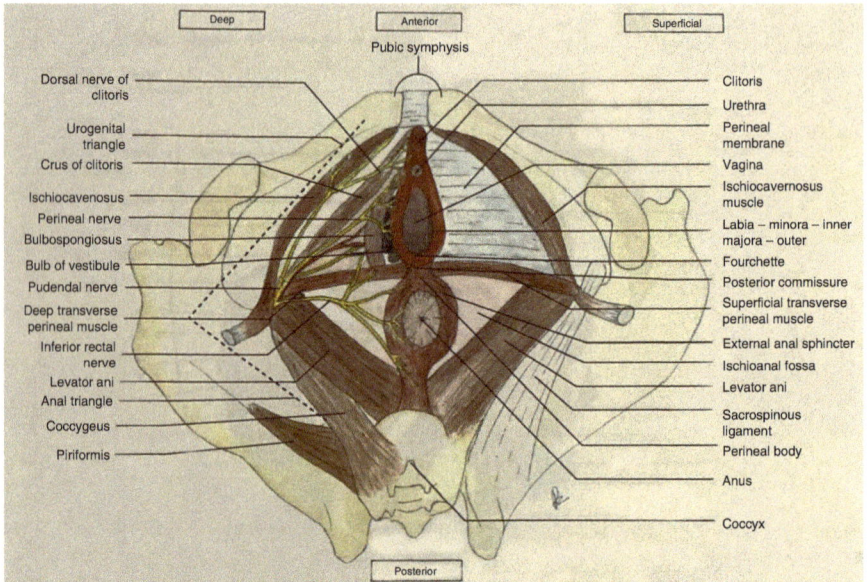

| Deep | Anterior | Superficial |

Pubic symphysis

Dorsal nerve of clitoris —
Urogenital triangle —
Crus of clitoris —
Ischiocavernosus —
Perineal nerve —
Bulbospongiosus —
Bulb of vestibule —
Pudendal nerve —
Deep transverse perineal muscle —
Inferior rectal nerve —
Levator ani —
Anal triangle —
Coccygeus —
Piriformis —

— Clitoris
— Urethra
— Perineal membrane
— Vagina
— Ischiocavernosus muscle
— Labia – minora – inner majora – outer
— Fourchette
— Posterior commissure
— Superficial transverse perineal muscle
— External anal sphincter
— Ischioanal fossa
— Levator ani
— Sacrospinous ligament
— Perineal body
— Anus
— Coccyx

Posterior

Fig. 2.4 Transverse diagram of female pelvis with deep (left) and superficial (right) structures

The Perineum

The perineum lies below the pelvis and is divided into two unequal triangles by a transverse line joining the anterior aspects of the tips of the ischial tuberosities, the larger posterior anal triangle and the smaller anterior urogenital triangle. The anal triangle contains the anus whilst the urogenital triangle contains the external genitalia in women (Fig. 2.4 and Box 2.1).

Box 2.1: The Muscles of the Female Perineum Fig. 2.4

The muscles of the female urogenital triangle are all innervated by the perineal branch of the pudendal nerve (S2, 3, and 4) and obtain their blood supply from the internal pudendal artery, a branch of the anterior division of the internal iliac artery:

1. The *superficial transverse perineal muscles* lie below (or superficial) to the perineal membrane. They originate from the ischial tuberosity on each side and insert onto and support the perineal body.
2. The *deep transverse perineal muscles lie above (or deep) to the perineal membrane*. They originate on the ischial tuberosity and ramus and insert into the perineal body providing additional support.
3. The *bulbospongiosus muscles* act as the vaginal sphincter and support erection of the clitoris (dorsal arterial branch to clitoris). They originate

from the perineal body in women and inserts into the fascia of the bulbs of the vestibule and the aponeurosis of the crura of the cavernosum.
4. The *ischiocavernosus muscles* originate from the ischial tuberosity and ramus and travel forward to encompass the corpora and inserts into the aponeurotic fascia over the corpus cavernosum of the clitoris. They aid with erection of the clitoris.
5. The *sphincter urethrae* originates on the pubic arch and inserts around the urethra. It allows voluntary urethral sphincter contraction.

The Deep Perineal Pouch, the Perineal Membrane, and the Perineal Body (Figs. 2.2 and 2.4)

The deep perineal pouch (DPP) lies inferior to the pelvic floor and superior to the perineal membrane. The vagina and the urethra perforate and pass through the DPP. It contains the muscles that support and close the urethra – the external sphincter muscle, the sphincter urethrovaginalis (which surrounds and supports the urethra and the vagina), and the compressor urethrae. Immediately inferior to it is the perineal membrane, which is a triangular-shaped thickened fascia which covers the urogenital triangle at the level of the hymen, and which is attached laterally to the pubic arch. It is an important support structure for the pelvic floor and has a hiatus through which the urethra and vagina pass into the perineum. It also provides support for the attachment of the external genitalia and the muscles of the superficial perineal pouch (SPP). The perineal membrane attaches the 'urethra, vagina, and perineal body to the ischiopubic rami' [9]. The perineal membrane has a posterior free edge at the level of a line between the ischial tuberosities. The perineal body (PB) is sited midway along this posterior free edge. The deep transverse perineal muscles are small paired muscles which originate from the ischial tuberosities (above the perineal membrane) and run horizontally within the DPP to insert into the perineal body. Their action is to stabilise the perineal body (see Box 2.1). The perineal body sits at the junction between the anterior urogenital triangle and the posterior anal triangle and is the site of insertion of many of the muscles of the pelvic floor and perineum and is thus a significant pelvic floor and perineal support structure. Damage to and consequent laxity of the perineal body and associated supports following vaginal childbirth can lead to pelvic organ prolapse.

Superficial Perineal Pouch (Figs. 2.2, 2.4, and 2.5)

The superficial perineal pouch lies inferior to the perineal membrane and superior to the superficial perineal fascia (of Colles). It contains the superficial transverse perineal muscles, the bulbospongiosus muscles, and the ischiocavernosus muscles. The superficial perineal muscles are small paired muscles originating from the ischial tuberosity and running horizontally inferior to the perineal membrane to insert into the perineal body. Their action is to stabilise the perineal body (see Box 2.1), and their nerve supply is from the deep branch of the perineal nerve (nerve roots S2, S3, and S4). The bulbospongiosus muscles are paired small muscles that arise from the perineal body and run forwards covering the bulb of the vestibule to insert into an aponeurosis attached to the undersurface of the crura of the clitoris. Their nerve supply is from the perineal branch of the pudendal nerve (nerve roots S2, S3, and S4), and they act to aid clitoral erection, vaginal contractions at orgasm, and closure of the vagina. The ischiocavernosus muscles are small paired muscles originating from the ischium and underside of the inferior pubic rami to run forwards and cover the crura of the clitoris. They insert into an aponeurosis attached to the undersurface of the clitoris and the bulbs of the vestibule. Their innervation is from the perineal branch of the pudendal nerve (nerve roots S2, S3, and S4) and their function is to aid clitoral erection and stabilise the vagina during orgasm.

The superficial perineal pouch also contains the two corpora cavernosa (which contain erectile tissue) of the clitoris. The crura of the corpora cavernosa originate in the region and are attached to the pubic arch. The distal free ends of the corpora travel anteriorly and medially and fuse to form the body of the clitoris. The bulbs of the vestibule contain additional erectile tissue and are situated around the vaginal introitus. They are attached to the perineal membrane and are covered with the bulbospongiosus muscle. The bulbs of the vestibule join anteriorly to form the glans clitoris in the midline, anterior to the urethral opening. The crura of the clitoris are covered by the ischiocavernosus muscles. The greater vestibular glands sit posterior to the bulb of the vestibule.

Features of Female External Genitalia (Fig. 2.4)

From anterior to posterior, the female perineum contains the mons pubis, the clitoris and clitoral hood, the external urethral meatus, the vaginal orifice, the posterior vaginal commissure (or fourchette), the perineum and perineal body, and most posteriorly the anus. The anterior vagina wall is very closely related to the urethra. The posterior vaginal wall is separated from the rectum by the perineal body. The vaginal orifice is also called the vestibule of the vagina and may be partially occluded by the thin membrane of the hymen in females who have never had sexual intercourse or used a tampon. The paired hairless labia minora enclose the clitoris and surround the vaginal vestibule. The paired labia majora (with an inner hairless and an outer hair-bearing surface) surround the labia minora laterally and fuse anteriorly with the mons pubis. Within the labia majora is a deep fat pad which has a dual blood supply from the internal pudendal artery posterolaterally and the external pudendal artery anteromedially. This dual blood supply allows the labial fat pad to be mobilised as a vascularised flap used in reconstruction as a modified Martius labial fat pad interposition flap, for example, following vesico-vaginal fistula closure, where it is placed between the closed bladder and the vaginal closure.

The Ischioanal Fossae (Fig. 2.4)

The ischioanal fossae are large fascial lined spaces filled with fat and loose connective tissue between the skin of the anal triangle region and the pelvic diaphragm. They communicate above the anococcygeal ligament which is located between the anal canal and tip of the coccyx. Laterally, they are bound by the ischium and obturator internus, medially by the anal canal, posteriorly by the sacrotuberous ligament and gluteus maximus, and anteriorly by the base of the urogenital diaphragm (the fibromuscular structures of the deep perineal pouch of the perineum).

Female Pelvic Organs

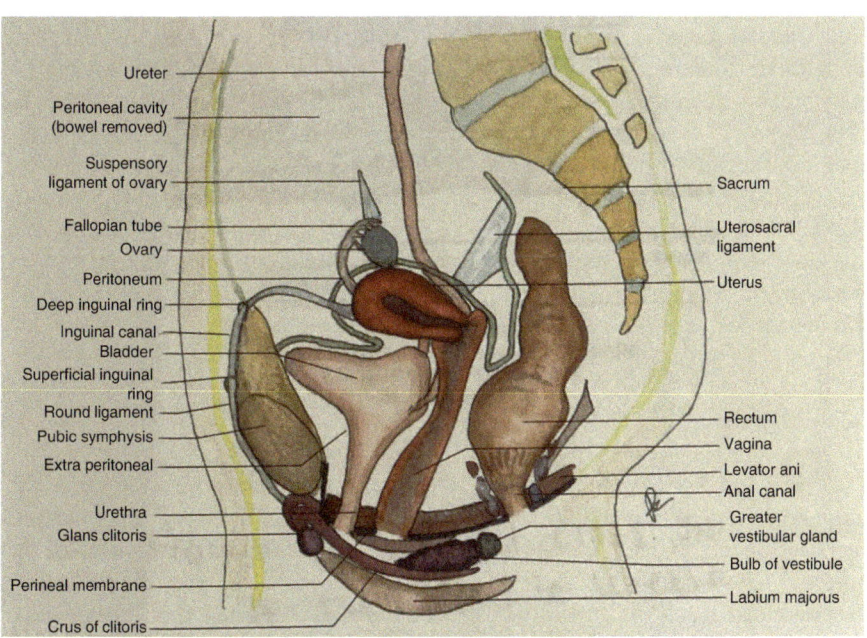

Fig. 2.5 Saggital section a female pelvis and lower abdomen

Reproductive Organs

Uterus and Cervix

The uterus is a thick-walled, pear-shaped organ formed predominantly from smooth muscle which sits in the pelvis posterior to the bladder and anterior to the rectum. The uterus has three parts, the fundus, the body, and the cervix. The fundus is superior to the body of the uterus. The body of the uterus forms the upper two-thirds of the organ. The fallopian tubes are connected to the uterine fundus superolateral and communicate with the uterine cavity. The peritoneum that passes over the uterus becomes the broad ligament laterally. The peritoneum that covers the fallopian tubes and suspends them from the is known as the mesosalpinx. The lowest third of the uterus is the cervix – which is the narrowest section of the uterus. The internal cervical opening (os) is continuous with the uterine cavity and the external cervical os opens into the upper vagina. The vaginal section of the cervix is within the vaginal fornix. The cervical canal is lined by columnar epithelium which transitions to the stratified squamous epithelium in the vagina. This cervical canal and the adjacent transition zone are the areas from where cervical smears are taken to screen for premalignant and malignant changes.

The peritoneum covers the fundus of the uterus, the posterior aspect of the uterus, and the anterior aspect of the rectum, and this area is known as the pouch of Douglas (rectouterine pouch). Fluid can collect in the pouch of Douglas consequent to any inflammation within the abdominal cavity such as following appendicitis, a ruptured ovarian cyst, or a tubo-ovarian abscess. Peritoneum also covers the anterior aspect of the uterine body and the posterior aspect of the upper part of the bladder and in so doing forms the vesicouterine pouch. The uterine artery crosses above the ureter as it traverses the round ligament very near to the cervix. Due to this close anatomical relationship, the distal ureter is at-risk of injury during hysterectomy. The pubocervical, cardinal, and uterosacral ligaments support the cervix and uterus.

Fallopian Tubes

The fallopian tubes are approximately 10 cm long and divided into three parts. The infundibulum is the fimbriated lateral part that curls over the top of the ovary on each side, in the midsection is the dilated ampulla, and the narrow isthmus joins the fallopian tube medially to the uterus and uterine cavity. The fallopian tubes allow the passage of eggs from the ovaries to the uterus for reproduction. Fertilisation usually occurs within the fallopian tubes whilst implantation usually occurs in the uterus. If implantation occurs within the fallopian tube, an ectopic pregnancy ensues which may cause a life-threatening emergency if the ectopic pregnancy causes fallopian tube rupture with associated bleeding.

Ovaries

There are two ovaries each sited laterally in the pelvis within the ovarian fossa. The obturator nerve, the internal, and external iliac vessels are in close proximity to the ovary, and care should be taken when performing oophorectomy not to damage these structures. The ovary is attached to the broad ligament by the mesovarium and the uterus by the suspensory ligament of the ovary, which is contiguous with the round ligament. The round ligament originates on the anterior superior aspect of the uterus in the parametrium and passes inferolaterally to exit the pelvis through the internal inguinal ring to insert into the subcutaneous tissues of the labia majora and the mons pubis.

Lower Urinary Tract Organs

Urinary Bladder

The urinary bladder is a hollow pear-shaped organ composed predominantly of smooth muscle. It allows low-pressure storage of urine without leakage and permits volitional emptying of the bladder when socially acceptable. The bladder has a dome superiorly, two lateral walls, an anterior wall, and a base. The urachus, which is the remnant of the foetal allantois, arises from the apex of the anterior wall of the bladder and travels to the umbilicus within the median umbilical ligament. The bladder base is densely attached by the pelvic fascia to the upper cervix and vaginal. This is a not uncommon site for fistula formation in patients who have had previous pelvic surgery or radiotherapy. Affected patients may present with a continuous form of urinary incontinence due to urine escaping continuously from the bladder into the vagina.

The bladder wall is composed of four layers, the fatty layer of the adventitia externally, the detrusor smooth muscle, the lamina propria (connective tissue), and the urothelium (transitional urothelial cells) internally. The trigone is a triangular flattened area on the posterior bladder wall at the base of the bladder adjacent to the bladder neck. Its superolateral margins are defined by the ureteric orifices, between which there is an inter-ureteric bar. The ureters enter the bladder through an oblique intramural tunnel, which prevents reflux of urine back up the ureters to the kidneys. If this antireflux tunnel is deficient, vesicoureteric reflux (VUR) can occur resulting in varying degrees of dilatation of the ureters, renal pelvis, and calyces (hydrone-phrosis). If VUR is associated with urinary tract infection or high bladder pressures, it can lead to pyelonephritis and/or loss of renal function. The bladder neck smooth muscle is continuous with the smooth muscle of the urethra and is thought to acts physiologically as an involuntary smooth muscle sphincter. This autonomic sphinc-ter helps to maintain closure of the upper urethra and bladder neck during bladder filling. The bladder and bladder neck are supported posteriorly by the endopelvic fascia. The retropubic space of Retzius is bounded by the transversalis fascia anteriorly and the peritoneum posteriorly. The urachus traverses this space within the median umbilical ligament. The urachus is the obliterated remnant of the foetal allantois which drains urine in utero from the bladder via the umbilical cord. Cysts very rarely adenocarcinoma may form within the urachal remnant and present as discharge from the umbilicus. The urachus can be used to aid dissection to the bladder and is generally identified, mobilised, tied, and divided during a cystectomy (removal of the bladder).

The peritoneum covers the anterolateral aspects of the rectum and the upper aspects of the posterior wall, dome, and anterior wall of the bladder. As the bladder fills and increases in size, the peritoneum covering its upper aspect and intraperitoneal contents such as bowel loops are pushed cranially by the enlarging dome of the bladder. In a patient with no previous abdominal surgery or peritoneal breach, this creates a peritoneal cavity free space that allows direct access to the bladder. The exposed bladder can be palpated two finger breadths cranially to the pubic symphysis and the direct access utilised to aspirate the bladder or place a percutaneous suprapubic catheter for bladder drainage in either an emergency setting for acute urinary retention, where it is not possible to catheterise the bladder urethrally or electively for the management of urinary incontinence in selected patients.

Urethra (Figs. 2.2, 2.4, 2.6, and 2.7)

The urethra in women is approximately 3.5 cm in length. It is a hollow tubular structure with an innermost urothelium lining with a rich submucosal vascular plexus surrounded by smooth then striated muscle fibres. The smooth muscle consists of an inner longitudinal and an outer circular layer which aid with urethral closure by autonomic unconscious constriction. The external urethral sphincter encircles the urethra at its midpoint. It is composed of two types of fibres, slow twitch, which is constantly active and slow to fatigue allowing for tone and contraction to be maintained over long periods, and the fast twitch fibres under somatic voluntary (the rhabdosphincter) control in the proximal part of the sphincter complex. This layering creates urethral wall tension and compression which aid in the maintenance of continence. The widest area of the rhabdosphincter is over the middle third of the urethra with the bulk of the fibres anterior to the urethra – giving it a horseshoe or omega shape. Distally, the sphincter muscle fibres insert into the vaginal wall under the pubic arch and merge with the perineal membrane. Urinary continence in females relies on the quality of this sphincter. Posterior to the urethra, there is an abundance of connective tissue with the striated sphincter being described as a horseshoe shape. Continence within the urethra is achieved by coaptation of the urethral lumen (active and passive), external compression from the wall, the ability to manage changes in pressure transmitted from the abdomen, neurovascular stimulation, and fascial and ligamentous support. The striated external urethral sphincter is said to contribute one-third of the urethral resting tone [9]. The pubourethral ligament runs from the proximal urethra to the pubis, lateral to the symphysis to aid

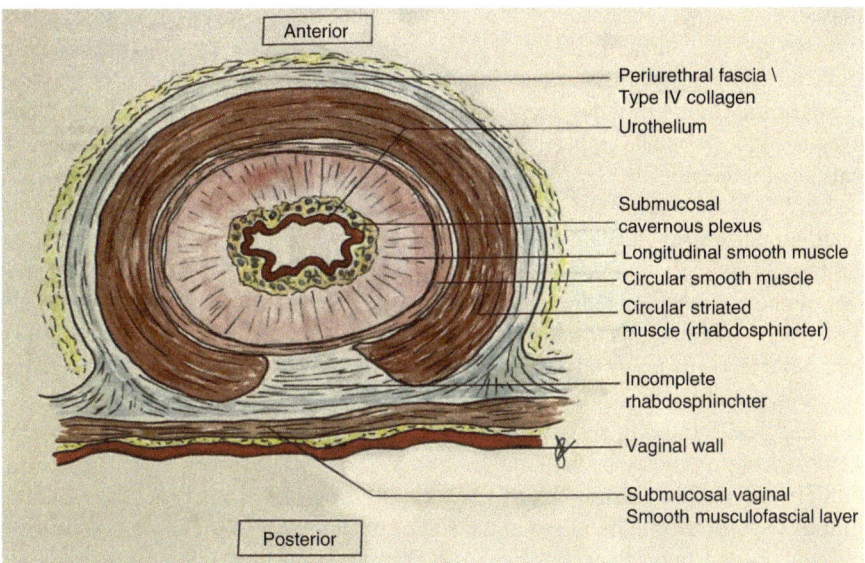

Fig. 2.6   Sagittal cross section of the female urethra

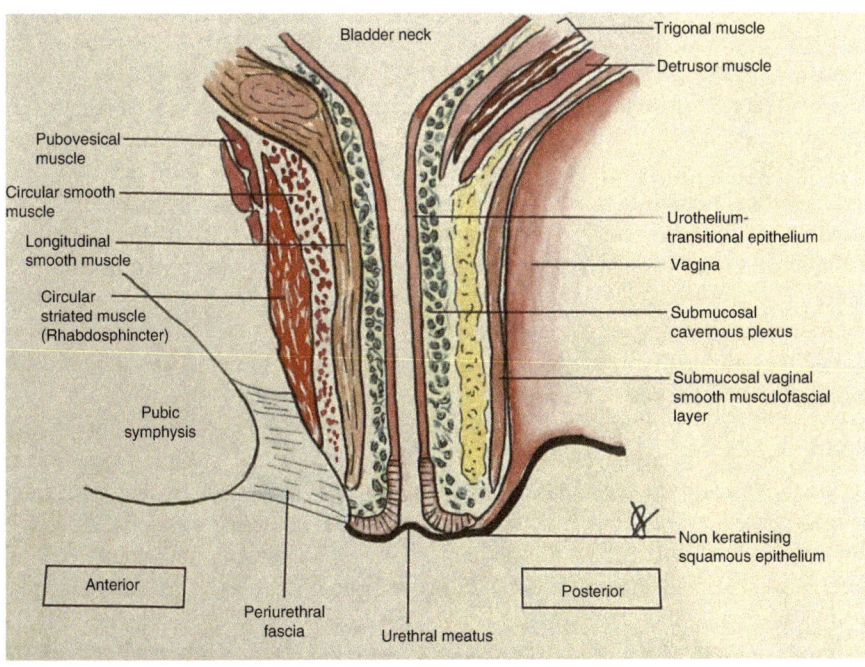

Fig. 2.7   Cross section of female urethra

urethral support. Hypermobility of the urethra (and bladder neck) due to ligamentous damage or connective tissue weakness or deficiency of the external urethral sphincter can lead to stress urinary incontinence (urinary leak with cough, sneeze, or exertion). The urethra has additional support from the endopelvic fascia and the muscles of the pelvic floor. In terms of contribution to urethral support, Rud reported that the striated muscle contributed 33% of the pressure, vascular factors contributed 28%, and the remaining 39% of support was from muscular and connective tissue support [10]. Once older than 25 years of age, there is an annual reduction in striated muscle cells causing progressive sphincter dysfunction with an estimated 15% reduction in maximum urethral closure pressure (MUCP) per decade [11]. However, in younger age groups vaginal delivery, sphincter dysfunction, and problems of urethral support are more equal contributors to stress incontinence. The contribution of the vascular plexus remains poorly understood; however, it is prominent and likely to aid in sealing the urethra. Urethral support appears to not be as important as previously believed in relation to urinary incontinence [1]. There are multiple submucosal glands which are located primarily in the distal and middle third of the urethra coinciding with the site of most urethral diverticula. The proximal urethra and bladder neck are seen to be mobile on fluoroscopic screening as opposed to the distal urethra which is seen to remain in a more fixed location [12].

The urethral closure pressure is the difference between the intravesical and intraurethral pressure. When intraurethral pressure is higher than intravesical pressure, then continence should be maintained. Urethral pressure profiles have been measured since 1967 when Toews, Brown, and Wickham (1969) described measuring pressures along the urethral length utilising catheters with side holes. The catheter position transducer was introduced in 1970 (Harrison and Constable) allowing consecutive readings to be superimposed. Prior to this, in 1948, pressure was measure with a vertical manometer (Bors) followed by balloon techniques which only measured over a finite length. In 1972, Malvern and Edwards described a mechanical withdrawal device to measure intraurethral pressure. From this measurement, the intravesical pressure was recorded, as well as the maximum urethral pressure (midurethral zone), urethral length, and maximal sphincter pressure [13].

The urethra has both fascial supports, which connect the anterior vaginal wall and periurethral tissues to the arcus tendinous, and muscular supports, connecting periurethral tissues to the levator ani on its medial border [9]. This support maintains the level of the bladder neck but allows for responsive dynamic movement during the micturition cycle. As abdominal pressure increases, for example, during coughing, the urethral support allows the urethra to be compressed against the anterior vaginal wall to facilitate urethral coaptation and maintain continence. Where there is weakness of the muscular and/or ligamentous support, there can be stress incontinence.

Surgery to treat stress urinary incontinence aims to provide support to the urethra and/or bladder neck by elevating the bladder neck via suture suspension of the lateral vaginal tissues to the iliopectineal ligaments of the superior pubic rami (Burch colposuspension) or a back plate for the urethra by placing a natural tissue or synthetic sling under the mid-portion of the urethra, passing it through the retropubic or transobturator space.

Ureters (Figs. 2.3 and 2.5)

Knowledge of the course of the ureters is important to avoid inadvertent injury during pelvic surgery. The ureters are hollow tubular structures that are approximately 25 cm long. They originate as the funnel-shaped renal pelvis and lie on the psoas muscle in the line of the vertebral transverse processes as they travel inferiorly to the bladder. They cross the genitofemoral nerve during this journey and in turn are crossed by the uterine artery distally as they pass under the round ligament close to the lateral border of the cervix (water under the bridge is a good aide memoir) and by the sigmoid arteries on the left side of the pelvis. They pass over the pelvic brim to enter the pelvis at the bifurcation of the common iliac artery, travel laterally around the pelvic side wall to enter the bladder medially via an intramural tunnel and exit as the ureteric orifices. Ureters move urine antegradely to the bladder using peristaltic (or bolus) muscular action. The narrowest points of the ureter are the pelvi-ureteric junction (PUJ), the pelvic brim, and the vesico-ureteric junction (VUJ). These are also the commonest locations for obstruction by ureteric stones.

Other Pelvic Organs

Rectum and Anus (Figs. 2.1, 2.2, 2.4, and 2.5)

The rectum is the penultimate part of the large intestine. It lies anterior to the sacrum. It has a distal distensible part called the ampulla that permits temporary storage of bowel contents (faeces) until it is appropriate and socially acceptable to volitionally defecate. The rectum begins at the level of the S3 vertebra and is in continuity with the sigmoid colon above and the anal canal below. It has a sacral flexure and an anorectal flexure which is formed by the puborectalis muscle, and which contributes to faecal continence. The rectum receives its arterial blood supply from the superior, middle, and inferior rectal arteries (which are branches of the inferior mesenteric, the internal iliac, and the internal pudendal arteries, respectively). Its venous drainage is via corresponding veins that follow the arteries. The upper third of the rectum is covered by the peritoneum on its anterior and lateral aspects, the mid rectum is covered by the peritoneum only on its anterior, and the lower third is below the level of the peritoneum and is not covered by any peritoneum at all. The peritoneum is continuous between the rectum and uterus and forms the rectouterine pouch (of Douglas).

The rectal ampulla becomes the anal canal at the level of the puborectalis muscle within the pelvic floor muscles (the anorectal junction). The anal canal is approximately 4 cm long and is located within the anal triangle of the perineum. At rest, it is empty, and the continence of faeces and flatus is maintained by the internal anal sphincter. The internal anal sphincter is composed of involuntary circular smooth muscle whilst the external anal sphincter is composed of striated muscle. Damage to the muscle or nerves of the anal sphincter can result in faecal incontinence. Damage may be consequent to pelvic radiotherapy, neurological conditions such as diabetes, multiple sclerosis or spinal cord injury, and vaginal childbirth. The mucosa lining the anus forms longitudinal folds called anal columns which coalesce distally at the pectinate line to form a circle of anal valves around the anal canal. The pectinate line is at the level of the anococcygeus membrane. The arterial supply above the pectineal line is from the superior (anastomosing with the middle) rectal arteries. The arterial blood supply below the pectineal line is from the inferior (anastomosing with the middle) rectal arteries. Below the pectineal line, the anal canal is lined by non-keratinised squamous epithelium (anal pecten) which terminates distally at the anocutaneous line (white line) and transitions into true skin at the external anal orifice.

Pelvic Blood Supply

Fig. 2.8 Saggital view of right side internal female pelvis with organs removed demonstrating neurovascular supply to pelvis

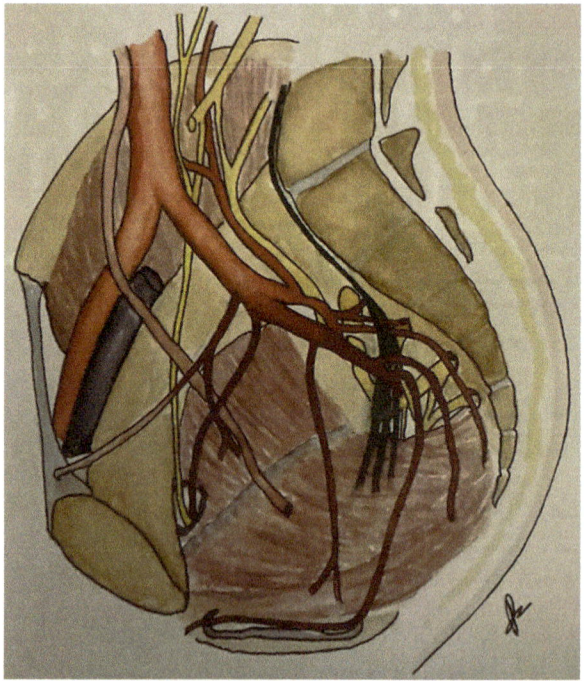

Arteries

The common iliac arteries take origin from the bifurcation of the abdominal aorta which occurs at the level of the T10 vertebra. Each common iliac artery is only approximately 3 cm long and almost immediately bifurcates at the sacroiliac joint (at the level of the L5/S1 vertebrae) into the internal and external iliac arteries. The female pelvis and perineum are both supplied by the internal iliac artery. The pelvic cavity venous system drains entirely into the internal iliac veins (Fig. 2.8).

Internal Iliac Artery

The internal iliac artery almost immediately divides into an anterior and posterior division The posterior division further branches into three muscular arteries, the iliolumbar, the lateral sacral, and the superior gluteal arteries. The iliolumbar artery is the first branch of the posterior division and ascends towards the sacroiliac joint. It supplies the iliacus, the psoas major, and the quadratus lumborum muscles and the cauda equina. The cauda equina (horse's tail) contains the nerve roots from the lumbosacral spine, and the coccygeal nerve after the spinal cord has terminated at the level of L1/L2 vertebra. The second branch of the posterior division is the lateral sacral artery which runs over the superficial aspect of piriformis to supply the piriformis muscle and the vertebral canal. The third branch of the posterior division is the superior gluteal artery which travels posteriorly to exit the pelvis above the piriformis muscle via the greater sciatic foramen to supply the muscles of the gluteal region.

The anterior division of the internal iliac artery gives seven branches which are in order of origin.

1. The obliterated umbilical artery, which may give rise to the superior vesical artery proximally whilst becoming obliterated distally. It lies within the medial umbilical ligament and is not always obliterated.
2. The superior vesical artery supplies the superior aspect of the urinary bladder.
3. The vaginal artery, which is the equivalent of the inferior vesical artery in men. It supplies the vagina, the inferior aspect of the bladder, and the rectum.
4. The obturator artery runs antero-inferiorly on the pelvic side wall to supply the ilium and femoral head.
5. The middle rectal artery supplies the rectum via extensive anastomoses with the superior rectal and the inferior rectal arteries.
6. The internal pudendal artery exits the pelvis through the greater sciatic foramen, turns around the sacrospinous ligament to enter the perineum through the inferior sciatic foramen, and supplies all the structures of the perineum.
7. The uterine artery runs medially on the surface of the levator ani, crosses above the ureter distally in the broad ligament, and supplies the uterus, with contributions to the vagina and ovary.

Arterial Blood Supply to Specific Structures and Organs in the Pelvis and Perineum

Ovary

The ovarian (gonadal) artery originates from the abdominal aorta at the level of the L1 vertebra, inferior to the renal artery. It crosses the external iliac vessels at the pelvic brim to enter the suspensory ligament of the ovary. It continues in the broad ligament and medially anastomoses with the uterine artery on the lateral wall of the uterus. It gives branches to the uterus and the fallopian tubes.

Vagina

The superior part of the vaginal is supplied by the uterine artery, whilst the remainder of the vagina is supplied by the middle rectal and pudendal arteries.

Urethra

The urethra is supplied by the internal pudendal artery.

Rectum and Anus

Rectal blood supply is from the superior rectal artery (a continuation of the inferior mesenteric artery), the middle rectal artery (a branch of the anterior division of the iliac artery), and the inferior rectal artery (a branch of the internal pudendal artery). The anal canal receives contributions from the inferior rectal vessels, which become superficial to supply the external anal sphincter and perianal skin.

Veins

The internal iliac vein carries venous blood from the pelvic organs, pelvic walls, perineum, and the external genitalia as well as from the lower limbs and the gluteal region. It is formed at the level of the greater sciatic notch in the pelvis, passes out of the pelvis over the pelvic brim to join with the external iliac vein on each side (which drains the lower limb), and becomes the common iliac vein which in turn join to form the inferior vena cava. The internal iliac vein runs posterior to the internal iliac artery on the psoas major muscle. The pelvic veins are paired with the branches of the internal iliac artery except for the iliolumbar artery and umbilical artery.

The rectum and uterus have surrounding venous plexus which, along with the lateral sacral veins, drain into the internal iliac vein. The venous plexuses are interconnected and surround the pelvic organs. The rectal venous plexus is a site of the portal-systemic venous system communication. The other sites are the distal oesophagus and the umbilicus. In clinical states causing portal hypertension such as chronic hepatic dysfunction, the portal hypertension results in back pressure into these collateral vessels at the sites of anastomoses. This causes venous dilation and clinically can be present with bleeding from oesophageal or anorectal varices. 'Caput medusae' may also be seen as dilated veins under the skin encircling the umbilicus.

The clitoris drains via a deep dorsal vein which enters the pelvis between the arcuate pubic ligament and the perineal membrane to join the vesical plexus. The clitoral skin venous drainage is into the great saphenous vein via the external pudendal veins.

The ovarian veins begin as a pampiniform plexus within the broad ligament. Initially, there are two ovarian veins on each side which merge into a single vein and follow the ovarian arteries retroperitoneally. The left ovarian (gonadal) vein drains into the left renal vein which then drains into the inferior vena cava. The right ovarian vein drains directly into the inferior vena cava. It is possible with renal tumours that extend down the renal veins especially on the left side and into the inferior vena cava to see ovarian varices on cross sectional imaging depending on severity of spread and/or labial varices.

Pelvic Plexuses and the Nerve Supply of the Pelvis and Perineum

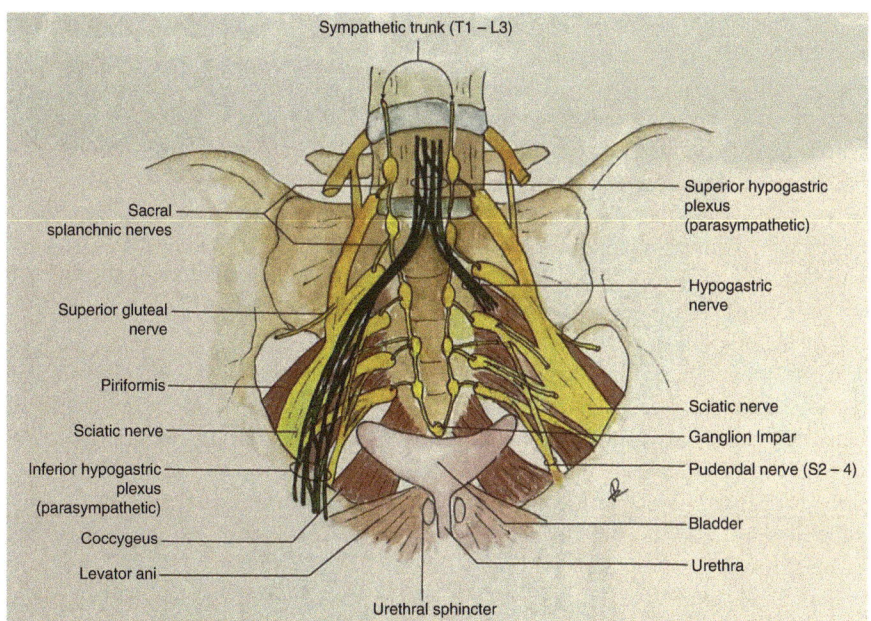

Fig. 2.9 Pelvis nerves anterior to sanctum – coronal view

Sacral Plexus, Coccygeal Plexus, and Somatic Nerves

The *sacral plexus* consists of motor and sensory nerves from the anterior rami of L4,5 and S1,2,3,4 spinal nerves. The sacral plexus is found on the surface of the piriformis muscle covered in fascia. The sacral sympathetic trunk has four ganglia (originating from T10-L2 segments of the spinal cord) and forms the ganglion impar on the anterior border of the coccyx. The nerves function to coordinate the control of voiding, defaecation, and orgasm. Branches of the sacral plexus include the sciatic nerve, the gluteal nerves to the lower limb, and the pudendal nerve. Other branches include motor nerves to the pelvic floor, the gluteal muscles, and the cutaneous sensory supply to the thigh. Somatic nerves are part of the peripheral nervous system and allow voluntary skeletal muscle control. Pelvic splanchnic nerves carry both fibres originating from the sympathetic nervous system and parasympathetic fibres. Pelvic splanchnic nerves are unique in that all others splanchnic nerves carry only sympathetic fibres.

The *coccygeal plexus* is formed mainly from the S5 nerve and the coccygeal nerve with some S4 nerve contribution. It provides cutaneous nerve supply to the coccygeal region.

Innervation of the Lower Urinary Tract: Visceral Plexuses

The lower urinary tract is supplied by *somatic*, *parasympathetic*, and *sympathetic* nerves. Function is coordinated by higher and local spinal centres allowing coordination of voiding and storage as well as voiding when socially acceptable.

The thoracolumbar spinal cord (T10-L2) gives rise to the *sympathetic nerves* which form the superior hypogastric plexus on the anterior aspect of L3-S1 vertebra. Stimulation of sympathetic nerves facilitates storage of urine by causing contraction of the smooth muscle within the urethra and the base of the bladder and inhibiting parasympathetic stimulation of detrusor contraction. This allows the bladder to fill and store urine under low pressure. Sympathetic nerve fibres are also responsible for smooth muscle contraction in the reproductive tract (ejaculation in particular), the internal urethral sphincter in males, and the internal anal sphincter in both sexes. The superior hypogastric plexus divides at the level of S1 to form the left and right hypogastric nerves.

The two hypogastric nerves enter the pelvis and travel laterally to form the prevertebral plexus carrying sympathetic, parasympathetic, and afferent fibres. The hypogastric nerves are joined by the pelvic splanchnic nerves carrying parasympathetic nerves (from S2-4) to form the inferior hypogastric plexus bilaterally in the retroperitoneal space either side of the rectum. This then progresses to creates three further plexuses: rectal, uterovaginal, and vesical. The erectile tissue of the clitoris is supplied by a terminal branch of the inferior hypogastric plexus after it enters and travels through the deep perineal pouch.

The sacral spinal cord (from segments S2-4) gives rise to *parasympathetic nerves* which travel in the pelvic nerves and when stimulated cause contraction of the detrusor to facilitate voiding. This is a type of local coordination centre known as the spinal micturition centre. The main control centre for bladder function is the pontine micturition centre in the brainstem. The parasympathetic nerves also stimulate erection and modulate the enteric nervous system.

The rectum has a sympathetic nerve supply from the hypogastric plexus and parasympathetic from the pelvic splanchnic nerves.

Somatic nerves from the sacral cord (Onuf's nucleus) run in the pudendal nerve (S2,3,4) to supply the striated urethral sphincter and cause sphincteric contraction when stimulated. The levator ani is supplied by direct sacral nerve fibres from branches of S4 and the pudendal nerve. The coccygeus muscle is supplied from S4 and S5. The piriformis muscle nerve supply originates from the ventral rami of nerve roots S1 and S2.

Other Important Nerves

Pudendal Nerve (Figs. 2.4 and 2.9)

The lateral walls of the ischioanal fossae contain the pudendal nerve which arises from S2,3,4 nerve roots. The pudendal nerve exits the pelvis via the greater sciatic foramen to enter the gluteal region. It then curves around the sacrospinous ligament at the ischial spine to enter the perineum via the lesser sciatic foramen. Once in the perineum, it enters Alcock's canal – which is a condensation of the obturator internus fascia and travels anteriorly along the lateral edge of the ischiorectal fossa in this canal. On exiting the pudendal canal, it branches to give the inferior rectal nerve which supplies the perianal skin and the external anal sphincter. At the posterior border of the perineal membrane, the pudendal nerve divides to form the perineal nerve which provides sensory supply to the vulva, the motor nerve supply to levator ani (mostly from S3 and S4 fibres) and the superficial perineal striated musculature, and a further branch – the dorsal nerve of the clitoris, to supply the clitoris.

Obturator Nerve

The obturator nerve (from nerve roots L2-4) is a branch of the lumbar plexus, which runs from the psoas muscle, along the pelvic side wall into the obturator canal on the superolateral border of the obturator foramen. It supplies the adductor compartment of the medial thigh.

Sensory Nerves

Sensory fibres that run back to L1 from the mons pubis and labia do so via the genitofemoral and ilioinguinal nerves. Sensation from the perineum runs via the small sciatic nerve to S1,2,3 via the posterior femoral cutaneous nerve. Sensory afferent nerves are important for detecting pain, temperature, and stretch within the bladder wall.

Lymphatics of the Female Pelvis

It is important to have knowledge of the lymphatic drainage sites from all pelvic organs particularly in relation to infection and malignancy. The main lymphatic drainage of the pelvic organs is to the internal and external iliac lymph nodes; however, there are also other lymphatics involved. From the iliac lymphatics, there is drainage via the common iliac nodes, para-aortic or lumbar nodes to the thoracic duct. The thoracic duct is found at the level of the 12th thoracic vertebra (T12). From there, it extends to the neck and drains into the venous system at the junction of left subclavian vein with the left internal jugular vein. The thoracic duct on the left drains most of the lymph from the body with exception of that from the right thorax, the right arm, the head, and neck, which drain to the right lymphatic duct. The right lymphatic duct drains into the venous system at the junction between right subclavian vein and the right internal jugular vein. Lymphadenopathy or lymphadenectomy can result in distal lymphoedema, seen most commonly in limbs.

Urinary Tract

The bladder lymphatics drain to the internal and external iliac lymph nodes. Removal of theses lymph nodes and vessels during lymphadenectomy performed for bladder (urothelial) cancer treatment at the time of radical cystectomy can result in the formation of a lymphocele due to leak from open lymphatics after removal of these nodes.

The urethral lymphatic drainage is to the internal iliac nodes and the superficial inguinal nodes. Primary urethral cancer is rare, however in a female patient with obstructive voiding symptoms and a 'woody' feeling urethra, urgent biopsy is essential. Radical surgery should include inguinal node as well as iliac node excision.

Reproductive Organs

The uterus and fallopian tube lymphatic drainage is into the external and internal iliac nodes plus the sacral nodes. The lower third of the vagina follows the vulval and urethra and drains into the superficial inguinal nodes. The upper two-thirds drain into the external and internal iliac nodes.

The ovarian lymphatic drainage is into the para-aortic regional lymph nodes consequent to the embryological origin of the ovaries. This means that metastatic lymphatic spread from an ovarian tumour is difficult to detect clinically unless huge and palpable abdominally.

The vulva and perineum on the medial aspect of the labiocrural skin fold drain upwards to the mons pubis and to superficial inguinal and femoral lymph nodes.

Rectum and Anus

The lymphatic drainage of the rectum follows the blood vessels back to the pre-aortic nodes surrounding the origin of the inferior mesenteric vessels. The lower anal canal drains to the superficial inguinal nodes along with the vagina and urethra. The remaining rectum drains to the inferior mesenteric nodes, the internal iliac nodes (middle rectal artery), the pararectal nodes, and the preaortic nodes.

Conclusions

The aim of this chapter has been to discuss normal female pelvic anatomy and physiology and relate to this to the possible causes of urinary incontinence and/or prolapse. This will allow a good foundation of understanding with regard to diagnosis of these conditions, help direct clinical examination and investigation, and highlight surgical landmarks. This chapter is important to help understanding throughout the rest of this book.

Take-Home Message

Pelvic organs are supported by muscles and ligaments. Any weakness in either can lead to pelvic organ prolapse or stress urinary incontinence. Pregnancy and vaginal delivery have significant effects on pelvic anatomy. History can point to a likely cause for the urinary incontinence and should include symptoms, duration, previous surgery, and/or treatment such as radiotherapy alongside a thorough, chaperoned, examination. In patients with continual urinary incontinence, overflow, congenital ectopic ureters, and fistula involving the urinary tract should be considered.

The levator ani consists of three muscles, and the main blood supply to the pelvic organs arises from the internal iliac artery.

Acknowledgement We would like to acknowledge the contribution of Ms. Suzanne Biers.

Further Reading
Gray's anatomy for students
Gynaecology by 10 teachers
Oxford handbook of clinical urology
Oxford textbook of urological surgery
Whats's new in the functional anatomy of pelvic organ prolapse? John O. L. Delancey. Curr Opin Obstet Gynecol. 2016;28(5):420–9

References

1. Delancey JO. Why do women have stress urinary incontinence? Neurourol Urodyn. 2010;29(Suppl 1):S13–7.
2. Enhorning G. Simultaneous recording of intravesical and intra-urethral pressure. A study on urethral closure in normal and stress incontinent women. Acta Chir Scand Suppl. 1961;Suppl 276:1–68.
3. Petros P. The integral system. Cent Eur J Urol. 2011;64(3):110–9.
4. DeLancey JO, Trowbridge ER, Miller JM, Morgan DM, Guire K, Fenner DE, et al. Stress urinary incontinence: relative importance of urethral support and urethral closure pressure. J Urol. 2008;179(6):2286–90; discussion 90
5. Blaivas JG, Olsson CA. Stress incontinence: classification and surgical approach. J Urol. 1988;139(4):727–31.
6. Abrams P, Cardozo L, Fall M, Griffiths D, Rosier P, Ulmsten U, et al. The standardisation of terminology in lower urinary tract function: report from the standardisation sub-committee of the International Continence Society. Urology. 2003;61(1):37–49.
7. Bonney V. On diurnal incontinence of urine in women. J Obstet Gynaecol Br Emp. 1923;30:358–65.
8. Berger MB, Doumouchtsis SK, DeLancey JO. Bony pelvis dimensions in women with and without stress urinary incontinence. Neurourol Urodyn. 2013;32(1):37–42.
9. Wei JT, De Lancey JO. Functional anatomy of the pelvic floor and lower urinary tract. Clin Obstet Gynecol. 2004;47(1):3–17.
10. Rud T, Andersson KE, Asmussen M, Hunting A, Ulmsten U. Factors maintaining the intraurethral pressure in women. Investig Urol. 1980;17(4):343–7.
11. Rud T. Urethral pressure profile in continent women from childhood to old age. Acta Obstet Gynecol Scand. 1980;59(4):331–5.
12. Muellner SR. The physiology of micturition. J Urol. 1951;65(5):805–13.
13. Edwards L, Malvern J. The urethral pressure profile: theoretical considerations and clinical application. Br J Urol. 1974;46(3):325–35.

Chapter 3
Diagnosis of Urinary Incontinence in Women

Elizabeth Dray and Haritha Pavuluri

Introduction

Urinary incontinence is a widely prevalent disorder in women which negatively impacts patient quality of life and leads to significant societal and personal costs [8]. On average, a symptomatic woman will spend $750 per year out of pocket on incontinence management [20]. This burden can be substantially reduced by treatment of a patient's incontinence [21]. In order to effectively treat, a clinician must first accurately diagnose. In this chapter, we will review the differential diagnosis of incontinence in women and how history and physical exam findings can help discriminate between these etiologies. We will review noninvasive tests that can strengthen this data. We will then identify when it is appropriate to pursue more invasive or resource-intensive studies for the characterization of incontinence.

Differential Diagnosis

The first step in determining the cause of urinary incontinence is establishing that the perceived wetness is, in fact, urine. Non-urinary causes of wetness include physiologic or pathologic vaginal discharge and peritoneal fluid or dialysate. The quantity and quality of normal vaginal discharge can vary widely amongst women. Increased vaginal discharge can be caused by infection or malignancy, and vaginal wet prep, STD testing, and imaging if indicated can be used to differentiate between

E. Dray (✉) · H. Pavuluri
University of South Carolina School of Medicine Greenville, Greenville, SC, USA
e-mail: elizabeth.dray@prismahealth.org

© The Author(s), under exclusive license to Springer Nature Switzerland AG 2022
A. P. Cameron (ed.), *Female Urinary Incontinence*,
https://doi.org/10.1007/978-3-030-84352-6_3

these sources. Some individuals may find normal discharge distressing, and, once infectious or other pathologic etiologies are ruled out, can be educated and reassured. In the setting of prior pelvic surgery, radiation, or malignancy, peritoneovaginal fistulae can form, leading to continuous leakage of peritoneal fluid per vagina. Rarely, patients may develop fistulae between the fallopian tube and the vagina as well. Ascites or the use of peritoneal dialysis should also raise suspicion for a non-urinary cause of wetness in the setting of continuous leakage.

An ectopic ureter beyond the continence mechanism or other congenital anatomic abnormality should be investigated in the setting of lifelong incontinence, specifically continuous urinary incontinence.

Transient causes of incontinence should always be considered in a patient's workup. Causes of transient incontinence can be remembered by the mnemonic DIAPPERS (Delirium, Infection, Atrophic vaginitis, Psychologic, Pharmacologic, Excess urine production, Restricted mobility, Stool impaction) [14]. History taking specifically correlating incontinence onset with other health events or new medications is integral in making these diagnoses. Often, these conditions do not require urologic intervention, but rather deductive reasoning and interspecialty communication (i.e., referral to endocrinology, stool disimpaction, etc.). Functional incontinence, while not always transient, is a prime example of a situation where a urologist can easily overtreat to a patient's detriment. Functional incontinence is when an individual has a normal urologic function but may experience incontinence due to decreased ability to access a bathroom in a timely fashion. This is typically secondary to underlying comorbidity, such as dementia or Parkinson's disease. The "treatment" may be as straightforward as providing the patient with a bedside commode or having them work with physical therapy to improve mobility.

Urinary incontinence should be classified as urgency urinary incontinence (UUI), stress urinary incontinence (SUI), or mixed incontinence (MUI). Overflow incontinence is the presence of incontinence in an overfull bladder [3]. Continuous leakage of urine, coital incontinence, and post-void dribbling are not in and of themselves discrete forms of incontinence but instead manifestations of urgency or stress incontinence, urinary retention, or anatomic abnormalities such as urologic fistula or urethral stricture/stenosis. All forms of incontinence require evaluation beyond history taking, and in the view of many experts, the leakage should be directly observed prior to the patient undergoing invasive therapies.

History and Physical Exam

When evaluating urinary incontinence in a female, taking a complete history is essential. Past medical history should include surgical history (specifically prior pelvic, obstetric, or back surgeries), medical history (neurologic conditions, endocrine dysfunction, connective tissue disorders, radiation, trauma), and gynecologic and obstetric history, including parity and pre- or postmenopausal status. Current medications, as well as any prior pharmacotherapies for incontinence, should be assessed. Exogenous hormones, sympathomimetics, sympatholytics, anticholinergics, and diuretics may all contribute to symptoms of urinary incontinence. When assessing the history of present illness, incontinence can be subjectively characterized by asking whether the patient leaks with activity or cough/sneeze, with urgency, or both. If the answer is both, the patient should be asked which is more bothersome to them. An attempt should be made to evaluate the severity and frequency of a patient's leakage, which can be determined by the number of pads or briefs a patient uses per day or the number of times they change clothes due to incontinence. It is important to ask the degree of saturation of a patient's briefs or pads as some patients may be bothered by relatively small amounts of urine loss and change pads frequently even if they are not saturated. Voiding frequency, both during the day and at night should be assessed, as well as the presence or absence of dysuria, pelvic pain, urinary tract infections, and hematuria. The patient should be evaluated for obstructive lower urinary tract symptoms (straining, subjective incomplete emptying, weak stream), gastrointestinal symptoms (i.e., fecal incontinence or constipation), and prolapse complaints, as pelvic floor disorders frequently coexist [9]. Patients should be asked about neurologic symptoms, particularly, if there is new-onset urge urinary incontinence in a young woman, as urinary incontinence may be the harbinger of a neurologic condition such as multiple sclerosis. Lastly, it is extremely important to assess the impact that incontinence has on a patient's quality of life. In the vast majority of cases, incontinence is not life-threatening and therefore should only be intervened on if it is bothersome to the patient.

The characteristics of a patient's urinary incontinence can also be assessed using a variety of validated questionnaires. Commonly used metrics include the Urogenital Distress Inventory short form [UDI-6], the Incontinence Impact Questionnaire short form [IIQ-7], the International Consultation on Incontinence Questionnaire Urinary Incontinence short form [ICIQ-SF], the King's Health Questionnaire [KHQ], Patient Global Impression of Severity Scale [PGI-S], and the Michigan Incontinence Symptoms Index (M-ISI). These questionnaires assess SUI, UUI, severity, and quality of life and appear to be mostly well-correlated [10]. In addition to incontinence symptoms, prolapse and colorectal symptoms can be assessed using the pelvic floor distress inventory (PFDI).

History alone is not entirely reliable in evaluating urinary incontinence, and a physical exam should always be performed. Age, weight, and debility should be evaluated, as these factors are correlated with incontinence and may affect whether the patient is an operative candidate [24]. An abdominal exam can provide important information, such as the presence of incisions and suprapubic fullness or tenderness. Every patient undergoing an initial evaluation of incontinence should have a pelvic exam. This should assess the external genitalia (including estrogenic status), urethra, uterus, and adnexa, and the presence or absence of pelvic organ prolapse (POP). The supine cough stress test (CST) is the gold standard for the diagnosis of stress urinary incontinence in women. This is performed with the patient in lithotomy position and the bladder filled to a comfortable degree and is considered positive if incontinence is shown with cough or Valsalva. If incontinence cannot be demonstrated in the supine position, the test can be repeated standing. The correlation of a positive CST with urodynamic-proven SUI is >90% [6]. Urethral position and mobility may be evaluated at rest and with straining and coughing to assess for urethral hypermobility. Mobility beyond 30° is generally considered abnormal. This may be aided by the "Q-tip test," where a lubricated Q-tip is placed in the urethra prior to Valsalva, which is only needed if there is uncertainty on the physical exam. While the presence of urethral hypermobility may help determine whether a patient is a good candidate for a specific surgical intervention, such as a midurethral sling, it does not appear to have any significant predictive value in diagnosing the presence of stress incontinence [5]. POP should be evaluated using a split speculum exam and documented using a standardized and reproducible classification technique, such as the Baden-Walker or Pelvic Organ Prolapse Quantification (POP-Q) system. If there is a known or suspected history of a neurologic condition, a brief neurologic exam can be performed to assess rectal sphincter tone and the presence or absence of the bulbocavernosus reflex (Table 3.1).

Noninvasive Testing

A variety of noninvasive tests can be used to gain further information and rule out potential causes of urinary incontinence. Urinalysis is usually the first lab test that is ordered in a patient with urinary incontinence. An abnormal urinalysis, such as the presence of blood, glucose, or leukocyte esterase (LE), can indicate secondary causes of incontinence. If unexplained hematuria is noted (≥ 3 rbc/hpf), cystoscopy should be pursued (AUA Guideline on hematuria). Glucosuria should prompt endocrine or internal medicine referral for diabetes workup if this has not yet been diagnosed or communication with the primary care provider regarding blood glucose control if this is known comorbidity. A urine culture should be sent if LE or nitrites are found, as a urinary tract infection may be the source of a patient's incontinence or an exacerbating factor in their symptoms.

A postvoid residual (PVR) should be obtained to rule out incomplete bladder emptying and to assess the appropriateness of interventions (i.e., urinary antispasmodics or sling). PVR may be obtained by noninvasive ultrasound or sterile in and out catheterization, as they are considered equivalent [22]. There is no universal definition of elevated PVR; however, the vast majority of women have a PVR <100 cc [22]. While PVRs greater than or equal to 300 cc may be acceptable in asymptomatic individuals without high-risk features, incontinence is, by definition, a symptom [18]. The author would therefore suggest that a PVR > 100 cc prompt a more invasive workup prior to irreversible interventions.

Bladder diaries, or frequency volume charts, are useful methods of both characterizing incontinence and revealing nonadaptive patient behaviors. These can be kept for 24–72 h. There is significant recall bias in patient-reported urinary frequency, nocturia, and incontinence, with patients often overestimating the severity of their symptoms [19]. Voiding diaries give objective evidence of excessive fluid or

Table 3.1 Common findings in the history of presenting symptoms, past medical history, physical exam, and diagnostic tests

	SUI	UUI	Overflow incontinence	Functional incontinence	Total/anatomic incontinence	Mixed
History	Leak with cough, sneeze, activity, laugh	Sudden urge followed by leakage, on way to the toilet, nocturia, unaware	Mixed symptoms of both SUI and UUI + obstructive symptoms	Cognitive or physical impairment, unable to void independently	Constant leakage	Symptoms of both SUI and UUI
Physical exam/diagnostic tests	Positive supine cough stress test Urethral hypermobility (Q-tip test)	Large volume, high-velocity incontinence triggered by bladder filling Occasionally provoked by cough (stress test)	Full bladder on palpation or PVR	Immobility or decreased independent tasks of living	Abnormal tampon test Urethral erosion Urinary leakage per vagina Ectopic ureter on pelvic imaging	Positive supine cough stress test Large volume, high-velocity incontinence
Past medical history	Increasing parity Obesity	Neurologic disorders Recurrent cystitis Pelvic radiation	History of sling procedure, neurological condition History of urethral instrumentation Anticholinergic medication	Dementia Immobility Mental illness	Previous pelvic surgery, trauma, radiation, or malignancy Chronic indwelling urethral catheter Incontinence since childhood	Increasing parity, obesity, age

bladder irritant consumption, allowing the clinician to provide a patient with personalized action items for behavioral intervention.

The role of pad weight tests is controversial and is largely used in academic settings for research purposes. Twenty-four-hour pad tests are more clinically relevant than one-hour pad tests and, while definitions vary, are typically considered positive if there is greater than 1.3 g of urine loss over that time period [2]. It should be noted, however, that studies have shown little difference between pad weight tests in self-reported "continent" and "incontinent" groups [15]. A more commonly used surrogate for the severity of incontinence is pads per day, which can be assessed through patient history. It is important to elicit the degree of pad saturation, as individuals may change their pads every time they urinate, even if they are relatively dry.

Dye testing is another useful test in assessing leakage—particularly in determining whether leakage is urine versus another fluid or in identifying the site of a fistula. In order to identify whether urine is the source of wetness, a patient can take 200 mg of oral Pyridium and wear a pad for several hours. If the fluid is urine, it will be orange in color. Sweat, peritoneal fluid, or vaginal discharge will remain clear. When looking for a fistula, a tampon is inserted, and dye, such as methylene blue, is instilled intravesically. Staining at the proximal aspect of the tampon is suggestive of a vesicovaginal fistula while distal staining may indicate urethral leakage. If there is concern for a ureterovaginal fistula, a double dye test is performed. In this case, the bladder is filled with a methylene blue solution, and oral Pyridium is concomitant. Orange staining of the tampon is pathognomonic of a ureterovaginal fistula while blue staining may be secondary to a vesicovaginal fistula or urethral incontinence [17].

Imaging has a limited role in the evaluation of urinary incontinence in women. If there is clinical suspicion for a urethral diverticulum or ectopic ureter, MRI pelvis is a sensitive, if potentially cost-prohibitive, means of definitive diagnosis. Renal ultrasonography is sensitive and specific for diagnosing hydronephrosis and should be obtained if high-risk features for upper tract deterioration are present. Translabial or transvaginal ultrasonography may be useful to visualize mesh that was previously placed for pelvic floor reconstruction if there is concern that this is a contributing factor in the patient's incontinence [16].

Advanced Testing

When the etiology of a patient's incontinence is unclear, two advanced testing modalities can be considered: a cystoscopy and urodynamic studies (UDS). Neither is indicated for the initial workup of the index patient (uncomplicated SUI or UUI AUA guidelines Gormley OAB Kobashi SUI). However, there are many circumstances in which one or both may be necessary to safely and thoroughly evaluate more complex presentations.

The role of cystoscopy is to directly visualize the patient's bladder and urethra, thus ruling out pathologies that may be causing or exacerbating the patient's symptoms. While routine cystoscopy does not appear to affect outcomes for most patients, there are clearly situations where cystoscopy is a commonsense adjunct to a patient's workup. For example, a lifelong smoker with urge urinary incontinence and dysuria with negative urine cultures should likely undergo a cystoscopy to rule out bladder cancer as the source of her irritative lower urinary tract symptoms. Furthermore, incontinence in the setting of prior transvaginal mesh, especially if there is a history of recurrent UTIs, should prompt a cystoscopy to exclude the diagnosis of mesh erosion. Cystoscopy and appropriate upper tract imaging should also be performed if the patient meets the diagnostic criteria for hematuria (AUA guideline hematuria).

Multichannel urodynamics (UDS) is the study of bladder storage and emptying. They consist of cystometry, which assesses pressure and volume during filling, and pressure-flow studies, which evaluate bladder pressure and urine flow rate during voiding. Multichannel UDS differs from uroflowmetry and simple cystometrics in that it objectively measures bladder pressures. Typically, it is accompanied by electromyography (EMG), which measures the activity of the striated urinary sphincter and pelvic floor musculature via a patch or needle electrode. In studies performed for the investigation of urinary incontinence, the primary goal is often the identification of urgency or stress incontinence. However, it is important to keep in mind that reduced compliance or incomplete bladder emptying can also contribute to leakage. Urgency urinary incontinence is often associated with detrusor overactivity (DO) on UDS. DO is a urodynamic observation of an involuntary detrusor contraction during bladder filling which may or may not be accompanied by incontinence. In the setting of a known neurologic condition, this is termed neurogenic DO [1]. It is important to keep in mind that up to 50% of individuals with urge urinary incontinence may not have DO on UDS. Furthermore, ~15% of patients *without* urge urinary incontinence can have "test-induced" DO [23]. Urodynamic findings do not outweigh a convincing history. Stress urinary incontinence is defined by the presence of an abdominal leak point pressure (ALPP) on UDS. ALPP is the intravesical pressure at which urine leakage occurs due to increased abdominal pressure in the absence of a detrusor contraction [1]. Patients without SUI do not have urinary incontinence at any abdominal pressure, and therefore do not have an ALPP. A lower ALPP is associated with worsening severity of SUI. By convention, an ALPP of <60 cm H2O is considered to be indicative of intrinsic sphincter deficiency. However, this does not take into account the presence or absence of urethral hypermobility on the exam and should therefore be interpreted with caution [11] (Table 3.2).

Patient selection and timing of UDS remains a controversial topic. Many experts have formerly advocated routine UDS prior to invasive or irreversible treatments for incontinence. This changed with the publication of the VALUE trial, a large, multicentered randomized control trial which showed no difference in outcomes between women with uncomplicated SUI who received UDS prior to sling placement and those who did not [13]. While similarly robust data does not exist for urge urinary incontinence, a recent meta-analysis did not show a clear benefit from UDS prior to third-line therapies for OAB [4]. Most experts would agree that UDS are indicated

Table 3.2 Findings on UDS as defined by the International Continence Society

	ICS definition
DO	Phasic contractions of detrusor muscle occurring during filling cystometry
	Waveform seen on cystometrogram
NDO	In patients with a clinically relevant neurologic disorder, phasic contractions of detrusor muscle occurring during filling cystometry
	Waveform seen on cystometrogram
Reduced compliance storage dysfunction (RCSD)	Non-phasic rise in detrusor pressure during filling cystometry
	Reduction in capacity/compliance
Reduced filling sensation	Perceived reduction in sensation during filling cystometry
Detrusor leak point pressure (DLPP)	Lowest pressure at which urinary leakage occurs in the absence of detrusor contraction or increased abdominal pressure
	>40 cm H_2O in females results in increased risk for morbidity
Abdominal leak point pressure (ALPP)	Absence of detrusor contraction, the lowest value of increased intrabdominal pressure that results in urine leakage at fixed bladder volume (200–300 mL)
	Valsalva (VLPP)
	<60 cm H_2O – Severe
	60–90 cm H_2O – Moderate
	>90 cm H_2O – Mild
	Cough (CLPP)

ICS Glossary. International Continence Society
McGuire EJ, Woodside JR, Borden TA, et al. Prognostic value of urodynamic testing in myelodysplastic patients. J Urol. 1981;126:205–9

before proceeding with invasive interventions in the setting of prior anti-incontinence or prolapse surgery, severe incontinence, poorly defined incontinence symptoms, elevated PVR or significant obstructive symptoms, neurologic lower urinary tract dysfunction, or inability to elicit SUI on a cough stress test or simple cystometrics [7].

Conclusions

At least one-quarter of women suffer from some degree of urinary incontinence [12]. All urologists and urogynecologists should be adept at evaluating these conditions. Workup should include a consideration of non-urologic sources of wetness and causes of transient incontinence, as well as an assessment of prior pelvic radiation or surgeries and gynecologic or obstetric history. Incontinence should be characterized by identifying the duration of symptoms, inciting and exacerbating factors, severity, and coexisting obstructive symptoms. All patients should undergo a pelvic and abdominal exam. At a minimum, a urinalysis should be performed and PVR assessed. Imaging and more invasive diagnostic tests should be obtained on an individualized basis.

References

1. Abrams P, Cardozo L, Fall M, Griffiths D, Rosier P, Ulmsten U, van Kerrebroeck P, Victor A, Wein A. Standardisation Sub-committee of the International Continence Society. The standardisation of terminology of lower urinary tract function: report from the Standardisation Sub-committee of the International Continence Society. Neurourol Urodyn. 2002;21(2):167–78. https://doi.org/10.1002/nau.10052. PMID: 11857671.
2. Al Afraa T, Mahfouz W, Campeau L, Corcos J. Normal lower urinary tract assessment in women: I. Uroflowmetry and post-void residual, pad tests, and bladder diaries. Int Urogynecol J. 2012;23(6):681–5. https://doi.org/10.1007/s00192-011-1568-z. Epub 2011 Sep 21. Review. PubMed PMID: 21935667.
3. D'Ancona C, Haylen B, Oelke M, Abranches-Monteiro L, Arnold E, Goldman H, Hamid R, Homma Y, Marcelissen T, Rademakers K, Schizas A, Singla A, Soto I, Tse V, de Wachter S, Herschorn S; Standardisation Steering Committee ICS and the ICS Working Group on Terminology for Male Lower Urinary Tract & Pelvic Floor Symptoms and Dysfunction. The International Continence Society (ICS) report on the terminology for adult male lower urinary tract and pelvic floor symptoms and dysfunction. Neurourol Urodyn. 2019;38(2):433–77. https://doi.org/10.1002/nau.23897. Epub 2019 Jan 25. PMID: 30681183.
4. Glass D, Lin FC, Khan AA, Van Kuiken M, Drain A, Siev M, Peyronett B, Rosenblum N, Brucker BM, Nitti VW. Impact of preoperative urodynamics on women undergoing pelvic organ prolapse surgery. Int Urogynecol J. 2020;31(8):1663–8. https://doi.org/10.1007/s00192-019-04084-8. Epub 2019 Aug 27. PMID: 31456030.
5. Holroyd-Leduc JM, Tannenbaum C, Thorpe KE, Straus SE. What type of urinary incontinence does this woman have? JAMA. 2008;299(12):1446–56. https://doi.org/10.1001/jama.299.12.1446. Review. PubMed PMID: 18364487.
6. Hsu TH, Rackley RR, Appell RA. The supine stress test: a simple method to detect intrinsic urethral sphincter dysfunction. J Urol. 1999;162(2):460–3. https://doi.org/10.1016/s0022-5347(05)68589-8. PubMed PMID: 10411057.
7. Kobashi KC, Albo ME, Dmochowski RR, Ginsberg DA, Goldman HB, Gomelsky A, Kraus SR, Sandhu JS, Shepler T, Treadwell JR, Vasavada S, Lemack GE. Surgical treatment of female stress urinary incontinence: AUA/SUFU guideline. J Urol. 2017;198(4):875–83. https://doi.org/10.1016/j.juro.2017.06.061. Epub 2017 Jun 15. PubMed PMID: 28625508.
8. Krhut J, Gärtner M, Mokris J, Horcicka L, Svabik K, Zachoval R, Martan A, Zvara P. Effect of severity of urinary incontinence on quality of life in women. Neurourol Urodyn. 2018;37(6):1925–30. https://doi.org/10.1002/nau.23568. Epub 2018 Mar 31. PubMed PMID: 29603780.
9. Lawrence JM, Lukacz ES, Nager CW, Hsu JW, Luber KM. Prevalence and co-occurrence of pelvic floor disorders in community-dwelling women. Obstet Gynecol. 2008;111(3):678–85. https://doi.org/10.1097/AOG.0b013e3181660c1b. PubMed PMID: 18310371.
10. Malik RD, Hess DS, Christie A, Carmel ME, Zimmern PE. Domain comparison between 6 validated questionnaires administered to women with urinary incontinence. Urology. 2019;132:75–80. https://doi.org/10.1016/j.urology.2019.07.008. Epub 2019 Jul 13. PubMed PMID: 31310769.
11. McGuire EJ, Fitzpatrick CC, Wan J, Bloom D, Sanvordenker J, Ritchey M, Gormley EA. Clinical assessment of urethral sphincter function. J Urol. 1993;150(5 Pt 1):1452–4. https://doi.org/10.1016/s0022-5347(17)35806-8. PubMed PMID: 8411422.

12. Minassian VA, Drutz HP, Al-Badr A. Urinary incontinence as a worldwide problem. Int J Gynaecol Obstet. 2003;82(3):327–38. https://doi.org/10.1016/s0020-7292(03)00220-0. Review. PubMed PMID: 14499979.
13. Nager CW, Brubaker L, Daneshgari F, Litman HJ, Dandreo KJ, Sirls L, Lemack GE, Richter HE, Leng W, Norton P, Kraus SR, Chai TC, Chang D, Amundsen CL, Stoddard AM, Tennstedt SL. Design of the Value of Urodynamic Evaluation (ValUE) trial: a non-inferiority randomized trial of preoperative urodynamic investigations. Contemp Clin Trials. 2009;30(6):531–9. https://doi.org/10.1016/j.cct.2009.07.001. Epub 2009 Jul 25. PubMed PMID: 19635587; PubMed Central PMCID: PMC3057197.
14. Resnick NM. Urinary incontinence in the elderly. Medical Grand Rounds 1984;3:281–90.
15. Ryhammer AM, Laurberg S, Djurhuus JC, Hermann AP. No relationship between subjective assessment of urinary incontinence and pad test weight gain in a random population sample of menopausal women. J Urol. 1998;159(3):800–3. PubMed PMID: 9474152.
16. Staack A, Vitale J, Ragavendra N, Rodríguez LV. Translabial ultrasonography for evaluation of synthetic mesh in the vagina. Urology. 2014;83(1):68–74. https://doi.org/10.1016/j.urology.2013.09.004. Epub 2013 Nov 12. PubMed PMID: 24231215.
17. Stamatakos M, Sargedi C, Stasinou T, Kontzoglou K. Vesicovaginal fistula: diagnosis and management. Indian J Surg. 2014;76(2):131–6. https://doi.org/10.1007/s12262-012-0787-y. Epub 2012 Dec 14. Review. PubMed PMID: 24891778; PubMed Central PMCID: PMC4039689.
18. Stoffel JT, Peterson AC, Sandhu JS, Suskind AM, Wei JT, Lightner DJ. AUA White Paper on Nonneurogenic Chronic Urinary Retention: Consensus Definition, Treatment Algorithm, and Outcome End Points. J Urol. 2017;198(1):153–60. https://doi.org/10.1016/j.juro.2017.01.075. Epub 2017 Feb 3. PMID: 28163030.
19. Stav K, Dwyer PL, Rosamilia A. Women overestimate daytime urinary frequency: the importance of the bladder diary. J Urol. 2009;181(5):2176–80. https://doi.org/10.1016/j.juro.2009.01.042. Epub 2009 Mar 17. PubMed PMID: 19296975.
20. Subak LL, Brubaker L, Chai TC, et al. High costs of urinary incontinence among women electing surgery to treat stress incontinence. Obstet Gynecol. 2008;111(4):899–907. https://doi.org/10.1097/AOG.0b013e31816a1e12.
21. Subak LL, Goode PS, Brubaker L, Kusek JW, Schembri M, Lukacz ES, Kraus SR, Chai TC, Norton P, Tennstedt SL. Urinary incontinence management costs are reduced following Burch or sling surgery for stress incontinence. Am J Obstet Gynecol. 2014;211(2):171.e1–7. https://doi.org/10.1016/j.ajog.2014.03.012. Epub 2014 Mar 11. PubMed PMID: 24631433; PubMed Central PMCID: PMC4349353.
22. Tseng LH, Liang CC, Chang YL, Lee SJ, Lloyd LK, Chen CK. Postvoid residual urine in women with stress incontinence. Neurourol Urodyn. 2008;27(1):48–51. https://doi.org/10.1002/nau.20463. PMID: 17563112.
23. van Waalwijk van Doorn ES, Meier AH, Ambergen AW, Janknegt RA. Ambulatory urodynamics: extramural testing of the lower and upper urinary tract by Holter monitoring of cystometrogram, uroflowmetry, and renal pelvic pressures. Urol Clin North Am. 1996;23(3):345–71. https://doi.org/10.1016/s0094-0143(05)70317-7. Review. PubMed PMID: 8701551.
24. Whitcomb EL, Lukacz ES, Lawrence JM, Nager CW, Luber KM. Prevalence and degree of bother from pelvic floor disorders in obese women. Int Urogynecol J Pelvic Floor Dysfunct. 2009;20(3):289–94. https://doi.org/10.1007/s00192-008-0765-x. Epub 2008 Nov 11. PubMed PMID: 19002365; PubMed Central PMCID: PMC4943873.

Chapter 4
Urodynamic Testing of Female Incontinence

Anne P. Cameron

Principles of Urodynamics

Pressure flow urodynamics (UDS) is one of the many tools that the continence care provider can employ to make a more precise diagnosis of a woman's urinary symptoms. They are not a substitute for a good history and physical exam, and their results in isolation without clinical context are difficult to interpret. In general, urodynamics should be used when the clinical diagnosis is unclear with a more basic assessment, and the results will change patient management.

A simple decision aid in determining if the urodynamics need to be performed is assessing the uncertainty in the diagnosis and multiplying this by the risk of the decision being made, either the risk of a missed important diagnosis or the risk of the procedure.

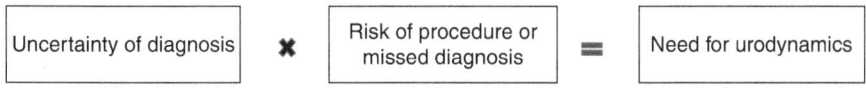

For example, if a patient has mixed incontinence on history (uncertainty of stress urinary incontinence (SU)I vs. urgency urinary incontinence (UUI) is high) and chooses pelvic floor physical therapy (risk is zero since this will help either condition), then the need for UDS is zero (high × 0 = 0) because it is not important to know if she indeed has SUI or UUI to proceed with her care since PFPT can treat both conditions. Another example would be a woman with urinary retention immediately after a sling procedure that has persisted for months who had no voiding

A. P. Cameron (✉)
Urology, University of Michigan, Ann Arbor, MI, USA
e-mail: annepell@med.umich.edu

symptoms and a low residual prior to the sling. In this case, the uncertainty of the diagnosis is zero even though the risk of the needed surgical procedure is high ($0 \times$ high = 0) and UDS are not needed.

Instances where the need for UDS has been well investigated are in the care of index cases of stress incontinence in women. The Value trial [1] randomized women with uncomplicated SUI undergoing sling placement to UDS or standard clinic assessment prior to surgery. The results of the UDS did not change management plans or the surgical outcome; hence, in this population, it is not needed. Studies on UDS testing trends have shown that the rate of preoperative testing has decreased since this study has been published [2]. A review of a 5% sample of Medicare beneficiaries with mixed incontinence found that regardless of the surgical approach in these women, preoperative UDS did not change the risk of re-intervention following surgery, further emphasizing that good clinical decision-making can be done without UDS, but with a good history and physical exam and potentially noninvasive testing [3].

The utility of urodynamics was assessed in a more complex population of patients, none of which were index cases of SUI, and among the 285 studies performed, the treatment plan changed in 43% of cases as a result of the UDS results, with 35% having a change in the surgical plan [4]. Fluoroscopy was used in most studies with helpful findings in 29.5% of cases.

Several studies have sought to assess the prognostic ability of UDS in predicting surgical outcomes for other incontinence procedures. Nobrega et al. assessed several urodynamic parameters in 99 patients with detrusor overactivity (DO) undergoing sacral neuromodulation and unfortunately did not find any urodynamics parameters that predicted the success of the staged procedure [5]. Similarly, the urodynamic diagnosis of DO prior to botulinum toxin injection did not alter patient-reported outcomes compared to those patients without DO [6]. In a series of male patients, however, higher BOOI (and elevated PVR) did predict a higher risk of urinary retention requiring self-catheterization [7].

Urodynamics, however, are often a cornerstone of urological diagnosis with many clinical scenarios where they are essential. Examples include assessments for safety compliance in neurogenic lower urinary tract dysfunction (NGLUTD) or differentiating between outlet obstruction or detrusor underactivity (DU) in a woman with retention. The AUA Guidelines discuss the use of UDS, and both the female stress incontinence and OAB guidelines state that UDS should not be used in the initial workup of the uncomplicated patient but recommend their use for diagnostic purposes and complex patients [8, 9]. In this chapter, the International Continence Society's (ICS) good urodynamic practices and terms will be referenced as the standard terminology [10].

Urodynamics Testing Alternatives

There are several noninvasive and cost-effective testing modalities that can be employed before or instead of formal pressure flow urodynamic studies.

A *post-void residual (PVR)* with either a bladder scanner (ultrasound) or a catheterized measurement of residual intravesical urine volume is an excellent screening tool to assess for incomplete bladder emptying or retention. This measurement is particularly helpful when it is very high or when there is a baseline value for that woman for comparison, such as a woman who had a residual of 0 ml before an incontinence procedure but now has a residual of 200 ml. There is no established "normal" value for residual urine [11]; a good rule of thumb in the context of expected deterioration of bladder contractility with age is that residual urine is totally normal if less than one's age. The method of collection should be specified since there are both false positives and negatives associated with each. Examples of a false-positive result with the ultrasound method include ascites, peritoneal dialysis, pregnancy, or an ovarian cyst where fluid outside the bladder is mistakenly measured. A false negative can result if the scanner is not directed towards the bladder or if the catheter used for collection is not placed completely within the lumen of the bladder or is withdrawn too soon.

A *uroflowmetry* (simple uroflow) measures the flow rate of the urine stream as a volume in milliliters per second and when combined with a post-void residual provides information on voiding dysfunction. This has the added benefit of physiological voiding in a private setting and should be performed in the patient's usual voiding position. A uroflowmetry is considered part of the ICS standard urodynamic test [10] where it is performed immediately before the study to obtain unintubated uroflow and residual urine results. Patients should arrive for the test with a comfortably full bladder and wait for their usual urge to void to be felt. A pitfall in uroflowmetry is having a woman void before her bladder is full often resulting in low voided volume (<150 cc) which is difficult to interpret since low volume voids are slower inflow and the male nomograms exclude these measurements. Conversely, uroflowmetry may be abnormal if voiding was postponed for too long before the test, with an overdistended bladder [10].

Measured values include the maximum flow rate (Qmax), average flow rate (Qave), and voided volume. The values for uroflowmetry in normal women vary considerably by voided volume, unlike in men where flow rates also decrease with age [12]. There is actually little data on normal uroflowmetry in women, unlike men where this measure has been widely utilized in the diagnosis of bladder outflow obstruction (BOO) from prostatic obstruction with clear normative values [13]. Women often void with very high flow (>30 ml/s = hyperflow), and the curve is bell-shaped, but voiding time is shorter than in men. Qave ranges from 17 to 24 ml/s in normal women and Qmax from 23 to 33 ml/s, with voided volume ranges between 250 and 550 ml and residual urine typically less than 15 ml [12]. The curve can be described as bell-shaped (normal), flat (very slow), flat peaked (evidence of obstruction), hyperflow (normal in women), and a straining pattern (use of abdominal muscle for voiding with sawtooth pattern) (Fig. 4.1).

Voiding diaries can give excellent physiologic information about bladder behavior outside of the testing environment where results can be altered by anxiety, discomfort, and a non-physiologic filling rate. Most measure fluid intake volume and fluid type as well as voided volume, sensation of urgency, and leakage

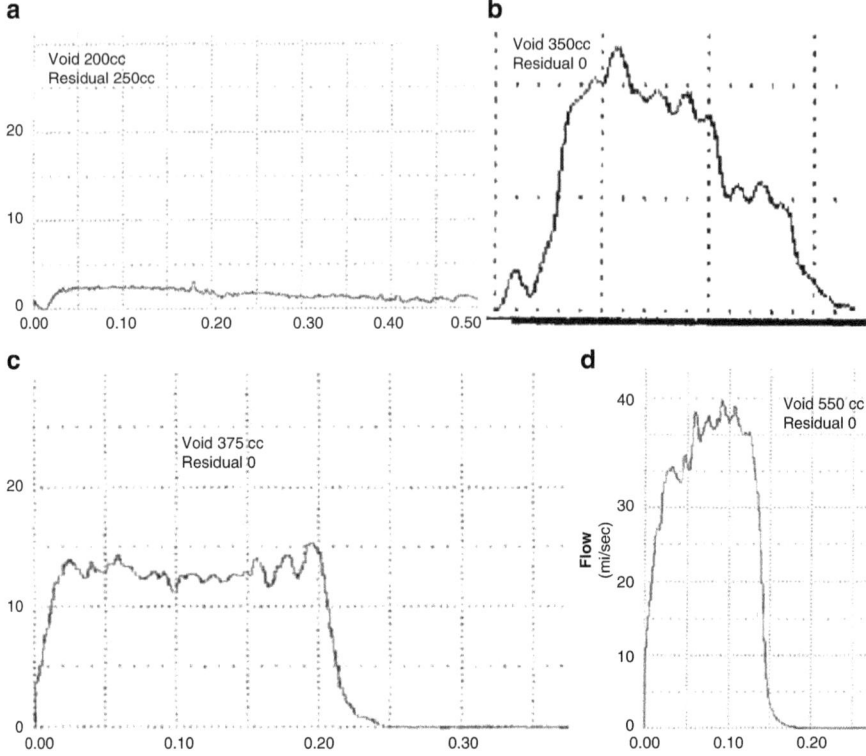

Fig. 4.1 (**a**–**c**) Uroflow tracings from the same female patient with (**a**) obstructing stricture with peak flow 3 ml/s, (**b**) after stricture dilation with the normal flow of 22 ml/s, (**c**) 1 year later after stricture recurrence max flow 15 ml/s with flat top flow pattern, and (**d**) hyperflow of a woman with SUI 45 ml/s

episodes during a set period of time. These provide an objective measure of daytime and nighttime frequency as well as more accurate bladder capacity that tends to be higher than in the testing environment. These results can serve to tailor conservative recommendations surrounding fluid intake [14] and can be used to measure the nocturnal polyuria index which is critical in diagnosing causes of nocturia.

Pad tests are a simple way of quantifying urine loss over a period of time. They are calculated by measuring the wet pad(s) minus the weight of the same number of dry products. In non-menstruating women, the pad net gain is mostly urine, but perspiration and vaginal discharge can contribute to the volume as well.

Short-term pad tests can be accomplished by drinking 500 ml of fluids in 15 min then wearing a pad in the office for 1 h accomplishing several prescribed physical activities such as walking and climbing stairs. Any value over 1 g is considered positive for urinary incontinence. A long-term pad test involves collecting all pads worn for 24–48 h. A net gain of 8 g in 24 h or 2 g on any individual pad is considered incontinence [12].

A *simple cystometric test*, also called "eyeball urodynamics," involves placement of a catheter and drainage of the urine content for a measured post-void residual followed by filling of the bladder with sterile saline using a cone tipped syringe and observing the fluid column. Any rise in the column accompanied by urgency is considered an episode of DO. Sensations are recorded similarly to a standard urodynamics study with first sensation, any urgency, and maximum capacity recorded. The catheter is then removed and a supine cough and Valsalva stress test performed with direct visualization of any leakage. If negative, the patient can be placed in a standing position and perform maneuvers (jumping/squats) and coughs with an absorbent paper towel on the perineum. Advantages of this approach are a much faster study than pressure flow UDS, and patients can perform more maneuvers than are possible when connected to UDS catheters. This test is well suited to the woman in whom you suspect SUI but require significant activity to provoke it. In a woman with prolapse in whom you want to assess for occult SUI, this is an ideal test to perform with both the prolapse reduced and not reduced since the presence of SUI with the prolapse reduced is helpful in counselling regarding the need for a prophylactic sling during the POP repair. If this test does not demonstrate SUI in a woman undergoing prolapse surgery, formal UDS are an excellent method if suspicion is high [15]. Simple cystometric testing does not provide any information on voiding pressures or robust information on DO, but is well suited to diagnose SUI.

Urodynamics Testing and Interpretation

If one is going to perform a test, you need a question that needs to be answered. The urodynamics testing can be best optimized if the technician performing the testing is aware of the question at hand. In general, most urodynamics are performed to answer one or more of the following questions [16]:

1. Is this incontinence stress, urgency, or both?
2. In a woman with persistent incontinence post sling or other procedure, does she have SUI, UUI, or obstruction?
3. In a woman with NGLUTD, is her urinary tract safe? (reflux, poor compliance, adequate capacity, DO)
4. In a woman with elevated residual urine, is it atonic bladder, voiding dysfunction, or obstruction?

If one frames the testing environment around answering one or more of these questions, it makes interpreting the test much easier and allows the technician to tailor testing accordingly. For example, in a woman with a question of incontinence who does not leak during the study, the technician can perform more Valsalva and cough maneuvers or change the woman's position to standing to try to elicit SUI, or in a woman with retention, you may allow to fill to higher volumes to give her the best possible chance of eliciting voiding. This simplified diagnostic organization also makes interpretation easy since your goal in interpretation surrounds answering the clinical question at hand and allows you to potentially ignore findings that are perhaps simply artifacts of the study such as incomplete bladder emptying during the pressure flow study on a woman with incontinence who has a normal pre-study PVR.

Antibiotics and Patient Preparation for UDS

Preparation for a urodynamic study should be straightforward. Patients should be encouraged to hydrate, take all prescribed medications, and eat regular meals on the day of testing. All patients should be asked about signs and symptoms of a UTI and at a minimum have a urinalysis performed on the day of the procedure to screen for urinary tract infection. The definition of a UTI varies across many studies but can be best defined as a positive urinalysis/dipstick plus symptoms suggestive of a UTI and a positive urine culture [17]. Dipstick urinalysis is the most readily available and is therefore most widely used [18]. A dipstick negative for blood, leucocyte esterase, nitrites and protein has a 98% predictive value [19]. However, it is not rare for women with LUTS to present with a positive LE or nitrites on a dipstick. A urine culture requires laboratory assessment, and results will not be available the same day; hence, urine microscopy could be performed in this situation (if available) to assess for bacteriuria. Symptom assessment is critical in these situations since bacteriuria alone is not a contraindication to urodynamics. A positive urine culture without symptoms is simply bacteriuria, not a UTI, and does not require treatment, nor should it alter the UDS results. If bacteriuria is suspected based on dipstick or microscopy, then the study can proceed, but with antibiotic prophylaxis [18]. In the event that a woman does present with symptoms of a UTI and a positive dipstick, she very likely has a UTI; hence, a culture should be sent, and the urodynamics should be delayed until she is treated [18].

A best practice policy statement on urodynamic antibiotic prophylaxis was published in 2017, and based on the available evidence, women with normal genitourinary anatomy and without risk factors do not require antibiotics at the time of UDS to prevent UTI. This comprises a large percentage of urodynamics patients, and avoidance of antibiotics in this population is a way that we can contribute to antibiotic stewardship and avoid the cost and side effects of these drugs. Risk factors where antibiotics are recommended either because of increased risk of UTI post-procedure or that their medical condition would result in a more serious complication should they get a UTI include patients with neurogenic lower urinary tract dysfunction, bladder outlet obstruction, or elevated post-void residual, age over 70, presence of current bacteriuria (known or suspected based on dipstick), immunosuppression/corticosteroid use and immune deficiency, chronic catheter use, and those patients who have recent total joint implants.

The antibiotic of choice should depend on your local antibiogram generated from regional resistance patterns, but in general, a single dose of double strength

Table 4.1 Antibiotics and risk factors for UTI after urodynamics

Need for peri-procedure antibiotics for urodynamics		Antibiotic of choice in order of safety and efficacy
Yes	No	
Neurogenic lower urinary tract dysfunction	Patients without genitourinary anomalies	1. Trimethoprim sulfamethoxazole DS PO
Elevated post-void residual	Diabetes	2. Cefalexin 500 mg PO or amoxicillin/clavulanate 875 mg PO
Asymptomatic bacteriuria	Prior genitourinary surgery	3. Levofloxacin 500 mg PO or ciprofloxacin 500 mg PO or gentamicin 80 mg IM
Immunosuppression	Recently hospitalized patients	
External urine collection device (condom catheter)	History of recurrent UTI (not current)	
Any form of indwelling catheter	Post-menopausal women	
Intermittent catheterization	Nutritional deficiencies/obesity	
Age over 70	Cardiac valvular disease	
Total joint wrisk factor or <2 years	Pins, plates or screws	

trimethoprim-sulfamethoxazole is the first choice. Other factors to consider include patient allergies and tolerance to antibiotics and prior urine cultures, particularly in those women who have recurrent UTIs or known bacteriuria where prior cultures can guide antibiotic selection. See the table for a list of antibiotics and risk factors requiring antibiotics which can be posted in your urodynamics suite as an easy reference guide (see Table 4.1) [18].

Other risks of urodynamics studies include urethral trauma from catheter insertion, which can be minimized with good technique and experience; dysuria, which can be managed with Pyridium or acetaminophen/ibuprofen as needed; transient urinary retention in those patients at risk for retention; and patient physical or emotional discomfort, which can be significantly mitigated with supportive staff.

The anxiety surrounding a UDS test for a patient and the impact of this emotional distress and physical discomfort on the test results are real. In a high anxiety state, it is more difficult to void, and patient satisfaction with your care will suffer. In an academic setting with a dedicated urodynamics nurse that surveyed 314 patients about their experience, 50.7% did not find the study either emotionally or physically uncomfortable, 55% of patients thought the study experience was better than expected, and 37% felt the study was as expected. However, 29% felt the physical component was the most uncomfortable with the urethral catheter being the worst part. Emotional discomfort was the worst part for 12% of patients with anxiety being the most commonly reported component (27%), followed by embarrassment (18%). Patient factors that predicted less physical discomfort were not surprisingly older age and the presence of a neurological condition [20]. Interventions to decrease pain and anxiety such as music and informational videos in a randomized trial did not decrease these symptoms compared to usual care [21]; however, satisfaction with the study has been associated with confidence in the technical ability of the provider and the maintenance of privacy [22].

Systematic Interpretation of a UDS Study

There are many references on standards in urodynamics that discuss the detailed nuance of study performance [10, 23–25] that are beyond the scope of this chapter but are nonetheless essential reading in good urodynamic performance. Like any other complex diagnostic study, having a systematic method of reading the test is important for quality control and to ensure findings are not missed.

The cystometrogram involves continuous fluid filling of the bladder with abdominal and intravesical pressure measurements. Cystometry ends with the permission to void or with incontinence of total bladder volume [10]. The filling solution and rate should be specified. There are two rates of filling possible. One is the maximum physiologic filling rate estimated by body weight in kilograms divided by four which is typically 20–30 ml/min. However, filling is often faster than this physiologic rate for convenience purposes. Also, the patient continues to produce urine during the test (up to 25% of the volume); hence, the cystometric capacity is the filling volume plus any urine produced. In women, the abdominal pressure can be measured with a rectal catheter or a vaginally placed catheter with no difference in discomfort or patient acceptability; however, vaginally placed catheters are more often lost or expelled [10] and are less reliable.

An easy-to-remember mnemonic for the cystometrogram portion is the 4Cs (capacity, compliance, contractions, coughs) and 2Ss (sensation, Sphincter function), followed by the pressure flow portion of the study.

The pressure flow study begins immediately after permission to void and ends when the detrusor pressure returns to baseline or the patient considers voiding complete. It is important to note that the values analyzed are only valid for a voluntary void and not a leak generated by an incontinence episode/DO. Values should be measured for maximum urine flow in ml/s (Qmax) and the detrusor pressure at the maximum flow (PdetQmax) as well as any abdominal straining during voiding detected in Pabd, the shape of the voiding curve, and sphincter relaxation noted as relaxation on electromyography (EMG). Pressure flows are often plotted with the flow on the x-axis and pressure on the y-axis in a time-based graph. The shape of the flow curve can be a smooth arc, flat, or fluctuating [26]. See Table 4.2 and Fig. 4.2 for examples of systematic reading of a UDS study.

Table 4.2 Systematic urodynamics reading guide

Systematic reading mnemonic	Measurement	Units	Normal value
Cystometrogram			
Capacity	Maximum cystometric capacity (MCC)	ml, only accurate within 10 ml	Approx. 500 ml in women
Compliance	Δvolume/Δpressure	ml/cmH2O	>20 associated with upper tract deterioration, but typically much higher
Contractions	Presence of DO during CMG portion of the study (can also be seen as an aftercontraction in PFS)	Present or absent Duration (seconds), amplitude Pdet (cmH2O), and concomitant leaks reported	Absent
Coughs	Both Valsalva leak point pressure (VLPP) and Cough leak point pressure (CLPP) maneuvers. Collectively, these are called abdominal leak point pressure ALPP	cmH2O	Absent
Sensation	Record: First sensation of filling (FSF) First desire to void (FDV) Strong desire to void (SDV) and any urgency episodes	ml	No specified values but identified as normal, absent, reduced, and increased Expect FSF at 30% of capacity and FDV at 60%
Sphincter function	Does EMG rise with maneuvers?	EMG measured with two surface electrodes on the perineum	EMG should rise with maneuvers
Pressure flow:			
PDetQmax	Detrusor pressure at maximum flow	cmH2O	Tends to be lower in women, and can be 0 in normal women
Qmax	Maximum flow	Ml/s	Can be very high in women, no upper limit of normal
Straining	Abdominal pressure rise and vesical pressure rise	Present or absent	Not always pathological, as some people augment voiding with abdominal contraction
Sphincter relaxation	EMG reading		Should decrease with void

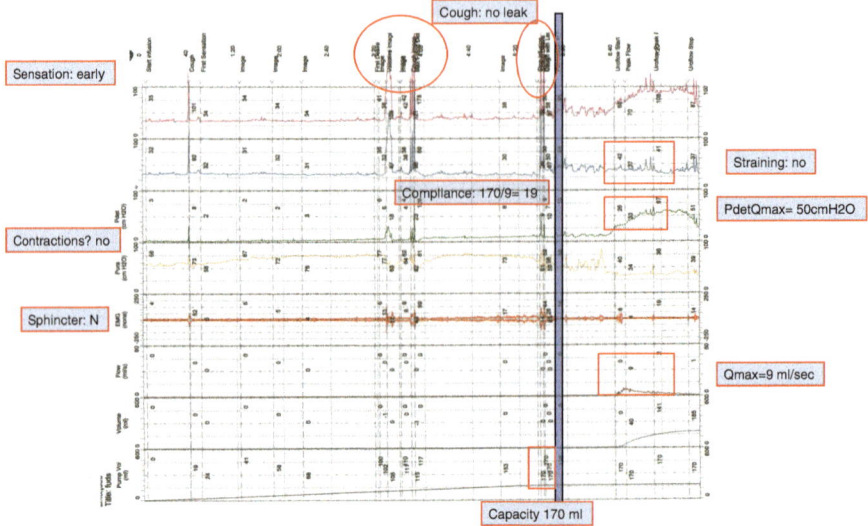

Fig. 4.2 Systematic reading of a urodynamic study. Female with new-onset urgency post sling. Diagnosis: small bladder capacity, borderline normal compliance, no DO, no SUI, early urgency, normal sphincter guarding with cough, and relaxation with void. With a flow of 9 ml/s and PdetQmax of 50 cmH2O, a diagnosis of BOO is made based on all definitions and fluoroscopic images show urine pooling in the urethra (Fig. 4.8b)

Urodynamic Diagnoses

In reality, there are only a handful of diagnoses that can be made with pressure flow urodynamics. These include SUI, DO, detrusor underactivity/atonic bladder, bladder outlet obstruction (functional or anatomic), and poor bladder compliance. The addition of fluoroscopy during the study can increase diagnostic information, but is not typically needed unless anatomic anomalies are suggested. During urodynamic interpretation, if one keeps this list of possible diagnoses in mind, it simplifies reading studies.

Stress Urinary Incontinence

Stress urinary incontinence is defined as "the complaint of involuntary loss of urine on effort or physical exertion or sneezing or coughing" [27]. It is diagnosed on urodynamics either with urine leakage demonstrated during cough maneuvers or Valsalva in the absence of a detrusor contraction. During the cystometrogram, a Valsalva and a series of three progressively stronger coughs are performed at 200 ml filling and again at bladder capacity. If there is leakage in the absence of detrusor overactivity, then SUI is diagnosed. If leakage is observed, a value is recorded as the cough leak point pressure (CLPP) or a Valsalva leak point pressure (VLPP), with the lowest recorded value being the abdominal leak point pressure (ALPP). There is

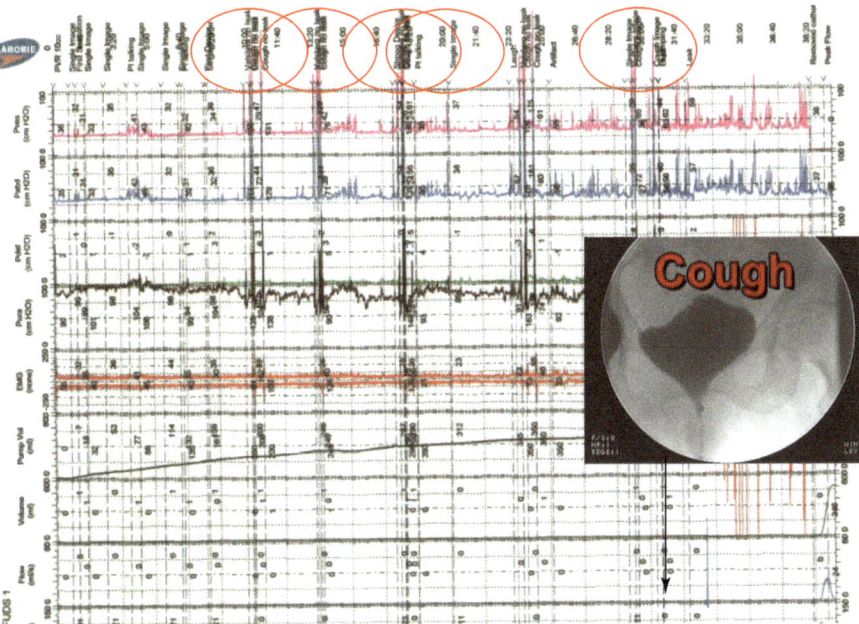

Fig. 4.3 SUI: Woman with symptoms of SUI not demonstrated on full bladder exam hence urodynamics performed. SUI was not demonstrated at 200c; hence, maneuvers were repeated at 250, 300, and 390 ml. Small volume leak not recorded on flow (black arrow), but a leak on fluoroscopy seen at 390 ml with cough

no standard pressure recording that is universally accepted with some recording, the abdominal pressure reading (Pabd), and others utilizing the vesical pressure recording (Pves). Cough LPP tend to have higher pressures than Valsalva [28], and the CLPP or VLPP pressure is recorded at the exact moment where the leakage is observed. A cough is so brief that this can be difficult to pinpoint. It has been observed that both of these values decrease with increased bladder volumes during the study and that those women with worse urinary incontinence tend to have lower recorded abdominal leak point pressures [28]. If clinical suspicion is very high for SUI and no leakage is observed, it is appropriate to repeat maneuvers at maximum cystometric capacity (see Fig. 4.3) and to have the woman do extra maneuvers such as going from sitting to standing or jumping if that is what causes her to leak at home.

A potential error in the diagnosis of SUI on urodynamics can occur if the maneuvers are performed with the urodynamics catheter in place. Even though it is of a small caliber (7F) and most women with SUI (>90%) will leak with the catheter in place, there are women with SUI on physical exam who fail to leak during UDS, and removing the catheter will "unmask" SUI. Up to 50% of women with SUI symptoms, but no leakage during UDS, will demonstrate SUI once the catheter is removed [29]. These women do not necessarily have high leak point pressures with the mean VLPP in this study being only 67 cmH2O. Hence, if a woman has SUI on history or this is seen on bedside examination, but not reproduced during UDS, the catheter should be removed and maneuvers repeated. To avoid the need for a new urodynamics catheter during the pressure flow portion of the procedure, the voiding portion of the test can be completed and then the bladder refilled and the catheter removed for stress maneuvers [9]. Attention should be paid to patient positioning; a woman who only leaks standing is not going to leak supine and will be unlikely to leak sitting. Hence, maneuvers should be repeated in the position she leaks.

Intrinsic sphincter deficiency is clinically important to diagnose prior to incontinence surgery since procedure success is diminished, particularly for transobturator synthetic slings [30]. This can be diagnosed with maximum urethral closure pressure, which is difficult to interpret due to varying measurement techniques and different reference values depending on the catheter type used [30]. As such, ALPP is more commonly utilized to diagnose ISD. ISD was most often cited with a cutoff value of <60 cm H20 [30], but the most recent definition of ISD has now evolved to an imprecise subjective diagnosis. The International Continence Society now defines ISD as a "very weakened urethral closure mechanism." [31]

Detrusor Overactivity

Detrusor overactivity is defined as a non-volitional rise in detrusor pressure during filling either spontaneous or provoked. Provocative maneuvers include a supraphysiologic filling rate, a change of position, cough, laugh, or handwashing/water running. It can be accompanied by a sensation of urgency, or the patient may be unaware (see Fig. 4.4).

The pressure rise can result in urine loss during the contraction. There is no minimum threshold of detrusor pressure considered diagnostic of DO (low amplitude DO example in Fig. 4.6), but the higher amplitude and longer duration of contractions imply worse disease and can predict renal deterioration in NGLUTD [32]. DO is considered idiopathic in patients without neurological disease and considered neurogenic DO in those with a clinical history of these conditions [31]. There is no visible difference between these two conditions on the tracing, and urodynamics cannot be utilized to diagnose a neurological disease. An "after contraction" is a continued or new detrusor pressure that rises immediately after the flow has ended [10] and is also diagnostic of DO. There is also a known phenomenon of "cough-associated detrusor overactivity," which is an onset of DO that occurs immediately following the cough maneuvers and can be mistaken by patients as SUI, but will be evident as DO on UDS [10]. See Fig. 4.5.

Common artifacts that can be confused with DO are rectal vault contractions or passage of gas during maneuvers that can cause a transient drop in Pabd [23]. Also, similarly to SUI, DO is more likely to occur in the upright position, so a woman should be at least in the seated position for the study [10].

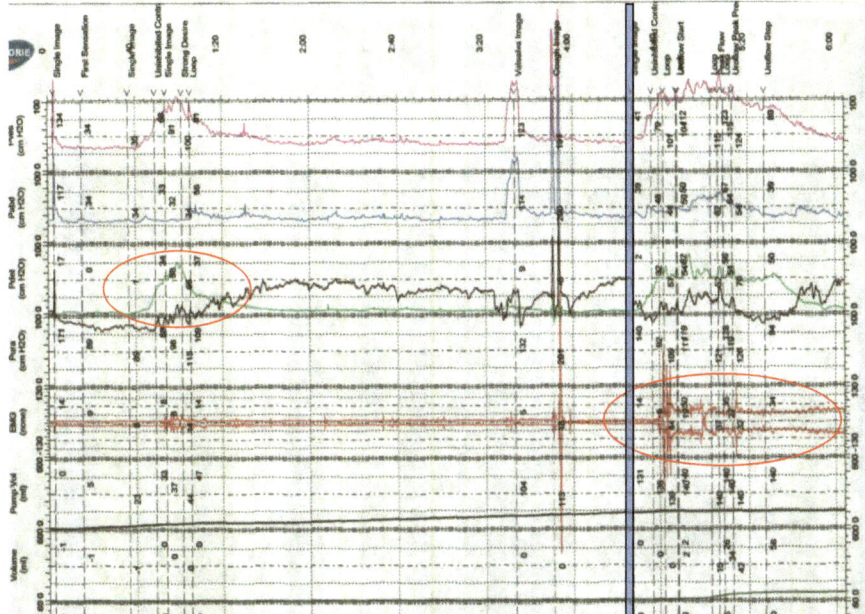

Fig. 4.4 Detrusor overactivity and functional obstruction: A woman with incontinence and pelvic pain. DO of high amplitude 80 cmH2O at 38 ml, no SUI, small bladder capacity 131 ml with a painful void with evidence of obstruction with PdetQmax of 56 and evidence of significant EMG firing. (Fig. 4.8e of spinning top appearance of the bladder)

Detrusor Underactivity or Atonic Bladder

Incomplete bladder emptying, straining to void, slow flow, or total urinary retention in women can be a result of bladder outlet obstruction or poor bladder contractility. These diagnoses are difficult to differentiate with anything but a pressure flow study during UDS. Further complicating this diagnostic dilemma is that some women will not be able to generate a bladder contraction or void during the UDS study due to anxiety or discomfort, and in these cases, a definitive diagnosis cannot be made. This is defined as "situational inability to void as usual" and should be discussed with the patient if they express that this voiding episode has not been representative [10].

Detrusor underactivity is a urodynamic diagnosis defined as a contraction of reduced strength and/or duration, resulting in prolonged bladder emptying and/or a failure to achieve complete bladder emptying within a normal time span. It is important to remember that many women void volitionally without any difficulty, with a very low detrusor contraction, or with augmented abdominal straining, and this is not pathological. There are varying criteria used to diagnose DU in women. Groutz defined it as a Qmax<12 ml/s with a void of at least 100 ml or a PVR of 150 ml on two or more free uroflow readings [33]. Abarbanel and Marcus use the criteria of

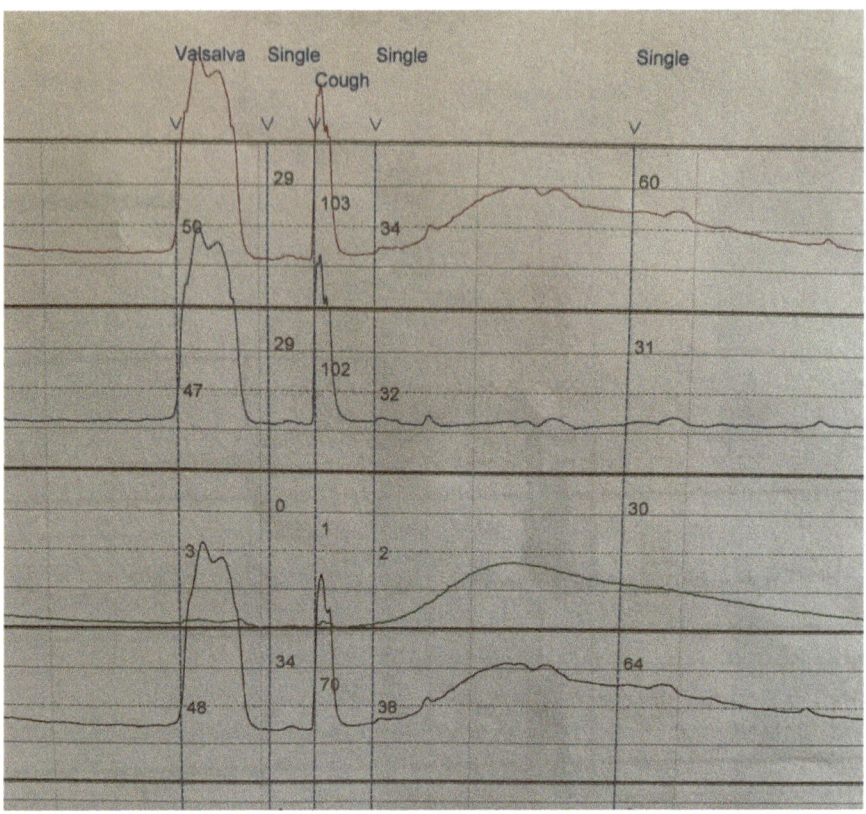

Fig. 4.5 Cough associated DO: episode of DO immediately following cough and Valsalva maneuvers "cough associated detrusor overactivity" in a woman with subjective symptoms of SUI based on leakage after coughing

PdetQmax<30 cmH2O and Qmax<10 ml/s during pressure flow study [34], and Gammie et al. [35] used PdetQmax <20 cmH2O and Qmax <15 ml/s voiding less than 90% without any clinical obstruction. In men, bladder contractility index has been used to define DU with a BCI < 100 being diagnostic [13]. See Fig. 4.6.

$$\text{Bladder contractility index} \left(\text{BCI}\right) = \text{pdetQmax} + 5\text{Qmax}$$
$$\text{Strong} = \text{BCI of} > 150$$
$$\text{normal contractility} = \text{BCI of } 100 - 150$$
$$\text{weak contractility} = \text{BCI of } < 100$$

$$\text{Bladder voiding efficiency, called voided percent} \left(\text{Void\%}\right)$$
$$= \text{amount voided / total bladder volume}$$
$$= \text{void} / \left(\text{void} + \text{PVR}\right) * 100$$

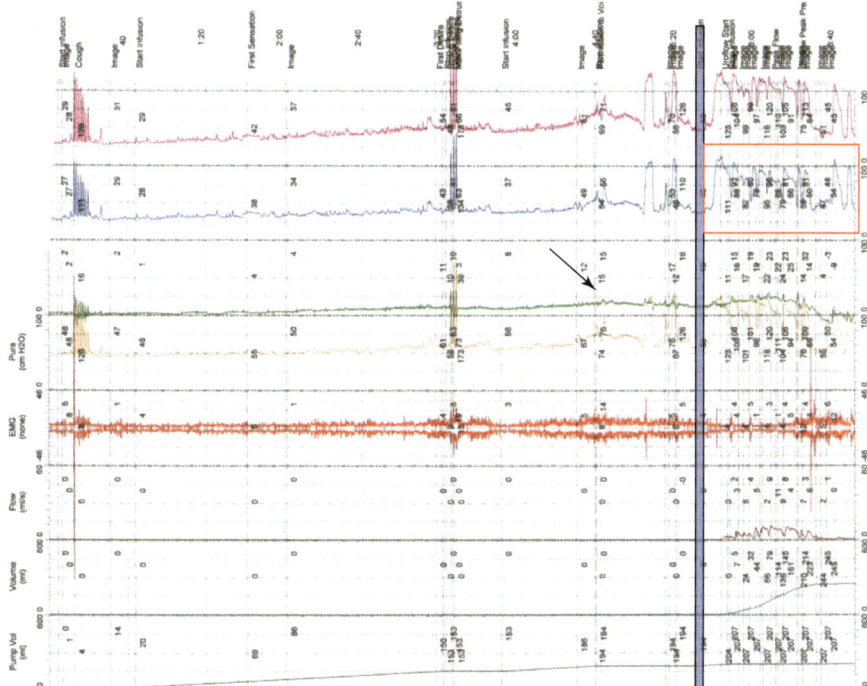

Fig. 4.6 Detrusor underactivity and DO: An 84-year-old with incontinence and straining to void after radiation treatment for cervical cancer 30 years ago. She has borderline compliance 194 ml/12 cmH2O = 16. There is a small DO episode black arrow with no leak. During pressure flow, PdetQmax = 22 cmH2O, Qmax = 9 ml/s., straining: yes- see red box BCI=PdetQmax+5Qmax = 22 + 9 * 5 = 67

In a large series of 1015 women with non-neurogenic LUTS evaluated urodynamically, 15% had DU utilizing the Groutz definition, 10% by the Ababarnel criteria, and 6% with the Gammie criteria. The latter two criteria are both deemed clinically significant at differentiating between those with and without DU [36]. Straining is seen as an increase in both the Pves and Pabd pressure. This can be observed during position changes or during attempts to void [10]. See Fig. 4.6.

Bladder Outflow Obstruction

Bladder outflow obstruction (BOO) is often called bladder outlet obstruction; however, the new correct terminology is bladder outflow obstruction [10]. The diagnosis of BOO in women is more difficult than in men due to a lack of consensus on a urodynamic diagnosis [37]. Several nomograms exist but all characterize BOO as an increased detrusor pressure and reduced urine flow rate.

Groutz et al. defined urethral obstruction as a persistently low free flow rate of less than 12 ml/s combined with a detrusor pressure at maximum flow greater than 20 cm H2O during the pressure-flow study [33]. Lemack & Zimmern suggested that women with voiding detrusor pressure of 25 cm H2O or more, together with a flow rate of 12 ml/s or lower, were obstructed [38]. Kuo defined bladder outflow obstruction as a voiding detrusor pressure of 50 cm H2O or greater together with a narrow urethra on voiding cystourethrography [39]. Blaivas and Groutz developed an often used obstruction nomogram based on statistical analysis of the maximum detrusor pressure during the pressure-flow study of voiding, together with the maximum flow rate Qmax in repeated free uroflow studies. Patients with pdetQmax greater than 57 cm H2O were classified as either moderately or severely obstructed. Those with pdet below 57 cm H2O were classified as either mildly obstructed or unobstructed, depending on the value of free Qmax. Among a group of 600 consecutive women, 6% were mildly obstructed, 2% were moderately obstructed, and fewer than 1% were severely obstructed [40]. Nitti et al. defined obstruction qualitatively as radiographic evidence of narrowing in the presence of a sustained detrusor contraction. For obstructed women, the mean values of pdetQmax and Qmax were 43 cm H2O and 9 ml/s, respectively [41].

Akikwala [42] compared the different approaches to diagnosis in a cohort of 91 women with 25 having likely obstruction and found that the definition proposed by Nitti had the greatest concordance [42]. Most recently, Solomon and Greenwell [43] created a new nomogram proposing a female BOOI calculated as PdetQmax-2.2Qmax. If fBOOI is <0, then there is a less than 10% chance of obstruction and if fBOOI>5 then 50% chance of obstruction. This nomogram was validated in a patient population of women undergoing surgery for relief of obstruction where the nomogram was accurate at predicting symptom relief following surgery [44]. See Fig. 4.2 for an example of BOO due to a sling (anatomic) and Fig. 4.4 for BOO due to voiding dysfunction (functional).

There are only a handful of possible etiologies that could cause BOO in women which include fixed anatomical obstructions such as an overtightened urethral sling, urethral stricture, pelvic organ prolapse, or malignancy. There is a suggestion that UDS are not needed in the case of a suspected obstruction following sling surgery since a clinical history of new significant voiding symptoms is essentially diagnostic of obstruction and UDS are only needed in those cases where there are exclusively storage symptoms [45]. The other large category of BOO is functional obstructions, which is a failure of the outlet to relax. These functional obstructions include dysfunctional voiding, which is "an intermittent and/or fluctuating flow rate due to involuntary intermittent contractions of the periurethral striated muscle during voiding in neurologically normal individuals," [27] or detrusor sphincter dyssynergia, which is "a detrusor contraction concurrent with an involuntary contraction of the urethral and/or periurethral striated muscle." Occasionally, the flow may be prevented altogether. The easiest way to differentiate between these conditions is clinical history as a person can only have DSD due to a neurological condition without exception.

The presence of the urodynamics catheter is proposed to possibly impact flow rate. Groutz looked at flow rates with a 7F catheter in place compared to a free flow study and found a decrease in flow with the catheter in place [46]; however, other studies have not found this same impact [47]. It does however seem prudent that if the urodynamicist has doubt of the validity of a uroflow during the UDS with a catheter in place, a free flow can be performed to ensure the catheter is not causing obstruction or discomfort preventing voiding.

NGB Safety or Poor Compliance

The detrusor leak point pressure (DLPP) is the lowest detrusor pressure at which urine leakage occurs in the absence of either a detrusor contraction or increased abdominal pressure [48]. Detrusor leak point pressure measurement was introduced in myelodysplastic children as an indicator of the risk of upper urinary tract deterioration [48]. In these patients and others with neurogenic lower urinary tract dysfunction, the detrusor leak point pressure is important because a high value is correlated with a higher risk of upper urinary tract pathology. The absolute value associated with worse risk has historically been 40 cmH2O [48] but may be higher in adult populations [32]. Non-neurogenic patients do not have a DLPP, and this term is often confused with ALPP or leaking occurring with an episode of DO.

The primary reason for performing UDS studies in patients with NGLUTD is that their upper urinary tract can be at risk from their disease and some of these urodynamic findings do not have obvious symptoms. In a large systematic review [32], those patients with spina bifida and spinal cord injury as their neurological diagnosis were at higher risk of upper tract deterioration, specifically hydronephrosis, than those with multiple sclerosis. Poor bladder compliance and high DLPP both put patients at risk.

Bladder compliance is defined as the change in volume over the rise in detrusor pressure during filling cystometry (see Fig. 4.7).

$$\text{Compliance} = \Delta \text{volume} / \Delta \text{pressure}$$

This calculation ignores any episodes of detrusor overactivity, and these can make the calculation more difficult. Also, a sustained bladder contraction can mimic loss of bladder compliance but will abate if filling cytometry is stopped. This is a good way to determine if the pressure rise is DO or loss of compliance. Cutoffs for normal compliance vary from <10 to <30 ml/cmH2O, but in most neurologically intact individual's compliance, it is well over 100 ml/cmH2O.

Detrusor overactivity is a common finding in patients with NGLUTD occurring in approximately 60% [32] and is a clear explanation for urinary incontinence. The Pdetmax of contractions ranges from 35 to 115 cmH2O and pressures above

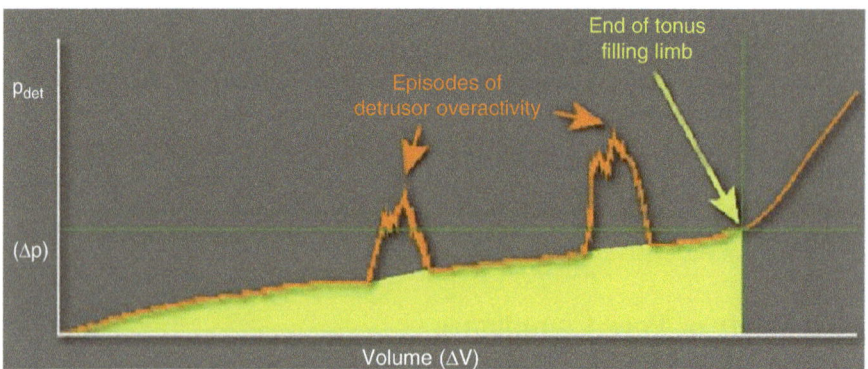

Fig. 4.7 Compliance calculation: solid yellow area represents best-fit pressure-volume relationship for calculation of compliance. Note only the initial compliance curve is used in the calculation and not terminal compliance or episodes of detrusor overactivity

75 cmH2O are an independent risk factor for UUTD [32]. The duration of the contraction ranges from 48 to 236 s with higher duration predicting hydronephrosis (236 vs 114 s). DSD is seen in up to 44% of patients with NGLUTD and is another predictor of UUTD.

Anatomic Diagnoses Seen on Fluoroscopy

Simultaneous fluoroscopy during UDS utilizing contrast-based bladder filling media provides additional anatomical information, with the added burden of fluoroscopic equipment and radiation exposure to the patient and urodynamicist. The additional information can be of great benefit particularly in the NGLUTD population [49] where vesicoureteric reflux and bladder neck abnormalities can be clearly visualized. Other populations where fluoroscopy can be of benefit are women with retention where the source of obstruction can be seen and assists in the diagnosis of sling obstruction location, pelvic organ prolapse as a source of obstruction, and the classic spinning top bladder of voiding dysfunction. Other findings can include urethral diverticulum, bladder diverticulum, or trabeculations (Figs. 4.8 and 4.9).

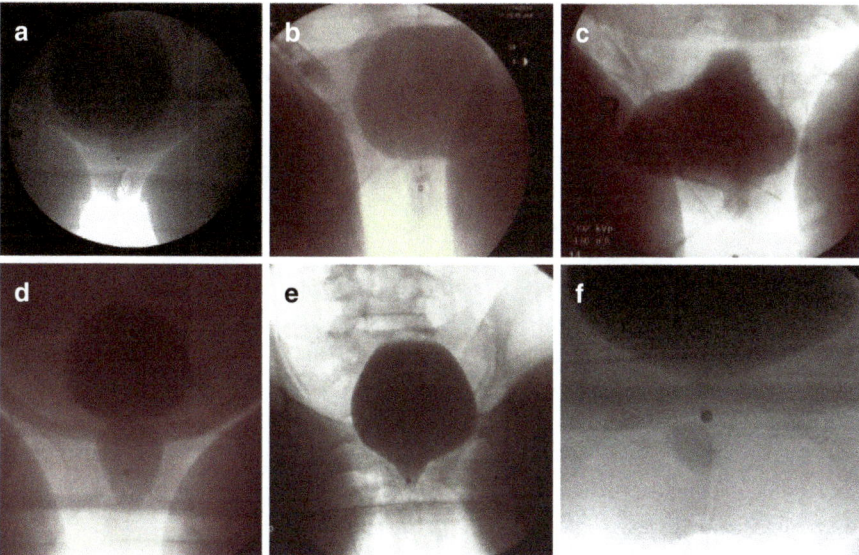

Fig. 4.8 Urethral findings on fluoroscopy: (**a**) primary bladder neck obstruction seen during voiding, (**b**) contrast held up at the level of a sling with pooling of the contrast, (**c**) DSD and trabeculated bladder in a woman with MS, (**d**) severe BOO with sling placed at the distal urethra causing massive obstruction and ballooning of urethra with the void, (**e**) voiding dysfunction with spinning top bladder with the void, (**f**) urethral diverticulum discovered incidentally

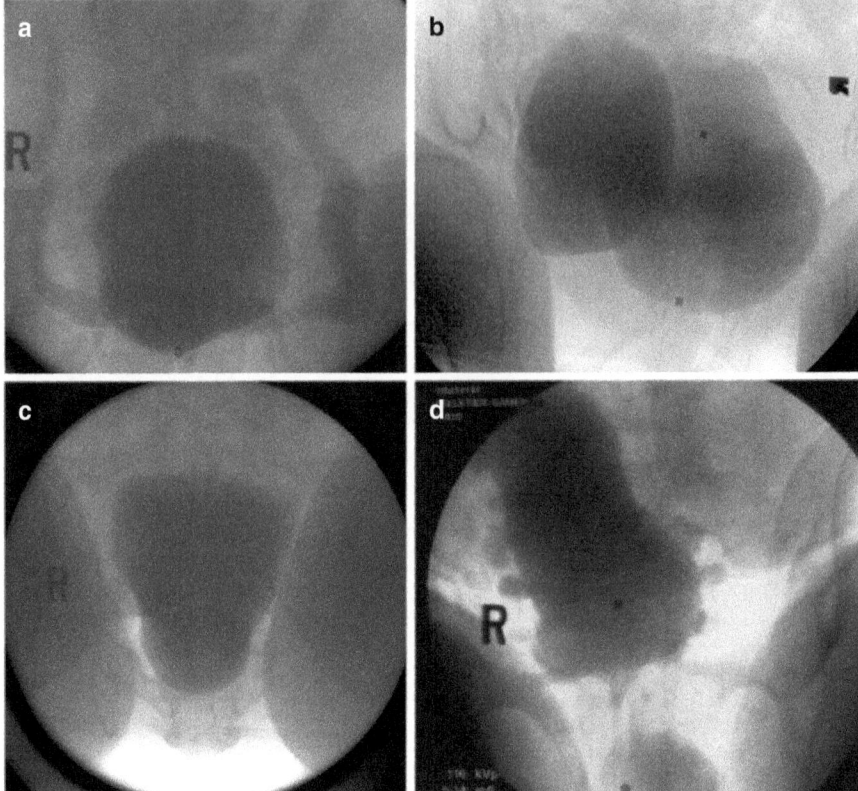

Fig. 4.9 Bladder and ureteral findings seen on fluoroscopy: (**a**) grade 4 bilateral reflux in a neurogenic bladder, (**b**) large bladder diverticulum, (**c**) cystocele causing BOO during the void, (**d**) severe bladder trabeculations causing a Christmas tree-shaped bladder associated with poor bladder compliance

Conclusion

Urodynamics is a powerful tool in the diagnosis of LUTD in women and are best used when less invasive investigations do not yield a diagnosis, and accurate diagnosis is important to the treatment of the patient. Urodynamics interpretation is best done systematically with a cautious eye for artifacts in the tracing and knowledge of the patient's clinical condition to ensure results are congruent. Urodynamics testing is also more useful when a clear and concise diagnostic question is formulated before undertaking the test to ensure the most accurate results are achieved. Urodynamics can reliably diagnose SUI, DO, DU, BOO, and poor bladder compliance, and the addition of fluoroscopy can further identify anatomical anomalies in those select patients where it is needed.

References

1. Nager CW, FitzGerald MP, Kraus SR, Chai TC, Zyczynski H, Sirls L, et al. Urodynamic measures do not predict stress continence outcomes after surgery for stress urinary incontinence in selected women. J Urol. 2008;179(4):1470–4.
2. Lloyd JC, Dielubanza E, Goldman HB. Trends in urodynamic testing prior to midurethral sling placement—what was the value of the VALUE trial? Neurourol Urodyn. 2018;37(3):1046–52.
3. Chughtai B, Hauser N, Anger J, Asfaw T, Laor L, Mao J, et al. Trends in surgical management and pre-operative urodynamics in female medicare beneficiaries with mixed incontinence. Neurourol Urodyn. 2017;36(2):422–5.
4. Suskind AM, Cox L, Clemens JQ, Oldendorf A, Stoffel JT, Malaeb B, et al. The value of urodynamics in an academic specialty referral practice. Urology. 2017;105:48–53.
5. Nobrega RP, Solomon E, Jenks J, Greenwell T, Ockrim J. Predicting a successful outcome in sacral neuromodulation testing: are urodynamic parameters prognostic? Neurourol Urodyn. 2018;37(3):1007–10.
6. Rachaneni S, Champaneria R, Latthe P. Does the outcome of botulinum toxin treatment differ in OAB patients with detrusor overactivity compared to those without detrusor overactivity?: a systematic review. Int Urogynecol J Pelvic Floor Dysfunct. 2015;26:S32–3.
7. Subak LL, Brown JS, Kraus SR, Brubaker L, Lin F, Richter HE, et al. The "costs" of urinary incontinence for women. Obstet Gynecol [Internet]. 2006;107(4):908–16. Available from: http://www.pubmedcentral.nih.gov/articlerender.fcgi?artid=1557394&tool=pmcentrez&rendertype=abstract
8. Gormley EA, Lightner DJ, Faraday M, Vasavada SP. Diagnosis and treatment of overactive bladder (non-neurogenic) in adults: AUA/SUFU guideline amendment. J Urol [Internet]. 2015;193(5):1572–80. Available from: https://doi.org/10.1016/j.juro.2015.01.087
9. Kobashi KC, Albo ME, Dmochowski RR, Ginsberg DA, Goldman HB, Gomelsky A, et al. Surgical treatment of female stress urinary incontinence: AUA/SUFU guideline. J Urol [Internet]. 2017;198(4):875–83. Available from: http://linkinghub.elsevier.com/retrieve/pii/S0022534717748574
10. Rosier PFWM, Schaefer W, Lose G, Goldman HB, Guralnick M, Eustice S, et al. International continence society good urodynamic practices and terms 2016: urodynamics, uroflowmetry, cystometry, and pressure-flow study. Neurourol Urodyn. 2017;36(5):1243–60.
11. Peterson AC, Smith AR, Fraser MO, Yang CC, JOL DL, Gillespie BW, et al. The distribution of post-void residual volumes in people seeking care in the symptoms of lower urinary tract dysfunction network observational cohort study with comparison to asymptomatic populations. Urology. 2019;130:22–8.
12. Al Afraa T, Mahfouz W, Campeau L, Corcos J. Normal lower urinary tract assessment in women: I. Uroflowmetry and post-void residual, pad tests, and bladder diaries. Int Urogynecol J. 2012;23(6):681–5.
13. Abrams P. Bladder outlet obstruction index, bladder contractility index and bladder voiding efficiency: three simple indices to define bladder voiding function. BJU Int. 1999;84(1):14–5.
14. Cameron AP, Wiseman JB, Smith AR, Merion RM, Gillespie BW, Bradley CS, et al. Are three-day voiding diaries feasible and reliable? Results from the symptoms of lower urinary tract dysfunction research network (LURN) cohort. Neurourol Urodyn. 2019;38(8):2185–93.
15. Glass D, Lin FC, Khan AA, Van Kuiken M, Drain A, Siev M, et al. Impact of preoperative urodynamics on women undergoing pelvic organ prolapse surgery. Int Urogynecol J. 2020;31(8):1663–8.
16. Suskind AM, Cox L, Clemens JQ, Oldendorf A, Stoffel JT, Malaeb B, et al. The value of urodynamics in an academic specialty referral practice. Urology [Internet]. 2017;105:48–53. Available from: https://doi.org/10.1016/j.urology.2017.02.049
17. Hooton TM, Bradley SF, Cardenas DD, Colgan R, Geerlings SE, Rice JC, et al. Diagnosis, prevention, and treatment of catheter-associated urinary tract infection in adults: 2009 international clinical practice guidelines from the Infectious Diseases Society of America. Clin Infect

Dis [Internet]. 2010;50(5):625–63. Available from: http://cid.oxfordjournals.org/lookup/doi/10.1086/650482

18. Cameron AP, Campeau L, Brucker BM, Clemens JQ, Bales GT, Albo ME, et al. Best practice policy statement on urodynamic antibiotic prophylaxis in the non-index patient. Neurourol Urodyn. 2017;36(4):915–26.

19. Litza JA, Brill JR. Urinary tract infections. Prim Care Clin Off Pract [Internet]. 2010;37(3):491–507. Available from: https://doi.org/10.1016/j.pop.2010.04.001

20. Suskind AM, Clemens JQ, Kaufman SR, Stoffel JT, Oldendorf A, Malaeb BS, et al. Patient perceptions of physical and emotional discomfort related to urodynamic testing: a questionnaire-based study in men and women with and without neurologic conditions. Urology. 2015;85(3):547–51.

21. Solomon ER, Ridgeway B. Interventions to decrease pain and anxiety in patients undergoing urodynamic testing: a randomized controlled trial. Neurourol Urodyn. 2016;35(8):975–9.

22. Shaw C, Williams K, Assassa PR, Jackson C. Patient satisfaction with urodynamics: a qualitative study. J Adv Nurs. 2000;32(6):1356–63.

23. Raz O, Tse V, Chan L. Urodynamic testing: physiological background, setting-up, calibration and artefacts. BJU Int. 2014;114(S1):22–8.

24. Mahfouz W, Al Afraa T, Campeau L, Corcos J. Normal urodynamic parameters in women: part II – invasive urodynamics. Int Urogynecol J. 2012;23(3):269–77.

25. D'Ancona CAL, Gomes MJ, Rosier PFWM. ICS teaching module: Cystometry (basic module). Neurourol Urodyn. 2017;36(7):1673–6.

26. Drake MJ. Fundamentals of terminology in lower urinary tract function. Neurourol Urodyn. 2018;37(July):S13–9.

27. Haylen BT, Freeman RM, Swift SE, Cosson M, Davila GW, Deprest J, et al. An international Urogynecological Association (IUGA) / International Continence Society (ICS) joint terminology and classification of the complications related directly to the insertion of prostheses (meshes, implants, tapes) & grafts in female pelvic flo. Int Urogynecol J. 2011;22(1):3–15.

28. Seo YH, Kim SO, Yu HS, Kwon D. Leak point pressure at different bladder volumes in stress urinary incontinence in women: comparison between Valsalva and cough-induced leak point pressure. Can Urol Assoc J. 2016;10(1-2):E23–7.

29. Maniam P, Goldman HB. Removal of transurethral catheter during urodynamics may unmask stress urinary incontinence. J Urol. 2002;167(5):2080–2.

30. Parrillo LM, Ramchandani P, Smith AL. Can intrinsic sphincter deficiency be diagnosed by urodynamics? Urol Clin North Am [Internet]. 2014;41(3):375–81. Available from: https://doi.org/10.1016/j.ucl.2014.04.006

31. D'Ancona C, Haylen B, Oelke M, Abranches-Monteiro L, Arnold E, Goldman H, et al. The International Continence Society (ICS) report on the terminology for adult male lower urinary tract and pelvic floor symptoms and dysfunction. Neurourol Urodyn. 2019;38(2):433–77.

32. Musco S, Padilla-Fernández B, Del Popolo G, Bonifazi M, Blok BFM, Groen J, et al. Value of urodynamic findings in predicting upper urinary tract damage in neuro-urological patients: a systematic review. Neurourol Urodyn. 2018;37(5):1522–40.

33. Groutz A, Blaivas JG, Chaikin DC. Bladder outlet obstruction in women: definition and characteristics. Neurourol Urodyn. 2000;19(3):213–20.

34. Abarbanel J, Marcus EL. Impaired detrusor contractility in community-dwelling elderly presenting with lower urinary tract symptoms. Urology. 2007;69(3):436–40.

35. Gammie A, Kaper M, Dorrepaal C, Kos T, Abrams P. Signs and symptoms of detrusor Underactivity: an analysis of clinical presentation and urodynamic tests from a large group of patients undergoing pressure flow studies. Eur Urol. 2016;69(2):361–9.

36. Jeong SJ, Lee JK, Kim KM, Kook H, Cho SY, Oh SJ. How do we diagnose detrusor underactivity? Comparison of diagnostic criteria based on an urodynamic measure. Investig Clin Urol. 2017;58(4):247–54.

37. Rademakers K, Apostolidis A, Constantinou C, Fry C, Kirschner-Hermanns R, Oelke M, et al. Recommendations for future development of contractility and obstruction nomograms for women. ICI-RS 2014. Neurourol Urodyn. 2016;35(2):307–11.
38. Defreitas GA, Zimmern PE, Lemack GE, Shariat SF. Refining diagnosis of anatomic female bladder outlet obstruction: comparison of pressure-flow study parameters in clinically obstructed women with those of normal controls. Urology. 2004;4(4):675–9.
39. Kuo HC. Videourodynamic characteristics and lower urinary tract symptoms of female bladder outlet obstruction. Urology. 2005;66(5):1005–9.
40. Blaivas JG, Groutz A. Bladder outlet obstruction nomogram for women with lower urinary tract symptomatology. Neurourol Urodyn. 2000;19(5):553–64.
41. Nitti VW, Tu LM, Gitlin J. Diagnosing bladder outlet obstruction in women. J Urol. 1999;161(5):1535–40.
42. Akikwala TV, Fleischman N, Nitti VW. Comparison of diagnostic criteria for female bladder outlet obstruction. J Urol. 2006;176(5):2093–7.
43. Solomon E, Yasmin H, Duffy M, Rashid T, Akinluyi E, Greenwell TJ. Developing and validating a new nomogram for diagnosing bladder outlet obstruction in women. Neurourol Urodyn. 2018;37(1):368–78.
44. Lindsay J, Solomon E, Nadeem M, Pakzad M, Hamid R, Ockrim J, et al. Treatment validation of the Solomon-Greenwell nomogram for female bladder outlet obstruction. Neurourol Urodyn. 2020;39(5):1371–7.
45. Aponte MM, Shah SR, Hickling D, Brucker BM, Rosenblum N, Nitti VW. Urodynamics for clinically suspected obstruction after anti-incontinence surgery in women. J Urol. 2013;190(2):598–602.
46. Groutz A, Blaivas JG, Sassone AM. Detrusor pressure uroflowmetry studies in women: effect of a 7Fr transurethral catheter. J Urol. 2000;164(1):109–14.
47. Harding C, Horsburgh B, Dorkin TJ, Thorpe AC. Quantifying the effect of urodynamic catheters on urine flow rate measurement. Neurourol Urodyn. 2012;31(1):139–42.
48. McGuire EJ. Urodynamics of the neurogenic bladder. Urol Clin N Am. 2010;37(4):507–16.
49. Winters JC, Dmochowski RR, Goldman HB, Herndon CDA, Kobashi KC, Kraus SR, et al. Urodynamic studies in adults: AUA/SUFU guideline. J Urol. 2012;188(6 SUPPL):2464–72.

Chapter 5
Historical Treatment of SUI and UUI in Women

Justina Tam and Una J. Lee

Introduction

Urinary incontinence in women is highly prevalent, affecting a reported 5–70% of the population, with increasing prevalence associated with increasing age [1]. With its high prevalence, the desire for effective treatments, and advancements in the pathophysiologic understanding of the continence mechanism, procedures for urinary incontinence have evolved over time. These procedures reflect various surgical techniques and the contemporaneous anatomic and functional understanding of urinary incontinence. Although many of these historical surgical procedures are no longer performed, a foundational understanding of these techniques is important to appreciate the current state of urinary incontinence surgery in women. Also, patients may have undergone prior anti-incontinence procedures that have resulted in altered anatomy or physiology, so an understanding of these procedures is essential to treating women with prior surgery. The objective of this chapter is to review historical treatments of stress urinary incontinence and urgency urinary incontinence in women.

The first written sources dealing with urinary incontinence were Egyptian manuscripts from the second millennium BC, which described devices for male urine collection and pessaries for women [2]. Since then, noninvasive treatments such as female urethral plugs, electrotherapy, surgical excision of part of the urethral wall to narrow the urethral diameter, and urethrolysis followed by torsion of the urethra are among some of the treatments described for the treatment of stress urinary incontinence [2]. Herein, we describe historical techniques for urinary incontinence that modern-day urologists may encounter.

J. Tam · U. J. Lee (✉)
Section of Urology and Renal Transplantation, Virginia Mason Medical Center, Seattle, WA, USA
e-mail: Justina.Tam@virginiamason.org; Una.Lee@virginiamason.org

© The Author(s), under exclusive license to Springer Nature Switzerland AG 2022
A. P. Cameron (ed.), *Female Urinary Incontinence*, https://doi.org/10.1007/978-3-030-84352-6_5

Native Tissue Plication

The Kelly plication, performed by Howard A. Kelly in 1900, was the first described surgical technique used in the management of female stress urinary incontinence (SUI) that became a routine clinical procedure. This technique involves anterior colporrhaphy, which was first described by Schultz at the end of the nineteenth century [3], and plication of the bladder neck using mattress sutures placed in the endopelvic fascia [2, 4], which narrows the posterior urethrovesical angle to improve continence [5]. In this procedure, a vertical incision is made in the vaginal wall and dissected free laterally, exposing the bladder neck and the paravaginal space [3]. The endopelvic fascia is sutured together to create a bridge of tissue in the midline to support the bladder neck and proximal urethra (Fig. 5.1).

The anterior colporrhaphy-Kelly plication was utilized and studied throughout the 1980s with multiple publications documenting the effectiveness; however, long-term outcomes have not been as successful with a 37% 5-year objective

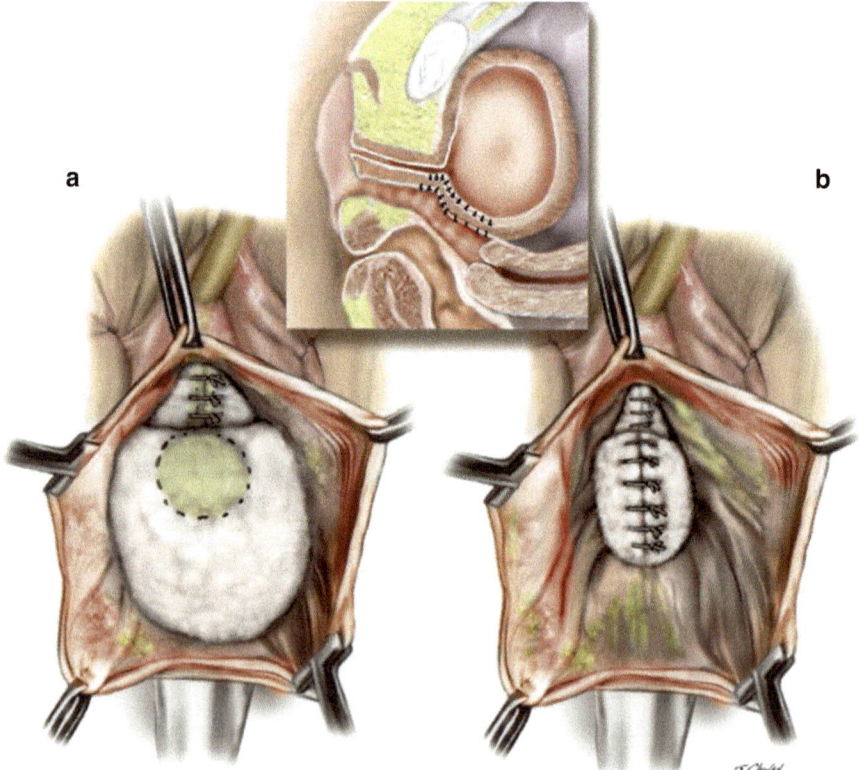

Fig. 5.1 Anterior colporrhaphy with Kelly plication. (**a**) The vaginal mucosa is opened, and interrupted sutures are placed under the urethra. (**b**) Completed colporrhaphy with midline plication using interrupted sutures. Preferential support is provided to the proximal urethra over that provided to the bladder neck. (Figure from Maher and Karram [6])

Table 5.1 Trends in the surgical management of stress urinary incontinence among female Medicare beneficiaries[a]

Procedure	2002	2003	2004	2005	2006	2007	Total
Pubovaginal sling	25,840 (5270)	28,580 (5749)	31,480 (6269)	31,640 (6185)	33,300 (6525)	33,880 (6693)	184,720
Injectable bulking agents	14,100 (2875)	12,100 (2434)	11,300 (2250)	10,160 (1986)	10,980 (2151)	11,320 (2236)	69,960
Urethropexy	4340 (885)	2480 (499)	1820 (362)	1360 (266)	1080 (212)	820 (162)	11,900
Hysterectomy with colpo-urethropexy	2900 (591)	3320 (668)	2740 (546)	2280 (446)	2440 (478)	3100 (612)	16,780
Raz-type suspension	1100 (224)	680 (137)	480 (96)	320 (63)	220 (43)	100 (20)	2900
Laparoscopic repair	680 (139)	600 (121)	540 (108)	480 (94)	500 (98)	560 (111)	3360
Pereyra procedure	240 (49)	140 (28)	100 (20)	160 (31)	40 (8)	40 (8)	720
Kelly plication	140 (29)	120 (24)	140 (28)	220 (43)	140 (27)	80 (16)	840
Total	49,340	48,020	48,600	46,620	48,700	49,900	291,180

Table from Rogo-Gupta et al. [10]
[a]Data are presented as counts, which were calculated from unweighted counts multiplied by 20, and the data in parenthesis are rates per 100,000 female Medicare beneficiaries with a primary diagnosis of urinary incontinence

success rate [7] and 46.81% rate of objective stress urinary incontinence at 5 years [8]. By the 2000s, the Kelly plication surgery had been largely replaced by other urinary incontinence surgeries [9, 10] (Table 5.1).

The Ingelman-Sundberg pubococcygeal repair, described in 1947 [11], used an arcuate incision below the external urethral meatus in the anterior vaginal wall, followed by suturing of bladder ligaments, pubococcygeal muscles, and bulbo-cavernosus muscles to the midline to support the urethra [12] (Fig. 5.2). Long-term outcomes at up to 3 years of a follow-up demonstrated a cure rate of 92% [14], and at 10–20 years of follow-up, patient-reported cure rates were 56.2–84% [12, 15]. There was a high rate (54.9%) of either recurrent rectocele after concurrent rectocele repair or development of rectocele during the follow-up period, which the author speculates may be due to cutting of the medial portion of the levator ani or related underlying insufficiency of the connective tissues [12].

Autologous Tissue Retropubic Slings

Retropubic slings using autologous tissue were first performed using muscle, with the belief that the muscle would contract like a sphincter [5]. The first of these was described by Van Giordano in 1907, who used gracilis muscle, followed by Goebell in 1910 using pyramidalis muscle, and Frangenheim in 1914 who used the

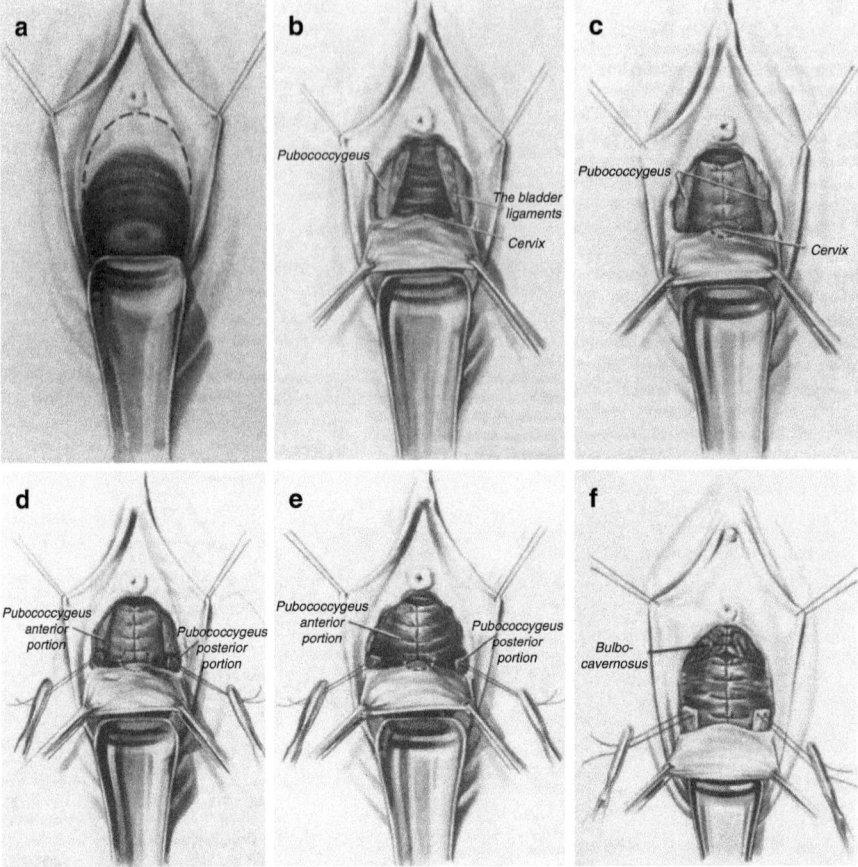

Fig. 5.2 Ingleman-Sundberg pubococcygeal repair. The anterior vaginal mucosa is opened (**a, b**) to allow the identification of bladder ligaments, pubococcygeal muscles, and bulbocavernosus muscles, which are then sutured to the midline to support the urethra (**c–f**). (Figure from Ingelman-Sundberg [13])

pyramidalis muscle and rectus fascia [2, 3, 5]. In 1917, Stoeckel suggested a combination of the pyramidalis muscle–rectus fascia sling with transvaginal muscular plication of the bladder neck; this procedure is now known as the Goebell-Frangenheim-Stoeckel operation [2]. In this procedure, a pedicled strip of vertical rectus fascia with attached pyramidalis muscle is split and rotated suburethral to encircle the urethra from either side. This technique has a reported 84–88% rate of success [16, 17], with a decrease in success at 2 years reported in one study [16] and between 91.5% and 96% continence at mean 68-month follow-up in another [17]. Moderate to very excellent results were reported by 73% of patients, and poor results were reported by 27%. Postprocedural complications for this procedure include temporary urinary retention requiring intermittent catheterization (60%), irritative symptoms (37.5%), and minor urethral obstruction (12.5%) [17].

A vaginal sling procedure using a strip of vaginal tissue including the vaginal epithelium has also been described [18]. This strip of tissue is placed posterior to the urethra with the ends of the strips passed to the anterior abdominal wall and sutured together, just superior to the pubic symphysis [18] (Fig. 5.3). The author reported that 16/19 patients were cured, 2 were improved, and 1 had subsequent abdominal trauma resulting in rupture of the sling and recurrence of incontinence [18].

While techniques utilizing muscle tissue and vaginal epithelium are no longer commonly in use, modifications of these procedures using fascia alone are currently in use, including autologous fascia lata which was described by Price in 1933 as a retropubic approach in which the fascia lata strip is passed under the urethra and the ends of the strip are secured to the rectus muscle [19], and the Aldridge modification described in 1942 which uses transverse strips of anterior rectus fascia that are anchored at the midline and passed through a retropubic approach beneath the urethra and sutured together [20, 21]. Rates of cure after an Aldridge-type fascial sling have been reported to vary between 78% and 86% [22–24], falling to 71% over a 16-year period [25]. The long-term outcomes and complications associated with retropubic autologous rectus fascia and fascia lata slings, which are currently still in use, will be described in Chap. 17.

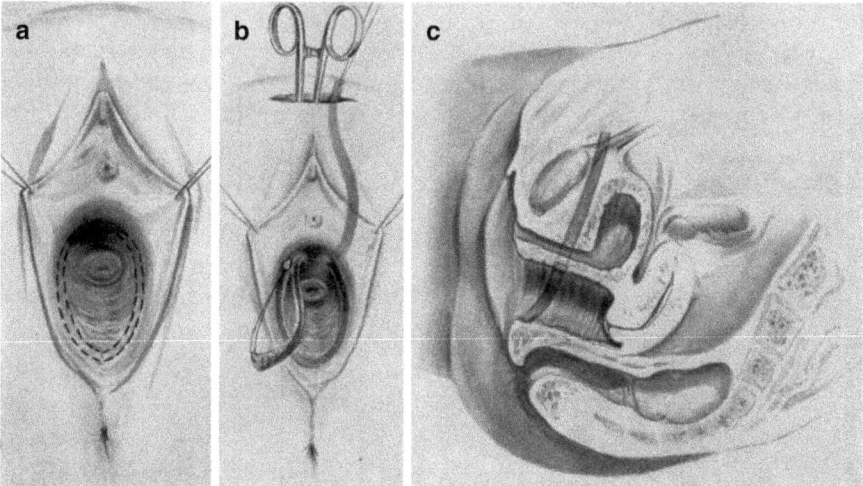

Fig. 5.3 Vaginal sling procedure described by Ingelman-Sundberg. (**a**) Two flaps about 15 mm wide are cut through all layers of the vagina. (**b**) After a catheter has been introduced into the bladder, a small incision is made just above the pubic symphysis; a clamp is then passed through the space of Retzius to meet the finger placed in the vagina in the tissue lateral to the urethra. The procedure is repeated on both sides. (**c**) Vaginal epithelium flaps are passed to the anterior abdominal wall, superior to the pubic symphysis, and sutured together. (Figure from Ingelman-Sundberg [18])

Cystourethropexy

The Marshall-Marchetti-Krantz cystourethropexy (MMK) was described in 1949 and is a retropubic procedure in which sutures are placed into the periurethral tissues and bladder neck and onto the periosteum of the pubis or cartilage of the pubic symphysis to displace the urethra and bladder neck superiorly and anteriorly [26] (Fig. 5.4). Additional sutures were also placed into the serosa of the bladder and rectus muscles to pull the bladder anteriorly into the space of Retzius, to help elevate the bladder along with the bladder neck during coughing or lifting [26]. Subjective continence rates after MMK were reported to be 92% and 84.5% in those with prior failed incontinence surgery [27]. Long-term subjective continence rates were reported to be 85.7% at 5 years and 75% at 15 years [28]. Reported complications of the MMK cystourethropexy include a reported 0.74–2.5% rate of osteitis pubis [27, 29] and ureteral obstruction secondary to suture placement causing ureterovesical junction obstruction [30].

The Burch procedure originated when John C. Burch reported difficulties with suture placement secondary to poor visualization and the periosteum of the posterior pubic symphysis not holding sutures in place during the MMK [31]. Initially, in the Burch colposuspension, sutures were placed in the paravaginal tissues lateral to the bladder neck and proximal urethra, and these tissues were suspended with sutures toward the tendinous arch of the fascia pelvis. This was later modified to utilize ipsilateral iliopectineal (Cooper's) ligaments on the pelvic sidewalls [32] (Fig. 5.5). Additional sutures could also be placed at the level of the lateral vaginal fornix and secured to the iliopectineal ligament to provide support to a lateral or paravaginal defect. A Cochrane analysis reported that overall continence with the Burch procedure was 85–90% within the first year and 70% after 5 years [34]. This procedure may be performed via both an open or a laparoscopic approach, and data from a Cochrane analysis suggest that open and laparoscopic colposuspension are

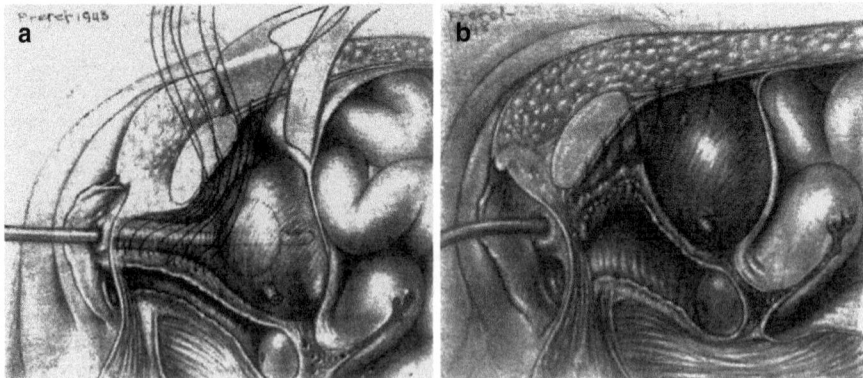

Fig. 5.4 Marshall-Marchetti-Krantz cystourethropexy (MMK). (**a**) Sagittal section demonstrating location paraurethral sutures on the left. (**b**) Sutures tied down demonstrating urethra, bladder neck, and bladder displaced superiorly and anteriorly. (Figure from Marshall et al. [26])

Fig. 5.5 Burch colposuspension. Figure of 8 sutures were placed on each side of the proximal urethra and bladder neck and brought up through ipsilateral iliopectineal (Cooper's) ligaments. (Figure from Baggish and Karram [33], Fig. 34.4)

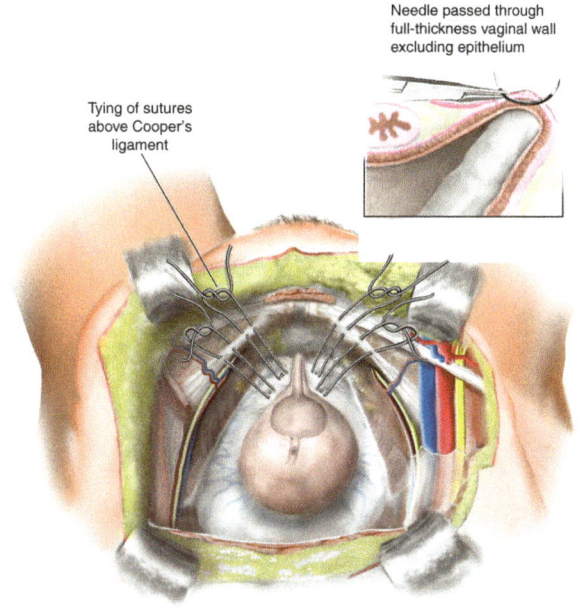

Needle passed through full-thickness vaginal wall excluding epithelium

Tying of sutures above Cooper's ligament

equally effective for treating incontinence in the short term [35]. Reported complications associated with Burch colposuspension include postoperative hematoma or transfusion in 2% [36], which is believed to be related to paravaginal vein injury due to inadequate tissue exposure prior to suture placement [32], bladder injury (up to 9.6%, more common with prior pelvic surgery), ureteral kinking (up to 2%), urinary tract infection (UTI) (up to 40% depending on how UTI was defined), wound infection (up to 10.8%), urinary retention (<3%), de novo detrusor instability (up to 8%), dyspareunia (up to 4%), and postoperative enterocele or other genital organ prolapses (7.6%–26.7%) [36–40]. With regard to genital organ prolapse related to Burch colposuspension, its etiology is unclear; however, this predisposition may be due to a mechanical change in the orientation of the vagina [40], may be related to the natural history of pelvic organ prolapse [32, 39], or may be due to neurologic damage of the pelvic floor muscles related to the procedure [41]. This procedure still in use is described in Chap. 15.

Needle Suspension Procedures

A number of needle suspension procedures have historically been performed, all with the goal of correcting SUI by returning the urethra to a well-supported position using sutures placed in the paraurethral tissues by passing a needle through small lower abdominal and vaginal incisions. In 1959, Pereyra described a technique involving the passage of a special needle through a small suprapubic incision

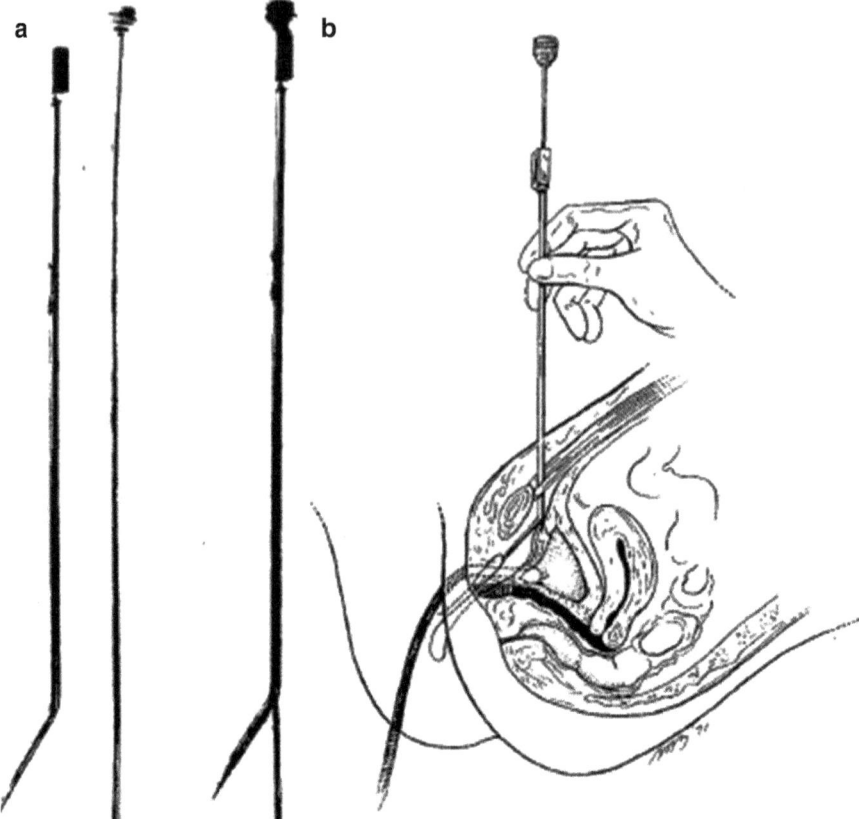

Fig. 5.6 Peyrera needle suspension. (**a**) The Peyrera cannula consists of an angled tip needle with a hollow shaft and a stylet which is inserted through the hollow shaft. Each pointed end is fitted with an eye for carrying a suture. (**b**) The Peyrera cannula is passed above the pubic symphysis and into the periurethral tissue lateral to the urethra. The stylet is then passed through the cannula and exits at a second point in the periurethral tissue. A similar suture is placed on the opposite side, and both sutures are tied over the rectus fascia to suspend the urethra. (Figure from Kursh et al. [43])

[42–44]. After the vaginal epithelium has been dissected away from the paraurethral tissues, the needle is passed behind the pubic bone and lateral to the urethra and guided out onto a finger through into the paraurethral tissue (Fig. 5.6). The original procedure described the passage of steel wire to support the tissues, resulting in two loops of wire, with each wire passing through the abdominal wall, the paraurethral tissues, and then back up to the abdominal wall. The wires are then tensioned to provide the appropriate elevation of the urethra and bladder neck and tied at the level of the rectus fascia. As these wires were expected to cut through the vaginal and paraurethral tissues over time, the support was expected to be maintained by the development of scar tissue while they were held in this position by the wires. Cautery was also applied along the proximal, lateral urethra, to aid in this goal of scar tissue development. Cystoscopy was not performed as part of this procedure, resulting in potential passage of the wire through the bladder. This procedure was eventually modified to include the use of chromic suture rather than steel wire. Further modifications to this technique involved exposure of pubourethral ligaments, which were then included in the suspension sutures [45, 46], as well as the Stamey and the Raz modifications of the procedure, which are described later in this chapter. Reported success rates have been variable, with Peyrera and Lebherz reporting a 94% cure or marked improvement rate during 12–24-month follow-up [44] and longer-term follow-up data demonstrating an 81.6% rate of complete absence of SUI in women with uncomplicated recurrent SUI, during a mean follow up of 36.3 months [47]. However, other authors reported lower cure rates of <50% at 1 year and 53.6% at an average follow-up of 23.2 months [43, 48]. Complications associated with the modified Pereyra needle suspension procedure included wound infection (5.5%), urinary tract infection (3.7%), vaginal-wall hematoma (3.7%), new-onset urge incontinence and de novo detrusor instability (11.1%), postoperative obstructive voiding requiring intermittent self-catheterization (9.3%), enterocele (5.6%), and recurrent cystocele or rectocele (5.6%) [47].

In 1973, the Stamey procedure was described, involving a vaginal incision and suspension of the urethra and bladder neck accomplished by placement of nylon monofilament suture with 1 cm of 5 mm diameter polyethylene terephthalate Dacron tube as buttresses on either side of the urethra (Fig. 5.7). The sutures were tied to themselves, ipsilaterally, without crossing the midline, with moderate tension [46]. Cystoscopic control of this type of procedure was first introduced by Stamey as a part of this procedure to assess suture placement and needle passage. Long-term follow-up evaluations suggest that the cure rate declines over time, with variable rates of success. The reported 10-year cure rate ranges from 33% to 76.4%, [50, 51] with a 15-year cure rate of 47.9% [52]. Another study with a mean follow-up of 66 months demonstrated that 50% of patients remained completely continent for the entire follow-up, 11.5% had initial failure, and 38.5% with initial complete continence developed recurrence 6–90 months after the procedure [53]. Patients were also asked about their satisfaction with the results of the procedure, with 35.7% reporting being completely cured, 27% with substantial improvement, 12.7% with minor improvement, 12.7% with no change, and 11.9% with worse results. Reported complications included peritoneal perforation with acute abdomen requiring laparotomy (1.1%), bleeding/hematoma (2.7%), infection (31.1%), prolonged suprapubic pain (6.5%), and obstruction to urine flow (8.2%) [53].

The Raz procedure, reported in 1981, utilized placement of a suprapubic catheter and an inverted U-shaped vaginal incision with perforation of the endopelvic fascia and development of the retropubic space through the vaginal incision [54]. Nonabsorbable polypropylene sutures are placed bilaterally in a helical fashion to include the pubocervical fascia, the medial cut edge of the urethropelvic ligament, and the vaginal wall without including vaginal epithelium (Fig. 5.8). A suprapubic incision is then made and dissected down to the anterior rectus fascia. A ligature carrier needle is passed through the suprapubic incision and into the vagina, and the vaginal sutures are then transferred to the suprapubic incision and tied together,

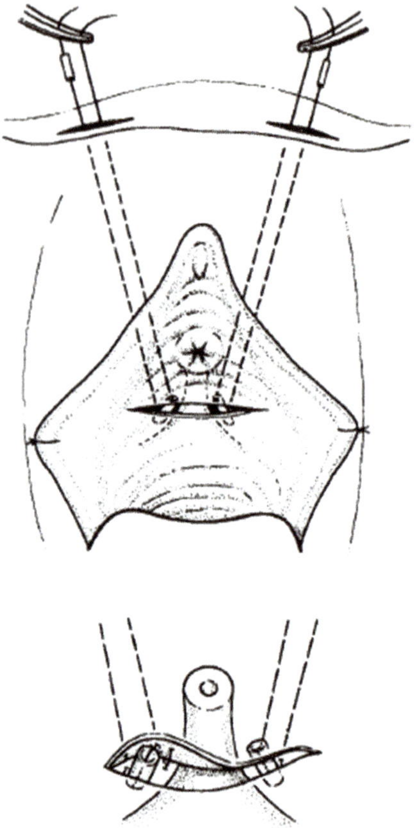

Fig. 5.7 Stamey needle suspension procedure. Sutures are placed bilaterally with buttresses on either side of the urethra. (Figure from Hilton and Mayne [49])

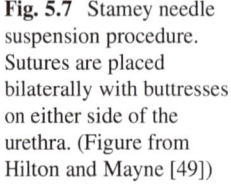

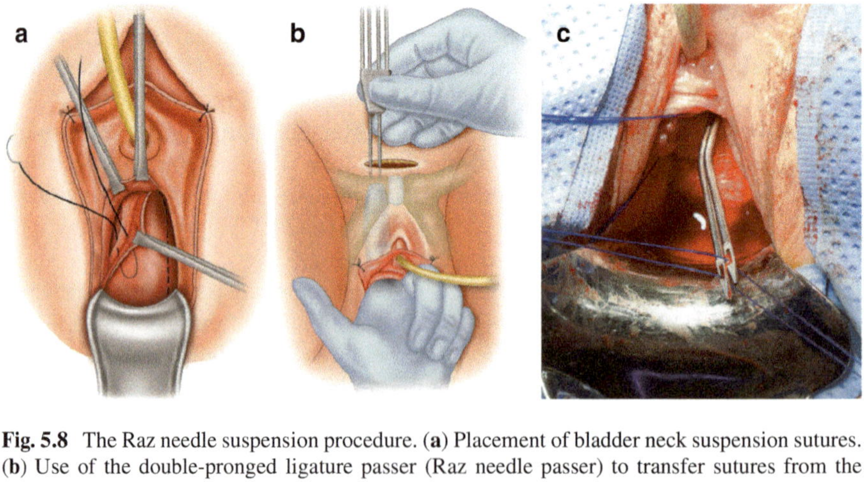

Fig. 5.8 The Raz needle suspension procedure. (**a**) Placement of bladder neck suspension sutures. (**b**) Use of the double-pronged ligature passer (Raz needle passer) to transfer sutures from the vagina to the suprapubic region. Under finger guidance, the tips of the passer are transferred from the suprapubic incision to the vaginal incisions. (**c**) Sutures are transferred through the eyes of the Raz needle passer and retracted to the suprapubic region. (Figure from Raz [55], p. 44, 46, 47, Fig. 2.13, 2.20, 2.21)

crossing the midline over the anterior rectus fascia, with minimal tension [46, 54]. Cystoscopy was performed as part of this procedure to evaluate for bladder or ureteral injury. Short-term results with a mean follow-up of 15 months have demonstrated 90.3% success, defined as cure or significant improvement in SUI [56]. These results were also stratified by severity of incontinence and demonstrated that success of the Raz bladder neck suspension depends upon the severity of SUI, as >90% success was reported in women mild to moderate SUI and 65% success in severe SUI [56]. However, longer-term studies have suggested variable success, with 20% of patients reporting no incontinence and 51% reporting SUI with or without urge incontinence at a mean follow-up of 9.8 years [57]. Despite recurrent or persistent SUI, 71% of patients reported significant improvement in incontinence, and 73% reported being satisfied with the results of the procedure [57]. The short-term results only included patients with stress incontinence with or without mild (grade 1) cystocele [56] who underwent the Raz procedure, suggesting that patient selection may play a role in the rate of success with the procedure. Reported complications of the Raz procedure included de novo urgency incontinence in 7.5%, secondary pelvic prolapse in 6%, prolonged retention in 2.5%, and suprapubic pain in 3% [56].

The Gittes procedure, developed in 1987, which uses no incisions, but only skin and vaginal perforations, involves the placement of monofilament suture to obtain deep bites of the vaginal wall and paraurethral tissues bilaterally [58]. A needle is passed through the anterior rectus fascia and into the vagina, where full-thickness bites of the vaginal wall including the epithelium are taken (Fig. 5.9). After the vaginal sutures are placed, the suture is passed back up to the anterior rectus fascia. The ipsilateral sutures were tied together and then tied across the midline with minimal tension [46]. Reported rates of complete and improved continence have been reported to range from 23.1% at 53 months [59], 14% at 5 years [60], 72.6% at

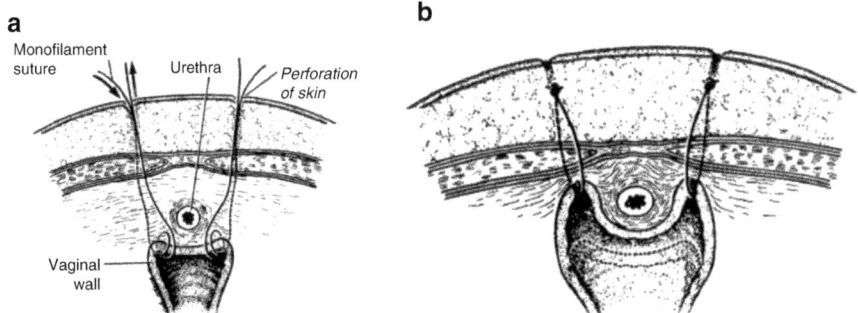

Fig. 5.9 The Gittes needle suspension procedure. (**a**) No incisions, only skin, and vaginal perforations. A needle is passed through the anterior rectus fascia and into the vagina, where full-thickness bites of the vaginal wall at the level of the bladder neck, including the epithelium, are taken. After the vaginal sutures are placed, the suture is passed back up to the anterior rectus fascia. (**b**) Sutures are tied down into the suprapubic fat to bury the knots. (Figure from Gittes and Loughlin. [58])

Fig. 5.10 Points of suture passage through the vaginal wall for the Benderev (Vesica) needle suspension procedure. (Figure from Bodell and Leach [46])

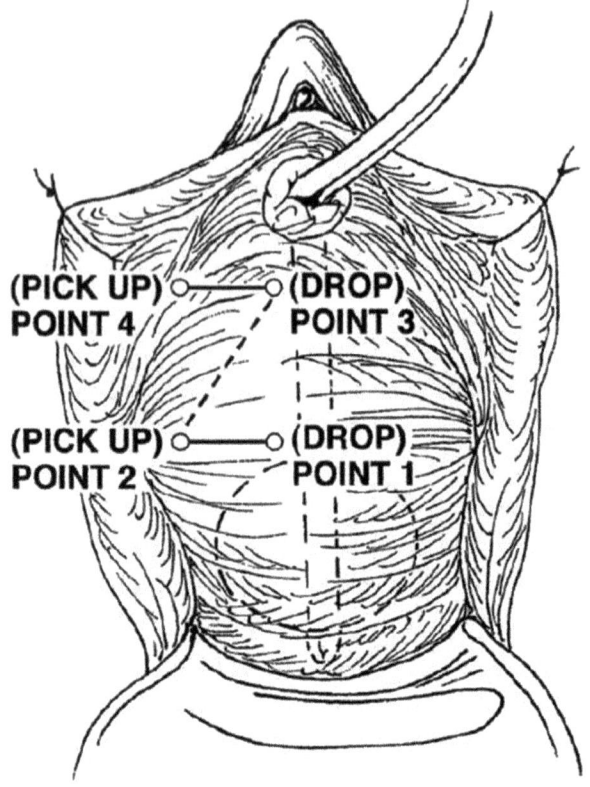

62.5 months [61], and 37% at 6.4 years [51]. Reported complications have included wound infection (2.3%), repeated UTIs (1.1%), persistent groin pain requiring suture removal (5.7%), and de novo postoperative urgency and/or urgency incontinence (20%) [59, 62].

The Benderev, or Vesica procedure, was developed in 1994 and used bone anchors placed in the bilateral pubic tubercles as well as a suture passer device [63, 64]. Either one incision or two small incisions were made to allow access to the bilateral pubic tubercles. A bone anchor was placed in each pubic tubercle, and an attached suture was passed using a suture passer from the suprapubic incision into the vagina at the level of the bladder neck. The sutures were placed into the vaginal epithelium in a Z configuration [46, 64] (Fig. 5.10) and then tied in the suprapubic region by placing a spacer device between the pubic bone and the knot of the suture. Reported rates of complete dryness were 85% at 6 months, 46–94% at 12 months [65, 66], and 31% at 5 years [66]. Based on these long-term outcomes, the study investigators no longer advocate this form of bladder neck suspension for stress urinary incontinence. Of those with recurrent incontinence, 70% were symptomatic enough to undergo further surgical treatment. Fraying and breakage of the Vesica suspensory sutures at the bone anchors were noted in those who underwent subsequent Burch colposuspension, and this is the proposed reason for poor success with this procedure. Reported complications include wound infection (16%), requiring temporary intermittent catheterization (4.7–10%), suture erosion into bladder (5%), suture erosion into vagina (2.56%), presumed osteitis pubis (1.2–5%), and transient de novo detrusor instability (7%) [65–67].

Urethral Bulking

Several transurethrally injected substances have been used to produce bulking of the urethra to improve urethral coaptation in an effort to improve stress urinary incontinence. Periurethral paraffin injection was first suggested by Gersuny at the end of the nineteenth century [2]. Cod liver oil injection was reported in 1938 with 60% cure and 25% improvement at 1 year [63]. The use of Teflon was first described in 1973 by Politano and Berg [69, 70], with a reported rate of cure or improvement at 24 months of 30–38% [71], and was noted to lead to fibrosis with urethral obstruction and Teflon migration to lymph nodes, causing granulomas [2, 3]. Autologous fat tissue injection was introduced in 1989 by Gonzalez de Gariby, with 3-month results demonstrating a 22.2% cure or improvement rate that was no different than saline injection and has been associated with the complication of fat pulmonary embolism [72, 73]. Collagen injection was introduced in 1989 by Shortliffe and found to have a 53% rate of cure or improvement during 9–23-month follow-up [74]. Although these agents are no longer used, a number of newer urethral bulking agents have since been described and will be discussed in greater detail in Chap. 14.

Bladder Denervation

Denervation of the bladder by unilateral or bilateral resection of inferior hypogastric plexus has been reported by Ingelman-Sundberg in 1959 as a treatment for urge incontinence due to a neurogenic cause or contracted bladders due to interstitial cystitis [75] (Fig. 5.11). Preoperative testing is required prior to proceeding with denervation. After performing cystometry, xylocaine solution with adrenalin is injected into the anterior fornix 1 cm lateral to the cervix and at a depth of 3 cm, unilaterally, to denervate the bladder. Repeat cystometry is performed at 5 min after injection, and a post void residual is checked. If uninhibited contractions and bladder capacity are improved on cystometry after unilateral injection, then unilateral resection is performed. However, if there is no improvement seen on cystometry, then the same injection is performed on the contralateral side with repeat cystometry and post void residual. If improvement is seen on cystometry after the second injection, then bilateral resection is performed. However, if the post void residual volume is elevated, only unilateral resection is performed. If residual urine is greater than 150 ml after unilateral anesthesia, then the procedure should not be performed.

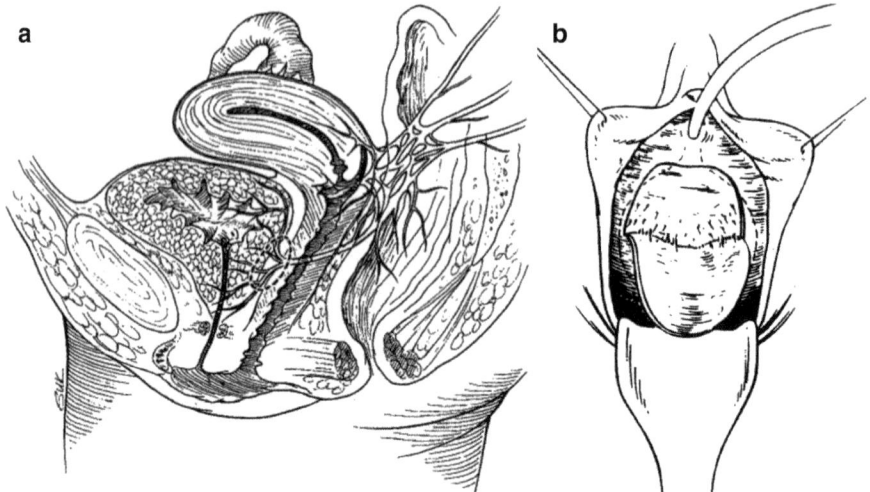

Fig. 5.11 Bladder denervation for treatment of urgency urinary incontinence. (**a**) Terminal branches of the pelvic nerve entering the bladder at the level of the trigone. (**b**) Dissection of the vaginal epithelium and perivesical fascia from bladder the level of the trigone. (Figure from Westney et al. [76])

The procedure is performed transvaginally, beginning with a transverse incision below the external urethral orifice. The anterior vaginal wall is dissected free from the urethral orifice up to the cervix, the bladder ligaments are bluntly separated from the levator ani, and the hypogastric plexus is exposed laterally to the rectum and following the inferior vesical vessels medially [76]. The nerves are then grasped and resected. Reported rates of complete or partial response to the procedure at a mean follow-up of 44.1 months were 67.8% (54% complete responders) [76], while Inglman-Sundberg reported long-term rates of 70% (mean follow-up time not reported) [77].

Transvesical phenol injection of the paravesical nerve plexuses has been described for refractory detrusor instability/detrusor hyperreflexia by damaging postganglionic fibers of the bladder. Poor response rates were described, with 11–82% response rate [78–80], and serious complications of the procedure have been described including detrusor acontractility and fistula formation [81, 82]. Prior pelvic radiation has been regarded as an absolute contraindication to this therapy [83]. Due to poor efficacy and risk of complications, this treatment is not recommended and is no longer used [78]. Given the potential long-term effects of a neuroablative procedure and denervated tissue potentially being in a more pathologic state than before performing the procedure [84], other neuromodulatory techniques may become more favored.

Detrusor Myectomy

Detrusor myectomy, also known as auto-augmentation, was first described in 1989 by Cartwright and Snow, to avoid the complications associated with bowel augmentation including electrolyte disturbances, enteric fistula, abscess, mucus production, and peritoneal adhesions [85]. In this procedure, a large, wide-mouthed, well-draining diverticular bulge of bladder epithelium is created by excising detrusor muscle over the dome of the bladder and leaving the bladder epithelium intact (Fig. 5.12). Long-term success rates have been reported to be 60–80% [86–88], with higher success rates in patients with idiopathic overactive bladder than those with neurogenic detrusor overactivity (70–79% vs 33–50%) [86, 87]. Complications of the procedure have included the need for intermittent catheterization (45%) and UTI (31.5%) [87]. Some authors have concluded that the procedure is not efficacious especially in the management of those with neurogenic voiding dysfunction and do not support the procedure [89]. However, others advocate that this still remains

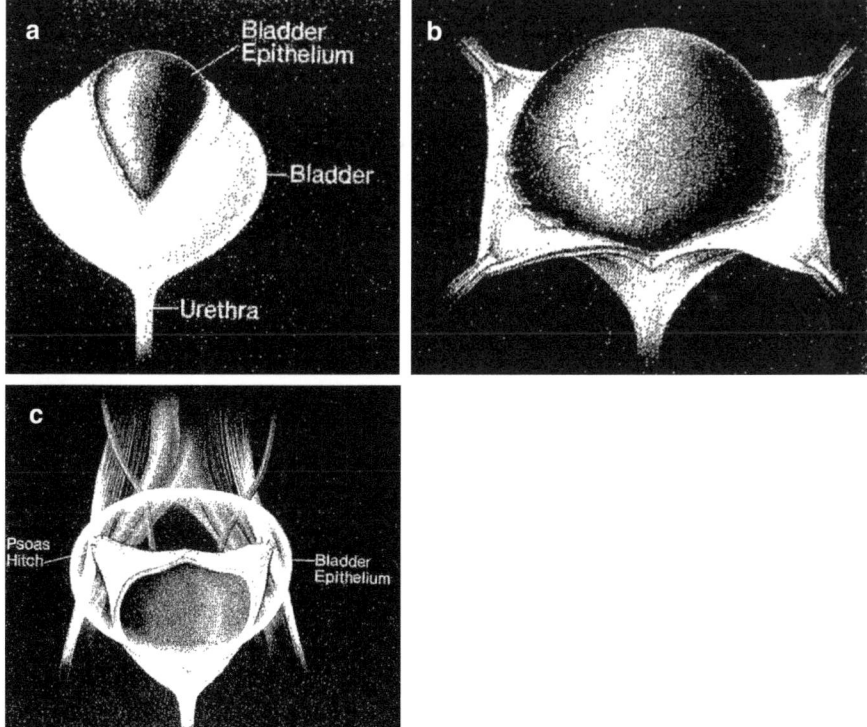

Fig. 5.12 Detrusor myectomy, also known as auto-augmentation. (**a**) Detrusor is incised, leaving the bladder epithelium intact. (**b**) Detrusor stripped from intact bladder epithelium. (**c**) Wide-mouthed diverticular bulge of the bladder with bladder filling. (Figure from Cartwright and Snow [85]; discussion 520–1)

useful in the armamentarium of the urologist due to ease of the procedure and decreased morbidity, and does not preclude the performance of enterocystoplasty in case of failure of detrusor myectomy/myotomy [90, 91].

Conclusion

Treatments for urinary incontinence have been documented as early as the second millennium BC and have ranged from less invasive treatments such as urethral plugs to plication of the urethra and bladder neck to various iterations of needle suspension procedures, colposuspension, to auto-augmentation and bladder denervation. For female stress urinary incontinence surgeries, this historical review highlights that various techniques were utilized to support and stabilize the urethra and the surrounding tissues, and the methods described above are not intended to be a complete list of every technique that has been used to treat SUI. The success rates quoted in the literature depend on the definition of success used and may differ from contemporary definitions of success which may be a composite of subjective and objective outcomes that are patient-reported and/or patient-centered.

While the prevalence of these techniques has decreased significantly with the introduction of the mid-urethral sling in 1998 [8], there is still a role for non-mesh-based surgical treatment options such as a Burch colposuspension and autologous slings in select properly counseled patients. An understanding of prior treatments is key to understanding the evolution and principles of current techniques. This historical background is also important for the surgeon's knowledge as patients who have had anti-incontinence procedures in prior decades may have had one of the above-described procedures. Surgical treatment of urinary incontinence will continue to evolve and improve as our understanding deepens and we build on prior knowledge and experience.

References

1. Milsom I, Gyhagen M. The prevalence of urinary incontinence. Climacteric. 2019;22:217.
2. Schultheiss D, Hofner K, Oelke M, et al. Historical aspects of the treatment of urinary incontinence. Eur Urol. 2000;38:352.
3. Hinoul P, Roovers JP, Ombelet W, et al. Surgical management of urinary stress incontinence in women: a historical and clinical overview. Eur J Obstet Gynecol Reprod Biol. 2009;145:219.
4. Kelly HA, D. W. Urinary incontinence in women without manifest injury to the bladder. Am Coll Surg. 1914;18:444.
5. Schreiner G, Beltran R, Lockwood G, et al. A timeline of female stress urinary incontinence: how technology defined theory and advanced treatment. Neurourol Urodyn. 2020;39:1862.
6. Maher CF, Karram M. Surgical management of pelvic organ prolapse, Chapter 8. p. 117–37.
7. Bergman A, Elia G. Three surgical procedures for genuine stress incontinence: five-year follow-up of a prospective randomized study. Am J Obstet Gynecol. 1995;173:66.
8. Thaweekul Y, Bunyavejchevin S, Wisawasukmongchol W, et al. Long term results of anterior colporrhaphy with Kelly plication for the treatment of stress urinary incontinence. J Med Assoc Thail. 2004;87:357.

9. Anger JT, Weinberg AE, Albo ME, et al. Trends in surgical management of stress urinary incontinence among female Medicare beneficiaries. Urology. 2009;74:283.
10. Rogo-Gupta L, Litwin MS, Saigal CS, et al. Trends in the surgical management of stress urinary incontinence among female Medicare beneficiaries, 2002-2007. Urology. 2013;82:38.
11. Ingelman-Sundberg A. Extravaginal plastic repair of the pelvic floor for prolapse of the bladder neck; a new method to operate for stress incontinence. Gynaecologia. 1947;123:242.
12. Obrink A. Pubococcygeal repair ad modum Ingelman-Sundberg. A retrospective investigation with 10-20 years time of observation. Acta Obstet Gynecol Scand. 1977;56:391.
13. Ingelman-Sundberg A. Urinary incontinence in women, excluding fistulas. Acta Obstet Gynecol Scand. 1952;31(3):266–91.
14. Gomes da Silveira G, Eduardo Piccoli C. Ingelman-Sundberg operation for urinary incontinence. Our experience. Acta Obstet Gynecol Scand. 1977;56:399.
15. Debodinance P. Comparison of the Bologna and Ingelman-Sundberg procedures for stress incontinence associated with genital prolapse: ten-year follow-up of a prospective randomized study. J Gynecol Obstet Biol Reprod (Paris). 2000;29:148.
16. Mazeman E, Wemeau L, Biserte J, et al. Bladder neck suspension for stress incontinence: long-term evaluation. Eur Urol. 1978;4:123.
17. Chefchaouni MC, Thiounn N, Conquy S, et al. Treatment of stress urinary incontinence in women using the Goebell-Stoeckel surgical method. Study of 59 operated patients. Long-term review. J Urol (Paris). 1995;101:215.
18. Ingelman-Sundberg A. A vaginal sling operation; for cases of stress incontinence and for women who cannot use a diaphragm due to prolapse of the anterior vaginal wall. J Obstet Gynaecol Br Emp. 1957;64:849.
19. Price P. Plastic operations for incontinence of urine and feces. Arch Surg. 1933;26:1043.
20. Aldridge AH. Transplantation of fascia for relief of urinary stress incontinence. Am J Obstet Gynecol. 1942;44:398.
21. Chai TC. Edward McGuire's influence in the field of stress urinary incontinence and bladder storage symptoms. Neurourol Urodyn. 2010;29 Suppl 1:S32.
22. Mc LH. Fascial slings for stress incontinence. J Obstet Gynaecol Br Emp. 1957;64:673.
23. Jeffcoate TN. The results of the Aldridge sling operation for stress incontinence. J Obstet Gynaecol Br Emp. 1956;63:36.
24. McIndoe GA, Jones RW, Grieve BW. The Aldridge sling procedure in the treatment of urinary stress incontinence. Aust N Z J Obstet Gynaecol. 1987;27:238.
25. McLaren HC. Late results from sling operations. J Obstet Gynaecol Br Commonw. 1968;75:10.
26. Marshall VF, Marchetti AA, Krantz KE. The correction of stress incontinence by simple vesicourethral suspension. Surg Gynecol Obstet. 1949;88:509.
27. Mainprize TC, Drutz HP. The Marshall-Marchetti-Krantz procedure: a critical review. Obstet Gynecol Surv. 1988;43:724.
28. McDuffie RW Jr, Litin RB, Blundon KE. Urethrovesical suspension (Marshall-Marchetti-Krantz). Experience with 204 cases. Am J Surg. 1981;141:297.
29. Kammerer-Doak DN, Cornella JL, Magrina JF, et al. Osteitis pubis after Marshall-Marchetti-Krantz urethropexy: a pubic osteomyelitis. Am J Obstet Gynecol. 1998;179:586.
30. Persky L, Guerriere K. Complications of Marshall-Marchetti-Krantz urethropexy. Urology. 1976;8:469.
31. Burch JC. Urethrovaginal fixation to Cooper's ligament for correction of stress incontinence, cystocele, and prolapse. Am J Obstet Gynecol. 1961;81:281.
32. Sohlberg EM, Elliott CS. Burch colposuspension. Urol Clin North Am. 2019;46:53.
33. Baggish MS, Karram MM, editors. Atlas of pelvic anatomy and gynecologic surgery. 5th ed. p. 421.
34. Lapitan MCM, Cody JD, Mashayekhi A. Open retropubic colposuspension for urinary incontinence in women. Cochrane Database Syst Rev. 2017;7:CD002912.
35. Freites J, Stewart F, Omar MI, et al. Laparoscopic colposuspension for urinary incontinence in women. Cochrane Database Syst Rev. 2019;12:CD002239.
36. Demirci F, Petri E. Perioperative complications of Burch colposuspension. Int Urogynecol J Pelvic Floor Dysfunct. 2000;11:170.

37. Kenton K, Oldham L, Brubaker L. Open Burch urethropexy has a low rate of perioperative complications. Am J Obstet Gynecol. 2002;187:107.
38. Wee HY, Low C, Han HC. Burch colposuspension: review of perioperative complications at a women's and children's hospital in Singapore. Ann Acad Med Singap. 2003;32:821.
39. Wiskind AK, Creighton SM, Stanton SL. The incidence of genital prolapse after the Burch colposuspension. Am J Obstet Gynecol. 1992;167:399.
40. Burch JC. Cooper's ligament urethrovesical suspension for stress incontinence. Nine years' experience--results, complications, technique. Am J Obstet Gynecol. 1968;100:764.
41. Kjolhede P. Genital prolapse in women treated successfully and unsuccessfully by the Burch colposuspension. Acta Obstet Gynecol Scand. 1998;77:444.
42. Pereyra AJ. A simplified surgical procedure for the correction of stress incontinence in women. West J Surg Obstet Gynecol. 1959;67:223.
43. Kursh ED, Wainstein M, Persky L. The Pereyra procedure and urinary stress incontinence. J Urol. 1972;108:591.
44. Pereyra AJ, Lebherz TB. Combined urethrovesical suspension and vaginourethroplasty for correction of urinary stress incontinence. Obstet Gynecol. 1967;30:537.
45. Pereyra AJ, Lebherz TB, Growdon WA, et al. Pubourethral supports in perspective: modified pereyra procedure for urinary incontinence. Obstet Gynecol. 1982;59:643.
46. Bodell DM, Leach GE. Needle suspension procedures for female incontinence. Urol Clin North Am. 2002;29:575.
47. Holschneider CH, Solh S, Lebherz TB, et al. The modified Pereyra procedure in recurrent stress urinary incontinence: a 15-year review. Obstet Gynecol. 1994;83:573.
48. Crist T, Shingleton HM, Roberson WE. Urethrovesical needle suspension: postoperative loss of vesical neck support demonstrated by chain cystography. Obstet Gynecol. 1969;34:489.
49. Hilton P, Mayne CJ. The Stamey endoscopic bladder neck suspension: a clinical and uro-dynamic investigation, including actuarial follow-up over four years. Br J Obstet Gynaecol. 1991;98(11):1141–9.
50. Mills R, Persad R, Handley Ashken M. Long-term follow-up results with the Stamey operation for stress incontinence of urine. Br J Urol. 1996;77:86.
51. Kondo A, Kato K, Gotoh M, et al. The Stamey and Gittes procedures: long-term followup in relation to incontinence types and patient age. J Urol. 1998;160:756.
52. Clemens JQ, Stern JA, Bushman WA, et al. Long-term results of the Stamey bladder neck suspension: direct comparison with the Marshall-Marchetti-Krantz procedure. J Urol. 1998;160:372.
53. Conrad S, Pieper A, De la Maza SF, et al. Long-term results of the Stamey bladder neck suspension procedure: a patient questionnaire based outcome analysis. J Urol. 1997;157:1672.
54. Raz S. Modified bladder neck suspension for female stress incontinence. Urology. 1981;17:82.
55. Raz S. Atlas of vaginal reconstructive surgery
56. Raz S, Sussman EM, Erickson DB, et al. The Raz bladder neck suspension: results in 206 patients. J Urol. 1992;148:845.
57. Trockman BA, Leach GE, Hamilton J, et al. Modified Pereyra bladder neck suspension: 10-year mean followup using outcomes analysis in 125 patients. J Urol. 1995;154:1841.
58. Gittes RF, Loughlin KR. No-incision pubovaginal suspension for stress incontinence. J Urol. 1987;138:568.
59. Elkabir JJ, Mee AD. Long-term evaluation of the Gittes procedure for urinary stress incontinence. J Urol. 1998;159:1203.
60. Nigam AK, Otite U, Badenoch DF. Endoscopic bladder neck suspension revisited: long-term results of Stamey and Gittes procedures. Eur Urol. 2000;38:677.
61. Kuo HC. Long-term results of surgical treatment for female stress urinary incontinence. Urol Int. 2001;66:13.
62. Theodorou C, Floratos D, Katsifotis C, et al. Transvaginal incisionless bladder neck suspension. A simplified technique for female genuine stress incontinence. Int Urol Nephrol. 1998;30:273.
63. Benderev TV. A modified percutaneous outpatient bladder neck suspension system. J Urol. 1994;152:2316.

64. Appell RA, Rackley RR, Dmochowski RR. Vesica percutaneous bladder neck stabilization. J Endourol. 1996;10:221.
65. Rackley RR, Winters JC, Appell RA. Percutaneous bladder neck/urethra stabilization with bone-anchor suture fixation for type II genuine stress urinary incontinence. Presented at the 91st Meeting of the American Urologic Association, 1996.
66. Reid SV, Parys BT. Long-term 5-year followup of the results of the vesica procedure. J Urol. 2005;173:1234.
67. Matkov TG, Hejna MJ, Coogan CL. Osteomyelitis as a complication of vesica percutaneous bladder neck suspension. J Urol. 1998;160:1427.
68. Murless BC. The injection treatment of stress incontinence. J Obstet Gynaecol Br Emp. 1938;45:67.
69. Politano VA, Small MP, Harper JM, et al. Periurethral teflon injection for urinary incontinence. Trans Am Assoc Genitourin Surg. 1973;65:54.
70. Berg S. Polytef augmentation urethroplasty. Correction of surgically incurable urinary incontinence by injection technique. Arch Surg. 1973;107:379.
71. Benshushan A, Brzezinski A, Shoshani O, et al. Periurethral injection for the treatment of urinary incontinence. Obstet Gynecol Surv. 1998;53:383.
72. Santiago Gonzalez de Garibay AM, Castro Morrondo J, Castillo Jimeno JM, et al. Endoscopic injection of autologous adipose tissue in the treatment of female incontinence. Arch Esp Urol. 1989;42:143.
73. Lee PE, Kung RC, Drutz HP. Periurethral autologous fat injection as treatment for female stress urinary incontinence: a randomized double-blind controlled trial. J Urol. 2001;165:153.
74. Shortliffe LM, Freiha FS, Kessler R, et al. Treatment of urinary incontinence by the periurethral implantation of glutaraldehyde cross-linked collagen. J Urol. 1989;141:538.
75. Ingelman-Sundberg A. Partial denervation of the bladder, a new operation for the treatment of urge incontinence and similar conditions in women. Acta Obstet Gynecol Scand. 1959;38:487.
76. Westney OL, Lee JT, McGuire EJ, et al. Long-term results of Ingelman-Sundberg denervation procedure for urge incontinence refractory to medical therapy. J Urol. 2002;168:1044.
77. Ingelman-Sundberg A. Partial bladder denervation for detrusor dyssynergia. Clin Obstet Gynecol. 1978;21:797.
78. Chapple CR, Hampson SJ, Turner-Warwick RT, et al. Subtrigonal phenol injection. How safe and effective is it? Br J Urol. 1991;68:483.
79. Blackford HN, Murray K, Stephenson TP, et al. Results of transvesical infiltration of the pelvic plexuses with phenol in 116 patients. Br J Urol. 1984;56:647.
80. Wall LL, Stanton SL. Transvesical phenol injection of pelvic nerve plexuses in females with refractory urge incontinence. Br J Urol. 1989;63:465.
81. Harris RG, Constantinou CE, Stamey TA. Extravesical subtrigonal injection of 50 per cent ethanol for detrusor instability. J Urol. 1988;140:111.
82. McInerney PD, Vanner TF, Matenhelia S, et al. Assessment of the long-term results of subtrigonal phenolisation. Br J Urol. 1991;67:586.
83. Cameron-Strange A, Millard RJ. Management of refractory detrusor instability by transvesical phenol injection. Br J Urol. 1988;62:323.
84. Petrou SP. Long-term results of Ingelman-Sundberg denervation procedures for urge incontinence refractory to medical therapy. Int Braz J Urol. 2002;28:491.
85. Cartwright PC, Snow BW. Bladder autoaugmentation: early clinical experience. J Urol. 1989;142:505.
86. Swami KS, Feneley RC, Hammonds JC, et al. Detrusor myectomy for detrusor overactivity: a minimum 1-year follow-up. Br J Urol. 1998;81:68.
87. Kumar SP, Abrams PH. Detrusor myectomy: long-term results with a minimum follow-up of 2 years. BJU Int. 2005;96:341.
88. Aslam MZ, Agarwal M. Detrusor myectomy: long-term functional outcomes. Int J Urol. 2012;19:1099.
89. Karsenty G, Vidal F, Ruffion A, et al. Treatment of neurogenic detrusor hyperactivity: detrusor myomectomy. Prog Urol. 2007;17:580.
90. Johnson EU, Singh G. Long-term outcomes of urinary tract reconstruction in patients with neurogenic urinary tract dysfunction. Indian J Urol. 2013;29:328.
91. Chen LC, Kuo HC. Current management of refractory overactive bladder. Low Urin Tract Symptoms. 2020;12:109.

Part II
Conservative Treatment

Chapter 6
Behavioral Therapy and Lifestyle Modifications for the Management of Urinary Incontinence in Women

Kimberly Kenne and Catherine S. Bradley

Introduction

Most clinical practice guidelines recommend behavioral therapies as initial treatments for women with urinary incontinence (UI). These interventions vary widely and may include fluid management, dietary changes, avoidance of bladder irritants, timed voiding, bladder training, management of bowel function, exercise, weight loss, and advice regarding absorptive products and skin protection. While the evidence for support of these interventions is often limited, they are generally low-risk and inexpensive. These factors support their inclusion early in treatment algorithms.

Evidence to support these treatments is lacking in many cases because these interventions are difficult to study. Behavioral therapy and lifestyle modification are difficult to standardize and monitor. High-quality prospective interventional studies are rare; thus, much of the literature around this topic is observational in nature. Outcomes tend to be reported for a combination of behavioral interventions, making interpretation of results difficult. Patient compliance represents a challenge as well, as it may be difficult to assess how well patients adhere to behavioral recommendations. Some evidence supports the use of behavioral therapies in conjunction with other treatments. For example, in the multicenter randomized trial BE-DRI, adding behavioral therapy (including bladder training and fluid management, as well as pelvic floor muscle training) to drug treatment in women with urgency-predominant UI had a beneficial effect on patient satisfaction, perceived improvement, and reduction of other bladder symptoms [1].

Guideline documents published by the American Urological Association (AUA), American Urogynecologic Society (AUGS), and American College of Obstetricians

K. Kenne (✉) · C. S. Bradley
Obstetrics and Gynecology: Female Pelvic Medicine and Reconstructive Surgery, University of Iowa, Iowa City, IA, USA
e-mail: kimberly-kenne@uiowa.edu; catherine-bradley@uiowa.edu

A. P. Cameron (ed.), *Female Urinary Incontinence*,
https://doi.org/10.1007/978-3-030-84352-6_6

and Gynecologists (ACOG) all recommend the use of behavioral therapy in the initial treatment of female UI, typically including pelvic floor muscle exercises and training programs in this category [2–4]. High-quality evidence does exist to support the use of pelvic floor muscle exercises and training for both stress and urgency incontinence (see Chap. 7).

In this chapter, we discuss other behavioral treatments for female UI, many of which may be considered lifestyle modifications. In the following sections, we review each behavioral intervention and summarize the available evidence supporting its use for the treatment of female UI and other urinary symptoms. Table 6.1 lists the interventions discussed in this chapter, the patients in whom they may be recommended, and a description of the evidence supporting each one. While it is important to understand what evidence is available related to behavioral treatments for UI, the treatments are generally low-risk and low-cost and may hold other health benefits for women. Thus, they can often be implemented immediately following initial

Table 6.1 Behavioral treatments recommended for urinary incontinence in women

Intervention	Target population	Description of evidence supporting intervention
Dietary modifications	All patients	Weak: inconsistent results from mostly observational studies suggest possible associations between diet and dietary components and urinary incontinence
Fluid management	All patients	Moderate: interventional studies show consistent benefit of fluid restriction for urinary incontinence and overactive bladder
Caffeine reduction	Patients consuming caffeine	Weak: inconsistent results from observational studies support association between caffeine and urinary incontinence; small interventional studies do not show benefit
Alcohol reduction	Patients consuming alcohol	Weak: inconsistent results from observational studies focused on association between alcohol and urinary incontinence
Tobacco cessation	Tobacco users	Weak: observational studies suggest association between tobacco use and urinary incontinence
Timed/prompted voiding	Infrequent voiders	Weak: interventional studies provide inconsistent evidence for benefit
Bladder training	Frequent voiders	Moderate: interventional studies show benefit of bladder training for urinary incontinence
Bowel management	Patients with constipation	Weak: inconsistent results from observational studies support association between constipation and urinary incontinence and other urinary symptoms
Exercise	All patients	Weak: limited interventional studies provide evidence for use
Weight loss	Overweight and obese patients	Strong: high-quality randomized trials show benefit for urinary incontinence
Absorbent products	All patients	Weak: limited interventional studies provide evidence for use
Skin protectants	All patients	Weak: limited interventional studies provide evidence for use

evaluation and prior to invasive or costly testing. Figure 6.1 demonstrates the educational handout we provide to patients after their initial evaluation for UI with instructions and recommendations related to many of these lifestyle modifications.

Things to do to help your bladder problem:

1. Avoid bladder irritants. There are some foods and liquids that may irritate the bladder.

Avoid or reduce these foods and drinks:

- Alcoholic beverages: liquor, wine and beer
- Caffeine: coffee, tea, dark sodas, darker herbal teas and chocolate
- Very acidic fruit or fruit juices: orange, grapefruit, lemon, lime, mango and pineapple
- Artificial sweeteners: Equal and Nutrasweet
- High doses of vitamins
- Carbonated beverages

The best beverage is water.

2. Drink 4–6 oz of fluid (small cup) every 3–4 hours, evenly spaced throughout the day. Limit your total fluid intake to 48–64 oz per day (~6–8 8 oz cups). The goal is pale yellow urine that does not have a strong odor.

3. Urinate by the clock-every 2–3 hours. Don't wait until you feel full or for a more convenient time. Try to relax when voiding. Do not strain or bear down to start a stream or empty your bladder more quickly.

4. Reduce nighttime awakenings to empty your bladder.

- Limit fluid intake after dinner to reduce nighttime urination.
- Avoid swelling in your lower legs by wearing support hose or elevating your legs when resting during the day.

5. Establish regular bowel habits.

Constipation affects bladder control. Dietary fiber supplements, stool softeners, or laxatives (such as Miralax) are options to help keep bowels regular and easy.

6. Watch your weight. Obesity makes bladder control more difficult.

7. If you smoke, here is one more reason to consider a quit plan. Smoking makes leakage worse because of chronic cough and irritation to the bladder.

8. Don't irritate your vulva area. Avoid colored and perfumed toilet tissue and sanitary napkins. Wash with warm water, wear all-cotton underwear, or small urine-loss pads.

Good bladder habits can be developed at any time. Old habits may be hard to break especially when we try to change too many things at once. Start slowly, changing one thing at a time until you become comfortable with your new healthy habits.

Good Luck!

Fig. 6.1 Patient educational handout describing behavioral treatments and lifestyle modifications for urinary incontinence and other urinary symptoms

Diet

Dietary and fluid modifications comprise a large portion of behavioral management of urinary incontinence. Much of the literature surrounding alterations in diet and implications on bladder function use diet as a proxy for weight loss, and this relationship will be further examined in a subsequent section. With regard to specific dietary components and their relationship to stress urinary incontinence, Dallosso et al. [5–7] found that consumption of saturated and monounsaturated fats may increase the risk of stress UI while intake of breads/starches and vegetables may decrease the risk. When looking at specific nutrients, a large epidemiologic study found consumption of both zinc and vitamin B12 was associated with stress incontinence in women [5–7].

Given the identification of estrogen receptors in the urogenital tissues (bladder, urethra, vaginal epithelium, muscles and fascia of the pelvis), the relationship between consumption of food rich in phytoestrogens has been examined with regard to stress UI, overactive bladder (OAB), and lower urinary tract symptoms (LUTS). However, a randomized trial evaluating a diet rich in soy, hypothesized to increase circulating estrogens via phytoestrogens, showed no improvement compared with a control diet in management of overall LUTS or UI [8]. Similarly, Waetjen et al. [9] found no association between the reported dietary intake of three phytoestrogen classes (isoflavones, coumestrol, or lignans) and developing any type of incontinence (stress or urgency) in women transitioning through menopause.

With regard to urinary urgency, frequency, urgency UI and OAB, many of the recommendations surrounding dietary modification involve avoidance of foods that may acidify the urine composition or irritate the bladder, for example, citrus products. In a longitudinal cohort study, Curto et al. [6] found supplemental vitamin C use above recommended daily intake was associated with higher odds of daytime urinary storage symptoms in women, but higher baseline vitamin C intake from foods and beverages was associated with a lower odds of urgency symptoms. Similar results were seen in an observational, population-based, epidemiologic study of 2060 women. In this study, high-dose intake of vitamin C and calcium were positively associated with UI symptoms, whereas vitamin C and β-cryptoxanthin from foods and beverages were inversely associated with voiding symptoms [10]. Overall, these studies suggest that vitamin C supplementation above moderate, absorbable doses (>250 mg/day) may irritate the bladder and should be avoided.

Dallosso et al. [6] reported in a longitudinal study that higher intake of vitamin D ($P = 0.008$), protein ($P = 0.03$), and potassium ($P = 0.05$) was significantly associated with decreased risk of new OAB. These results were not confirmed in a pilot randomized double-blind, placebo-controlled trial of postmenopausal women with urgency UI and vitamin D insufficiency, versus placebo. In this trial, a 43% decrease in urgency UI episodes was seen with 50,000 IU vitamin D3 treatment weekly, but this did not reach statistical significance compared to placebo (where 28% reduction in urgency UI episodes was seen), except in the subset of Black women (who had 63% reduction compared to 23% with placebo) [11]. To further evaluate vitamin D's involvement in the regulation of detrusor muscle contractions, Markland et al. [12] performed an analysis of nearly 73,000 older and middle-aged women in the Nurses' Health Study I and II and found little evidence of a relationship between vitamin D intake and the development of UI. From a macronutrient level, Dallosso et al. [6] found a reduced risk of OAB onset with higher consumption of vegetables, bread, and chicken.

Most of the research findings related to specific dietary components and UI are epidemiologic and represent associations that may not be causal. Thus, it is difficult to make specific dietary recommendations for the treatment and/or prevention of UI and likely best to advise patients to consume a well-balanced diet to promote general health and wellness.

Fluid and Caffeine Management

Perhaps the most widely recommended behavioral modifications for the management of UI and other urinary symptoms focus on fluid and caffeine management. Both the AUA and AUGS/ACOG recommend fluid management as a first-line behavioral modification [2–4]. Recommendations generally emphasize overall management of volume of fluid consumed and avoidance of irritative fluids, in particular, caffeine. Despite these recommendations and consensus among experts about the importance of fluid management, the literature available is varied. For example, when reviewing the Nurses' Health Study cohorts, Townsend et al. [13], found no association between total fluid intake and risk of incident UI (hazard ratio 1.04, 95% CI 0.98–1.10 comparing top versus bottom quintile of fluid intake). In analyses of incontinence type, total fluid intake was not associated with risk of incident stress, urgency, or mixed incontinence.

With regard to stress UI specifically, Dallosso et al. [6], reported that carbonated drinks were a significant risk factor for the onset of stress UI and OAB in a prospective cohort study. A 4-week randomized, prospective, crossover study aimed to determine the effect of caffeine restriction and change in volume of fluid intake on urinary symptoms in women with stress UI. In this trial, Swithinbank et al. [14] determined that decreasing fluid intake reduced incontinence and frequency episodes when comparing the week of decreased fluids with baseline or the week of increased fluids. There was, however, no increase in incontinence episodes when the week of increasing fluids was compared with baseline. The authors concluded that decreasing fluids improved urinary symptoms, and while women must maintain adequate daily fluid intake to avoid dehydration, they should be advised to drink less fluid to improve symptoms as part of conservative treatment [14].

Studies in patients with OAB and urgency UI generally show a positive association between fluid intake and symptoms [15]. Women experience increased frequency and urgency symptoms with fluid increase and decreased frequency and urgency with fluid reductions. With regard to incontinence specifically, results tend to be more mixed, and in general, most patients have a difficult time adhering to fluid protocols [15]. In a systematic review of ten interventional and observational studies, Callan et al. [16] reported reducing fluid intake was beneficial in reducing OAB symptoms. These authors also found that increasing fluid intake was associated with worsening OAB symptoms in observational studies but that no difference in symptoms was seen in interventional studies.

Caffeine, which is consumed more than any other stimulant in the world, has diuretic effects and may also affect the bladder by increasing detrusor pressure and promoting detrusor excitability [17]. A significant body of literature has been published regarding the effect of caffeine intake on urinary symptoms and reduction of caffeine is generally considered part of the behavioral management of UI. In several studies, caffeine reduction was associated with reduced urinary frequency, urgency, and OAB quality-of-life scores [15]. And while there is some conflicting literature, a systematic review by Bradley et al. [15] states, "Overall evidence suggests a weak positive association between caffeine and UI, but there are conflicting results for urinary incontinence types."

The Nurses' Health Studies prospectively investigated the association between total caffeine intake (as determined by food frequency questionnaires) and incidence of UI, including stress, urgency, and mixed UI. Over 4 years of follow-up in 65,176 women, a modest, but significantly increased, risk of weekly incontinence was seen among women with the highest versus lowest caffeine intake (RR 1.19, 95% CI 1.06–1.34, comparing >450 vs. <150 mg/day), as was a significant trend of increasing risk with increasing intake (P for trend = 0.01). Higher daily caffeine intake (roughly equivalent to ≥ 4 cups of coffee or ≥ 10 cups/cans of caffeinated tea or soda per day), but not lower levels, was associated with a modest increased risk of urgency UI in women [18]. When examining the Nurses' Health Studies longitudinally, longer-term caffeine intake was not associated with risk of UI progression over 2 years among women with moderate incontinence [19].

The National Health and Nutrition Examination Survey, a cross-sectional national representative survey, found that caffeine intake in the highest quartile (204 mg/day) was associated with any UI (prevalence odds ratio (POR) 1.47, 95% CI 1.07–2.01), but not moderate/severe UI (POR 1.42, 95% CI 0.98–2.07). Authors concluded moderation of caffeine intake remains a reasonable part of the multicomponent treatment for UI [17]. Similarly, Maserejian et al. [20] found that women who increased coffee intake by at least 2 servings per day compared with categories of decreased or unchanged intake had 64% higher odds of progression of urgency (P = 0.003). Women with recently increased soda intake, particularly caffeinated diet soda, had higher symptom scores, urgency, and LUTS progression. These findings support recommendations to limit caffeinated beverage intake. In a small cystometric study, caffeine intake of 4.5 mg/kg 30 min prior to examination caused diuresis, a lower threshold of sensation during filling, and increased flow rate and voided volume, suggesting caffeine can promote early urgency and frequency [21]. There may be a dose-dependent positive relationship between caffeine intake and OAB [22].

A question which remains is whether general fluid restriction or caffeine restriction specifically is of greater consequence for women with UI. Zimmern et al. [23]

suggested that general fluid management instructions (intake of 50 to 70 ounces of liquid per day) can contribute to the reduction of urgency UI symptoms for women taking anticholinergic medications, but additional individualized instructions along with other behavioral therapies did little to further improve outcomes. Segal et al. [24] found a significant relationship between quartiles of total fluid intake and increasing number of daily voids ($P < 0.001$) and quartiles of caffeinated fluid intake and increasing severity of urgency UI ($P = 0.038$). The type and volume of fluid intake were significantly associated with symptoms of urinary frequency and urgency UI. They concluded consumption of increasing amounts of total fluid was significantly associated with urinary frequency, and intake of large amounts of caffeinated fluids was associated with urgency UI.

Conversely, two small randomized trials did not find a benefit to caffeine restriction over general fluid reductions for UI. A small randomized, crossover study tested caffeine restriction as well as fluid intake changes in women with stress and urgency UI and found changing from caffeinated to decaffeinated beverages had no impact on symptoms, while overall fluid intake reductions resulted in reduced frequency and incontinence episodes [14]. Lastly, Schimpf et al. [25] completed a randomized trail designed to test the common clinical advice of treating OAB by eliminating potentially irritating beverages (those including caffeine, artificial sweeteners, citrus, and alcohol) while keeping volume of intake stable. The authors reported that reduction in intake of potentially irritating beverages did not result in reduced voiding frequency compared to a control group [26]. Urgency symptoms and bother scores were also unchanged. Together, current evidence suggests that reducing potentially irritating beverage intake (including caffeinated beverages) may be less influential than reducing total fluid intake volume for UI and OAB symptoms.

Alcohol and Tobacco

Alcohol consumption has also been examined as a modifiable behavior in the management of UI given its sedative effects, ability to impair mobility, and diuresis [27]. A systematic review published in 2017 reports there is limited information and inconsistent results related to alcohol and urinary symptoms [15]. Whereas alcohol may impact urgency and frequency symptoms among current drinkers, findings are inconsistent by intake level and symptom subtype. No association was found between type of UI and alcohol intake [15].

Tobacco use and its effect on LUTS have also been examined, and smoking cessation remains a recommended behavioral modification for the management of urinary symptoms. Some studies provide evidence of a positive association between tobacco use and stress [28, 29], urgency and mixed incontinence [30], and incontinence of any (unspecified) type [30–32]. Six studies found no association, and one found a negative association between occasional UI and current smoking [15]. Hannested et al. [31] showed mixed results between current, former, and heavy smoking and various measures of incontinence. Former and current smoking was associated with incontinence, but only for those who smoked more than 20 cigarettes per day. Severe incontinence was weakly associated with smoking regardless of number of cigarettes.

Dallosso et al. [6] found a significant association between smoking and risk of OAB with current smokers 1.44 times more likely to develop OAB than nonsmokers. Within the broad category of evidence for OAB or LUTS in general (rather than incontinence specifically), there are some consistent and some inconsistent findings. A small amount of evidence suggests former and/or current smoking is related to frequency in women. Two studies showed a positive association between urgency and current tobacco use [33, 34], while two did not [35, 36]. Maserejian et al. [37] found that women smokers were twice as likely to develop LUTS, particularly storage symptoms (OR = 2.15, 95% CI: 1.30–3.56, $P = 0.003$), compared to never-smokers and recommended smoking cessation.

Single studies showed a positive association between smoking and women's maximum cough spike [28], cough leak point pressure, and maximal intravesical pressure generated by cough [38]. The two studies that examined severe UI showed a positive association [15]. Taken together, research suggests a relationship between tobacco and urinary symptoms may be present. Although not definitive, given the additional health benefits to smoking cessation, it is reasonable to include this among behavioral recommendations for UI.

Timed Voiding

In addition to modification of fluid intake, a common behavioral modification for the management of UI is timed or prompted voiding. The goal of this modification unlike bladder training (described below) is not to increase time between voids, voided volume, or bladder capacity, but rather to encourage regular bladder emptying in order to reduce UI that more often happens at higher bladder volumes [39]. Most evidence related to this practice is for "prompted voiding," a type of timed voiding frequently used in patients with cognitive dysfunction and in assisted-living situations, where a caregiver or family member prompts a patient to void at a regular interval.

In a review of nine trials examining 674 patients (mostly women) comparing prompted voiding to unprompted voiding, there was limited evidence whether either approach had improved incontinence [40]. Authors theorized that an increase in prompted voids decreased incontinent episodes in the short term. In a more recent Cochrane review examining fixed interval or timed voiding for the management of UI in elderly women with reduced cognition and impaired mobility, two trials consisting of 298 women provided insufficient evidence supporting this treatment. However, given the low risk of potential harm and the high likelihood of risk (such as medication side effects) in this population from other treatments, prompted voiding was still deemed a reasonable treatment option [41]. Alternatively,

Holroyd-Leduc et al. [42] reported that several randomized trials examining the role of prompted voiding initiated by a caregiver revealed better outcomes than usual incontinence-related care (including regular checking and changing of wet garments and bedding).

While evidence is lacking, most experts recommend timed or scheduled voiding for patients with urgency UI and OAB, particularly in those who do not report significant frequency, or whose bladder diaries suggest longer voiding intervals or incontinence that regularly occurs just prior to voids.

Bladder Training

Bladder training is a behavioral therapeutic strategy which encourages patients with urgency and frequency symptoms, as well as mixed and stress UI, to gradually increase the amount of time between voids, thereby increasing their bladder capacity and potentially reducing leakage and the sensation of urinary urgency [39]. This technique was first described in 1966, and patients were initially instructed to void at a set interval of every 1–2 h. According to the severity of their symptoms, the interval between voids was increased by half-hour increments until 3.5 h was achieved [43]. Bladder training generally requires intact cognition, highly motivated patients, and a fixed voiding schedule, regardless of a sense of urge to void. Exact training techniques vary between studies, but all involve strategies to increase the time interval between voids progressively. In the protocol for the ESTEEM trial, bladder training was described as a "multicomponent intervention that involved patient education regarding lower urinary tract function, setting incremental voiding schedules, and teaching urge control techniques to postpone voiding and adhere to a schedule" [44].

In 1996, Davies et al. [43] performed an inpatient study of 50 consecutive patients with urinary frequency, urgency, and urgency incontinence. At the time of discharge, they reported that 80% of women were subjectively cured and satisfactorily improved. However, this success deteriorated to 32% in patients who replied to a postal survey 12–29 months later. Echoing the difficulty in maintaining a rigorous voiding schedule, Visco et al. [45] concluded bladder training success in the real world may be substantially lower than described in intensive clinical trials as 55% of study subjects never started bladder training or were noncompliant with treatment. Newman et al. [44] reported that randomized trials using intention-to-treat models show a mean reduction in UI of 60–80% after bladder training. A Cochrane review in 2004 reported that bladder training may help people who are physically and mentally able to use this method, but it may take months to achieve results [46]. Authors tentatively concluded that the limited evidence suggested bladder training may be helpful for the treatment of UI; this recommendation was tempered because the trials had variable quality and small size and thus results were less certain [46].

One study examined changes in urodynamic parameters following bladder training, and no measurable change was identified. Based on this, Elser et al. [47]

concluded the mechanism by which clinical improvement occurs remains unknown. Possible mechanisms for the effectiveness of bladder training include (1) improving central control over bladder sensations and urethral closure and/or (2) changing an individual's behavior in ways that increase the lower urinary system's "reserve capacity" as knowledge of circumstances that cause bladder leakage is gained [44]. Patients with UI, particularly with urgency, often void frequently to avoid this symptom. This behavior can lead to a reduction in functional bladder capacity, which in turn may perpetuate urgency symptoms.

Many investigators have examined bladder training together with other management strategies for the treatment of UI. For example, Mattiasson et al. [48] reported the median percentage reduction in voiding frequency was greater in patients taking tolterodine and performing bladder training than in patients taking tolterodine alone (33% vs 25%, $P < 0.001$). The combined therapy group also had a larger median percentage increase in volume per void (31% vs 20% $P < 0.001$). Wyman et al. [49] examined whether bladder training, pelvic muscle exercises with biofeedback, or combination therapy was more beneficial for the treatment of UI and found combination therapy had the greatest immediate efficacy in management regardless of urodynamic diagnosis. However, at 3 months following treatment, all three interventions had similar results, suggesting the specific treatment may not be as important as a structured intervention program. In a Cochrane review, authors reported there was not enough evidence to determine whether bladder training was useful as a supplement to other therapies [46].

Benefits of voiding strategies, including both timed or prompted voiding and bladder training, include their minimal risk, low cost, and potential efficacy for all UI types (stress, urgency, and mixed). Thus, they remain an ideal first-line therapy and should be considered prior to more invasive and/or costly diagnostic testing or therapeutic measures.

Bowel Management

A common behavioral recommendation for the treatment of UI and other LUTS is the management/regulation of bowel function. The co-occurrence of constipation with urinary symptoms is well established in the pediatric population, called dysfunctional elimination syndrome [50, 51]. In fact, treatment of constipation relieved 90% of daytime incontinence in children and eliminated the recurrence of urinary tract infections [50]. While this link is not as well established in adult women, the literature generally supports the theory that normal bowel function contributes to normal bladder function. In a secondary analysis of 2812 community-dwelling women, Cameron et al. [52] found that women with defecation difficulties had an increased rate of LUTS [52]. Specifically, women with difficult defecation were more likely to experience nocturia (mean 1.8 ± 0.1 vs. 1.3 ± 0.0), urgency (47.6 vs. 29.2%), increased daytime frequency (mean 8.2 ± 0.3 vs. 7.2 ± 0.1), dysuria (22.9% vs. 13.7%), and a sensation of incomplete bladder emptying (55.6% vs. 28.2%).

The exact pathophysiology of the relationship between bladder and bowel function remains somewhat unclear. One proposed mechanism is that delaying fecal evacuation requires contraction of the external anal sphincter and puborectalis until fecal urgency subsides. If this behavior is maintained over time, the rectum becomes overdistended and the pelvic floor musculature hypertonic, which itself contributes to the development of urinary symptoms [53]. Additionally, a full rectum and sigmoid may exert extrinsic pressure on the bladder, decreasing functional capacity or possibly stimulating the stretch receptors of the bladder wall, triggering a detrusor contraction [53, 54]. Finally, it is also possible that signals related to defecation dysfunction occurring in shared neurologic pathways in the spinal cord or pelvic nerves may lead to alterations in the central nervous system regulating bladder function [55]. The theory of a common neurologic pathway impacting function (or dysfunction) in both organs is supported by the success seen in treatment of both bowel and bladder symptoms via sacral nerve stimulation with identical lead placement in the S3 foramina [56].

While further studies are needed to confirm that treatment of bowel symptoms in adult women improves bladder symptoms, these measures remain part of initial treatment recommendations and are certainly not harmful. Most often, this involves recommending a bowel regimen for constipation, such as regular use of stool softeners, fiber supplements, or laxatives, tailored to the individual patient's condition and symptoms. Women with bothersome LUTS should be asked about defecatory symptoms, and these should be addressed concurrently given their likely interrelation.

Exercise

Most evidence related to the use of exercise to manage UI involves exercise programs to achieve weight loss and thus improve incontinence symptoms. However, research also suggests that individuals who describe themselves as less active than others of the same age are more likely to develop stress incontinence, and a low physical activity level has been significantly associated with an increased risk of development of OAB [6]. Alternatively, at the other extreme, women who participate in high-intensity physical activities such as powerlifting or CrossFit may experience higher rates of UI [57–59]. These women report using preventative measures for protection from incontinence during exercise, such as emptying their bladder before workouts, wearing dark-colored pants, and performing Kegel exercises during workouts [59].

The use of pelvic floor muscle exercises for the treatment of UI is reviewed in Chap. 7. However, several studies have examined the performance of a modified Pilates or yoga programs which incorporate pelvic floor strengthening to improve compliance and motivation to complete a pelvic floor exercise regimen. Hein et al. [60], in a 12-week pilot study, proposed that the performance of a pelvic floor strengthening Pilates program may be beneficial given the difficulty to maintain a pelvic floor routine in isolation. They reported improved incontinence scores and high levels of compliance with the program. Similarly, in a pilot randomized trial, Lausen et al. [61] reported benefit in making pelvic floor muscles exercises part of a modified Pilates class to increase motivation in performing these exercises. Lastly, weight training in combination with pelvic floor muscle training provided earlier improvement in UI compared with pelvic floor muscle training alone in a small randomized trial of elderly women with stress UI [62].

In a single-center randomized pilot trial, Huang et al. [63] found that community-dwelling women with UI were successful in implementing a yoga-based intervention through group classes and home practice. Women who completed the 3-month yoga program saw an average of 76% reduction in frequency of incontinence, while women who completed a time-equivalent muscle stretching and strengthening program saw a 56% decrease. They concluded that yoga has the potential to provide community-based management of UI in women, although unclear if this is superior to other physical activity. Despite these promising studies, a recent Cochrane review concluded that the role of yoga or a modified Pilates regimen for the management of UI remains uncertain, as most trials are small and at high risk of bias [64].

Weight Loss

Obesity is a serious public health concern with implications on many aspects of a woman's life, including continence. Obesity is a well-established risk factor for the onset of stress UI [6]. In fact, across adult life, higher body mass index (BMI) for women is linked with symptoms of stress and severe incontinence. Women who are overweight or obese since their early adult life have more than double the risk of severe incontinence [65]. It is therefore important to encourage women to maintain a normal weight at all ages both as a means of preventing the development of incontinence and as a means of management of incontinence after it presents.

The association between obesity and urgency UI is not as well-understood, but the mechanism of action linking obesity and stress UI is likely the positive relationship between BMI and abdominal circumference and several urodynamic measures. Richter et al. [66] demonstrated incremental increases in intra-abdominal pressure and intravesical pressure with increasing BMI or abdominal circumference in an overweight and obese cohort with stress UI. With increasing weight women appear to move closer to their continence threshold during stress events. Fuganti et al. [38] demonstrated that obese women had higher maximal intravesical peak pressures with cough, compared to women with lower BMI. These studies suggest that weight loss may reduce incontinence by reducing intravesical pressures during cough and other activities.

The impact of weight loss on UI was demonstrated in the landmark Program to Reduce Incontinence by Diet and Exercise (PRIDE) trial [66]. In PRIDE, overweight and obese women with at least ten UI episodes per week were randomized to a 6-month weight loss program or to a structured education program. At 6 months, the intervention group had a mean weight loss of 8% (7.8 kg) and experienced a 47% decrease in mean weekly incontinence episodes, as compared with the control group who had a weight loss of 1.6% (1.5 kg) and a 28% reduction of incontinence episodes ($P = 0.01$). The intervention group also had a greater reduction in frequency of stress UI episodes, but not urgency incontinence episodes, compared to the control group. The authors concluded that behavioral weight loss intervention reduced the frequency of self-reported UI episodes among overweight and obese women [67].

The link between weight loss and improvement in UI was maintained in the PRIDE study population through 18-month follow-up [67]. At 12 months, the intervention group reported a greater percent reduction in weekly stress UI episodes (65% vs 47%, $P < 0.001$), and a greater proportion achieved at least a 70% decrease in weekly total and stress UI episodes compared to baseline. At 18-months, a greater proportion of women in the intervention group had more than 70% improvement in urgency incontinence episodes as well, but the differences between the groups for improvement in stress and total UI episodes were not significant. The authors concluded weight loss intervention reduced both the frequency of stress incontinence episodes through 12 months and improvement in patient satisfaction with regard to incontinence through 18 months [68].

While falling outside of the realm of behavioral modifications, weight loss that is the result of bariatric surgery has also proven to improve UI in obese women. Several studies have supported that weight loss after bariatric surgery improved clinically significant UI [69–71], and this improvement appears to be maintained from 1 to 5 years following bariatric surgery [72, 73].

The AUGS Systematic Review Group studied the impact of weight loss intervention on LUTS and UI in overweight and obese women [74]. They identified high-certainty evidence that behavioral weight loss decreases the prevalence of stress UI 15% to 18% and overall UI 12% to 17% at 1 to 2.9 years. This improvement is seen after a 5% to 10% reduction in body weight with further weight loss having minimal additional benefit. The certainty of evidence on the long-term impact of these interventions was lower: the effect seems to diminish over time, which may be attributable to weight re-gain. The certainty of the evidence was moderate to low regarding the benefit of behavioral weight loss on urgency UI and OAB symptoms. No randomized trials evaluated the impact of surgical weight loss on urinary symptoms, and the level of evidence on this matter was low [74].

Absorbent Products and Skin Protection

For women who continue to experience UI despite treatment, absorbent products and skin protection are important to maintain quality of life and avoid incontinence-associated dermatitis. About 9% of the annual cost of incontinence treatment is for absorbent products [75, 76], and 87% of community-living women 60 years and older use pads to manage their incontinence [77]. These products need to be dependable and inconspicuous [77, 78]. Women obtain information about such products from many sources but most ultimately resort to a trial-and-error approach to product selection. Thus, healthcare providers should provide information about absorbent products during their assessment of incontinence [79].

Women who experience mild UI can select from four main designs of absorbent products: disposable insert pads, disposable menstrual pads, washable undergarments with an integral pad, and washable inserts [80]. A Cochrane review found limited data comparing these products but concluded based on one eligible study that for leakage prevention, overall acceptability, and preference, disposable inserts are better than menstrual pads, which are better than washable undergarments with integral pads, which are better than washable inserts. There was no clear difference with regard to skin health between washable or disposable options. Most women prefer disposable pads, but these are often the more expensive option [80].

Women who experience moderate to heavy incontinence, based on a Cochrane review with two eligible trials, may benefit most from disposable "pull-up" style products, despite the expense. Disposable inserts are a cheaper alternative but may not provide as much protection. Again, no particular design seemed better or worse for skin health. Ultimately, women have different options and preferences for absorbent product design and using a combination of options may be most suitable and cost-effective [81].

Consideration should also be given to cleaning, moisturizing, and protecting the vulvar and perineal skin for incontinent women. Incontinence-associated dermatitis, ranging from redness, swelling, oozing, crusting, and scaling changes to loss of skin integrity, occurs when urine (or stool) is in contact with the skin [39]. Secondary infections may occur, such as topical candidiasis. To avoid such complications, a skin care regimen should be recommended for patients with incontinence. A skin care regimen involves cleansing after each incontinence episode with a perineal cleanser (not bar or hand soap), moisturizing (with glycerine, lanolin, or mineraloil), and application of a moisture barrier (e.g. petrolatum, lanolin, zinc oxide) to shield against irritants and moisture [39].

Limited studies have examined skin care products for the prevention of incontinence-associated dermatitis in adults [82]. In a review by Pather et al. [83], the authors concluded skin care regimens that include the use of a topical barrier product are beneficial in preventing and treating dermatitis related to UI, but there was no evidence to indicate superior outcomes from any specific product. Another systematic review suggested that perineal skin cleansers may be effective at preventing incontinence-associated dermatitis and maintaining skin barrier function compared to traditional soap and water [84]. Regardless of the limited evidence, a regimen to clean, moisturize, and protect vulvar and perineal skin for women who experience incontinence is an important aspect of incontinence care.

Conclusion

A wide variety of behavioral and lifestyle modifications are recommended as initial treatments for women with UI. The evidence base supporting these recommendations is overall weak and largely observational in nature, with few randomized trials contributing to this area.

References

1. Burgio KL. Behavioral therapy to enable women with urge incontinence to discontinue drug treatment: a randomized trial. Ann Intern Med. 2008;149:161.
2. Lightner DJ, Gomelsky A, Souter L, Vasavada SP. Diagnosis and treatment of overactive bladder (non-neurogenic) in adults: AUA/SUFU guideline amendment 2019. J Urol. 2019;202:558–63.
3. Kobashi KC, Albo ME, Dmochowski RR, et al. Surgical treatment of female stress urinary incontinence: AUA/SUFU guideline. J Urol. 2017;198:875–83.
4. ACOG practice bulletin no. 155: urinary incontinence in women. Obstet Gynecol. 2015;126:e66–81.
5. Dallosso HM, McGrother CW, Matthews RJ, Donaldson MMK, The Leicestershire MRC Incontinence Study Group. Nutrient composition of the diet and the development of overactive bladder: a longitudinal study in women. Neurourol Urodyn. 2004;23:204–10.
6. Dallosso HM, McGrother CW, Matthews RJ, Donaldson MMK, the Leicestershire MRC Incontinence Study Group. The association of diet and other lifestyle factors with overactive bladder and stress incontinence: a longitudinal study in women. BJU Int. 2003;92:69–77.
7. The Leicestershire MRC Incontinence Study Group, Dallosso H, Matthews R, McGrother C, Donaldson M. Diet as a risk factor for the development of stress urinary incontinence: a longitudinal study in women. Eur J Clin Nutr. 2004;58:920–6.
8. Manonai J, Songchitsomboon S, Chanda K, Hong JH, Komindr S. The effect of a soy-rich diet on urogenital atrophy: a randomized, cross-over trial. Maturitas. 2006;54:135–40.
9. Waetjen LE, Leung K, Crawford SL, Huang M-H, Gold EB, Greendale GA. Relationship between dietary phytoestrogens and development of urinary incontinence in midlife women. Menopause. 2013;20(4):428–36.
10. Maserejian NN, Giovannucci EL, McVary KT, McKinlay JB. Intakes of vitamins and minerals in relation to urinary incontinence, voiding, and storage symptoms in women: a cross-sectional analysis from the Boston Area Community Health Survey. Eur Urol. 2011;59:1039–47.
11. Markland AD, Tangpricha V, Mark Beasley T, Vaughan CP, Richter HE, Burgio KL, Goode PS. Comparing vitamin D supplementation versus placebo for urgency urinary incontinence: a pilot study. J Am Geriatr Soc. 2019;67:570–5.
12. Markland AD, Vaughan C, Huang A, Tangpricha V, Grodstein F. Vitamin D intake and the 10-year risk of urgency urinary incontinence in women. J Steroid Biochem Mol Biol. 2020;199:105601.
13. Townsend MK, Jura YH, Curhan GC, Resnick NM, Grodstein F. Fluid intake and risk of stress, urgency, and mixed urinary incontinence. Am J Obstet Gynecol. 2011;205:73.e1–6.
14. Swithinbank L, Hashim H, Abrams P. The effect of fluid intake on urinary symptoms in women. J Urol. 2005;174:187–9.
15. Bradley CS, Erickson BA, Messersmith EE, et al. Evidence of the impact of diet, fluid intake, caffeine, alcohol and tobacco on lower urinary tract symptoms: a systematic review. J Urol. 2017;198:1010–20.

16. Callan L, Thompson DL, Netsch D. Does increasing or decreasing the daily intake of water/ fluid by adults affect overactive bladder symptoms? J Wound Ostomy Continence Nurs. 2015;42:614–20.
17. Gleason JL, Richter HE, Redden DT, Goode PS, Burgio KL, Markland AD. Caffeine and urinary incontinence in US women. Int Urogynecol J. 2013;24:295–302.
18. Jura YH, Townsend MK, Curhan GC, Resnick NM, Grodstein F. Caffeine intake, and the risk of stress, urgency and mixed urinary incontinence. J Urol. 2011;185:1775–80.
19. Townsend MK, Resnick NM, Grodstein F. Caffeine intake and risk of urinary incontinence progression among women. Obstet Gynecol. 2012;119:950–7.
20. Maserejian NN, Wager CG, Giovannucci EL, Curto TM, McVary KT, McKinlay JB. Intake of caffeinated, carbonated, or citrus beverage types and development of lower urinary tract symptoms in men and women. Am J Epidemiol. 2013;177:1399–410.
21. Lohsiriwat S, Hirunsai M, Chaiyaprasithi B. Effect of caffeine on bladder function in patients with overactive bladder symptoms. Urol Ann. 2011;3:14.
22. Selo-Ojeme D, Pathak S, Aziz A, Odumosu M. Fluid and caffeine intake and urinary symptoms in the UK. Int J Gynecol Obstet. 2013;122:159–60.
23. Zimmern P, Litman HJ, Mueller E, Norton P, Goode P. Effect of fluid management on fluid intake and urge incontinence in a trial for overactive bladder in women. BJU Int. 2009;105:1680–5.
24. Segal S, Saks EK, Arya LA. Self-assessment of fluid intake behavior in women with urinary incontinence. J Women's Health. 2011;20:1917–21.
25. Schimpf MO, Smith AR, Miller JM. Fluids affecting bladder urgency and lower urinary symptoms (FABULUS): methods and protocol for a randomized controlled trial. Int Urogynecol J. 2020;31:1033–40.
26. Schimpf MO, Smith AR, Hawthorne K, Garcia C, Miller JM. Fluids affecting bladder urgency and lower urinary symptoms (FABULUS): results from a randomized controlled trial. Female Pelvic Med Reconstr Surg. 2020;26((105)Supplement 1):S5.
27. Karram MM, Walters MD, Elsevier (Amsterdam). Urogynecology and reconstructive pelvic surgery. Philadelphia: Elsevier/Saunders; 2015.
28. Bump RC, McClish DK. Cigarette smoking and urinary incontinence in women. Am J Obstet Gynecol. 1992;167:1213–8.
29. Richter HE, Burgio KL, Brubaker L, et al. Factors associated with incontinence frequency in a surgical cohort of stress incontinent women. Am J Obstet Gynecol. 2005;193:2088–93.
30. Tampakoudis P, Tantanassis T, Grimbizis G, Papaletsos M, Mantalenakis S. Cigarette smoking and urinary incontinence in women—a new calculative method of estimating the exposure to smoke. Eur J Obstet Gynecol Reprod Biol. 1995;63:27–30.
31. Hannestad YS, Rortveit G, Daltveit AK, Hunskaar S. Are smoking and other lifestyle factors associated with female urinary incontinence? The Norwegian EPINCONT Study. BJOG Int J Obstet Gynaecol. 2003;110:247–54.
32. Danforth KN, Townsend MK, Lifford K, Curhan GC, Resnick NM, Grodstein F. Risk factors for urinary incontinence among middle-aged women. Am J Obstet Gynecol. 2006;194:339–45.
33. Tähtinen RM, Auvinen A, Cartwright R, Johnson TM, Tammela TLJ, Tikkinen KAO. Smoking and bladder symptoms in women. Obstet Gynecol. 2011;118:643–8.
34. Nuotio M, Jylhä M, Koivisto A-M, TLJ T. Association of smoking with urgency in older people. Eur Urol. 2001;40:206–12.
35. Aydin Y, Hassa H, Oge T, Yalcin OT, Mutlu FŞ. Frequency and determinants of urogenital symptoms in postmenopausal Islamic women. Menopause. 2014;21:182–7.
36. de Boer TA, Slieker-ten Hove MCP, Burger CW, Vierhout ME. The prevalence and risk factors of overactive bladder symptoms and its relation to pelvic organ prolapse symptoms in a general female population. Int Urogynecol J. 2011;22:569–75.
37. Maserejian NN, Kupelian V, Miyasato G, McVary KT, McKinlay JB. Are physical activity, smoking and alcohol consumption associated with lower urinary tract symptoms in men or women? Results from a population based observational study. J Urol. 2012;188:490–5.

38. Fuganti PE, Gowdy JM, Santiago NC. Obesity and smoking: are they modulators of cough intravesical peak pressure in stress urinary incontinence? Int Braz J Urol. 2011;37:528–33.
39. Cameron AP, Jimbo M, Heidelbaugh JJ. Diagnosis and office-based treatment of urinary incontinence in adults. Part two: treatment. Ther Adv Urol. 2013;5:189–200.
40. Eustice S, Roe B, Paterson J. Prompted voiding for the management of urinary incontinence in adults. Cochrane Database Syst Rev. 2000; https://doi.org/10.1002/14651858.CD002113
41. Ostaszkiewicz J, Johnston L, Roe B. Timed voiding for the management of urinary incontinence in adults. In: The Cochrane Collaboration, editor. Cochrane Database Syst. Rev. Chichester: Wiley; 2000. p. CD002802.
42. Holroyd-Leduc JM, Straus SE. Management of urinary incontinence in women: scientific review. JAMA. 2004;291:986.
43. Davies JA, Hosker G, Lord J, Smith ARB. An evaluation of the efficacy of in-patient bladder retraining. Int Urogynecol J. 2000;11:271–6.
44. Newman DK, Borello-France D, Sung VW. Structured behavioral treatment research protocol for women with mixed urinary incontinence and overactive bladder symptoms. Neurourol Urodyn. 2018;37:14–26.
45. Visco AG, Weidner AC, Cundiff GW, Bump RC. Observed patient compliance with a structured outpatient bladder retraining program. Am J Obstet Gynecol. 1999;181:1392–4.
46. Wallace SA, Roe B, Williams K, Palmer M. Bladder training for urinary incontinence in adults. Cochrane Database Syst Rev. 2004; https://doi.org/10.1002/14651858.CD001308.pub2
47. Elser DM, Wyman JF, McClish DK, Robinson D, Fantl JA, Bump RC. The effect of bladder training, pelvic floor muscle training, or combination training on urodynamic parameters in women with urinary incontinence. Continence Program for Women Research Group. Neurourol Urodyn. 1999;18:427–36.
48. Mattiasson A, Blaakaer J, Høye K, Wein AJ, The Tolterodine Scandinavian Study Group. Simplified bladder training augments the effectiveness of tolterodine in patients with an overactive bladder. BJU Int. 2003;91:54–60.
49. Wyman JF, Fantl JA, McClish DK, Bump RC. Comparative efficacy of behavioral interventions in the management of female urinary incontinence. Continence Program for Women Research Group. Am J Obstet Gynecol. 1998;179:999–1007.
50. Loening-Baucke V. Urinary incontinence and urinary tract infection and their resolution with treatment of chronic constipation of childhood. Pediatrics. 1997;100:228–32.
51. Feng WC, Churchill BM. Dysfunctional elimination syndrome in children without obvious spinal cord diseases. Pediatr Clin N Am. 2001;48:1489–504.
52. Cameron A, Fenner DE, DeLancey JOL, Morgan DM. Self-report of difficult defecation is associated with overactive bladder symptoms: difficult defecation in OAB. Neurourol Urodyn. 2010;29:1290–4.
53. Franco I. Overactive bladder in children. Part 2: management. J Urol. 2007;178:769–74; discussion 774
54. Fernandes E, Vernier R, Gonzalez R. The unstable bladder in children. J Pediatr. 1991;118:831–7.
55. Warne SA, Godley ML, Wilcox DT. Surgical reconstruction of cloacal malformation can alter bladder function: a comparative study with anorectal anomalies. J Urol. 2004;172:2377–81; discussion 2381
56. Jarrett MED. Neuromodulation for constipation and fecal incontinence. Urol Clin North Am. 2005;32:79–87.
57. Hagovska M, Švihra J, Buková A, Dračková D, Horbacz A. The impact of different intensities of exercise on body weight reduction and overactive bladder symptoms- randomised trial. Eur J Obstet Gynecol Reprod Biol. 2019;242:144–9.
58. Wikander L, Cross D, Gahreman DE. Prevalence of urinary incontinence in women powerlifters: a pilot study. Int Urogynecol J. 2019;30:2031–9.

59. Yang J, Cheng JW, Wagner H, Lohman E, Yang SH, Krishingner GA, Trofimova A, Alsyouf M, Staack A. The effect of high impact crossfit exercises on stress urinary incontinence in physically active women. Neurourol Urodyn. 2019;38:749–56.

60. Hein JT, Rieck TM, Dunfee HA, Johnson DP, Ferguson JA, Rhodes DJ. Effect of a 12-week pilates pelvic floor-strengthening program on short-term measures of stress urinary incontinence in women: a pilot study. J Altern Complement Med. 2020;26:158–61.

61. Lausen A, Marsland L, Head S, Jackson J, Lausen B. Modified Pilates as an adjunct to standard physiotherapy care for urinary incontinence: a mixed methods pilot for a randomised controlled trial. BMC Womens Health. 2018;18:16.

62. Virtuoso JF, Menezes EC, Mazo GZ. Effect of weight training with pelvic floor muscle training in elderly women with urinary incontinence. Res Q Exerc Sport. 2019;90:141–50.

63. Huang AJ, Chesney M, Lisha N, Vittinghoff E, Schembri M, Pawlowsky S, Hsu A, Subak L. A group-based yoga program for urinary incontinence in ambulatory women: feasibility, tolerability, and change in incontinence frequency over 3 months in a single-center randomized trial. Am J Obstet Gynecol. 2019;220:87.e1–87.e13.

64. Wieland LS, Shrestha N, Lassi ZS, Panda S, Chiaramonte D, Skoetz N. Yoga for treating urinary incontinence in women. Cochrane Database Syst Rev. 2019; https://doi.org/10.1002/14651858. CD012668.pub2

65. Mishra GD, Hardy R, Cardozo L, Kuh D. Body weight through adult life and risk of urinary incontinence in middle-aged women: results from a British prospective cohort. Int J Obes. 2008;32:1415–22.

66. Richter HE, Creasman JM, Myers DL, Wheeler TL, Burgio KL, Subak LL, for the Program to Reduce Incontinence by Diet and Exercise (PRIDE) Research Group. Urodynamic characterization of obese women with urinary incontinence undergoing a weight loss program: the Program to Reduce Incontinence by Diet and Exercise (PRIDE) trial. Int Urogynecol J. 2008;19:1653–8.

67. Subak LL, Wing R, West DS, et al. Weight loss to treat urinary incontinence in overweight and obese women. N Engl J Med. 2009;360:481–90.

68. Wing RR, West DS, Grady D, et al. Effect of weight loss on urinary incontinence in overweight and obese women: results at 12 and 18 months. J Urol. 2010;184:1005–10.

69. Ait Said K, Leroux Y, Menahem B, Doerfler A, Alves A, Tillou X. Effect of bariatric surgery on urinary and fecal incontinence: prospective analysis with 1-year follow-up. Surg Obes Relat Dis. 2017;13:305–12.

70. O'Boyle CJ, O'Sullivan OE, Shabana H, Boyce M, O'Reilly BA. The effect of bariatric surgery on urinary incontinence in women. Obes Surg. 2016;26:1471–8.

71. Whitcomb EL, Horgan S, Donohue MC, Lukacz ES. Impact of surgically induced weight loss on pelvic floor disorders. Int Urogynecol J. 2012;23:1111–6.

72. Anglim B, O'Boyle CJ, O'Sullivan OE, O'Reilly BA. The long-term effects of bariatric surgery on female urinary incontinence. Eur J Obstet Gynecol Reprod Biol. 2018;231:15–8.

73. Gabriel I, Tavakkoli A, Minassian VA. Pelvic organ prolapse and urinary incontinence in women after bariatric surgery: 5-year follow-up. Female Pelvic Med Reconstr Surg. 2018;24:120–5.

74. Yazdany T, Jakus-Waldman S, Jeppson PC, et al. American Urogynecologic Society systematic review: the impact of weight loss intervention on lower urinary tract symptoms and urinary incontinence in overweight and obese women. Female Pelvic Med Reconstr Surg. 2020;26:16–29.

75. Hu T-W, Wagner TH, Bentkover JD, Leblanc K, Zhou SZ, Hunt T. Costs of urinary incontinence and overactive bladder in the United States: a comparative study. Urology. 2004;63:461–5.

76. Wilson L. Annual direct cost of urinary incontinence. Obstet Gynecol. 2001;98:398–406.

77. Fader M, Bliss D, Cottenden A, Moore K, Norton C. Continence products: research priorities to improve the lives of people with urinary and/or fecal leakage. Neurourol Urodyn. 2010;29:640–4.

78. Teunissen TAM, Lagro-Janssen ALM. Sex differences in the use of absorbent (incontinence) pads in independently living elderly people: do men receive less care? Int J Clin Pract. 2009;63:869–73.
79. Smith N, Hunter KF, Rajabali S, Milsom I, Wagg A. Where do women with urinary incontinence find information about absorbent products and how useful do they find it? J Wound Ostomy Continence Nurs. 2019;46:44–50.
80. Fader M, Cottenden AM, Getliffe K. Absorbent products for light urinary incontinence in women. Cochrane Database Syst Rev. 2007; https://doi.org/10.1002/14651858. CD001406.pub2
81. Fader M, Cottenden AM, Getliffe K. Absorbent products for moderate-heavy urinary and/or faecal incontinence in women and men. Cochrane Database Syst Rev. 2008; https://doi.org/10.1002/14651858.CD007408
82. Beeckman D, Van Damme N, Schoonhoven L, et al. Interventions for preventing and treating incontinence-associated dermatitis in adults. Cochrane Database Syst Rev. 2016; https://doi.org/10.1002/14651858.CD011627.pub2
83. Pather P, Hines S, Kynoch K, Coyer F. Effectiveness of topical skin products in the treatment and prevention of incontinence-associated dermatitis: a systematic review. JBI Database Syst Rev Implement Rep. 2017;15:1473–96.
84. Lachance CC, Argaez C. Perineal skin cleansers for adults with urine incontinence in long-term care or hospital settings: a review of the clinical effectiveness and guidelines. Ottawa: Canadian Agency for Drugs and Technologies in Health; 2019.

Chapter 7
Physical Therapy and Continence Inserts

Paige De Rosa, Ilana Bergelson, and Elizabeth Takacs

Introduction

Urinary incontinence (UI) has a reported prevalence of 25–45% in women [1], increasing incidence as a woman ages, during pregnancy, and postpartum, and has a significant impact on quality of life. Pelvic floor muscle training (PFMT) and other conservative treatments such as pessaries have often been underutilized or believed to be ineffective. PFMT was first described in 1936 by Margaret Morris in Britain but became more widespread after Arthur Kegel presented successful treatment of 64 patients in 1948 [2]. Kegel exercises are, essentially, a form of PFMT As originally described, correct isolation and contraction of the pelvic floor was confirmed by a perineometer; however, over time, Kegels evolved into a home treatment regimen without confirmation of correct contraction and with resultant often incorrect performance of the exercises and thus deemed ineffective [3]. Preventative measures and conservative treatment regimens for urinary incontinence are similar to other medical conditions in that they require both motivated patients and providers. Providers must take the time to educate patients on the different options and ensure the correct performance of PFME if being utilized. Supervised training requires a physical therapist with specialized training and certification in pelvic floor therapy, and this may be a challenge, for instance, in rural areas. Further, patients must be willing to accept that results are not immediate, and the therapies

Supplementary Information The online version of this chapter (https://doi.org/10.1007/978-3-030-84352-6_7) contains supplementary material, which is available to authorized users.

P. De Rosa · I. Bergelson · E. Takacs (✉)
Department of Urology, University of Iowa, Iowa City, IA, USA
e-mail: elizabeth-takacs@uiowa.edu

need to be continued to maintain their effect. In addition to the barriers to utilization, there is no substantiative research showing the effectiveness and outcomes of the conservative measures as either preventative or therapeutic. Consistent across meta-analyses and systematic reviews is the conclusion that no recommendations can be provided given the heterogenous nature of trial designs and interventions in the otherwise sparse literature.

Primary Prevention of Incontinence

Most research on urinary incontinence has focused on treatment, often surgical or procedural intervention. This has resulted in a purposeful paradigm shift in UI research with a conscientious focus on the prevention of UI and promotion of continence [4]. Within this paradigm, a key is understanding both risk factors and protective factors at different levels in social ecology [5]. A multilevel prevention model has been outlined for both individual and population-based outcomes that incorporates education, identification of cases, intervention, embedded change, and outcome measures [4]. A review of the 6th International Consultation on Incontinence (ICI) Primary Prevention of UI concluded that, to date, there is limited data for interventions focused on prevention except for older adult women and pregnant and postpartum women [4].

Prevention of UI in Older Women

It is well established that UI prevalence increases as the population ages. Several studies have focused on preventative interventions for women over age 55 including in the areas of general education about pelvic floor disorders including incontinence [6], development of a tool for identification of at-risk individuals [7], and impact of both group and individual education of behavioral training [8, 9]. Based on these and other studies, the ICI concluded that there is Level 1 evidence supporting that a Grade A recommendation of education designed for older women should be provided [4].

UI Prevention During Pregnancy and Postpartum

During pregnancy, the prevalence of UI ranges from 18.6% to 75% increasing with gestational age [10]. In the multilevel prevention model, identification risk factors are essential to understanding who is at risk for the development of incontinence, and interventions could be targeted to at-risk populations or events that increase risk. Modifiable risk factors for the development of UI during pregnancy and postpartum can be categorized by maternal and prenatal risk factors, intrapartum and fetal factors, and type of birth. Commonly identified risk factors include maternal age, increased body mass index, smoking, and UI prior to pregnancy [10, 11], weight gain during pregnancy [10], and gestational DM [10]. The 6th ICI provided Grade B recommendation to stop smoking, achieve a normal postpartum body weight, and avoid constipation during pregnancy [4]. Data is less clear and conflicting on associating intrapartum factors like perineal laceration/episiotomy, prolonged second stage, and high neonatal birth weight and UI [11]. Mode of delivery, specifically vaginal versus elective cesarean section, remains a controversial topic and is beyond the scope of this chapter.

Furthermore, pelvic floor muscle strength, prior SUI, newborn weight, and new-onset SUI during pregnancy have been identified as risk factors for postpartum UI [12]. Prior SUI and new-onset SUI are directly related to pelvic floor muscle strength and may be a target for intervention to prevent UI from developing. The overarching goal of PFME to improve support and minimize risk is to increase PFM strength to the bladder, bladder neck, and urethra [10, 12]. Both the 2020 Cochrane Database Systematic Review and the 6th ICI concluded that there is sufficient evidence to support the use of structured PFMT in early pregnancy for continent women as a way to prevent onset of UI late in pregnancy and postpartum [4, 13] and PFM exercises should be provided to all pregnant women [4].

Vaginal and Urethral Devices

Conservative management for stress urinary incontinence includes the use of intravaginal devices such as pessaries. While pessaries have often been used for pelvic organ prolapse (POP), there are several types of pessaries that can be used for SUI. Pessaries can be thought of as support pessaries with a central opening versus space-occupying pessaries, which have a solid or perforated design. Support pessaries such as the Mar-land pessary, incontinence dish (Fig. 7.1), or ring pessary with or without support knob may adequately treat stress urinary incontinence. Pessary devices for SUI stabilize the urethra by elevating the bladder neck and compressing the urethra against the pubic symphysis and minimizing urethral hypermobility [14, 15]. This has been demonstrated by magnetic resonance imaging (MRI) images during Valsalva and demonstrated increased urethral length while the posterior urethro-vesical angles were decreased [16]. Urodynamic studies (UDS) with a pessary in place have demonstrated increase in detrusor pressure with a decrease in maximal flow rate and suggest indicting that pessaries increase urethral resistance [15].

Pessaries are not a one-size-fits-all, and improvement in symptoms, satisfaction, and continued use of a pessary are dependent on successful pessary fitting [15]. It is important that an individualized approach is taken for pessary fittings as discomfort, bleeding, and repeated expulsions are common reasons for discontinuation [17]. Pessaries are a low-cost, low-risk, nonsurgical option that can be offered to almost

Fig. 7.1 (**a**) MILEX incontinence dish with and without support. (**b**) Poise® Impressa® bladder support. (**c**) Uresta® bladder support

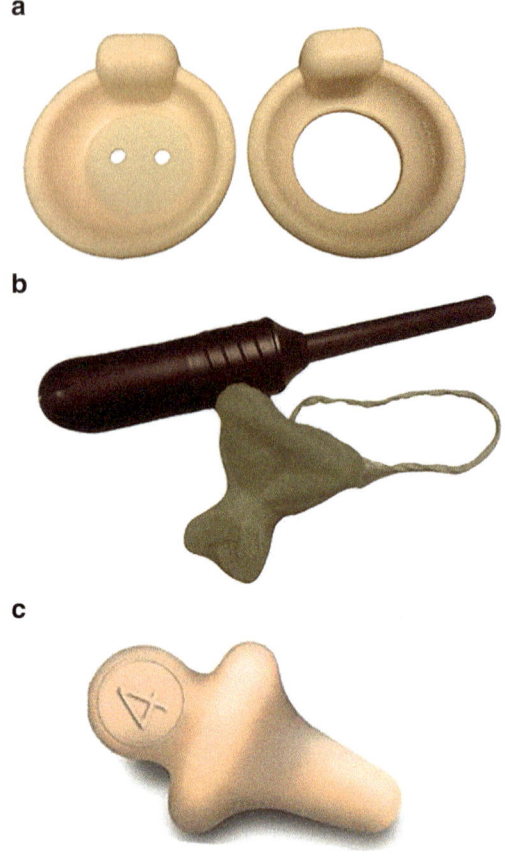

all patients. Specific contraindications to use include patients with active pelvic or vaginal infection, severe ulceration, allergy to silicone or rubber, and patients who will likely not return for appropriate follow-up [15]. Use of vaginal estrogen is recommended for postmenopausal women who are candidates. It has been demonstrated that those that use vaginal estrogen cream are more likely to continue the use of the pessary with less discharge, but it is not protective from erosions [18]. Minor complications of pessary use include changes in vaginal discharge and odor, spontaneous expulsion, voiding difficulty, and vaginal epithelial erosion [14, 15]. Severe complications include bleeding, severe vaginal discharge, constipation, pain, impaction, fibrosis, and erosion into adjacent organs, which are more often associated with longer duration of use (6–10 years), pessaries utilized for POP, or forgotten or neglected pessaries. Outcomes demonstrate that greater than 50% of women using pessaries for incontinence will be satisfied with their symptomatic improvement [17, 19, 20]. When comparted behavioral therapy, which includes supervised PFMT, there was no difference between pessary and behavioral therapy groups at 3 and 12 months [19, 20]. Higher failure rates of pessaries have been associated with prior incontinence surgery [17].

Limitations to the use of pessaries have been identified as the lack of knowledge on pessary fitting and patient difficulty correctly positioning and inserting the device. Uresta is a medical-grade, rubber bell-shaped pessary specifically for SUI that is inserted into the vaginal canal to provide urethral support at the bladder neck [21]. It is inserted by holding the handle and directing the tapered portion (with lubricant if necessary) into the vagina (Fig. 7.1). The patient determines the appropriate size by purchasing the starter kit and tries progressively larger sizes. The correct size is the one that does not cause discomfort, that provides reduction or resolution of SUI symptoms, and with which she experiences no difficulty in urination or defecation (https://www.uresta.com/pages/support). Reasons for discontinuing of Uresta are similar to other pessaries including inadequate symptom control and expulsion of the device, which may be attributed to the inappropriate fit of the pessary [21]. Studies have not documented other adverse events or significant discomfort noted by the patients [21, 22]. (https://myuresta.com/wp-content/uploads/2019/08/023099-Uresta-IFU-NA-2018-PRF.pdf). Outcome studies are limited to a single prospective study and single in-office assessment with pad test. In the first study, 66% of patients with SUI or SUI predominate MUI who were successfully fitted for the device and followed prospectively, significant reduction in all types of UI was noted, and 76% continued to use the device at 1 year [21]. The second study, an office pad test, was performed with Uresta or a placebo vaginal silastic ring with 50% or greater reduction in pad weight after placement of the Uresta in comparison to the placebo [22]. Longer-term studies or studies with larger patient populations are not available.

Impressa is another vaginal insert for incontinence. This device has an applicator that is similar to a tampon that is used to place a nylon mesh-covered resin core (Fig. 7.1). The Impressa applicator is placed within the vaginal canal and, once the core is deployed, provides sub-urethral support in a tension-free manner with a string is attached to the distal end and grasped for removal [23]. Like Uresta, the Impressa patient purchases a sizing kit in which the appropriate size is based on comfort and reduction or resolution of leakage. Risks of the device include vaginal spotting, vaginal pain, vaginal and urinary tract infections, and possible toxic shock syndrome. The device is recommended to be in place no more than 12 h per day (https://www.poise.com/-/media/poise/files/poise-impressa-instructions-for-use.pdf). In the literature, it was noted that urinary flow rates and post-void residuals did not differ significantly with device usage. The most common side effects are discomfort, pain, and spotting [23]. In limited short-term studies, women using Impressa achieved >/= 70% pad weight gain reduction, and only 8% reported feeling incontinent at the conclusion of the 28-day study period [23]. In addition, mean quality-of-life scores and other questionnaire data demonstrated significant improvement [24].

Of historical note, the urethral insert FemSoft had also been utilized for female stress urinary incontinence. This device involved a tube with a bulbous tip inserted into the urethra with a balloon that filled with mineral oil to stay in place. While studies had found that there were statistically significant reductions in pad weights and episodes of incontinence, adverse events included urinary tract infections, trauma from insertion, and even migration of device with the need for cystoscopy for device retrieval. This device has since been discontinued by the manufacturer [25].

Pelvic Floor Muscle Therapy

Pelvic floor muscle therapy (PFMT) with the goal to increase the strength of the pelvic floor has become an essential component of the treatment approach for patients with stress urinary incontinence (SUI), urgency urinary incontinence (UUI), and mixed urinary incontinence (MUI), but strengthening exercise programs are contraindicated in patients with pelvic floor muscle dysfunction, high-tone pelvic floor, or pelvic pain. In 2010, the 4th International Consultation on incontinence made the following recommendations: initial treatment of UI should include appropriate lifestyle advice, physical therapy, scheduled voiding regimens, behavioral therapies, and medications. Specifically, Grade A recommendation was provided for supervised PFT for women with SUI and supervised bladder training for OAB.

One of the greatest challenges with PFMT is that there is significant variability in how often and in what form patients receive education and assessment, techniques, tools and devices used to assist training, and the exercise programs themselves. The frequency at which nonpregnant patients receive instruction on PFMT is variable estimated to be between 42% and 73% with verbal or written instruction occurring most often and physical exam instruction occurring only 7–28% of the time [26, 27]. Pregnant or postpartum patients are aware of the importance of PFME; however, most education is through verbal or written instructions, and few receive physical exam instruction [28, 29]. There is variability in the ability of women to perform correct contractions. In a digital assessment of antenatal women, 66% were unable to perform an appropriate contraction at baseline [30], and in women over the age of 55 or greater, 23–60% of women were able to generate a squeeze Oxford Scale 3 or higher, 8–16% were not able to perform a contraction, 9–44% used accessory muscles, and 6–12% performed a Valsalva [26, 27]. Therefore, it is important as a first step to ensure that the patients are able to identify the appropriate pelvic floor muscles and perform contractions correctly by digital palpation [31].

Assessment of Pelvic Floor Contraction

Vaginal digital palpation is commonly used for the assessment of pelvic floor muscle strength. It is inexpensive, and due to its minimally invasive nature, it is well tolerated for patients and easy to incorporate into routine pelvic examination, and no special equipment is required. Three common assessment scales have been developed and used for assessment of the pelvic floor: the modified oxford scale

Table 7.1 Comparison of the common assessment scales for pelvic floor contraction

Modified Oxford Scale[a]	Brink Scale[b]	PERFECT Scheme[c]
Pressure	*Pressure*	**P** *Pressure/power*
0 – No response	1 – No response/cannot perceive squeeze	0 – No response
1 – Flicker	2 – Weak squeeze/felt as flick	1 – Flicker
2 – Weak squeeze	3 – Moderate squeeze/felt all around the finger	2 – Weak squeeze
3 – Moderate squeeze	4 – Strong squeeze/full finger compression	3 – Moderate squeeze
4 – Good squeeze		4 – Good squeeze
5 – Strong squeeze		5 – Strong squeeze
	Displacement	**E** *Endurance*
	1 – None	How long can they hold max voluntary contraction (Up to 10 s)
	2 – Fingertips move anteriorly	
	3 – Whole length of fingers more anterior	
	4 – Whole fingers move anteriorly	
	Duration	**R** *Repetitions*
	None	How many maximum volume contractions the patient can hold with a rest between (max to 10 reps)
	≥1 s and ≤3 s	
	> 3 s	
		F *Fast contractions* The number of 1 s maximum volume contractions patient can perform in a row (max of 10 contractions)
		ECT Every contraction timed

[a]Schüssler et al. [32]
[b]Brady et al. [5]
[c]Laycock and Jerwood [34]

(MOS) [32], Brink scale [33], and PERFECT Scheme [34] (Table 7.1). The MOS assessment is completed by single digital palpation of the vagina with squeeze, and strength of squeeze is rated on a scale of 0 (no squeeze) to 5 (strong). Several authors have reported that the MOS has only fair to moderate inter-rater reliability [31, 35, 36]. The Brink Scale reports the assessment of three components of the contraction, pressure, duration, and displacement of the vertical plane, and a total score [33]. Assessment is performed by two-finger palpation with the index finger resting on the middle finger in the anteroposterior plane [34]. All components of the Brink scale have demonstrated good interrater reliability with the lowest correlation in the squeeze duration [33, 37, 38] and good test-retest reliability [33]. When compared to perineometer maximum pressure squeeze, the Brink total score and pressure score have moderate correlation (0.67–0.71) [37]. In contrast to the MOS and the Brink scale, the PERFECT Scheme was designed to assess both fast- and slow-twitch fibers of the pelvic floor muscles. In this assessment model, power (or pressure), endurance, repetition, and fast contractions are assessed using single finger palpation vaginally in women or rectally in men [34].

Perineometery and ultrasound are additional tools used in the assessment of pelvic floor muscle strength. The perineometer is a vaginal manometer that can measure the pressure of vaginal squeeze, resting pressure, and endurance [30]. Manometry has demonstrated high inter-rater and intra-rater reliability [36, 37] and is more often used for research purposes than in clinical practice. Transabdominal ultrasound imaging is currently used predominately in the research setting; however, with the increase in availability, it is an emerging technology in clinic practice. US enables assessment of the squeeze and lift through visualization of the patient's posterior bladder wall elevation [39]; however, it cannot assess strength.

Education on Pelvic Floor Muscle Contraction

The second key element to the successful implementation of PFME and PFMT is educating women on how to perform pelvic floor exercises correctly through written and verbal communication with or without palpation, midstream interruption, or use of tools and devices in biofeedback. Historically education has been provided to patients in class settings, videos, and paper. The TULIP project demonstrated that there was no difference between groups educated via a 2-h class or a 20-min video for urgency and incontinence [40]. As information technology and the Internet have progressed, there has been increased interest in the use of web-based or mobile application for education on PFME. A series of studies were performed to assess the impact of education materials that included information on SUI, PFMT exercises, a tutorial on the Knack maneuver, exercises with graphics, and a three-times-a-day exercise program in women with self-reported SUI. Internet-based education materials were as effective as mailed materials with both groups reporting significant improvement in symptoms and conditions, specific quality-of-life questions, and being sustained at 2 years [41, 42]; these findings were similar when the educational materials were provided to all women regardless of the diagnosis of SUI [43]. The web-based educational material from the above studies is now a mobile app called Tät(®), which also includes reminders. Assessment of the impact of the app demonstrated that it was effective in improving participants' QOL and symptom severity and increased compliance [44]. The acceptance of web-based pelvic floor treatment programs has also been supported by a second independent study [45]. It has been identified that women who reported improvements had high treatment expectations, weight control, and self-rated improvement in muscle strength [46].

Teaching correct contraction is important for outcomes in all types of incontinence. Incorrect contraction includes those who are not able to generate any contraction, use of accessory muscles, or Valsalva effort. A correct contraction consists of a squeeze around the vaginal opening followed by an inward and cranial lift [30], and on exam vaginal muscles should be pulled upward and inward without the use of accessory muscles including abdominal and gluteal muscles [27]. Qualitative research with a focus group of physiotherapists and one continence nurse identified that training-specific cues and verbal prompts are unique in pelvic floor therapy and communication skills need to indicate understanding and safety to the patient. Most participants agreed that there is a need for an "information bank" of cues and verbal prompts and that cues may require different language for men and women [47]. One study identified that patients most often responded with a correct squeeze to "squeeze your vaginal muscles you use to hold your urine" and the direction of "lift your vaginal muscles inward and upward" least often elicited the correct squeeze [27]. Table 7.2 lists verbal cues that may be useful in helping your patients elicit a correct contraction.

The midstream interruption technique has been used to help women verify that they are engaging the correct pelvic floor muscles and to perform PFME correctly [26]. In this technique, women are instructed to stop the flow of urine while voiding. A recent study demonstrated that stopping the stream sequentially during voiding resulted in statistically higher PVR (36.7 m vs 8.2 ml) and less efficient micturition with lower maximum flow rate (17.8 ml/min vs 26.9 ml/min), and the authors concluded this should not be used in the current practice of PFMT [48]. There are hypothetical concerns that when performed regularly, interrupting the urine stream may be interrupting the normal micturition cycle with the potential to promote voiding dysfunction, which has led this technique to be used less frequently. It has been recommended that women not routinely interrupt their urine stream when performing PFME [48, 49].

Though vaginal palpation is classically used to evaluate and teach appropriate contractions, biofeedback has emerged as an adjunct and/or alternative method. In the broadest sense, biofeedback can be both cognitive visualization or more commonly considered use of various tools, computer analysis, and physical visual imagery to assist in the identification and correct performance of the desired exercises. The use of biofeedback and specifically the techniques used depend on the physical therapist. Though small individual studies have demonstrated superior strength of pelvic floor muscles and outcomes in incontinence [50, 51], a 2019 meta-analysis of RCTs for the use of biofeedback with PFMT concluded that biofeedback did not offer therapeutic benefits overall [52].

Outcomes

There are numerous methods in which patients can perform PFME and PFMT including supervised or unsupervised settings, group versus individual therapy, and use of adjuncts like electrical stimulation and biofeedback. Data available on the success of unsupervised programs is conflicting. Early studies suggested that unsupervised treatment programs were inferior to supervised programs when assessing by pad test, diaries, questionnaires, and subjectively reported improvements with low satisfaction in outcomes for the nontreatment groups [53–56]. More recent publications that confirm the appropriate performance of PFME prior to the start of treatment have demonstrated improvement in outcomes measures in patients performing home regimens [57, 58]. This emphasizes the importance of patients

Table 7.2 Cues[a]

Generic cues	Female-specific cues
Verbal cues:	*Verbal cues:*
"Squeeze and lift"	"Squeeze and lift"
"Squeeze and lift your pelvic floor"	"Lift your vaginal muscles inward and
"Think of close and lift, so you're drawing	upward"
your tailbone up to the pubic bone"	"What you sit on, between your anus and
Imagery cues:	vagina, imagine your saddle is drawing up
"So elevator.... going up the lift"	inside"
"Imagine you're stopping yourself from	"Swing the tailbone forward to stop a wee
passing water as a cue that I think helps	and close the vagina"
most people"	"If you're sitting, lift away from the chair,
"Imagine you're in a crowded elevator,	squeeze and lift away from the chair and then
you've got some wind and you're trying to	let go and sink down into it, once if they're
hold it in because you don't want anyone to	sitting"
hear or smell what you're about to let go."	"Sucking up through a straw so it's a longer,
"Think of the ocean, or thinking about	slower contraction"
seeing that wave come in and then feeling it	"Squeeze the vaginal muscles you use to
go and releasing out and moving away"	hold your gas or air"
"Using the description of a clock face,	"Squeeze the vaginal muscles you use to
imagine 12's at the top, six is where your	hold your urine"
tail bone is, three and nine are the sides, and	*Digital cues:*
if you imagine you're sitting at a certain	"Can you feel my finger? Can you imagine
sized clock now and draw all those numbers	there's a tampon there?"
together and draw it up inside, and then you	"Can you feel my finger? Can you push/pull
take it down you're trying to get people to	against my finger?"
relax, so starting with a wristwatch and let	"Okay squeeze here" as palpating internally
those numbers drift out to a wall clock."	"Squeeze the muscles of your vagina around
"Pulling a straw up inside, pull everything	my fingers"
up and in"	*Imagery cues:*
"Plane taking off often if you want some	"Imagine a cotton ball sitting on the
more forward movement"	underwear and trying to lift up the cotton
	ball off and hold it inside and let it go, so
	very gentle, very soft references or peeling it
	away from the underwear"
	"Imagine you're trying to lift the vagina
	away from your underwear"
	"Imagine a lift going up, a lift coming down"
	"Imagine you're drawing a pea up and
	through the vagina toward your head."
	"Imagine that you're drawing that tampon
	further in"
	"Imagine someone is trying to pull on
	tampon string, and you're trying to resist
	against it"
	"That idea of having something inside and
	drawing it up"

[a]Slade et al. [47]

undergoing unsupervised programs to be able to correctly perform PFME. For sustained improvement in symptoms, patients will need to continue to perform PFMT even after the completion of supervised programs highlighting PFMT requires commitment from patients [59].

PFMT appears to be equally effective in reducing symptom severity when administered in individual therapy (IT) sessions or group therapy (GT) sessions [60–62] and may be potentially more cost-effective [61]. There has been some variation in the reported literature about differences in objective assessments. Figueiredo et al. reported improved PFM function in those that received at least some component of IT compared to those that received only GT [62]. In contrast, de Oliveira et al. did not demonstrate differences in PFM strength or pad test between IT and GT [60].

When considering the outcomes of PFMT, even if patients do not have a significant improvement in pelvic floor muscle strength, they still may have improvement in quality of life [57]. Specific recommendations of the International Consultation on Incontinence are outlined in Table 7.3.

Counterbracing and Urge Suppression

Counterbracing or "the Knack maneuver" consists of timing a pelvic muscle contraction with the moment of expected leakage. Originally described in 1986 by Burgio et al., the Knack is a purposeful contraction of the pelvic floor muscles before and during stress maneuvers [63, 64]. It has been demonstrated to displace the bladder neck and decrease mobility during cough [65]. The knack has been shown to decrease leakage 71–98.2% with 18.8% eliminating leakage all together [64, 66, 67]. Behavioral modification and bladder retraining are mainstays of conservative treatment for urinary urgency incontinence. In bladder training, patients are instructed on lower urinary tract function, setting incremental voiding schedules, and urge suppression techniques or the "freeze and squeeze"(Supplementary Fig. 7.1). PFMT is important in bladder retraining to promote urge suppression and minimize leaking [68]. It has been demonstrated that contraction of the PFM increases intraurethral pressures, decreases detrusor pressure, and suppresses the micturition reflex [69]. Based on currently available published studies, there is evidence that PFMT may reduce OAB symptoms and UUI; however, due to heterogeneity in studies, it is possible to clearly determine the effect [70].

Creating Individualized Programs

Patients entering PFMT programs are going to have different baseline knowledge, skills, and expectations. It is critical to recognize these differences and understand the patient's perspective to develop a training program individualized to the

Table 7.3 Recommendations of the 5th International Consultation on Incontinence[a]

	Grade of recommendation	Recommendation
PFMT		
Continent primiparas – prevention of UI	A	Should be offered a supervised, high-intensity strengthening antepartum program to prevent postpartum UI
Treatment of UI > 3 months postpartum	A	Offered as 1st line conservative therapy
	B	Intensive PFMT is likely to increase effect of treatment
Prevention AND treatment in childbearing women	B	Consider cost/benefit or population-based approaches to health professionals taught antepartum or postpartum PFMT
UI – general	A	Offered as 1st line conservative therapy for SUI, UUI, or MUI. Provide the most intensive PFMT program possible
	A	Supervised and taught by trained health professionals are better than self-directed programs
Biofeedback-assisted PFMT		
Clinic biofeedback	A	No clear benefit
	B	No clear benefit
Vaginal weighted cones		
SUI	B	Training sessions supervised by trained health professionals can be 1st line for women who are able and prepared to use VWC
Bladder training		
UI – general	A	May be an appropriate 1st line therapy
UUI or MUI	B	Effective 1st line conservative therapies
SUI	B	PFMT is better than BT
DO, or UUI	B	BT or anticholinergic drugs may be effective

[a]Dumoulin et al. [76]
PFMT pelvic floor muscle training, *UI* urinary incontinence, *SUI* stress urinary incontinence, *UUI* urge urinary incontinence, *MUI* mixed urinary incontinence, *DO* detrusor overactivity, *BT* bladder training, *VWC* vaginal weighted cones

patient, and for that reason, the utility of generic management is limited [47]. Effective education can occur through traditional classroom environment, written material, videos, and web-based programs, and mobile apps. Training can take place in individualized or in group settings, but the assessment of the patient's ability to perform pelvic floor muscle contraction and corrective direction is essential. Adjuncts with supervision, biofeedback, and other devices may be necessary to help patients correctly perform exercises. Providing exercise regimens is further compounded by the literature, and due to the lack of standardized protocols across studies, it is challenging to form conclusions on what is most effective [34]; however, we do provide a general strengthening regimen in Supplementary Fig. 7.2. After assessment and confirmation of correct pelvic floor squeeze, the provider can use the general strengthening regimen to set starting parameters and goals for the patient. If, however, a patient cannot correctly perform a contraction in the office, referral to a physical therapist should be considered prior to abandoning PFMT as an option. Patients undergoing supervised PFMT with a physical therapist will have individually directed home programs based on repetitive reassessments.

Conclusion

UI has a tremendous economic burden on both the health care system and patients, and with the aging population, the economic impact will only continue to increase. In 2007, the total burden (including lost work productivity) from OAB alone was $65.9 billion with an estimated $82.6 billion in 2020 [5]. With the rising cost of healthcare and economic burden of UI, it is important to continue to consider non-surgical intervention. Cost-analysis studies have demonstrated that based on willingness to pay, surgical intervention is the most cost-effective for those with high monetary thresholds, but for the lowest willingness to pay threshold, the pessary is the most cost-effective [71]. Within the gamut of nonsurgical intervention, PFMT appears to have the greatest monetary benefit [72], and for surgical failures, conservative management should be considered [73]. The success of conservative, nonsurgical treatment options for UI is dependent on patient selection. It has been identified that menopause, higher education, no prior incontinence procedure, and lower frequency of leakage were predictors for success with nonsurgical interventions in SUI [74] and that long-term success is greater for older patients and those that perform the PFMT regularly [75]. These factors may need to be considered when offering nonsurgical interventions to patients.

References

1. Altman D, Cartwright R, Lapitan MC, Milsom I, Nelson R, Sjöström S, Tikkinen KAO. Epidemiology of urinary incontinence (UI) and other lower urinary tract symptoms (LUTS), pelvic organ prolapse (POP) and anal incontinence (AI). In: Abrams P, Cardozo L, Wagg A, Wein A, editors. Incontinence: 6th international consultation on incontinence, Tokyo, September 2016. Bristol: International Continence Society; 2017. p. 1–141.
2. Price N, Dawood R, Jackson SR. Pelvic floor exercise for urinary incontinence: a systematic literature review. Maturitas. 2010;67(4):309–15.
3. Lamin E, Parrillo LM, Newman DK, Smith AL. Pelvic floor muscle training: underutilization in the USA. Curr Urol Rep. 2016;17(2):10.
4. Palmer MH, Cockerell R, Griebling TL, Rantell A, van Houten P, Newman DK. Review of the 6th international consultation on incontinence: primary prevention of urinary incontinence. Neurourol Urodyn. 2020;39(1):66–72.
5. Brady SS, Bavendam TG, Berry A, Fok CS, Gahagan S, Goode PS, et al. The Prevention of Lower Urinary Tract Symptoms (PLUS) in girls and women: developing a conceptual framework for a prevention research agenda. Neurourol Urodyn. 2018;37(8):2951–64.

6. Geoffrion R, Robert M, Ross S, van Heerden D, Neustaedter G, Tang S, et al. Evaluating patient learning after an educational program for women with incontinence and pelvic organ prolapse. Int Urogynecol J Pelvic Floor Dysfunct. 2009;20(10):1243–52.
7. Diokno AC, Ogunyemi T, Siadat MR, Arslanturk S, Killinger KA. Continence Index: a new screening questionnaire to predict the probability of future incontinence in older women in the community. Int Urol Nephrol. 2015;47(7):1091–7.
8. Diokno AC, Newman DK, Low LK, Griebling TL, Maddens ME, Goode PS, et al. Effect of group-administered behavioral treatment on urinary incontinence in older women: a randomized clinical trial. JAMA Intern Med. 2018;178(10):1333–41.
9. Tannenbaum C, Agnew R, Benedetti A, Thomas D, van den Heuvel E. Effectiveness of continence promotion for older women via community organisations: a cluster randomised trial. BMJ Open. 2013;3(12):e004135.
10. Sangsawang B. Risk factors for the development of stress urinary incontinence during pregnancy in primigravidae: a review of the literature. Eur J Obstet Gynecol Reprod Biol. 2014;178:27–34.
11. Kissler K, Yount SM, Rendeiro M, Zeidenstein L. Primary prevention of urinary incontinence: a case study of prenatal and intrapartum interventions. J Midwifery Womens Health. 2016;61(4):507–11.
12. Baracho SM, Barbosa da Silva L, Baracho E, Lopes da Silva Filho A, Sampaio RF, Mello de Figueiredo E. Pelvic floor muscle strength predicts stress urinary incontinence in primiparous women after vaginal delivery. Int Urogynecol J. 2012;23(7):899–906.
13. Woodley SJ, Lawrenson P, Boyle R, Cody JD, Mørkved S, Kernohan A, et al. Pelvic floor muscle training for preventing and treating urinary and faecal incontinence in antenatal and postnatal women. Cochrane Database Syst Rev. 2020;5(5):CD007471.
14. Jones KA, Harmanli O. Pessary use in pelvic organ prolapse and urinary incontinence. Rev Obstet Gynecol. 2010;3(1):3–9.
15. Al-Shaikh G, Syed S, Osman S, Bogis A, Al-Badr A. Pessary use in stress urinary incontinence: a review of advantages, complications, patient satisfaction, and quality of life. Int J Women's Health. 2018;10:195–201.
16. Komesu YM, Ketai LH, Rogers RG, Eberhardt SC, Pohl J. Restoration of continence by pessaries: magnetic resonance imaging assessment of mechanism of action. Am J Obstet Gynecol. 2008;198(5):563 e1–6.
17. Farrell SA, Singh B, Aldakhil L. Continence pessaries in the management of urinary incontinence in women. J Obstet Gynaecol Can. 2004;26(2):113–7.
18. Dessie SG, Armstrong K, Modest AM, Hacker MR, Hota LS. Effect of vaginal estrogen on pessary use. Int Urogynecol J. 2016;27(9):1423–9.
19. Richter HE, Burgio KL, Brubaker L, Nygaard IE, Ye W, Weidner A, et al. Continence pessary compared with behavioral therapy or combined therapy for stress incontinence: a randomized controlled trial. Obstet Gynecol. 2010;115(3):609–17.
20. Kenton K, Barber M, Wang L, Hsu Y, Rahn D, Whitcomb E, et al. Pelvic floor symptoms improve similarly after pessary and behavioral treatment for stress incontinence. Female Pelvic Med Reconstr Surg. 2012;18(2):118–21.
21. Farrell SA, Baydock S, Amir B, Fanning C. Effectiveness of a new self-positioning pessary for the management of urinary incontinence in women. Am J Obstet Gynecol. 2007;196(5):474 e1–8.
22. Lovatsis D, Best C, Diamond P. Short-term Uresta efficacy (SURE) study: a randomized controlled trial of the Uresta continence device. Int Urogynecol J. 2017;28(1):147–50.
23. Ziv E, Stanton SL, Abarbanel J. Efficacy and safety of a novel disposable intravaginal device for treating stress urinary incontinence. Am J Obstet Gynecol. 2008;198(5):594 e1–7.
24. Ziv E, Stanton SL, Abarbanel J. Significant improvement in the quality of life in women treated with a novel disposable intravaginal device for stress urinary incontinence. Int Urogynecol J Pelvic Floor Dysfunct. 2009;20(6):651–8.

25. Sirls LT, Foote JE, Kaufman JM, Lightner DJ, Miller JL, Moseley WG, et al. Long-term results of the FemSoft urethral insert for the management of female stress urinary incontinence. Int Urogynecol J Pelvic Floor Dysfunct. 2002;13(2):88–95; discussion
26. Moen MD, Noone MB, Vassallo BJ, Elser DM, Urogynecology N. Pelvic floor muscle function in women presenting with pelvic floor disorders. Int Urogynecol J Pelvic Floor Dysfunct. 2009;20(7):843–6.
27. Kandadai P, O'Dell K, Saini J. Correct performance of pelvic muscle exercises in women reporting prior knowledge. Female Pelvic Med Reconstr Surg. 2015;21(3):135–40.
28. Ismail SI. An audit of NICE guidelines on antenatal pelvic floor exercises. Int Urogynecol J Pelvic Floor Dysfunct. 2009;20(12):1417–22.
29. Fine P, Burgio K, Borello-France D, Richter H, Whitehead W, Weber A, et al. Teaching and practicing of pelvic floor muscle exercises in primiparous women during pregnancy and the postpartum period. Am J Obstet Gynecol. 2007;197(1):107 e1–5.
30. Ahlund S, Nordgren B, Wilander EL, Wiklund I, Friden C. Is home-based pelvic floor muscle training effective in treatment of urinary incontinence after birth in primiparous women? A randomized controlled trial. Acta Obstet Gynecol Scand. 2013;92(8):909–15.
31. Bo K, Finckenhagen HB. Vaginal palpation of pelvic floor muscle strength: inter-test reproducibility and comparison between palpation and vaginal squeeze pressure. Acta Obstet Gynecol Scand. 2001;80(10):883–7.
32. Schüssler B, Laycock J, Hesse U, Hilton P, Kölbl H, Debus-Thiede G, et al. Evaluation of the pelvic floor. In: Schüssler B, Laycock J, Norton PA, Stanton SL, editors. Pelvic floor re-education. London: Springer; 1994.
33. Brink CA, Wells TJ, Sampselle CM, Taillie ER, Mayer R. A digital test for pelvic muscle strength in women with urinary incontinence. Nurs Res. 1994;43(6):352–6.
34. Laycock J, Jerwood D. Pelvic floor muscle assessment: the PERFECT scheme. Physiotherapy. 2001;87(12):631–42.
35. Ferreira CH, Barbosa PB, de Oliveira SF, Antonio FI, Franco MM, Bo K. Inter-rater reliability study of the modified Oxford Grading Scale and the Peritron manometer. Physiotherapy. 2011;97(2):132–8.
36. Navarro Brazalez B, Torres Lacomba M, de la Villa P, Sanchez Sanchez B, Prieto Gomez V, Asunsolo Del Barco A, et al. The evaluation of pelvic floor muscle strength in women with pelvic floor dysfunction: a reliability and correlation study. Neurourol Urodyn. 2018;37(1):269–77.
37. Hundley AF, Wu JM, Visco AG. A comparison of perineometer to brink score for assessment of pelvic floor muscle strength. Am J Obstet Gynecol. 2005;192(5):1583–91.
38. Boyles SH, Edwards SR, Gregory WT, Denman MA, Clark AL. Validating a clinical measure of levator hiatus size. Am J Obstet Gynecol. 2007;196(2):174 e1–4.
39. Sherburn M, Murphy CA, Carroll S, Allen TJ, Galea MP. Investigation of transabdominal real-time ultrasound to visualise the muscles of the pelvic floor. Aust J Physiother. 2005;51(3):167–70.
40. Sampselle CM, Newman DK, Miller JM, Kirk K, DiCamillo MA, Wagner TH, et al. A randomized controlled trial to compare 2 scalable interventions for lower urinary tract symptom prevention: main outcomes of the TULIP study. J Urol. 2017;197(6):1480–6.
41. Sjostrom M, Umefjord G, Stenlund H, Carlbring P, Andersson G, Samuelsson E. Internet-based treatment of stress urinary incontinence: a randomised controlled study with focus on pelvic floor muscle training. BJU Int. 2013;112(3):362–72.
42. Sjostrom M, Umefjord G, Stenlund H, Carlbring P, Andersson G, Samuelsson E. Internet-based treatment of stress urinary incontinence: 1- and 2-year results of a randomized controlled trial with a focus on pelvic floor muscle training. BJU Int. 2015;116(6):955–64.
43. Bokne K, Sjostrom M, Samuelsson E. Self-management of stress urinary incontinence: effectiveness of two treatment programmes focused on pelvic floor muscle training, one booklet and one internet-based. Scand J Prim Health Care. 2019;37(3):380–7.

44. Asklund I, Nystrom E, Sjostrom M, Umefjord G, Stenlund H, Samuelsson E. Mobile app for treatment of stress urinary incontinence: a randomized controlled trial. Neurourol Urodyn. 2017;36(5):1369–76.
45. Barbato KA, Wiebe JW, Cline TW, Hellier SD. Web-based treatment for women with stress urinary incontinence. Urol Nurs. 2014;34(5):252–7.
46. Nystrom E, Asklund I, Sjostrom M, Stenlund H, Samuelsson E. Treatment of stress urinary incontinence with a mobile app: factors associated with success. Int Urogynecol J. 2018;29(9):1325–33.
47. Slade SC, Hay-Smith J, Mastwyk S, Morris ME, Frawley H. Strategies to assist uptake of pelvic floor muscle training for people with urinary incontinence: a clinician viewpoint. Neurourol Urodyn. 2018;37(8):2658–68.
48. Chesnel C, Charlanes A, Tan E, Turmel N, Breton FL, Ismael SS, et al. Influence of the urine stream interruption exercise on micturition. Int J Urol. 2019;26(11):1059–63.
49. Lukacz ES, Santiago-Lastra Y, Albo ME, Brubaker L. Urinary incontinence in women: a review. JAMA. 2017;318(16):1592–604.
50. Bertotto A, Schvartzman R, Uchoa S, Wender MCO. Effect of electromyographic biofeedback as an add-on to pelvic floor muscle exercises on neuromuscular outcomes and quality of life in postmenopausal women with stress urinary incontinence: a randomized controlled trial. Neurourol Urodyn. 2017;36(8):2142–7.
51. Aksac B, Aki S, Karan A, Yalcin O, Isikoglu M, Eskiyurt N. Biofeedback and pelvic floor exercises for the rehabilitation of urinary stress incontinence. Gynecol Obstet Investig. 2003;56(1):23–7.
52. Nunes EFC, Sampaio LMM, Biasotto-Gonzalez DA, Nagano R, Lucareli PRG, Politti F. Biofeedback for pelvic floor muscle training in women with stress urinary incontinence: a systematic review with meta-analysis. Physiotherapy. 2019;105(1):10–23.
53. Felicissimo MF, Carneiro MM, Saleme CS, Pinto RZ, da Fonseca AM, da Silva-Filho AL. Intensive supervised versus unsupervised pelvic floor muscle training for the treatment of stress urinary incontinence: a randomized comparative trial. Int Urogynecol J. 2010;21(7):835–40.
54. Wong KS, Fung BKY, Fung LCW, Ma S. Pelvic floor exercises in the treatment of stress urinary incontinence in Hong Kong Chinese women. September 1997; Yokohama Japan. In: Proceedings of the 27 Annual Meeting of the International Continence Society; 1997. p. 23–6.
55. Sugaya K, Owan T, Hatano T, Nishijima S, Miyazato M, Mukouyama H, et al. Device to promote pelvic floor muscle training for stress incontinence. Int J Urol. 2003;10(8):416–22.
56. Zanetti MR, Castro Rde A, Rotta AL, Santos PD, Sartori M, Girao MJ. Impact of supervised physiotherapeutic pelvic floor exercises for treating female stress urinary incontinence. Sao Paulo Med J. 2007;125(5):265–9.
57. Al Belushi ZI, Al Kiyumi MH, Al-Mazrui AA, Jaju S, Alrawahi AH, Al Mahrezi AM. Effects of home-based pelvic floor muscle training on decreasing symptoms of stress urinary incontinence and improving the quality of life of urban adult Omani women: a randomized controlled single-blind study. Neurourol Urodyn. 2020;39(5):1557–66.
58. Cavkaytar S, Kokanali MK, Topcu HO, Aksakal OS, Doganay M. Effect of home-based Kegel exercises on quality of life in women with stress and mixed urinary incontinence. J Obstet Gynaecol. 2015;35(4):407–10.
59. Kruger AP, Luz SC, Virtuoso JF. Home exercises for pelvic floor in continent women one year after physical therapy treatment for urinary incontinence: an observational study. Rev Bras Fisioter. 2011;15(5):351–6.
60. de Oliveira CF, Rodrigues AM, Arruda RM, Ferreira Sartori MG, Girao MJ, Castro RA. Pelvic floor muscle training in female stress urinary incontinence: comparison between group training and individual treatment using PERFECT assessment scheme. Int Urogynecol J Pelvic Floor Dysfunct. 2009;20(12):1455–62.

61. Lamb SE, Pepper J, Lall R, Jorstad-Stein EC, Clark MD, Hill L, et al. Group treatments for sensitive health care problems: a randomised controlled trial of group versus individual physiotherapy sessions for female urinary incontinence. BMC Womens Health. 2009;9:26.
62. Figueiredo VB, Nascimento SL, Martinez RFL, Lima CTS, Ferreira CHJ, Driusso P. Effects of individual pelvic floor muscle training vs individual training progressing to group training vs group training alone in women with stress urinary incontinence: a randomized clinical trial. Neurourol Urodyn. 2020;39(5):1447–55.
63. Burgio KL, Robinson JC, Engel BT. The role of biofeedback in Kegel exercise training for stress urinary incontinence. Am J Obstet Gynecol. 1986;154(1):58–64.
64. Miller JM, Ashton-Miller JA, DeLancey JO. A pelvic muscle precontraction can reduce cough-related urine loss in selected women with mild SUI. J Am Geriatr Soc. 1998;46(7):870–4.
65. Miller JM, Perucchini D, Carchidi LT, DeLancey JO, Ashton-Miller J. Pelvic floor muscle contraction during a cough and decreased vesical neck mobility. Obstet Gynecol. 2001;97(2):255–60.
66. Miller JM, Sampselle C, Ashton-Miller J, Hong GR, DeLancey JO. Clarification and confirmation of the Knack maneuver: the effect of volitional pelvic floor muscle contraction to preempt expected stress incontinence. Int Urogynecol J Pelvic Floor Dysfunct. 2008;19(6):773–82.
67. Miller JM, Hawthorne KM, Park L, Tolbert M, Bies K, Garcia C, et al. Self-perceived improvement in bladder health after viewing a novel tutorial on knack use: a randomized controlled trial pilot study. J Womens Health (Larchmt). 2020;29(10):1319–27.
68. Burgio KL. Update on behavioral and physical therapies for incontinence and overactive bladder: the role of pelvic floor muscle training. Curr Urol Rep. 2013;14(5):457–64.
69. Shafik A, Shafik IA. Overactive bladder inhibition in response to pelvic floor muscle exercises. World J Urol. 2003;20(6):374–7.
70. Bo K, Fernandes A, Duarte TB, Brito LGO, Ferreira CHJ. Is pelvic floor muscle training effective for symptoms of overactive bladder in women? A systematic review. Physiotherapy. 2020;106:65–76.
71. Von Bargen E, Patterson D. Cost utility of the treatment of stress urinary incontinence. Female Pelvic Med Reconstr Surg. 2015;21(3):150–3.
72. Simpson AN, Garbens A, Dossa F, Coyte PC, Baxter NN, McDermott CD. A cost-utility analysis of nonsurgical treatments for stress urinary incontinence in women. Female Pelvic Med Reconstr Surg. 2019;25(1):49–55.
73. Kavanagh A, Sanaee M, Carlson KV, Bailly GG. Management of patients with stress urinary incontinence after failed midurethral sling. Can Urol Assoc J. 2017;11(6Suppl2):S143–S6.
74. Schaffer J, Nager CW, Xiang F, Borello-France D, Bradley CS, Wu JM, et al. Predictors of success and satisfaction of nonsurgical therapy for stress urinary incontinence. Obstet Gynecol. 2012;120(1):91–7.
75. Lindh A, Sjostrom M, Stenlund H, Samuelsson E. Non-face-to-face treatment of stress urinary incontinence: predictors of success after 1 year. Int Urogynecol J. 2016;27(12):1857–65.
76. Dumoulin C, Hunter KF, Moore K, Bradley CS, Burgio KL, Hagen S, Imamura M, Thakar R, Williams K, Chambers T. Conservative management for female urinary incontinence and pelvic organ prolapse review 2013: Summary of the fifth International Consultation on Incontinence. Neurourol Urodyn. 2016;35(1):15–20. https://doi.org/10.1002/nau.22677. Epub 2014 Nov 15. PMID: 25400065.

Part III
Medical and Surgical Treatment of UUI

Chapter 8
Medical Therapy with Antimuscarinics and ß3-Agonists

Sophia Delpe Goodridge and Leslie M. Rickey

Introduction

Overactive bladder (OAB) is a benign lower urinary tract condition which affects between 10% and 17% of the population with an increase in prevalence as patients age [1, 2]. In North America alone, OAB conditions impact 34 million people and are associated with a large economic burden. In the United States, it is estimated that $12 billion annually is spent on the management of overactive bladder [3]. Non-life-threatening lower urinary tract dysfunction can be debilitating with consequential impacts on quality of life including impaired mobility, decreased domestic and work-related productivity, social isolation, sleep disturbance, depression, and impaired sexual function [4–6]. Though the overall prevalence among men and women is similar, women report greater severity of symptoms and experience a higher incidence of urgency urinary incontinence [4].

Overactive bladder is defined by the International Continence Society as urinary urgency or the sudden need to urinate in the presence or absence of urgency urinary incontinence (UUI) and may also include daytime urinary frequency and nocturia [7]. Several theories exist regarding the underlying pathology associated with overactive bladder, including neurogenic and myogenic etiologies [8]. Age, infection, and inflammation can impact detrusor permeability and neuronal function, and individual microbiome appears to contribute to overactive bladder symptoms as well [9–11]. These theories are likely interrelated with the etiology of OAB being multilevel and heterogeneous across various patient phenotypes.

S. D. Goodridge
Wellstar Urology, Roswell, GA, USA

L. M. Rickey (✉)
Departments of Urology and Obstetrics, Gynecology & Reproductive Sciences, Yale School of Medicine, New Haven, CT, USA
e-mail: leslie.rickey@yale.edu

© The Author(s), under exclusive license to Springer Nature Switzerland AG 2022
A. P. Cameron (ed.), *Female Urinary Incontinence*,
https://doi.org/10.1007/978-3-030-84352-6_8

Oral pharmacotherapy is the second line of treatment for bothersome overactive bladder in the AUA/SUFU Guidelines once behavioral modification and pelvic muscle interventions have been considered [12]. Two drug classes have been identified for use in the treatment of overactive bladder: antimuscarinics and ß3-agonists. The aim of this chapter is to review the pharmacology of medications used for overactive bladder as well as side effect profiles and comparative efficacy.

Medication Pharmacology

Bladder function is regulated by the parasympathetic and sympathetic nervous systems. In the absence of pathology, the sympathetic nervous system facilitates bladder wall relaxation and storage of urine, while the parasympathetic nervous system mediates bladder wall contraction for bladder emptying [8].

Antimuscarinic medication functions by inhibiting the parasympathetic pathway via cholinergic muscarinic receptor blockade in the detrusor muscle, thus reducing or eliminating the severity of detrusor contraction. There are five identified muscarinic receptor subtypes (M1-M5), and [13] detrusor smooth muscle contains primarily M2 and M3 receptors. M3 receptors mediate cholinergic induced bladder contractions, while the role of M2 receptors is less well defined but is thought to act synergistically with M3 [14–16]. M2 and M3 receptors have been identified throughout the urothelium and on nerve fibers, and there are likely effects on the afferent pathways as well via A-delta and C-fiber nerves [17]. Currently available antimuscarinic therapies have varying levels of M3 affinity over other receptor subtypes which affects the side effect profile [18]. Muscarinic receptors are also abundant in the mouth, eyes, and gut, which account for the common side effects of dry mouth, constipation, and visual disturbances. Muscarinic receptors are present in the central nervous system, where M1 and M2 appear to be important for higher cognitive processes [19].

Adrenergic receptors are the targets of catecholamines including norepinephrine and epinephrine, with stimulation of the ß3 receptor resulting in detrusor relaxation. Three ß adrenoreceptors have been described: ß1, ß2, and ß3. ß3 receptors are predominantly found in the detrusor and urothelium and are activated by adrenergic stimulation. Ninety-seven percent of ß adrenergic receptors that are expressed on the mucosal and muscular layer of the detrusor are ß3 receptors [20].

Antimuscarinic Effectiveness

Six antimuscarinic oral agents are recognized by the AUA/SUFU Guidelines for use in patients with overactive bladder (Table 8.1) [12]. These agents include oxybutynin, tolterodine, darifenacin, solifenacin, fesoterodine, and trospium. Oxybutynin immediate release (IR) is the oldest currently used formulation of this drug class. A

Table 8.1 Antimuscarinic medications used in the treatment of overactive bladder

Oral anti-muscarinic agents used for overactive bladder	Dose	Formulation	Side effect	Specific population use
Darifenacin	7.5 mg once daily Can increase to 15 mg once daily max based on response and tolerance	Extended-release tablet	7.5 mg: Dry mouth 20.5% Constipation 14.8% UTI 4.7% 15 mg: Dry mouth 35.3% Constipation 21.3% Dyspepsia 8.4% UTI 4.5%	Do not exceed 7.5 mg in those with moderate hepatic impairment (Child-Pugh B) or taking potent CYP3A4 inhibitors Not recommended in those with severe hepatic impairment (Child-Pugh C) No dose adjustment recommended for patients with renal impairment
Fesoterodine	4 mg once daily Can increase to 8 mg once daily max based on response and tolerance	Extended-release tablet	4 mg: Dry mouth 18.8% Constipation 4% 8 mg: Dry mouth 19% Constipation 6%	Do not exceed 4 mg in those with severe renal impairment (CrCl <30 mL/min) or taking potent CYP3A4 inhibitors Not recommended in those with severe hepatic impairment. (Child-Pugh C) No dose adjustment recommended in those with moderate hepatic impairment (Child-Pugh B)
Oxybutynin	Adult: 5–15 mg once daily Do not exceed 30 mg daily Pediatric (age 6 and older): 5 mg once daily. Do not exceed 20 mg per day	Extended-release tablet	Dry mouth 71.4% Constipation 15.1% Headache 7.5% Somnolence 14.0% Dizziness 16.6%	Use not established in those with renal or hepatic impairment Use in pediatrics established but not recommended on those who cannot swallow without chewing Caution when administering with CYP3A4 inhibitors. Oxybutynin levels were ~2× higher when administered with ketoconazole

(continued)

Table 8.1 (continued)

Oral anti-muscarinic agents used for overactive bladder	Dose	Formulation	Side effect	Specific population use
Solifenacin	5 mg once daily Can increase to 10 mg once daily based on response and tolerance	Film-coated tablet	5 mg: Dry mouth 10.9% Constipation 5.4% 10 mg: Dry mouth 27.6% Constipation: 13.4% UTI 4.8%	Do not exceed 5 mg in those with severe renal impairment (CrCl <30 mL/min), moderate hepatic impairment (Child-Pugh B), or taking potent CYP3A4 inhibitors
Tolterodine	Immediate-release: 1–2 mg BID Extended-release: 2–4 mg once daily	Immediate-release and extended-release capsules	Dry mouth 30% Constipation 7% Headache 7% Vertigo/dizziness 5% Abdominal pain 5%	Immediate-release: Reduce dose to 1 mg BID in those with severe renal impairment (CrCl 10–30 mL/min) Reduce dose to 1 mg BID in those with severe hepatic impairment Extended-release: Reduce dose to 2 mg once daily in those with severe renal impairment (CrCl 10 to 30 mL/min). Not recommended in those with CrCl <10 mL/min Reduce dose to 2 mg once daily in those with mild to moderate hepatic impairment (Child-Pugh class A or B). Not recommended in those with Child-Pugh class C See dosing regarding coadministration with CYP3A4 inhibitors

Table 8.1 (continued)

Oral anti-muscarinic agents used for overactive bladder	Dose	Formulation	Side effect	Specific population use
Trospium	Immediate-release: 20 mg BID Extended-release: 60 mg once daily in the morning	Immediate-release and extended-release capsules	Dry mouth 5.8% Constipation 4.6%	Immediate-release: Reduce dose to 20 mg once daily at bedtime in those with severe renal impairment (CrCl <30 mL/min) There is no recommendation for use in those with hepatic impairment Geriatric patients >75 years old may titrate down to 20 mg once daily based on tolerability Extended-release: Not recommended in those with severe renal impairment (CrCl <30 mL/min) There is no recommendation for use in those with hepatic impairment

From: [21–28]
Included are all side effects measured at prevalence ≥4%

multitude of studies have been done comparing these drugs to placebo and to one another to assess efficacy and side effect profiles. In terms of general improvement of overactive bladder symptoms, the proportion of people that report resolution of urgency incontinence symptoms with medication is 49% (interquartile range, 35.6–58%) [29]. Improvement of urgency, frequency, and nocturia in patients without incontinence tends to be lower, in the 15–35% range [30, 31].

A recent meta-analysis compared outcomes in 128 eligible randomized studies. Overall, those taking active treatments were more likely to report subjective improvement in number of leakage episodes and voids compared to placebo (OR range 1.42–2.20), while differences between active treatments were not significant [32]. Another systematic review and meta-analysis in women in antimuscarinic trials found a reduction in two voids per day and 1.73 incontinence episodes per day, and similarly, there was no difference between medications in terms of superior efficacy [33]. Of note, 82% of the studies that met criteria for inclusion in the analysis were industry sponsored. Increased cytometric bladder capacity (54 mL, range 43–66) and volume at first contraction (52 mL, range 38–67 mL) was noted in treatment groups compared to placebo. Average increases in post void residual volumes were not clinically significant (0.1–6.8 mL) [18].

Patient assessed changes in symptom bother and impact as measured by the Incontinence Impact Questionnaire, King's Health Questionnaire, and Overactive Bladder Questionnaire (OAB-q) Bother Score also showed improvements in lower urinary tract symptoms (LUTS) related quality of life over placebo, without differences among antimuscarinic agents [34].

The most commonly reported side effect of all antimuscarinic medications was dry mouth (OR generally between 3–5 compared to placebo), with the highest rates found with oxybutynin IR (OR 9.5) [32]. The next most common side effects are constipation and vision changes. Adverse event reporting is variable across available clinical trials, but a systematic review reported dry mouth in 6.3–13.6%, constipation in 2.2–5.1%, and blurred vision in 0.8–6.2% of trial participants [35].

It should also be noted that despite effectiveness, OAB medication adherence varies greatly. In clinical trials rates of discontinuation range from 4% to 31%, while medical claim studies show higher rates of discontinuation ranging from 43% to 83%. Most patients discontinue medications within 30 days, with rates of discontinuation increasing over time, primarily driven by both lack of efficacy and medication side effects [36, 37].

It is well recognized that subjective outcomes that capture overall improvement and satisfaction from a patient standpoint are important in measuring treatment effect [38]. Patient assessed improvement in quality of life and global outcome measures likely take both symptom improvement and side effects into account and may be a superior indicator of successful treatment and medication adherence compared to bladder diary data alone.

Comparative Effectiveness

A number of randomized controlled trials of the six aforementioned antimuscarinic agents have been conducted, most of which are industry sponsored. A 2012 Cochrane Review was recently updated by Hsu et al. and outlined the comparative data, which confirmed that while there are differences in side effects, efficacy is similar among antimuscarinic medications [35].

In studies assessing efficacy of tolterodine versus oxybutynin chloride, no statistical differences were noted in incontinence episodes per day, micturition frequency, or quality of life. Tolterodine was found to have fewer adverse events resulting in a decreased rate of medication discontinuation (RR 0.52, 95% confidence interval 0.40–0.66) and fewer reported episodes of dry mouth (RR 0.65, 95% CI 0.60–0.71) [39]. One trial did find that patients taking oxybutynin 10 mg extended release (ER) were more likely to report no incontinence compared to those taking tolterodine 4 mg ER (23% vs 17%, $p = 0.03$) [40].

The immediate release formulations of trospium and oxybutynin have similar rates of improvement in symptoms; however subjects taking trospium were less likely to report dry mouth (RR 0.64, CI 0.52–0.77) which likely affected the lower withdrawal rate in this group. One included trial that compared solifenacin to oxy-butynin IR also showed lower rates of dry mouth and withdrawals in the solifenacin-treated subjects.

Another small trial compared darifenacin 7.5 mg to trospium ER 60 mg and found similar improvements in all of the Overactive Bladder Symptom Score (OABSS) subscales (urgency, frequency, nocturia, and UUI) and similar rates of increased constipation.

In trials comparing solifenacin 5 mg to tolterodine 4 mg, patients in the solifenacin group reported greater improvement in quality of life and fewer leakage episodes, while there was no difference in 24-h micturitions. Pooled results from two trials showed better improvement or cure with solifenacin (RR 1.25, CI 1.13–1.39). No differences were noted in withdrawal due to side effects and adverse events. It appears that dry mouth rates are lower with solifenacin compared to tolterodine IR but are higher with solifenacin compared to tolterodine ER. One new trial compared fesoterodine 4 mg to solifenacin 5 mg and reported similar improvement in the OABSS. Though the higher rates of constipation (5.1% vs 1.7%) and dry mouth (13.6% vs 5.0%) with fesoterodine were not statistically significant, there were more subjects that withdrew in the fesoterodine group (10.2% vs 0%) [35].

When comparing fesoterodine 8 mg to tolterodine ER 4 mg, subjects in the fesoterodine group reported increased improvement in quality of life (QOL), leakage episodes, frequency, and urgency. Though rates of improvement/cure were higher with fesoterodine (RR 1.11, CI 1.06–1.16), there were also higher rates of dry mouth and withdrawal due to adverse effects [39].

Reynolds et al. did a systematic review assessing comparative effectiveness of tolterodine IR/ER, trospium, darifenacin, solifenacin, and fesoterodine in women. All medications were found to be modestly effective in improving one or more OAB symptoms. Overall, there was marginal superiority with ER formulations. Ultimately, no one drug outperformed another, consistent with other systematic reviews and meta-analyses [40].

Transdermal Use of Antimuscarinics

Oxybutynin is the most widely prescribed antimuscarinic in the US market and has evolved over the past 40 years from oral formulations to transdermal patches and gels. This was largely influenced by the side effect profile of the oral immediate release form of oxybutynin [41]. Oxybutynin IR undergoes first-pass liver metabolism resulting in an active primary metabolite which has a higher affinity for salivary gland M3 receptors than detrusor muscle antimuscarinic receptors [42]. Endeavors to improve pharmacokinetics and lower incidence of adverse events led to development of transdermal antimuscarinic therapy.

Transdermal oxybutynin (OXY-TDS) enters the systemic circulation via small capillaries in the dermis with steady state maintained for 96 h. It avoids first pass through the liver reducing its primary metabolite resulting in decreased dry mouth (7.0%) and constipation (2.1%) [43]. Skin site reactions were the most commonly reported adverse events including erythema (8.3%) and itchiness (14.0%). Skin-related adverse events were reduced by application site rotation and largely resolved on their own. Randomized controlled trial studies comparing OXY-TDS to extended-release tolterodine showed equal efficacy in reducing incontinence episodes and urinary frequency, and both were superior to placebo [44].

Oxybutynin chloride topical gel (OTG) is a once-daily formulation which utilizes ethanol as a skin permeation enhancer. Steady-state plasma levels are achieved within 1 week of application. The pharmacokinetic profile is not negatively affected by showering or sunscreen application. Overall, urinary frequency and urgency incontinence episodes decreased significantly with the use of OTG with reported dry mouth rates of 6.9%. Application site reactions were infrequently observed (5.4%) [45–47]. Limited data is available comparing OTG to placebo or antimuscarinics. To date, there is no therapeutically equivalent version of OTG available in the United States.

ß3-Agonist Effectiveness

Mirabegron

ß3-agonists were developed as an alternative treatment option to antimuscarinics for the treatment of overactive bladder (Table 8.2). The first of two FDA-approved ß3-agonists is mirabegron, approved in 2012.

When compared to placebo, mirabegron 50 and 100 mg resulted in improved urgency incontinence episodes (-1.13 [-1.35, -0.91], -1.47 [-1.69, -1.25], -1.63 [-1.86, -1.40]) and 24 h voids (-1.05 [-1.31, -0.79], -1.66 [-1.92, -1.40] and -1.75 [-2.01, -1.48]) ($p < 0.05$). At 12 months, responders with $\geq 50\%$ decrease from baseline in the mean number of incontinence episodes were 63.7% and 66.3% in the mirabegron 50 mg and mirabegron 100 mg groups, respectively. Treatment satisfaction and patient reported improvement using the OAB-q and the Patient Perception of Bladder Condition (PPBC) showed significant improvement as well compared to placebo control groups [50].

In subjects receiving 50 mg and 100 mg doses, <2% reported constipation and dry mouth, and urinary retention was not reported. UTI (non-culture documented) was reported by 2.7% and 3.7% of subjects in the 50 mg and 100 mg arms, respectively, compared to 1.8% in the placebo group. Overall, the risk of dry mouth, constipation, and blurred vision was similar between mirabegron and placebo [51].

ß3-agonist receptors are found in the cardiovascular system, and activation may result in positive inotropic effects on the atrial tissue and negative inotropic effects on the ventricular tissue [20]. A meta-analysis evaluating the effect of mirabegron on the cardiovascular system found that hypertension was identified in 12% of participants in the 25 mg arm, 8.7% in the mirabegron 50 mg arm, and 8.5% of the placebo arm at 12 weeks of treatment, with a mean increase of systolic blood pressure and diastolic blood pressure of 1 mmHg. Increases in blood pressure were reversible after discontinuation of the medication [52]. A dose-dependent increase

Table 8.2 ß3-agonist medications used in the treatment of overactive bladder

Oral ß3-agonists used for overactive bladder	Dose	Formulation	Side effect	Specific population use
Mirabegron	25 mg daily 50 mg daily	Extended release	25 mg: HTN 11.3% UTI 4.2% 50 mg: HTN 7.5%	Avoid in patients with poorly controlled hypertension (systolic blood pressure $\geq$180 mmHg or diastolic blood pressure $\geq$110 mmHg, or both) Do not exceed 25 mg in patients with severe renal impairment (CLcr 15 to 29 mL/min or eGFR 15 to 29 mL/min/1.73 m^2) No dose adjustment is necessary in patients with mild or moderate renal impairment (CLcr 30 to 89 mL/min or eGFR 30 to 89 mL/min/1.73 m^2) Do not exceed 25 mg in patients with moderate hepatic impairment (Child-Pugh B) Monitor drugs metabolized by CYP2D6 enzyme No dosage adjustment for GEMTESA is recommended for patients with mild, moderate, or severe renal impairment (eGFR 15 to <90 mL/min/1.73 m^2) No dosage adjustment for GEMTESA is recommended for patients with mild to moderate hepatic impairment (Child-Pugh A and B)
Vibegron	75 mg daily	Extended release	Headache 4%	

From: [48, 49]
Included are all side effects measured at prevalence $\geq$4%

in heart rate of <3 beats per minute was noted in the 100 mg group. It is admittedly difficult to separate out drug effect from natural history of disease in some instances. When looking at shifts between hypertensive states, the proportion of subjects that went from a normotensive to hypertensive was detected in 2.6% of placebo, 2.6% of mirabegron 25 mg, and 6.4% of mirabegron 50 mg users. Worsening hypertension in those patients with a diagnosis at baseline occurred in 18.3% of placebo, 16.3% of mirabegron 25 mg, and 21% of mirabegron 50 mg subjects [53].

In a population-based cohort study, the 1-year incidence of arrythmia or tachycardia was similar between new users of mirabegron and antimuscarinic agents (3.6% vs 3.8%). There was no increased risk of myocardial infarction (MI) or stroke detected in the mirabegron group (HR 1.06; 95% CI 0.89–1.27) [54]. In a secondary analysis of patients $\geq$65 years, cardiac disorders were reported in five (1.1%) placebo patients and nine (2.0%) mirabegron patients [55]. Major adverse cardiac events were similar (0.4%) between patients in the mirabegron and placebo groups, with nonfatal stroke reported in three patients (two in placebo group and one in mirabegron 50 mg group) and one nonfatal MI in the mirabegron 50 mg group [53]. More research is necessary to elucidate whether there are higher risk patient groups that would influence decisions around ß3-agonist use for OAB.

Vibegron

Vibegron is a new ß3-agonist approved by the Federal Drug and Food Administration in December of 2020 for a once-daily 75 mg dose for the treatment of OAB. Notably, the medication does not have an effect on hepatic CYP enzymes, which should decrease risk of drug-drug interactions with medications metabolized by CYP2D6 [56]. In the Phase III EMPOWUR study comparing vibegron 75 mg to placebo with tolterodine extended-release 4 mg as an active control, there were greater improvements in voiding frequency and incontinence episodes in the vibegron group at 12 weeks (-1.8 vs -1.3 voids, $p < 0.001$ and -2.0 vs -1.4 episodes, $p < 0.0001$, respectively) [57]. In subjects with incontinence, 52% of vibegron-treated patients had a $\geq 75\%$ reduction in daily UUI compared to 37% in the placebo group ($p < 0.0001$), with improvement maintained at 52 weeks in an extension study [58]. Adverse events that were higher with vibegron versus placebo were headache, nasopharyngitis, diarrhea, and nausea. Hypertension was similar in both groups (1.7%), and blood pressure increase was also similar (0.7% for vibegron and 0.9% for placebo). Finally, discontinuation rates were 1.7% in the vibegron group, 1.1% in the placebo group, and 3.3% in the tolterodine group.

Efficacy of ß3-Agonist Compared to Antimuscarinic Monotherapy

Kelleher et al. performed a meta-analysis of antimuscarinic therapy compared to mirabegron 50 mg that included 64 studies. Regarding voiding frequency, no significant differences were found between mirabegron 50 mg and antimuscarinic monotherapies except for solifenacin 10 mg which was found to be more effective. Greater reductions in UUI were found with fesoterodine 8 mg compared to mirabegron; however, the remaining agents were equally effective. Achieving at least 50% reduction in incontinence episodes was similar across all medications, while trospium 60 mg (OR 1.62), solifenacin 10 mg (OR 1.28), and fesoterodine 8 mg (OR 1.27) were all more efficacious in achieving dry rates compared to mirabegron 50 mg [59].

Side effects which were analyzed in this meta-analysis included dry mouth, constipation, blurred vision, hypertension, and urinary retention. Dry mouth was significantly lower with mirabegron compared to all other active treatments except for oxybutynin IR 5 mg (OR 2.99; 0.68, 13.75). The risk of constipation and urinary retention was also significantly lower in the mirabegron group compared to most antimuscarinic agents. No significant differences were appreciated between the two drug classes with regard to blurred vision and hypertension [59].

In summary, this meta-analysis suggests that mirabegron has similar efficacy for OAB treatment compared to antimuscarinics with increased tolerability in some instances. A large database study of clinical practices in the United Kingdom showed a longer time to medication discontinuation for mirabegron compared to antimuscarinics (169 days vs 30–78 days) and greater persistence at 12 months

(38% vs 8.3–25%, $p < 0.0001$) [60]. A US database analysis showed similar low adherence rates over 12 months in both mirabegron (44%) and antimuscarinic (31%) users [61].

In terms of medication switching, 30% of patients previously maintained on antimuscarinic medication (for at least 3 months) reported moderate to marked improvement after switching to mirabegron, while 25% reported mild improvement, 31% reported no change, and 10% reported worsening outcomes [62]. Finally, in women who had previously failed therapy with at least one antimuscarinic agent, 37% of those treated with mirabegron 50 mg as second-line therapy were considered responders compared to 75% in the treatment naïve group ($p < 0.00001$) [63].

There is limited data on predictors of treatment outcome for the various OAB therapies across first-, second-, and third-line treatments. The Symptoms of Lower Urinary Tract Dysfunction Research Network (LURN) network is developing more discrete patient subtypes within the OAB spectrum of symptoms which may help improve patient-specific management recommendations. Additionally, effects of frailty, age, biology, comorbidities, and lifestyle factors should be considered in models seeking to inform risk stratification [64].

Combination Therapy

The OAB Guidelines were amended in 2019 to include consideration of combination therapy with antimuscarinic and beta-agonist formulations for patients with unsatisfactory symptom improvement with monotherapy alone. Various combinations of solifenacin and mirabegron have been trialed, and in general the combination regimens tend to have greater improvements in voiding frequency and incontinence episodes compared to placebo and monotherapy. Overall "dry" rates are higher as well (46–52% vs 38–46%) [65, 66].

In the BESIDE trial, subjects with continued incontinence while on solifenacin 5 mg were randomized to solifenacin 5 mg, solifenacin 10 mg, or combination therapy with solifenacin 5 mg + mirabegron 25 mg. Compared to solifenacin 10 mg monotherapy, the combination group had greater reductions in urgency incontinence episodes (-1.82 vs -1.63, $p = 0.014$), and more subjects demonstrated "zero incontinence" on 3-day diary [46% vs 40%, OR 1.28 (1.02–1.61, $p = 0.033$)] [66]. A randomized control trial evaluated the efficacy of mirabegron 50 mg versus solifenacin 10 mg versus combination mirabegron 50 mg and solifenacin 10 mg as compared to placebo. Response to treatment was measured by urodynamic evaluation as well as pre- and post-treatment OAB questionnaires. Efficacy was similar between the two monotherapy groups, and the combination therapy group had a greater improvement in UUI, frequency, and urgency without an increase in side effects [67]. In the combination group, 29% of the subjects reported side effects versus 33% in the mirabegron group, 21% in the solifenacin group, and 24% of the placebo subjects. The SYNERGY study further supported this data by demonstrating that combination therapy not only improved objective outcomes but also improved subjective, patient-relevant outcomes [68].

OAB Treatment and Cognitive Impairment

Emerging evidence has documented the risk of cognitive impairment in people taking medications with anticholinergic properties [69]. As described earlier, there are muscarinic receptors in the CNS, and OAB medications have the potential to cross the blood-brain barrier. Antimuscarinic medications used to treat OAB include both tertiary and quaternary amines. Tertiary amines are smaller, lipophilic, and neutral and thus able to cross the blood-brain barrier. Known tertiary amines are darifenacin, fesoterodine, oxybutynin, solifenacin, and tolterodine. Quaternary amines, such as trospium, have a net positive charge, are hydrophilic, and have decreased lipophilicity, therefore making it less likely to cross the blood-brain barrier [70]. Studies have also shown that drugs that are part of the permeability-glycoprotein (P-gp) system can actively be transported out of the brain. Darifenacin, fesoterodine, and trospium are P-gp system substrates and have been shown to have poor penetration across the blood-brain barrier in animal studies [71]. Several factors can increase the permeability of the blood-brain barrier including trauma, Parkinson's disease, Alzheimer's disease, diabetes, multiple sclerosis, hypertension, epilepsy, migraines, stress, and age [72].

In a large case-control study published in JAMA in 2019, cumulative anticholinergic drug exposure was a risk factor for a new diagnosis of dementia in subjects over 55 years during the 11-year study period. The adjusted odds ratio of dementia for bladder antimuscarinic drugs was 1.20–1.65, and this finding seems consistent with an earlier study that showed an OR of 1.2 for bladder antimuscarinic medication users 4–20 years prior to dementia diagnosis [69, 73]. Though the evidence associating anticholinergic use and risk of cognitive impairment (CI) is established, individual risk and causation are less well understood. Patients with OAB have more systemic neurologic, psychologic, cardiopulmonary, and musculoskeletal conditions and are more likely to have CNS and cardiovascular comorbidities that can increase their baseline risk of CI [74, 75]. However, a population-based cohort study showed an increased risk of dementia in new OAB antimuscarinic users versus new ß3-agonist users (HR 1.23, CI 1.12–1.35), though the overall risk was low [76]. Interestingly, gender appeared to play a role as the increased risk was seen primarily in males, with no significant difference in females in the subgroup analysis.

In short-term studies conducted in clinical populations taking antimuscarinic medication for OAB, there has been a varying effect on cognitive measures. In a randomized study of the vulnerable elderly, there was significant improvement in the PPBC and high satisfaction in patients randomized to fesoterodine versus placebo. Mini Mental State Exam (MMSE) remained stable in both groups at 12 weeks, though two patients in the fesoterodine group reported subjective memory impairment and one patient withdrew due to mild confusion [77]. In a small study of patients ≥75 years with mild cognitive impairment who were randomized to solifenacin, oxybutynin, or placebo, only oxybutynin was associated with decreases in attention measures [55]. When comparing cognitive tests in subjects ≥60 years randomized to darifenacin, oxybutynin ER, or placebo, only oxybutynin was associated with memory impairment after 3 weeks of use [78]. One prospective study assessing women ≥55 years with OAB found an initial decline in cognitive function after starting trospium ER based on the Hopkins Verbal Learning Test-Revised. Cognitive function returned to baseline by week four of treatment and remained stable until week 12 when the study was completed [79]. The authors did a follow-up randomized controlled study and did not see any difference in cognitive function between the trospium and placebo groups over a 4-week period [80].

Few ß3-agonist receptors exist in the central nervous system making ß3-agonist medications a potential treatment choice for patients who are at risk for development of cognitive impairment. Mirabegron is also a known substrate for the P-gp system. A recent study assessing safety and tolerability of mirabegron found that cognitive impairment was similar between treatment and placebo groups with no significant adjusted mean scores in Montreal Cognitive Assessment from baseline [81].

Many medications, both prescribed and over the counter, have anticholinergic effects. Polypharmacy increases in the elderly population, and anticholinergic load can increase the risk of cognitive impairment in elderly patients [80]. Though several anticholinergic load scales exist [82], no ideal scale is available for use in clinical practice, and existing scales vary with respect to ratings of anticholinergic activity and burden [83]. The Beers Criteria best practice guidelines for geriatric patients recommended that antimuscarinics should be avoided in the elderly or used minimally if necessary, and geriatrics societies have advised cessation of use of antimuscarinics in patients with dementia [83]. However, it is important to weigh the potential risks of medical therapy with the risks of not treating OAB, including anxiety and depression, increased of falls and fractures, and worse physical function [84]. Elderly patients treated for OAB report better health-related QoL and less activity impairment; therefore shared decision-making is critical [85]. The American Urogynecologic Association recommends considering alternate medications (currently ß3-agonists), avoiding antimuscarinic medications in women over 70 years, considering antimuscarinics with lower potential for crossing the blood-brain barrier, and discussion of third-line therapy with onabotulinum toxin A or neuromodulation [86]. The AUA/SUFU Guidelines similarly recommends using caution when using either class of medications in the frail elderly patient [87].

Summary

Overactive bladder becomes more prevalent as people age and significantly impacts quality of life, physical functioning, and mental health. OAB has both individual burden and societal costs and should be addressed in all patients who report bother regardless of their age. However, the side effects of antimuscarinics must be carefully considered. The potential for neurocognitive changes should be weighed in elderly patients in particular, as even a modest decline in cognitive function can result in loss of independence in this population [88].

In patients who have incomplete symptom improvement with first-line OAB interventions, pharmacotherapy can reduce symptoms and have important quality of life impact [89]. Medication for overactive bladder treatment in the United States has been comprised primarily of antimuscarinics, though ß3-agonists are increasingly available to patients with two formulations now FDA approved. Combination therapy may have superior benefit to monotherapy in some patients without compounding side effects. Assessment of side effect risk, including cognitive impairment, and shared decision-making is important to optimize the benefit to risk balance [90]. Further research into more patient-specific outcomes and development of predictive tools is necessary to help providers better counsel their patients and ultimately reduce the quality of life burden associated with overactive bladder conditions.

References

1. Irwin DE, Kopp ZS, Agatep B, Milsom I, Abrams P. Worldwide prevalence estimates of lower urinary tract symptoms, overactive bladder, urinary incontinence and bladder outlet obstruction. BJU Int. 2011;108(7):1132–8.
2. Stewart WF, Van Rooyen JB, Cundiff GW. Prevalence and burden of overactive bladder in the United States. World J Urol. 2003;20(6):327–36. https://doi.org/10.1007/s00345-002-0301-4.
3. Hu TW, Wagner TH, Bentkover JD. Costs of urinary incontinence and overactive bladder in the United States: a comparative study. Urology. 2004;63(3):461–5.
4. Milsom I, Kaplan SA, Coyne KS. Effect of bothersome overactive bladder symptoms on health-related quality of life, anxiety, depression, and treatment seeking in the United States: results from EpiLUTS. Urology. 2012;80(1):90–6. https://doi.org/10.1016/j.urology.2012.04.004.
5. Kinsey D, Pretorius S, Glover L. The psychological impact of overactive bladder: a systematic review. J Health Psychol. 2014; https://doi.org/10.1177/1359105314522084.
6. Stuart Reynolds W, et al. The burden of overactive bladder on US public health. Curr Bladder Dysfunct. 2016;11:8–13. https://doi.org/10.1007/s11884-016-0344-9.
7. Abrams P, Cardozo L, Fall M, et al. The standardization of terminology in lower urinary tract function: report from the standardization sub-committee of the international continence society. Urology. 2003;61:37–49.
8. Abrams P, Anderson KE. Muscarinic receptor antagonists for overactive bladder. BJUI. 2007;100(5):987–1006. https://doi.org/10.1111/j.1464-410X.2007.07205.x.
9. Pratt TS, Suskind AM. Management of overactive bladder in older women. Curr Urol Rep. 2018;19:92. https://doi.org/10.1007/s11934-018-0845-5.
10. Fok CS, Gao X, Lin H. Urinary symptoms are associated with certain urinary microbes in urogynecologic surgical patients. Int Urogynecol J. 2018;29:1765–71. https://doi.org/10.1007/s00192-018-3732-1
11. Curtiss N, Balachandran A, Krska L. A case-controlled study examining the bladder microbiome in women with Overactive Bladder (OAB) and healthy controls. Eur J Obstet Gynecol Reprod Biol. 2017;214:31–5. https://doi.org/10.1016/j.ejogrb.2017.04.040.
12. Gormley EA, Lightner DJ, Burgio KL, Chai TC, American Urological Association; Society of Urodynamics, Female Pelvic Medicine & Urogenital Reconstruction, et al. Diagnosis and treatment of overactive bladder (non-neurogenic) in adults: AUA/SUFU guideline. 2012; amended 2014. http://www.auanet.org/guidelines/overactive-bladder-(oab)-(aua/sufu-guideline-2012-amended-2014).
13. Andersson KE, Cardozo L, Cruz F, et al. Pharmacological treatment of urinary incontinence. In: Abrams P, Cardozo L, Wagg A, editors. Incontinence. 6th ed; 2017. p. 805–97.

14. Fetscher C, Fleichman M, Schmidt M. M(3) muscarinic receptors mediate contraction of human urinary bladder. Br J Pharmacol. 2002;136:641–3.
15. Igawa Y, Zhang X, Nishizawa O. Cystometric findings in mice lacking muscarinic M2 or M3 receptors. J Urol. 2004;172:2460–4.
16. Andersson KE. Antimuscarinics for treatment of overactive bladder. Lancet Neurol. 2004;3:46–53.
17. Mukerji G, Yiangou Y, Grogono J. Localization of M2 and M3 muscarinic receptors in human bladder disorders and their clinical correlations. J Urol. 2006;176:367–73.
18. Herbison P, Hay-Smith J, Moor K. Effectiveness of anticholinergic drugs compared with placebo in the treatment of overactive bladder: a systematic review. BMJ. 2003;326:841–4.
19. Kay GG, Granville LJ. Antimuscarinic agents: implications and concerns in the management of overactive bladder in the elderly. Clin Ther. 2005;27(1):127–38.
20. Goodridge SD, Dmochowski RR. B3-agonist for overactive bladder. In: Cox L, Rovner E, editors. Contemporary pharmacotherapy of overactive bladder. Cham: Springer; 2019. p. 115–31.
21. Darifenacin [prescribing information]. India: Jubilant Cadista Pharmaceuticals Inc; September 2017.
22. TOVIAZ (fesoterodine fumarate) [prescribing information]. Ireland: Pfizer Inc; October 2020.
23. Oxybutynin chloride [prescribing information]. Philadelphia: Lannett Company Inc; October 2019.
24. Solifenacin succinate [prescribing information]. Israel: Teva Pharmaceuticals USA, Inc; June 2020.
25. DETROL LA (tolterodine tartrate extended release) [prescribing information]. New York: Pharmacia and Upjohn Company LLC; 2020.
26. Tolterodine tartrate [prescribing information]. Peapack: Greenstone LLC; 2017.
27. Trospium chloride extended release [prescribing information]. Chantily: BluePoint Laboratories; 2020.
28. Trospium chloride [prescribing information]. Warren: Cipla USA Inc; 2020.
29. Riemsma R, Hagen S, Kirschner-Hermanns R. Can incontinence be cured? A systematic review of cure rates. BMC Med. 2017;15:63. https://doi.org/10.1186/s12916-017-0828-2.
30. Lukacz ES, Santiago-Lastra Y, Albo ME. Urinary incontinence in women: a review. JAMA. 2017;318(16):1592–604. https://doi.org/10.1001/jama.2017.12137.
31. Abrams P, Swift S. Solifenacin is effective for the treatment of OAB dry patients: a pooled analysis. Eur Urol. 2005;48(3):483–7. https://doi.org/10.1016/j.eururo.2005.06.007.
32. Herbison P, McKenzie JE. Which anticholinergic is best for people with overactive bladders? A network meta-analysis. Neurourol Urodyn. 2019;38(2):525–34. https://doi.org/10.1002/nau.23893.
33. Reynolds WS, McPheeters M, Blume J. Comparative effectiveness of anticholinergic therapy for overactive bladder in women. Obstet Gynecol. 2015;125(6):1423–32. https://doi.org/10.1097/AOG.0000000000000851.
34. Khullar V, Chapple C, Gabriel Z. The effects of antimuscarinics on health-related quality of life in overactive bladder: a systematic review and meta-analysis. Urology. 2006;68(2):38–48. https://doi.org/10.1016/j.urology.2006.05.043.
35. Hsu FC, Weeks CE, Selph SS. Updating the evidence on drugs to treat overactive bladder: a systematic review. Int Urogynecol J. 2019;30:1603–17. https://doi.org/10.1007/s00192-019-04022-8.
36. Sexton CC, Notte SM, Maroulis C. Persistence and adherence in the treatment of overactive bladder syndrome with anticholinergic therapy: a systematic review of the literature. Int J Clin Pract. 2011;65(5):567–85. https://doi.org/10.1111/j.1742-1241.2010.02626.x.
37. Benner JS. Patient-reported reasons for discontinuing overactive bladder medication. BJUI. 2010;105(9):1283–90.
38. Akino H, Namiki M, Suzuki K. Factors influencing patient satisfaction with antimuscarinic treatment of overactive bladder syndrome: results of a real-life clinical study. Int J Urol. 2014;21(4):389–94. https://doi.org/10.1111/iju.12298.

39. Madhuvrata P, Cody JD, Ellis G. Which anticholinergic drug for overactive bladder symptoms in adults. Cochrane Database Syst Rev. 2012; https://doi.org/10.1002/145618.CD005429.pub2.
40. Diokno AC, Appell RA, Sand PK. Prospective, randomized, double-blind study of the efficacy and tolerability of the extended-release formulations of oxybutynin and tolterodine for overactive bladder: results of the OPERA trial. Mayo Clin Proc. 2003;78(6):687–95.
41. Thuroff JW, Chartier-Kastler E, Corcus J. Medical treatment and medical side effects in urinary incontinence in the elderly. World J Urol. 1998;16(suppl 1):S248–61.
42. Waldeck K, Larsson B, Andersson KE. Comparison of oxybutynin and its active metabolite N-desethyloxybutynin in the human detrusor and parotid gland. J Urol. 1997;157(3):1093–7.
43. Dmochowski RR, Davila GW, Zinner NR. Efficacy and safety of transdermal oxybutynin in patients with urge and mixed incontinence. J Urol. 2002;168:580–6.
44. Dmochowski RR, Sand PK, Zinner NR. Comparative efficacy and safety of transdermal oxybutynin and oral tolterodine versus placebo in previously treated patients with urge and mixed urinary incontinence. Urology. 2003;62:237–42.
45. Staskin DR, Dmochowksi RR, Sand PK. Efficacy and safety of oxybutynin chloride topical gel for overactive bladder: a randomized, double-blind, placebo controlled, multicenter study. Adult Urol. 2009;181(4):1764–72.
46. Caramelli KE, Staskin DR, Volinn W. Steady-state pharmacokinetics of an investigational oxybutynin gel in comparison with oxybutynin transdermal system. Poster presented at: Annual Meeting of the American Urological Association; May 17–22, 2008.
47. Caramelli KE, Stanworth S, Volinn W, Hoel G. Pharmacokinetics of oxybutynin topical gel: effects of showering, sunscreen application, and person-to-person transference. Poster presented at: Annual Meeting of the American College of Clinical Pharmacy; October 19–22, 2008; Louisville.
48. Mybetriq (Mirabegron extended-release tablets) [prescribing information]. Northbrook. Astella Pharma; 2012.
49. Gemtesa (Vibegron) [prescribing information]. Irvine. Urovant Sciences, Inc.; 2020.
50. Chapple CR, Kaplan SA, Mitcheson D. Randomized double-blind, active-controlled Phase 3 study to assess 12-month safety and efficacy of Mirabegron, a β3-adrenoceptor agonist, in overactive bladder. Eur Urol. 2013;63(2):296–305. https://doi.org/10.1016/j.eururo.2012.10.048.
51. Nitti VW, Auerbach S, Martin N. Results of a randomized phase III trial of mirabegron in patients with overactive bladder. J Urol. 2013;189(4):1388–95.
52. Chapple CR, Dvorak V, Radziszewski P, Dragon Investigator Group. A phase II dose-ranging study of mirabegron in patients with overactive bladder. Int Urogynecol J. 2013;24(9):1447–58.
53. Herschorn S, Staskin D, Schermer CR. Safety and tolerability results from the PILLAR study: a Phase IV, double-blind, randomized, placebo-controlled study of mirabegron in patients ≥ 65 years with overactive bladder-wet. Drugs Aging. 2020;37:665–76. https://doi.org/10.1007/s40266-020-00783-w.
54. Tadrous M, Matta R, Greaves S. Association of mirabegron with the risk of arrhythmia in adult patients 66 years or older- a population-based cohort study. JAMA Int Med. 2019;179(10):1436–9.
55. Wagg A, Staskin D, Engel E. Efficacy, safety, and tolerability of mirabegron in patients aged ≥65yr with overactive bladder wet: a phase IV, double-blind, randomized, placebo-controlled study (PILLAR). Eur Urol. 2020;77(2):211–20. https://doi.org/10.1016/j.eururo.2019.10.002.
56. Rutman MP, King JR, Bennet N. Once-daily vibegron, a novel oralB3 agonist does not inhibit CYP2D6, a common pathway for drug metabolism in patients on OAB medications. J Urol. 2019;201:4S.
57. Staskin D, Frankel J, Varano S. International phase III, randomized, double-blind, placebo and active controlled study to evaluate the safety and efficacy of vibegron in patients with symptoms of overactive bladder: EMPOWUR. J Urol. 2020;204(2):316–24.
58. Staskin D, Frankel J, Varano S. Once-daily vibegron 75 mg for overactive bladder: double-blind 52-week results from an extension study of the international phase 3 trial (EMPOWUR). J Urol. 2021;205(5):1421–9.

59. Kelleher C, Hakimi Z, Zur R, et al. Efficacy and tolerability of Mirabegron compared with antimuscarinic monotherapy or combination therapies for overactive bladder: a systematic review and network meta-analysis. Eur Urol. 2018;74:334–5.
60. Chapple CR, Nazir J, Hakimi Z. Persistence and adherence with mirabegron versus antimuscarinic agents in patients with overactive bladder: a retrospective observational study in UK clinical practice. Eur Urol. 2017;72(3):389–99. https://doi.org/10.1016/j.eururo.2017.01.037.
61. Sussman D, Yehoshua A, Kowalksi J. Adherence and persistence of mirabegron and anticholinergic therapies in patients with overactive bladder: a real-world claims data analysis. Int J Clin Pract. 2017;71:3–4.
62. Liao CH, Kuo HC. High satisfaction with direct switching from antimuscarinics to mirabegron in patients receiving stable antimuscarinic treatment. Medicine. 2016;95(45):e4962. https://doi.org/10.1097/MD.0000000000004962.
63. Serati M, Leone Roberti Maggiore U, Sorice P, et al. Is mirabegron equally as effective when used as first- or second-line therapy in women with overactive bladder? Int Urogynecol J. 2017;28:1033–9. https://doi.org/10.1007/s00192-016-3219-x.
64. Adreev VP, Liu G, Yang C. Symptoms based clustering of women in the LURN observational cohort study. J Urol. 2018;200(6):1323–31.
65. Herschorn S, Chapple CR, Abrams P. Efficacy and safety of combinations of mirabegron and solifenacin compared with monotherapy and placebo in patients with overactive bladder. (SYNERGY study). BJU. 2017;120(4):562–75.
66. Drake JM, Chapple C, Esen AA. Efficacy and safety of mirabegron add-on therapy to solifenacin in incontinent overactive bladder patients with an inadequate response to initial 4-week solifenacin monotherapy: a randomized double-blind multicenter phase 3B study (BEDSIDE). Eur Urol. 2016;70(1):136–45. https://doi.org/10.1016/j.eururo.2016.02.030.
67. Kosilov K, Loparev S, Ivanovskaya M, Kosilova L. A randomized, controlled trial of effectiveness and safety of management of OAB symptoms in elderly men and women with standard-dosed combination of solifenacin and mirabegron. Arch Gerontol Geriatr. 2015;61(2):212–6.
68. Robinson D, Kelleher C, Staskin D, Mueller ER, Falconer C, Wang J, et al. Patient-reported outcomes from SYNERGY, a randomized, double-blind, multicenter study evaluating combinations of mirabegron and solifenacin compared with monotherapy and placebo in OAB patients. Neurourol Urodyn. 2018;27(1):394–406.
69. Coupland CAC, Hill T, Dening T. Anticholinergic drug exposure and the risk of dementia: a nested case-control study. JAMA Intern Med. 2019;179(8):1084–93. https://doi.org/10.1001/jamainternmed.2019.0677.
70. Rosenberg GA. Neurological diseases in relation to the blood-brain barrier. J Cereb Blood Flow Metab. 2012;32(7):1139-1151. https://doi.org/10.1038/jcbfm.2011.197.
71. Griebling TL, Campbell NL, Mangel J, et al. Effect of mirabegron on cognitive function in elderly patients with overactive bladder: moCA results from a phase 4 randomized, placebo-controlled study (PILLAR). BMC Geriatr. 2020;20(1):1. https://doi.org/10.1186/s12877-020-1474-7.
72. Chancellor, M.B., Staskin, D.R., Kay, G.G. et al. Blood-Brain Barrier Permeation and Efflux Exclusion of Anticholinergics Used in the Treatment of Overactive Bladder. Drugs Aging 2012;29:259–273.
73. Richardson K, Fox C, Maidment I. Anticholinergic drugs and risk of dementia: case-control study. BMJ. 2018;25(361):K1315.
74. Lai HH, Vetter J, Jain S. Systemic nonurological symptoms in patients with overactive bladder. J Urol. 2016;196(2):467–72.
75. Asche CV, Kim J, Kulkarni AS. Presence of central nervous system, cardiovascular and overall co-morbidity burden in patients with overactive bladder disorder in a real-world setting. BJUI. 2012;109(4):572–80.
76. Welk B, McArthur E. Increased risk of dementia among patients with overactive bladder treated with an anticholinergic medication compared to a beta-3 agonist: a population-based cohort study. BJUI. 2020;126(1):183–90.

77. Dubeau CD, Kraus SR, Griebling TL. Effect of fesoterodine in vulnerable elderly subjects with urgency incontinence: a double-blind, placebo controlled trial. J Urol. 2014;191(2):395–404. https://doi.org/10.1016/j.juro.2013.08.027.
78. Kay G, Crook T, Rekeda L. Differential effects of the antimuscarinic agents darifenacin and oxybutynin ER on memory in older subjects. Eur Urol. 2006;20(2):317–26.
79. Arklalitis G, Robminson D, Cardozo L. Cognitive effects of anticholinergic load in women with overactive bladder. Clin Interv Aging. 2020;15:1493–503.
80. Geller EJ, Crane AK, Wells EC. Effect of anticholinergic use for the treatment of overactive bladder on cognitive function in postmenopausal women. Clin Drug Investig. 2012;32(10):697–705.
81. Geller EJ, Dumond JB, Bowling JM, et al. Effect of trospium chloride on cognitive function in women aged 50 and older: a randomized trial. Female Pelvic Med Reconstr Surg. 2017;23(2):118–23.
82. Villalba-Moreno AM, Alfaro-Lara ER, Perez-Guerrero MC. Systematic review on the use of anticholinergic scales in poly pathological patients. Arch Gerontrol Geriatr. 2016;62:1–8. https://doi.org/10.1016/j.archger.2015.10.002.
83. Welsh TJ, van der Wardt V, Ojo G, et al. Anticholinergic drug burden tools/scales and adverse outcomes in different clinical settings: a systematic review of reviews. Drugs Aging. 2018;35:523–38.
84. Challegari E, Malotra B, Bungay PJ. A comprehensive non-clinical evaluation of the CNS penetration potential of antimuscarinic agents for the treatment of overactive bladder. Br J Clin Pharmacol. 2011;72(2):235–46.
85. Fick, D. M., T. P. Semla, and J. Beizer. "American Geriatrics Society 2015 Beers Criteria Update Expert Panel. American Geriatrics Society 2015 updated beers criteria for potentially inappropriate medication use in older adults." J Am Geriatr Soc 63.11 (2015):2227–46.
86. Chiarelli PE, Mackenzie LA, Osmotherly PG. Urinary incontinence is associated with an increase in falls: a systematic review. Aust J Pysiother. 2009;55(2):89–5. https://doi.org/10.1016/s0004-9514(09)70038-8.
87. Lee LK, Goren A, Zou KH. Potential benefits of diagnosis and treatment on health outcomes among elderly people with symptoms of overactive bladder. Int J Clin Pract. 2016;70(1):66–81.
88. Thomas TN, Walters MD. Clinical consensus statement: association of anticholinergic medication use and cognition in women with overactive bladder. Female Pelvic Med Reconstr Surg. 2021;27(2):69–71.
89. Lightner DJ, Gomelsky A, Souter L. Diagnosis and treatment of overactive bladder (non-neurogenic) in adults: AUA/SUFU guideline amendment 2019. J Urol. 2019;202:558–63.
90. Gray SL, Anderson ML, Dublin S, et al. Cumulative use of strong anticholinergics and incident dementia: a prospective cohort study. JAMA Intern Med. 2015;175(3):401–7.

Chapter 9
Posterior Tibial Nerve Stimulation for Female Urge Urinary Incontinence

Giulia Lane

In traditional acupuncture technique, the skin overlying the common peroneal and posterior tibial nerves is associated with treatment for pelvic disorders [1, 2]. In 1983, Dr. Ed McGuire and colleagues demonstrated that electrical stimulation over the posterior tibial nerve, which he termed posterior tibial nerve stimulation (PTNS), could inhibit detrusor contractions and treat urgency incontinence (UUI) due to detrusor instability [1–3]. Subsequently, Dr. Marshall Stoller developed early animal models and a commercial device [1–3]. Since that time, there has been robust evidence evaluating the efficacy of PTNS in women with urinary urgency incontinence. A 2016 systematic review and meta-analysis of non-implantable electrical stimulation for overactive bladder, including PTNS, found nearly twofold improvement or cure in OAB symptoms among those undergoing therapy compared to those undergoing no therapy [4]. The 2019 AUA Guidelines on OAB consider PTNS to be third-line therapy for the treatment of overactive bladder, and the treatment has FDA approval for this indication [5]. This chapter will review the mechanism of action, techniques, evidence, and adverse effects of PTNS for the treatment of overactive bladder and urgency urinary incontinence in women.

Mechanism of Action

The tibial nerve is the largest distal branch of the sciatic nerve, originating at the L4, L5, S1, S2, and S3 nerve roots and carries both motor and sensory fibers [6] (Fig. 9.1). The portion of the tibial nerve that runs posterior to the medial malleolus

G. Lane (✉)
Department of Urology, University of Michigan, Ann Arbor, MI, USA
e-mail: giuliala@med.umich.edu

© The Author(s), under exclusive license to Springer Nature Switzerland AG 2022
A. P. Cameron (ed.), *Female Urinary Incontinence*,
https://doi.org/10.1007/978-3-030-84352-6_9

Fig. 9.1 Origin of the
tibial nerve. The tibial
nerve is a branch of the
sciatic nerve. Both nerves
derive their origin from the
L4, L5, S1, S2, and S3
nerve roots. (Adapted from
Rigoard [33])

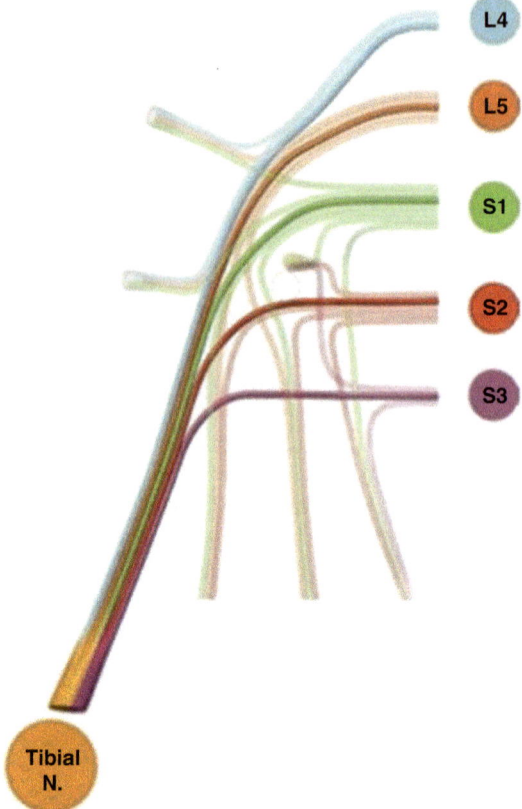

is termed the posterior tibial nerve, as such the posterior tibial nerve is not a branch of the tibial nerve [6]. The tibial nerve continues to the foot and branches and terminates as the medial plantar, lateral plantar, and calcaneal nerves [6]. The branches of the tibial nerve provide sensation to the plantar aspect of the foot [6]. The motor fibers of the terminal tibial nerve branches innervate the muscles controlling the phalanges and the plantar muscles of the foot [6] (Fig. 9.2).

The mechanism by which neuromodulation improves symptoms of overactive bladder and urgency incontinence is unknown. In the original 1983 publication, McGuire described that detrusor reflex responses to filling in animals can be delayed by acupuncture applied over the posterior tibial nerve [1]. Several recent hypotheses have been suggested, of these are either motor stimulation stimulating Onuf's nucleus, central inhibition via afferent nerves, or activation of sensory nerves [7]. In concordance with this, animal studies have found changes ranging from the bladder tissue level (protein expression and cell recruitment) to central cortical reorganization [8].

Fig. 9.2 The course of the tibial nerve. The tibial nerve is the largest distal branch of the sciatic nerve. It courses in the popliteal fossa and terminates as the medial plantar, lateral plantar, and calcaneal nerves. The arrow indicates the portion of the tibial nerve that runs posterior to the medial malleolus. (Adapted from Rigoard [33]. https://doi-org.proxy. lib.umich.edu/10.1007/978-3-319-43089-8_16)

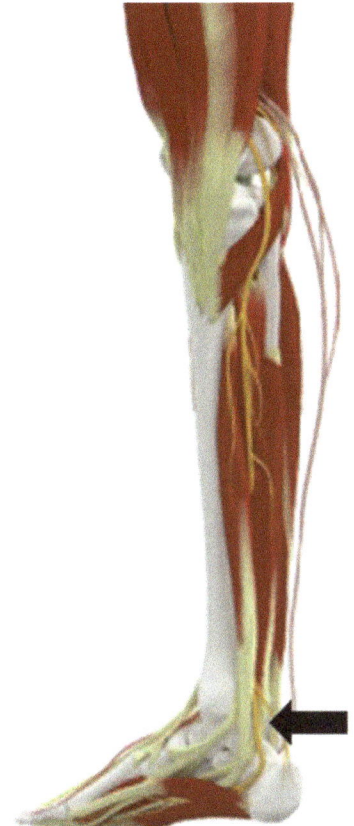

Techniques

Posterior tibial nerve stimulation can be delivered via percutaneous or transcutaneous approaches. PTNS is most commonly delivered unilaterally; however, there are studies examining bilateral PTNS therapy [4, 9].

In the percutaneous approach a 34 gauge solid needle is inserted at a 60° angle slightly posterior to the tibia and about 5 cm cephalad to the medial malleolus [10, 11]. An electrode from the stimulator is attached to the needle. An accompanying surface electrode is placed on the ipsilateral calcaneus [10, 11] (Fig. 9.3).

Transcutaneous posterior tibial nerve stimulation (T-PTNS) is delivered using surface electrodes rather than needles, applied over the posterior tibial nerve at the same area, and connected to transcutaneous electrical nerve stimulators (TENS) [12] (Fig. 9.4).

Fig. 9.3 Percutaneous posterior tibial nerve placement. A 34 gauge solid needle is inserted at a 60° angle slightly posterior to the tibia and about 5 cm cephalad to the medial malleolus. An electrode from the stimulator is attached to the needle. An accompanying surface electrode is placed on the ipsilateral calcaneus. (Image courtesy of Dr. Priyanka Gupta and Dr. Kenneth Peters)

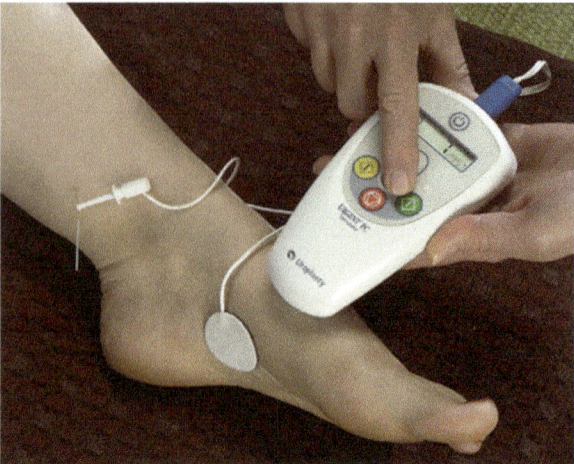

Fig. 9.4 Transcutaneous posterior tibial nerve stimulation. Transcutaneous posterior tibial nerve stimulation is delivered using surface electrodes applied over the posterior tibial nerve and the plantar aspect of the foot and connected to transcutaneous electrical nerve stimulator as demonstrated. (Image courtesy of Dr. Giulia Lane)

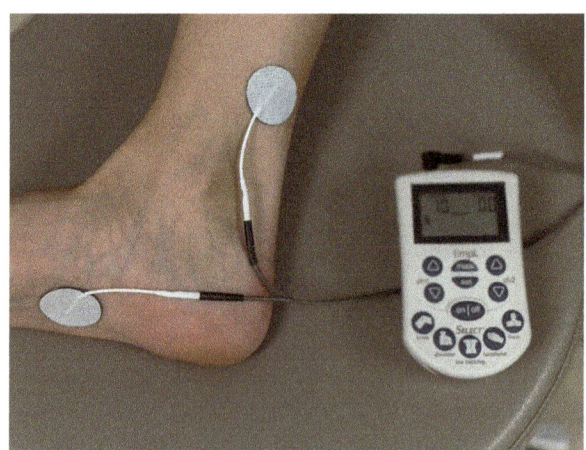

In both percutaneous and transcutaneous approaches, stimulation is delivered with low voltage stimulators. The range of voltage is 0.5–0 mA for percutaneous PTNS and 10–50 mA for transcutaneous PTNS; both are delivered with a square waveform for a duration of 200 μs at 20 Hz [4, 8, 10, 11, 13, 14]. The voltage is increased to confirm appropriate sensory and motor response. Motor responses consistent with accurate needle flexion include flexion of the great toe or fanning of the digits, whereas sensory responses include sensation over the sole of the foot. Once an appropriate response is achieved, the stimulation is gradually increased to a level of tolerable intensity for the patient [2, 11, 15].

Therapy for PTNS is commonly delivered for 30 min once a week for 12 consecutive weeks [8, 10, 11]. However, alternative schedules of therapy frequency and duration have been described [4, 16, 17]. Patients who have improvement in symptoms may continue therapy with maintenance sessions. Maintenance PTNS therapy is commonly delivered monthly; however, the frequency and duration of mainte-nance sessions described in the literature is variable [18, 19]. In the United States, two commercial stimulators for percutaneous PTNS exist: Urgent PC (Cogenix, Minneapolis, MN) and Nuvo (Medtronic, Minneapolis, MN). Many commercially available TENS stimulators are available for transcutaneous PTNS but are not FDA approved for this purpose.

Evidence for Effectiveness

Percutaneous Posterior Tibial Nerve Stimulation

A 2016 systematic review and meta-analysis of external electrical stimulation for treatment of overactive bladder found that there was moderate quality evidence to show that percutaneous tibial nerve stimulation was more effective than sham or placebo at improving overactive bladder symptoms (RR 3.19, 95% CI 2.22–4.58) [4]. The same review found that women who were treated with PTNS had over twice the improvement in UUI symptoms compared to sham (RR 2.23, 95% CI 1.46–3.40) [4]. The randomized controlled trials that provide the bulk of evidence for efficacy of percutaneous posterior tibial nerve stimulation are summarized below.

In 2010 Peters and colleagues published results of a multicenter, randomized controlled trial of 12 weekly 30 min sessions of percutaneous tibial nerve stimula-tion or sham therapy, termed the SUmmiT trial [11]. The trial included ambulatory adult men and women older with more than 3 months of severe symptoms of UUI as measured by four or more points on the OAB-q short form (SF) for urgency and an average urinary frequency of ten or more voids per day. Patients had failed con-servative care and had a 2 week washout period of antimuscarinic therapy prior to treatment. The study excluded patients with neurogenic bladder and those with use of third-line therapies for OAB, current urinary, or vaginal infections and those with pacemakers or implantable defibrillators. The primary outcome was the efficacy of PTNS compared to sham therapy as measured by a seven level global response assessment (GRA) at week 13 after completing 12 consecutive weekly intervention sessions lasting 30 min each. Patients who reported bladder symptoms as moder-ately or markedly improved on the GRA were considered responders.

A total of 220 adults were randomized (110 to each group), at 13 weeks using intention to treat analysis, 55% of patients in the PTNS group reported moderately or markedly improved GRA compared to 21% in the sham group ($p < 0.001$) [11]. The study evaluated outcomes on voiding diary, GRA subset symptom components, OAB-q SF, and SF-36 questionnaire as secondary outcomes. These were analyzed on a per-protocol outcome, with 103 patients analyzed in the PTNS group and 106 in the sham group. The study found significant improvement in GRA subset symptom components of bladder, urinary urgency, frequency, and urge incontinence symptoms between the sham and intervention group. There was a mean decrease (improvement) in OAB-q SF severity score of 36.7 (SD 21.5) points in the PTNS group compared to 29.2 (SD 20.7) points in the sham group ($p = 0.01$). Prior research has found that the minimally important difference for the OAB-q SF is 11 points, indicating that this difference is not only statistically but also clinically significant [20]. Statistically significant improvement in the PTNS group compared to sham was also found in the mean difference between baseline and 13 weeks in the OAB-q health-related quality of life scores. However, the mean difference between baseline and 13 weeks on the SF-36 physical and mental domain scales was not different between those undergoing PTNS therapy versus sham. Voiding diary results showed that PTNS decreased mean voids by −2.4 (SD 2.5) episodes per day, compared to 1.5 (SD 2.4) decrease per day with sham ($p = 0.01$) [11].

The Sustained Therapeutic Effects of Percutaneous Tibial Nerve Stimulation (STEP) study by Peters and colleagues enrolled 50 participants who were randomized to PTNS therapy and met the primary outcome of efficacy in the SUmmiT trial [18]. Patients in the STEP study underwent the following tapered protocol of five PTNS treatments: every 14 days for 28 days (two treatments), every 21 days for 42 days (two treatments), and one treatment after 28 days. Based on the OAB symptom changes with the varying intervals between treatments, patients were continued on regular PTNS therapy that sustained therapeutic benefits. GRA assessments were collected every 3 months for 36 months. The primary outcome was moderate or marked improvement on GRA at 36 months.

After the tapering protocol, study participants underwent a median of one therapy per month (IQR 1.0–1.6), based on the interval where they maintained therapeutic effect [18]. Voiding diary parameters were all improved at every 6 month follow-up time point through 36 months, with a median decrease from 12 to 8.7 voids per day at 36 months. At 36 months, 29 patients remained in the study, of these 28 (97%) met the primary endpoint for response to therapy. Although the study had a large amount of attrition, the authors noted that only 2 of 50 patients withdrew from the study due to difficulty attending treatment sessions [18].

In 2010 Finazzi-Agrò and colleagues published results of a randomized controlled trial comparing percutaneous PTNS with a placebo treatment. The study included adult women with urgency incontinence and urodynamically diagnosed detrusor overactivity incontinence that was refractory to conservative therapy and anticholinergic medications. They excluded those with pacemakers or defibrillators, active or recurrent urinary tract infections, diabetes mellitus, neurogenic bladder, bladder capacity <100 mL, and women with other urologic diagnoses. Women in the PTNS group received three 30 min treatments per week for a total of 12 sessions, while women in the sham group received the same frequency and duration of treatment but had the PTNS needle placed at the head of the gastrocnemius muscle. The primary outcome measure was the proportion of women who achieved at least a 50% reduction in UUI episodes on a 3 day voiding diary between baseline and follow-up (4 weeks). The study randomized 35 women and found that 71% of women in the PTNS arm met criteria for response compared to no women in the sham group ($p = 0.001$); median UI episodes over 3 days decreased from 4.1 to

1.8 in the PTNS group versus 4.2 to 3.8 in the sham group. The median number of voids per day decreased from 13.6 to 9.5 in the PTNS group versus 14.7 to 13.9 in the sham group. There was a significant increase in quality of life, measured by the urinary incontinence quality of life scale (I-QOL), in the PTNS group.

Transcutaneous Posterior Tibial Nerve Stimulation

There are at least three randomized controlled trials of transcutaneous posterior tibial nerve stimulation for the treatment of UUI. The authors of each conclude that there are statistically significant improvements in urinary symptoms among patients randomized to T-PTNS.

In 2010 Lucas Schreiner and colleagues randomized 51 women over the age of 60 with UUI to 12, 30 min, weekly sessions of T-PTNS and bladder training with Kegels versus bladder training with Kegels alone [14]. The number of daytime voids, nocturia episodes, and number of UUI episodes on 3 day voiding diary were improved in both groups; the T-PTNS had a more marked improvement compared to the control group in all three (number of voids: mean difference -1.4 vs -0.2, $p = 0.013$; nocturia mean difference: -1.6 vs 0.4, $p < 0.001$; UUI episodes mean difference -6.3 vs -1.3, $p < 0.001$) [14]. The investigators found that both groups had significant improvement on the International Consultation on Incontinence Questionnaire-Urinary Incontinence Short Form (ICIQ-UI-SF); however, the improvement in the T-PTNS was greater than the control arm (7.2 vs 2.6, $p < 0.001$) [14]. Prior researchers have found that the minimally important difference for this questionnaire is a five point decrease at 12 months [21]. The researchers reported that those undergoing T-PTNS had statistically greater improvement in the King's Health Questionnaire domains of impact on urinary incontinence, limitations of daily activities, physical limitations, emotions, sleep/provision, and measures of severity [14].

Booth and colleagues randomized 30 adults over 65 years with bladder or bowel dysfunction in residential care homes to transcutaneous PTNS versus sham treatment for 30 min, twice weekly for 6 weeks (12 total sessions) [22]. They measured results at 6 weeks and found that the total American Urological Association Symptom Index (AUA-SI) score decreased by a median of seven points in the T-PTNS group compared to a one point increase in the sham group ($p < 0.001$). Based on the AUA-SI, they found that 13 out of 15 patients in the T-PTNS arm reported improved symptoms compared to only four in the sham arm. The investigators did not find a difference in ICIQ-UI-SF score change from baseline to post intervention between the two arms. Patients in the T-PTNS arm had a mean reduction of 60 mL in post void residual as measured by ultrasound compared to only 4.8 mL in the sham arm ($p = 0.048$) [22].

In 2019, Baoretto and colleagues randomized 65 women to either transcutaneous tibial nerve stimulation ($n = 22$), perineal exercises ($n = 22$), or oxybutynin 10 mg daily (n = 13). There was a significant decrease in the number of voids on a 3-day voiding diary (pre vs post: 7.8 vs 7.1, p = 0.015) and in the number of UUI episodes (1.7 vs. 0.05, p = 0.015) in the T-PTNS group. The authors did find significant improvement in OABq SF scores in all three groups, but there was no significant difference in improvement between arms [23].

Recently Inés Ramírez-García and colleagues randomized 68 men and women to either transcutaneous versus percutaneous PTNS, each 30 min weekly sessions for 12 weeks. They performed a non-inferiority analysis and found that transcutaneous PTNS is non-inferior to percutaneous PTNS [12].

These studies provide consistent, level I evidence that percutaneous PTNS significantly improves overactive bladder symptoms compared to sham interventions, as evidenced by patient-reported outcome measures and quantitative analysis of voiding diaries.

Side Effects/Complications

One of the advantages of PTNS is that it can be performed in outpatient settings and poses minimal health risks, and there are few exclusion criteria. However, PTNS is contraindicated in patients with pacemakers or implantable defibrillators, pregnant patients, or patients planning to become pregnant during the treatment duration. Percutaneous PTNS is also contraindicated in patients prone to excessive bleeding.

Adverse events of percutaneous PTNS are rare and, if present, are mild and temporary. Most adverse events are associated with pain or discomfort at the needle entry site. In the study of percutaneous PTNS versus sham by Peters et al. (2010), six PTNS subjects (of 110) reported nine mild or moderate treatment-related adverse events. These consisted of ankle bruising (n = 1, 0.9%), discomfort at needle site (n = 2, 1.8%), bleeding at needle site (n = 3, 2.7%), and tingling in the leg (n = 1, 0.9%) [11]. The sham-controlled trial by Finazzi Agro found that no patients had serious complications, but transient pain at the needle insertion site was reported [16]. One study reported a 4 week, self-limited neuropathy corresponding to the distribution of the medial plantar branch of the tibial nerve with no associated conduction delay or ultrasonographic evidence of nerve injury [19]. Transcutaneous PTNS may have less adverse events; however in head-to-head comparisons of the two therapies, there were no serious adverse events reported in either group [12].

Access to treatment and treatment adherence may pose a significant barrier to PTNS. Patients must be able to travel to weekly appointments given the need for a medical provider to place the needle. Researchers have evaluated PTNS in residential care homes, which may decrease the burden of travel on patients. Newer technologies have evaluated implantable devices that would also alleviate this burden. However, of those who start therapy, treatment overall adherence is high and has not shown to be different between percutaneous or transcutaneous approaches [12].

Failed PTNS Pathophysiology and Treatment

In the initial randomized trials, only 5–6% of patients withdrew prior to the end of 12 weeks of percutaneous PTNS therapy [11, 24]. Outside of RCTs, rates of attrition prior to completing initial therapy as high as 22% have been reported [25]. Among patients who complete initial PTNS therapy, 48–76% of patients continue on to monthly maintenance sessions, with median duration of maintenance found to be about 1 year in large retrospective studies [18, 19, 25, 26]. A retrospective study of 400 patients undergoing PTNS at a single center in the Netherlands found that the median treatment duration among all patients was about 4 months [26]. This is consistent with the fact that about half of patients stop therapy after the initial 3 month treatment. However, the median treatment duration was considerably longer, about 4 years, among those who underwent PTNS with good therapeutic response and who did not drop out for other reasons [26]. In modeling, the authors found that the risk of quitting PTNS therapy due to logistic reasons (problems traveling to appointment) or physical reasons (pain at ankle site) was over 40% at 6 years for follow-up [26].

There is a paucity of literature on predictors of successful percutaneous PTNS outcomes among patients with OAB. Brandon and colleagues performed a prospective, open-label study to evaluate whether progression to maintenance PTNS is related to overall perceived improvement (measured by patient global impression of improvement, PGII) rather than symptom-specific improvement as measured by the OABq-SF [25]. Of 90 men and women who began PTNS, 70 (78%) completed therapy, 38 (54%) continued to monthly maintenance sessions, and less than half of these ($n = 17$, 45%) completed 12 months of monthly maintenance sessions, representing 19% of the initial patients who began therapy [25]. The authors found no differences in demographics, distance traveled to the office, health status, and urinary symptom scores between those who completed therapy and those who did not. They did find that patients who completed and elected monthly maintenance treatment had lower BMI (24 vs 28, $p < 0.01$) and lower PGII scores at week 12 (3.0 vs 4.0, $p < 0.01$) but not baseline or 12 week OABq-SF scores, compared to those who did not proceed to monthly maintenance [25].

Two studies elucidated reasons for discontinuing monthly percutaneous PTNS therapy [25, 26]. In one, nearly half of patients cited dissatisfaction with treatment therapy (10/21, 48%), while a large proportion did not list why they discontinued PTNS (8/21, 38%) [25]. Similarly, a large retrospective study of patients undergoing percutaneous PTNS found that 9% stopped therapy for no reason, while 40% stopped because of logistic reasons or pain at the ankle [26].

Patients who do not have significant benefit from initial percutaneous PTNS therapy can be offered first-, second-, or alternate third-line therapies [5]. However, literature shows that these patients often do not pursue further treatment. For example, in a study of 402 Dutch patients who started PTNS, 228 did not pursue maintenance PTNS, and of these the majority elected for no further therapy (57%), followed by medication therapy (27%) [26]. Similarly, Brandon et al. found that those who elected against monthly maintenance PTNS, the largest group pursued pharmacotherapy (19%, $n = 13$) followed by 15% who were lost to follow-up or elected no treatment [25]. Only 11% ($n = 7$) of patients elected to undergo other third-line therapies such as sacral neuromodulation (4%, $n = 3$) or onabotulinum toxin A (7%, $n = 5$) [25]. Women with urgency incontinence who stop percutaneous PTNS therapy or do not proceed to monthly PTNS may be at high risk of ceasing to pursue further intervention for their UUI symptoms and may benefit from closer follow-up.

New Technology in Posterior Tibial Nerve Stimulation

Implantable devices for posterior tibial nerve stimulation are at the cutting edge of neuromodulation for urge incontinence in women. These devices are placed overlying the posterior tibial nerve in office-based procedures utilizing local anesthesia only. There are three technologies available: fully implanted devices, leadless receiver devices, and devices with implanted leads that are powered by external stimulators [27, 28].

Implanted leads that are powered by external pulse transmitters, such as the Stimrouter® Peripheral Nerve Stimulation system (Bioness, United States), have been used for neuromodulation in patients with chronic pain [28]. However, there are ongoing trials to evaluate this technology for patients with urinary urge incontinence (NCT02873312) [29]. Leadless devices, such as the BlueWind RENOVA™ (BlueWind Medical, Herzliya, Israel), involve implanting a receiver "antenna" which is then powered by a cuff placed around the ankle [27, 30]. The fully implanted devices (eCoin™, Valencia Technologies, California) require no external energy source [27, 31].

In addition to implantable devices, ambulatory transcutaneous tibial nerve stimulation devices are currently being developed (geko™, Firstkind Ltd., United Kingdom) [28, 32]. These devices are attached to the skin overlying the posterior nerve by patients while at home. The device delivers 27 mA of current at 1 Hz and has seven settings corresponding to between 70 and 560 µs of pulse width [32].

Conclusion

Posterior tibial nerve stimulation is a viable option of the treatment of urge urinary incontinence in women. It can be delivered through transcutaneous or percutaneous approaches; however, percutaneous approaches have more robust outcome data. These approaches pose minimal risk of adverse events. Newer technologies are emerging to improve the convenience of therapy to women at home.

References

1. Mcguire EJ, Shi-chun Z, Horwinski ER, Lytton B. Treatment of motor and sensory detrusor instability by electrical stimulation. J Urol. 1983;129:78–9.
2. Heesakkers J, Blok B. Electrical stimulation and neuromodulation in storage and emptying failure. In: Partin AW, Dmochowski RR, Kavoussi LR, Peters CA, editors. Campbell Walsh Wein urology. Elsevier; 2021. p. 2739–2755.e3.
3. Stoller ML, Copeland S, Millard RJ, Murnaghan GF. The efficacy of acupuncture in reversing the unstable bladder in pig-tailed monkeys. J Urol. 1987;137(6):104A.
4. Stewart F, Gameiro OLF, El Dib R, Gameiro MO, Kapoor A, Amaro JL. Electrical stimulation with non-implanted electrodes for overactive bladder in adults. Cochrane Database Syst Rev. 2016;4:CD010098. https://doi.org/10.1002/14651858.cd010098.pub3.
5. Lightner DJ, Gomelsky A, Souter L, Vasavada SP. Diagnosis and treatment of overactive bladder (non-neurogenic) in adults: AUA/SUFU guideline amendment 2019. J Urol. 2019;202:558–63.
6. Granger CJ, Cohen-Levy WB. Anatomy, bony pelvis and lower limb, posterior tibial nerve. StatPearls; 2020.
7. van der Pal F, Heesakkers JPFA, Bemelmans BLH. Current opinion on the working mechanisms of neuromodulation in the treatment of lower urinary tract dysfunction. Curr Opin Urol. 2006;16:261–7.
8. Gaziev G, Topazio L, Iacovelli V, Asimakopoulos A, Di Santo A, De Nunzio C, Finazzi-Agrò E. Percutaneous Tibial Nerve Stimulation (PTNS) efficacy in the treatment of lower urinary tract dysfunctions: a systematic review. BMC Urol. 2013;13:61.
9. Takano S. Bilateral transcutaneous posterior tibial nerve stimulation for functional anorectal pain. 2014 IEEE 19th International Functional Electrical Stimulation Society Annual Conference (IFESS). 2014. https://doi.org/10.1109/ifess.2014.7036731
10. MacDiarmid SA, Peters KM, Shobeiri SA, Wooldridge LS, Rovner ES, Leong FC, Siegel SW, Tate SB, Feagins BA. Long-term durability of percutaneous tibial nerve stimulation for the treatment of overactive bladder. J Urol. 2010;183:234–40.
11. Peters KM, Carrico DJ, Perez-Marrero RA, Khan AU, Wooldridge LS, Davis GL, Macdiarmid SA. Randomized trial of percutaneous tibial nerve stimulation versus Sham efficacy in the treatment of overactive bladder syndrome: results from the SUmmiT trial. J Urol. 2010;183:1438–43.
12. Ramírez-García I, Blanco-Ratto L, Kauffmann S, Carralero-Martínez A, Sánchez E. Efficacy of transcutaneous stimulation of the posterior tibial nerve compared to percutaneous stimulation in idiopathic overactive bladder syndrome: randomized control trial. Neurourol Urodyn. 2019;38:261–8.
13. Nuhoğlu B, Fidan V, Ayyildiz A, Ersoy E, Germiyanoğlu C. Stoller afferent nerve stimulation in women with therapy resistant overactive bladder; a 1-year follow up. Int Urogynecol J Pelvic Floor Dysfunct. 2006;17:204–7.
14. Schreiner L, dos Santos TG, Knorst MR, da Silva Filho IG. Randomized trial of transcutaneous tibial nerve stimulation to treat urinary incontinence in older women. Int Urogynecol J. 2010;21:1065–70.
15. van Balken MR, Vandoninck V, Gisolf KW, Vergunst H, Kiemeney LA, Debruyne FM, Bemelmans BL. Posterior tibial nerve stimulation as neuromodulative treatment of lower urinary tract dysfunction. J Urol. 2001;166:914–8.
16. Finazzi Agrò E, Campagna A, Sciabica F, Petta F, Germani S, Zuccalà A, Miano R. Posterior tibial nerve stimulation: is the once-a-week protocol the best option? Minerva Urol Nefrol. 2005;57:119–23.
17. Yoong W, Ridout AE, Damodaram M, Dadswell R. Neuromodulative treatment with percutaneous tibial nerve stimulation for intractable detrusor instability: outcomes following a shortened 6-week protocol. BJU Int. 2010;106:1673–6.

18. Peters KM, Carrico DJ, Wooldridge LS, Miller CJ, MacDiarmid SA. Percutaneous tibial nerve stimulation for the long-term treatment of overactive bladder: 3-year results of the STEP study. J Urol. 2013;189:2194–201.
19. Yoong W, Shah P, Dadswell R, Green L. Sustained effectiveness of percutaneous tibial nerve stimulation for overactive bladder syndrome: 2-year follow-up of positive responders. Int Urogynecol J. 2013;24:795–9.
20. Blanker MH, Alma HJ, Devji TS, Roelofs M, Steffens MG, van der Worp H. Determining the minimal important differences in the International Prostate Symptom Score and Overactive Bladder Questionnaire: results from an observational cohort study in Dutch primary care. BMJ Open. 2019;9:e032795.
21. Sirls LT, Tennstedt S, Brubaker L, Kim H-Y, Nygaard I, Rahn DD, Shepherd J, Richter HE. The minimum important difference for the International Consultation on Incontinence Questionnaire-Urinary Incontinence Short Form in women with stress urinary incontinence. Neurourol Urodyn. 2015;34:183–7.
22. Booth J, Hagen S, McClurg D, Norton C, MacInnes C, Collins B, Donaldson C, Tolson D. A feasibility study of transcutaneous posterior tibial nerve stimulation for bladder and bowel dysfunction in elderly adults in residential care. J Am Med Dir Assoc. 2013;14:270–4.
23. Boaretto JA, Mesquita CQ, Lima AC, Prearo LC, Girão MJBC, Sartori MGF. Comparison of oxybutynin, electrostimulation of the posterior tibial nerve and peroneal exercises in the treatment of overactive bladder syndrome. Fisioter Pesqui. 2019;26:127–36.
24. Finazzi-Agrò E, Petta F, Sciabica F, Pasqualetti P, Musco S, Bove P. Percutaneous tibial nerve stimulation effects on detrusor overactivity incontinence are not due to a placebo effect: a randomized, double-blind, placebo controlled trial. J Urol. 2010;184:2001–6.
25. Brandon C, Oh C, Brucker BM, Rosenblum N, Ferrante KL, Smilen SW, Nitti VW, Pape DM. Persistence in percutaneous tibial nerve stimulation treatment for overactive bladder syndrome is best predicted by patient global impression of improvement rather than symptom-specific improvement. Urology. 2021;148:93–9. https://doi.org/10.1016/j.urology.2020.12.009.
26. Te Dorsthorst MJ, Heesakkers JPFA, van Balken MR. Long-term real-life adherence of percutaneous tibial nerve stimulation in over 400 patients. Neurourol Urodyn. 2020;39:702–6.
27. Yamahiro J, de Riese W, de Riese C. New implantable tibial nerve stimulation devices: review of published clinical results in comparison to established neuromodulation devices. Res Rep Urol. 2019;11:351–7.
28. Te Dorsthorst M, van Balken M, Heesakkers J. Tibial nerve stimulation in the treatment of overactive bladder syndrome: technical features of latest applications. Curr Opin Urol. 2020;30:513–8.
29. Overactive bladder treatment using StimRouter neuromodulation system: a prospective randomized trial. https://clinicaltrials.gov/ct2/show/NCT02873312?term=stimrouter&cond=oab&draw=2&rank=1. Accessed 28 Jan 2021.
30. Heesakkers JPFA, Digesu GA, van Breda J, Van Kerrebroeck P, Elneil S. A novel leadless, miniature implantable Tibial Nerve Neuromodulation System for the management of overactive bladder complaints. Neurourol Urodyn. 2018;37:1060–7.
31. MacDiarmid S, Staskin DR, Lucente V, et al. Feasibility of a fully implanted, nickel sized and shaped tibial nerve stimulator for the treatment of overactive bladder syndrome with urgency urinary incontinence. J Urol. 2019;201:967–72.
32. Seth JH, Gonzales G, Haslam C, Pakzad M, Vashisht A, Sahai A, Knowles C, Tucker A, Panicker J. Feasibility of using a novel non-invasive ambulatory tibial nerve stimulation device for the home-based treatment of overactive bladder symptoms. Transl Androl Urol. 2018;7:912–9.
33. Rigoard P. The tibial nerve. In: Rigoard P, editor. Atlas of anatomy of the peripheral nerves. Cham: Springer; 2017.

Chapter 10
Sacral and Pudendal Neuromodulation (SNM)

Priyanka Gupta

Introduction

Neuromodulation is the electrical or chemical modulation of a nerve that is used to influence the physiologic behavior of the end-organ innervated by that nerve [1]. In the area of voiding dysfunction, neuromodulation is a minimally invasive third-line therapy that can be used in the management of refractory overactive bladder (OAB) symptoms, fecal incontinence, and nonobstructive urinary retention. For the purposes of this chapter, we will focus on refractory OAB symptoms.

Mechanism of Action of Sacral and Pudendal Neuromodulation

The initial investigations into electrical stimulation for bladder dysfunction were pioneered by Tanagho and Schmidt in the 1970s [2]. In their widely cited study from 1988, they performed a dorsal rhizotomy and selective ventral neurotomy in a canine model. They then performed sacral nerve stimulation which led to restoration of normal bladder emptying [3]. Their studies ultimately led to the development of an implantable neuroprosthesis for the treatment of urge incontinence. The first device was the Pisces Quad foramen electrode which was placed into the S3 foramen through a paraspinous incision with splitting of the lumbodorsal fascia and paraspinous musculature. The electrode had to be sutured to the posterior sacral periosteum and tunneled to the generator which was implanted into the abdominal

P. Gupta (✉)
University of Michigan, Ann Arbor, MI, USA
e-mail: guptapr@med.umich.edu

© The Author(s), under exclusive license to Springer Nature
Switzerland AG 2022
A. P. Cameron (ed.), *Female Urinary Incontinence*,
https://doi.org/10.1007/978-3-030-84352-6_10

177

wall. This ultimately led to FDA approval of the device for the treatment of urge incontinence in 1997 [4]. The operative technique and device have subsequently undergone modifications to allow for more minimally invasive placement techniques and newer generators with longer battery lives.

The mechanism by which neuromodulation works is not completely understood. There are multiple neural pathways that influence responses of the bladder, gastrointestinal tract, and pelvic floor. The lumbar, pelvic, and pudendal nerves are comprised of afferent and efferent axons. During the storage phase, the sympathetic nervous system is active in allowing for bladder relaxation for storage and contraction of the urethral sphincter to prevent incontinence. In normal voiding the sensation of bladder fullness is sent to the sacral spinal cord via afferent axons to the pontine micturition center. An efferent signal is then sent through the parasympathetic nervous system through the S2–S4 nerve roots leading to bladder contraction and urethral relaxation to allow for voiding to occur. During the voiding phase, the pudendal nerve is activated to allow for relaxation of the external sphincter [5].

Sacral neuromodulation (SNM) is thought to be involved in the suppression of interneuronal transmission of the bladder reflex pathway. The two widely proposed mechanisms of action for SNM are (1) selective activation of afferent fibers that leads to inhibition of intraspinal and supraspinal signals for micturition and (2) direct activation of efferent fibers to the striated urethral sphincter which leads to inhibition of detrusor contraction [5, 6].

Pudendal neuromodulation (PNM) has been studied and employed as another method for addressing voiding dysfunction through peripheral nerve stimulation. The pudendal nerve is composed of fibers from S1 to S3 and is integral in bladder storage and emptying, defecatory function, and pelvic sensation as it provides innervation to the external urethral sphincter, anal sphincter, and pelvic floor muscles [7]. Similarly, pudendal nerve simulation is thought to affect both the spinal and cortical centers of storage and control. Specifically, in animal studies, it has been found that PNM suppresses nociceptive and non-nociceptive bladder signals [8, 9]. Due to the composition of the pudendal nerve, it is thought to have a broader sacral nerve root stimulation and has been studied as a potential target for patients that have failed SNM treatment.

Operative Techniques for Sacral and Pudendal Neuromodulation

Sacral Neuromodulation

This procedure is performed in two stages. The first stage can be an office-based procedure called a percutaneous nerve evaluation (PNE) or in the operating room as a first-stage lead placement (FSLP). Both methods allow for a trial period for the patient to test the clinical effectiveness of the therapy prior to proceeding with the implantation of the full device and battery. The operative steps for PNE and FSLP are detailed below.

Percutaneous nerve evaluation (PNE) [10]

1. Position the patient prone.
2. Identify the S3 foramen using anatomic landmarks if fluoroscopy is not available by measuring 10 cm from the coccyx along the midline of the spine and then 2 cm lateral and 3 cm superior to this point.[1]
3. Inject a local anesthetic at the needle insertion point.
4. Insert the needle at a 30–60° angle.
5. Confirm lead placement by asking the patient to report the location of the sensation of stimulation. Stimulation should be felt in the vaginal, scrotal, or rectal area. They may exhibit flexion of the big toe.
6. A temporary electrode is passed through the needle and taped to the skin.
7. Connect the lead to an external temporary pulse generator for 3–7 days while completing voiding diaries and symptom scores.

First-stage lead placement (FSLP) [10]

1. Position the patient prone.
2. Intravenous sedation is administered.
3. With the assistance of fluoroscopy, a directional guidewire is used to locate the midline which is marked with a vertical line. The intersection of the sacroiliac joint and the spinous process is then identified and marked with a transverse line. This defines the area of the S3 foramen (Fig. 10.1).

Fig. 10.1 Identification of FSLP landmarks. (Picture Credit: Kenneth Peters MD)

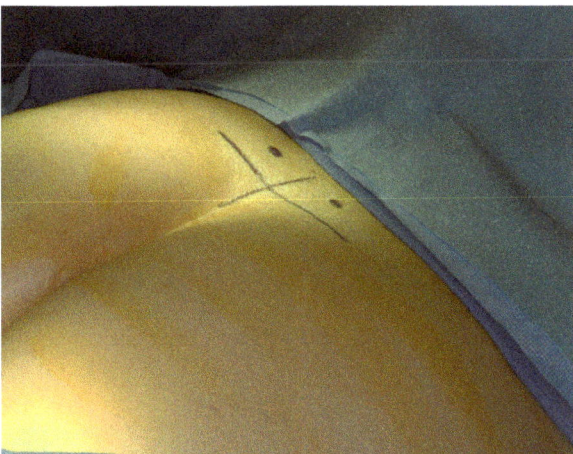

---

[1] This method can be used for the FSLP below if the surgeon prefers rather than using fluoroscopy, and the 3 cm rise in measurement is highly dependent on body habitus with thicker tissue requiring more distance.

4. If the S3 foramen is clearly visible on fluoroscopy in the anterior/posterior view, then mark the upper medial aspect of the foramen (Fig. 10.2).
5. If the S3 foramen is not identified due to overlying bowel contents, then start approximately 2 cm lateral and 3 cm (depending on body habitus) superior to the point where the two lines cross (see step #3). Mark this on the right and left sides (Fig. 10.2).
6. Pass the needle at a 60° angle into the entrance point to access the foramen and advance it to the edge of the inferior sacral bone plate (Fig. 10.3).

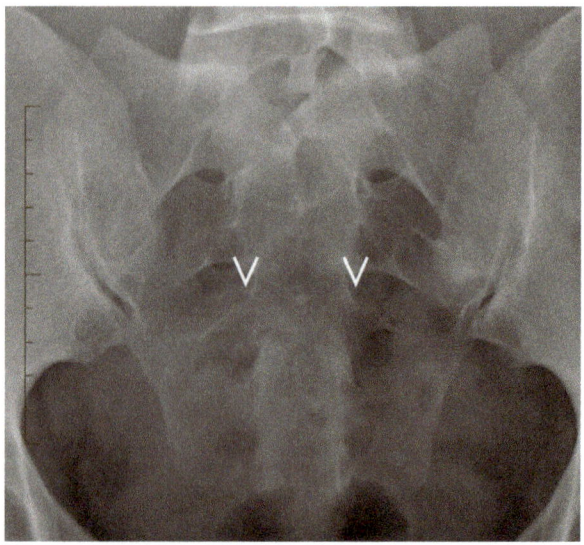

Fig. 10.2 Identifying the medial aspect of the S3 foramen. (Picture Credit: Medtronic)

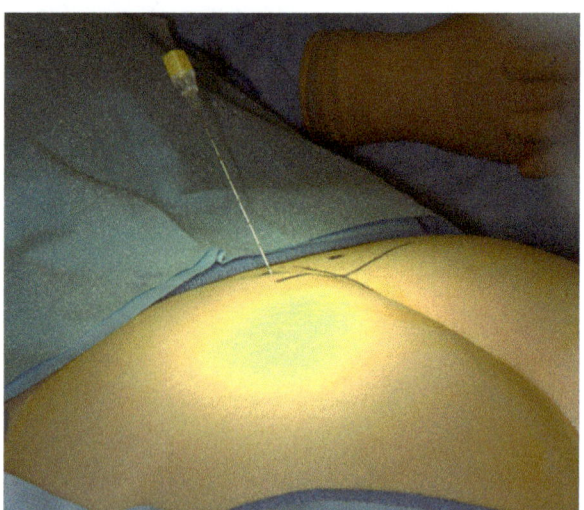

Fig. 10.3 Placement of the needle. (Picture Credit: Kenneth Peters MD)

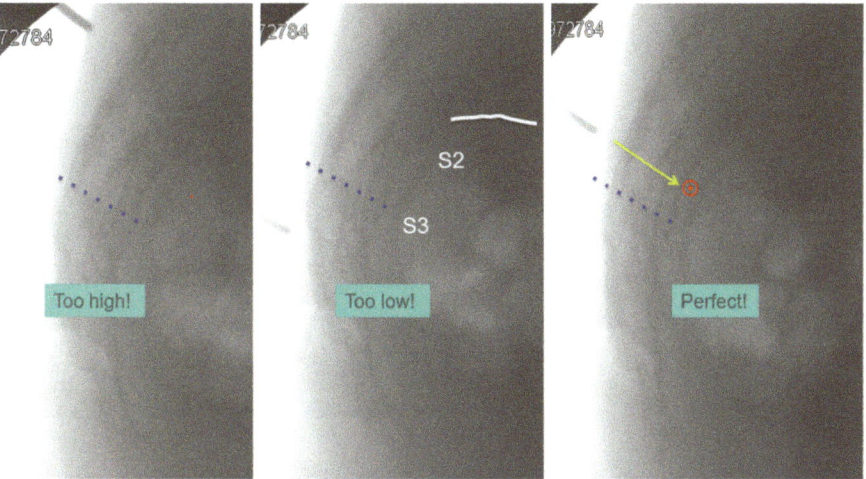

Fig. 10.4 Ideal lateral placement. (Credit: Medtronic (will need to obtain permission))

7. Perform electrical stimulation. The ideal response is a bellow contraction of the pelvic floor followed by flexion of the great toe that occurs with less than 2 volts of stimulation. A S2 stimulation would be suggested by plantar flexion of the entire foot with heel rotation, and a S4 stimulation would result in a bellows contraction alone.

8. Fluoroscopy with motor response can help confirm the appropriate foramen. In Fig. 10.4, imaging first shows the skin location to be too high, then too low, then just right. On the lateral view the target area should be about 1 cm above the S3 hillock. The hillock is the anterior protrusion of the bone from the anterior surface of the sacrum at the level of S3 as seen on the lateral x-ray (Fig. 10.4).

9. The directional guide wire is then placed through the cannula, and the tract is dilated using an introducer sheath. The introducer should not be advanced beyond the inferior bone plate.

10. The tined lead with the curved stylet positioned inferior and lateral is then deployed under fluoroscopic guidance. It has four cylindrical electrodes numbered 0–3. Leads 2 and 3 should straddle the bone edge. Each electrode is then stimulated individually. The motor responses are assessed with the goal to achieve response on all four electrodes under low voltage (ideally less than 2 volts).

11. Lead position is confirmed with fluoroscopy in the lateral and anterior–posterior positions (Figs. 10.5 and 10.6).

12. The potential site of the IPG is identified on the ipsilateral buttock, and a 2 cm incision is made and a subcutaneous pocket created. The IPG will be placed here if the test stage is successful.

Fig. 10.5 Ideal lateral
X-ray. (Credit: Medtronic)

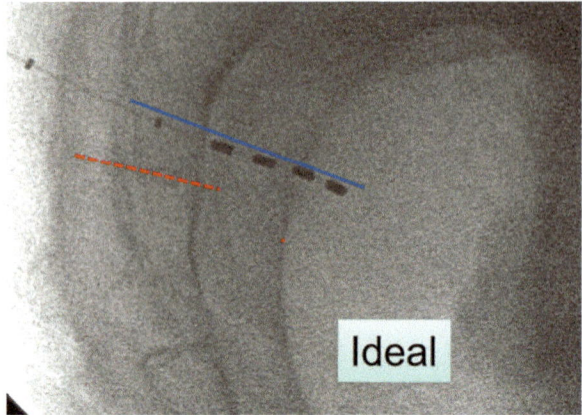

Fig. 10.6 Ideal anterior-
posterior X-ray. (Credit:
Medtronic)

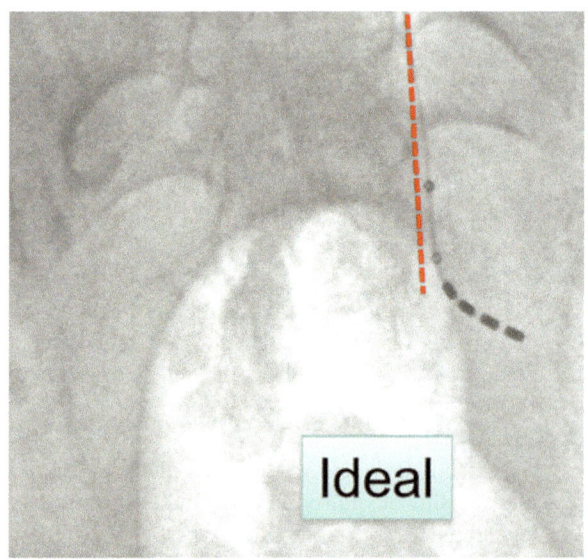

13. The percutaneous extension lead is connected to the tined lead, which is tun-
    neled out of the contralateral buttock and connected to the external neuromodu-
    lation system (ENS) and programming parameters are set.
14. The incision is closed, and the external portions of the leads are secured with
    sterile 4 × 4 dressings and a bandage.
15. Using the ENS, the patient trials various stimulation parameters during the
    14 day test period and maintains voiding diaries and symptom scores to assess
    improvement.

Second-stage placement of permanent implantable pulse generator (IPG) [10]

1. Patients experiencing a greater than 50% improvement in their symptoms and who are satisfied with the response are considered responders and should undergo a Stage II implant.
2. The previous pocket site is reopened, and the incision is enlarged. The lead is then connected to the permanent IPG. This can be a non-rechargeable or rechargeable IPG.
3. The device connections are tested and confirmed in the operating room. The pocket incision is closed with absorbable sutures.
4. Specific stimulation programs are tested and then programmed into the device postoperatively to achieve optimal device settings.

Pudendal Neuromodulation

Pudendal neuromodulation is also performed in two stages. This must be done with an FSLP due to the technique of placement and the length of the lead required. The technique requires the addition of electromyography monitoring and is described below, and the optimal point of stimulation of the pudendal nerve is at the level of the ischial spine. The stage II placement is similar to SNM, but the lead has to be tunneled to the IPG site from the incision site on the lower buttocks to the lower back.

First-stage lead placement [10]

1. Place the patient in a prone position, making sure to pad all pressure points appropriately.
2. Administer IV sedation, prep and drape the patient using sterile technique, and inject local anesthetic at the proposed puncture sites.
3. Place needle electrodes into the anal sphincter at the 3 o'clock and 9 o'clock positions. These will be used for intraoperative electromyography (EMG) monitoring.
4. Access the pudendal nerve percutaneously through the ischiorectal space, passing a foramen needle just medial to the ischial tuberosity in a medial-to-lateral direction toward the ischial spine (Fig. 10.7). As the needle is passed, perform stimulation at 5 Hz and 5 volts to identify the nerve. The nerve can be identified by seeing a compound muscle action potential (CMAP) on EMG and an anal wink on exam.
5. Advance the needle along the nerve while stimulating to confirm that it is running parallel to the nerve and not perpendicular. This will allow multiple electrodes on the permanent lead to stimulate the nerve.
6. Verify the position of the needle under fluoroscopy (Fig. 10.8). Then place a directional guide wire and lead introducer, in a similar fashion to the sacral neuromodulation procedure.

Fig. 10.7 Pudendal needle insertion. (Credit: Kenneth Peters MD)

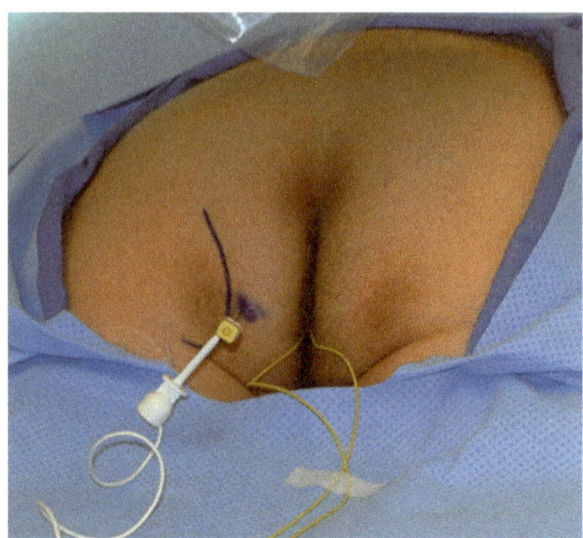

Fig. 10.8 Needle position on fluoroscopy. (Credit: Kenneth Peters MD)

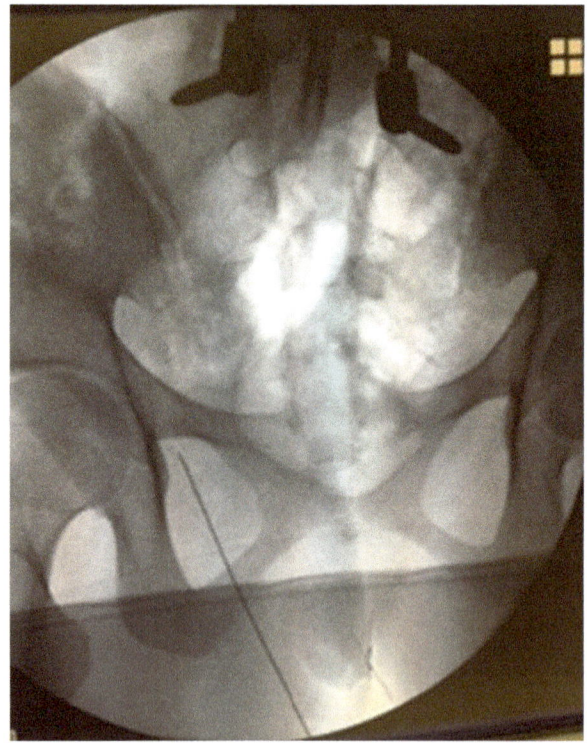

7. Advance a tined lead into position under fluoroscopy. Due to the longer trajectory from the lead to the neurostimulator site, the longer 41 cm lead is used. Stimulate each electrode and record the voltage required to obtain a motor and EMG response; ideally at CMAP and anal wink should be seen at less than 2 volts of stimulation on all four electrodes. When a satisfactory response is achieved at each electrode, deploy the tines.
8. Lead position should be confirmed with fluoroscopy in the anterior-posterior (Fig. 10.9) and lateral (Fig. 10.10) position.

Fig. 10.9 Anterior-posterior lead position. (Credit: Kenneth Peters MD)

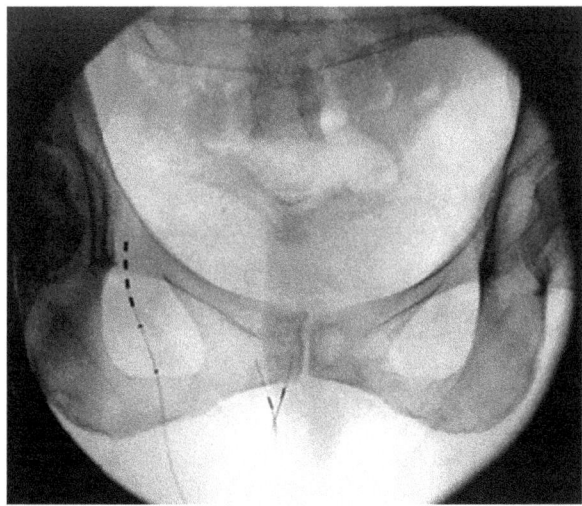

Fig. 10.10 Lateral lead position. (Credit: Kenneth Peters MD)

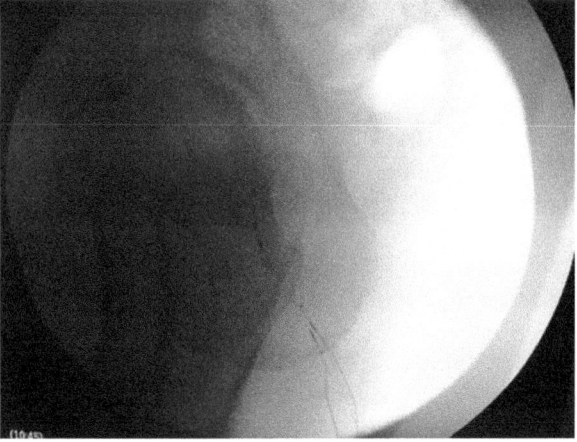

9. The potential site of the neurostimulator is identified on the ipsilateral buttock, and a 1 cm incision is made and a subcutaneous pocket created. The neurostimulator will be placed here if the test stage is successful.
10. The lead is tunneled to the neurostimulator site, and the percutaneous extension lead is connected and tunneled out of the contralateral buttock for temporary external stimulation.
11. The incision is closed, and the external cords are secured with dressing and a bandage.

Recent Technological Advances

Currently two SNM devices are FDA approved and available in the United States and Europe: the Interstim® Medtronic device and Axonics® sacral neuromodulation system. Both systems utilize a percutaneous quadripolar tined lead. They bring recent upgrades to the technology in that both are MRI compatible and offer a rechargeable battery option. The non-rechargeable implantable pulse generator (IPG) typically has a 3–5 year life span, and the new rechargeable IPG has 10–15 year life span and requires regular charging.

The MRI compatibility will expand the ability to use the device for patients that may require MRI for other conditions. It is estimated that at least half of patients that have neurostimulator or pacemaker devices may require an MRI examination in their lifetime [11]. In addition, approximately 23% of SNM explanations were performed due to the need for MRI examination [12]. The use of SNM as a therapeutic option for patients with neurologic disease such as multiple sclerosis and incomplete spinal cord injury as well as those with low back pain has previously been limited due to their need for regular MRI examinations [12]. This advance in technology will allow these patients to be able to trial the therapy for their urinary symptoms. Future studies will be needed to assess the efficacy and utility in these special populations.

The second advancement in SNM is the rechargeable IPG. The advantage of a rechargeable battery is it allows for a smaller volume IPG which can be more comfortable and a longer battery life which may decrease the need for reoperation. The currently available systems are the recharge-free Interstim II system (12.5 cm^3 volume), rechargeable Interstim Micro system (2.8 cm^3 volume), and rechargeable Axonics system (5.5 cm^3 volume). The smaller volume IPG may be desirable for patients with a lower BMI who are more conscious about the appearance of the device and comfort. However, for the majority of patients with average or above average BMI, the difference in size is not likely to be appreciable once implanted under the skin. In addition, in order to recharge the device, the belt and charger have to be positioned close to the IPG, and this may be more challenging for obese patients to be able to do this reliably. In elderly patients this may be an issue as well due to dexterity and memory issues that may inhibit a patient's ability to reliably charge the device. Finally, confidence with technology may be an important factor to consider as some patients may not be comfortable with performing the charging process.

The longevity of the IPG is another consideration as the theoretic advantage may be decreased number of operations needed for battery replacement. However, this may not be applicable in all situations. In a longitudinal study of 325 patients with SNM for fecal incontinence with a mean follow-up of 7.1 years, 21.7% had the device removed due to lack of efficacy, device problems, or infections [13]. Therefore, the reoperation rate may be driven by other factors related to device function rather than battery life alone. At this time, it is also unknown if battery fade may occur overtime. Some devices are known to experience battery fade, and it is possible that the life span may be shorter than 10–15 years.

In order to decide between recharge-free or rechargeable IPGs, clinicians must engage in a shared decision-making process with patients to ensure that these factors are considered and to help choose the therapy that will allow for the best outcomes for the patient. In a multicenter study of 352 patients with spinal cord stimulators, they found that patients with rechargeable devices ended their therapy sooner than those with recharge-free [14]. Studies in the spinal cord stimulator and deep brain stimulator space suggest that rechargeable systems carry a higher burden of therapy management which may lead to earlier discontinuation by patients [12]. This remains to be studied in the SNM space in the years to come.

Outcomes of SNM

Several studies have been published establishing the efficacy of SNM for refractory OAB-wet and OAB-dry patients. The InSite trial was a prospective, multicenter trial comparing SNM to standard medical therapy at 6 months. Patient were then followed to assess outcomes of SNM at 5 years. There were 340 patients who underwent test stimulation, and 272 were implanted. In the OAB-wet patients, they had a baseline of 3.1 ± 2.7 leaks/day. With SNM they had a mean reduction of 2.2 ± 2.7 leaks/day. In the OAB-dry patients, they had a baseline of 12.6 ± 4.5 voids/day and with SNM had a mean reduction of 5.1 ± 4.1 voids/day which was statistically significant. Eighty percent of subjects reported improvement in their urinary symptoms at 12 months [15]. In 5 year follow-up of the same cohort of patients, the therapeutic success was 67% using modified completers analysis and 82% using completers analysis. Patients showed improvement in all quality of life measures [16]. In a worldwide, multicenter trial of SNM, OAB-dry patients in the stimulation group demonstrated a significant improvement in number of voids from 16.9 ± 9.7 at baseline to 9.3 ± 5.1 at 6 months ($p < 0.0001$) after stimulation. In this study, 88% of the stimulation group had improvement in degree of urgency of urination. Interestingly in this study patients also had the device turned off after 6 months of therapy and had worsening of their symptoms back to baseline. All patients in this group had the therapy reactivated at the conclusion of the test [17]. Thereby the active stimulation from SNM is therapeutic in improving refractory OAB symptoms, but does not cure them permanently.

The literature also strongly supports the efficacy of SNM in improving incontinence and pad use in OAB-wet patients. In a randomized trial by Schmidt et al., 75% of patients were clinically successful, of which out of 34 patients, 16 (47%) were completely dry and 10 (29%) had greater than 50% reduction in incontinence episodes. Fifty-seven percent of patients no longer required diapers or pads [18]. In a retrospective review by Sutherland et al., they observe a decrease in mean daily incontinence episodes from 5.0 to 1.0 and mean daily pad use from 2.3 to 0.3 ($p < 0.05$) [19]. In a randomized trial by Weil et al., the noted a decrease in major leakage episodes of 3.8 per day ($p = 0.0039$) and a mean decrease in daily pad use of 4.4 ($p = 0.0011$) per day [20].

Although it is not currently an FDA-approved indication for the treatment, SNM has also been shown to be effective in patients with interstitial cystitis and pelvic pain. In a 2020 meta-analysis of SNM for pelvic pain syndromes, six prospective cohort studies and four retrospective case series were examined. They found that a mean of 69% of patients proceeded to implantation (range 52–91%). All of the studies included reported a decrease in pain score with SNM [21]. In a study by Peters of 26 patients with refractory IC, 71% had improvement in pelvic pain, 68% in urgency, and 72% in frequency symptoms. Ninety-six percent of patients stated they would undergo the implant again and would recommend the therapy to a friend [22]. In a retrospective study by Marinkovic, they noted similar success with SNM for treatment of IC as measured on the VAS scale with scores improving from 6.5 to 2.4 ($p < 0.01$), with a mean follow-up of 89 months [23].

Outcomes of PNM

Pudendal neuromodulation is currently not FDA approved for the treatment of voiding disorders and therefore is an off-label therapy for the treatment of OAB, urinary retention, and pelvic pain. In a 2005 prospective randomized control trial of SNM versus PNM, more patients chose PNM. During the trial phase both sacral and pudendal leads were implanted. Each lead was trialed for 7 days, and patients were blinded to which lead was being stimulated. Data regarding symptom improvement was collected for each lead. Patients were then able to choose which lead to have the IPG connected to. Out of 24 patients, 19 chose PNM, and five chose SNM. PNM was superior for overall symptom improvement ($p = 0.02$), urgency ($p = 0.005$), frequency ($p = 0.007$), and bowel function ($p = 0.049$) [24]. In another trial of SNM versus PNM for patients with refractory interstitial cystitis, a similar design as above was performed with both sacral and pudendal lead placement. In this study of 22 patients, 77% underwent permanent lead implantation, 59% chose the pudendal lead, and 18% chose the sacral lead. Overall reduction in symptoms was 59% in PNM and 44% in SNM [25]. In another study of 19 patients with pudendal neuralgia that underwent PNM, 36% of patients had complete or almost complete relief, 52% had significant pain relief, and 15% reported small pain relief. All of the patients underwent IPG placement [26]. In these small studies of PNM, it appears to be effective for the treatment of voiding dysfunction and pelvic pain.

Failed SNM

Some studies estimate that between 10% and 25% of patients fail SNM [15, 27]. PNM is particularly effective in patients that have failed SNM as few therapeutic options remain for this challenging population. In a study of patients who were refractory to SNM treatment for OAB and IC/PBS, 93% (41 out of 44) responded to PNM. At 1 year of follow-up, 83% of patients were still using their device, and 74% stated they would have the procedure again [28]. Carmel reported on three patients that underwent PNM after failed SNM for chronic pelvi-perineal pain who reported significant improvement in their symptoms after 2 years of follow-up [29]. PNM is an effective therapy for patients that have been refractory to SNM and should be considered for the treatment of voiding dysfunction and pelvic pain.

Adverse Events/Complications

SNM and PNM can be associated with device-related adverse events (AEs). We will focus on events related to the contemporary device which is a percutaneous quad-ripolar tined lead with a curved stylet. However, some earlier studies may discuss other implantation techniques. The InSite trial reported an adverse event rate of 30.5% [30]. The most common adverse event is pain, either from stimulation from the device or site related at the IPG or lead. The majority of adverse events were resolved with conservative management. Thirteen percent required surgical intervention; this included pain at the surgical site (4%), lack/loss of efficacy (4%), and infection (3%) [31]. In a multicenter study from France, they also noted a 33% AE rate with the majority of events resolved with reprogramming. The most frequent AEs included implant site pain (5%; 16/301) and implant site infections (4%; 13/301) [32].

IPG site complications tend to be the most common and can occur due to trauma at the site of the IPG or suboptimal placement during surgery. It is important to take into account patient factors including body habitus, location of bony landmarks, and the typical location of the patient's pants. If the placement is over a bony landmark or too superficial, this can cause pain. Additionally, if patients have changes in their weight, this can affect the location of the IPG as well which may lead to need for revision.

Lead migration is another potential complication. The incidence of this has greatly decreased since the introduction of the tined lead. In a study by Peters et al., they noted that lead migration decreased from 42% with the open placement technique to 15% with the percutaneous tined lead placement which was statistically significant [33]. More commonly this tends to occur if patients experience a fall or trauma to the site which can disrupt the lead. Improvement in surgical technique with the tined lead has greatly reduced this event from occurring.

Infection of the device is less common given the antibiotic prophylaxis that is typically administered at the time of device implantation. In the literature the rate of infection is estimated at less than 10% [33, 34]. Most infections present early after implantation. In the InSite trial 5/10 infections presented in the first 3 months after implantation [34]. As with any device infection, the recommendation is to remove the implanted device. After adequate treatment and resolution of the infection, one can consider replacement.

PNM has similar device-related complications including pain either at the lead or IPG site and risk of infection. PNM is more susceptible to lead migration as the lead is placed through soft tissue and not secured through a bony foramen. This makes the lead more susceptible to displacement through falls or trauma to the buttocks area. Peters et al. reported lead migration in three out of 84 patients and infection in one out of 84 patients [28].

Conclusions

Sacral and pudendal neuromodulation are effective therapies for refractory overactive bladder symptoms. With the introduction of MRI compatibility and rechargeable devices, the application of this therapy will be expanded in the upcoming years and will likely improve therapy for other conditions including neurogenic bladder and pelvic pain. This therapy is associated with a low risk of adverse events and provides sustained improvement in symptoms overtime.

References

1. Peters KM. Alternative approaches to sacral nerve stimulation. Int Urogynecol J. 2010;21(12):1559–63.
2. Tanagho EA, Schmidt RA, Orvis BR. Neural stimulation for control of voiding dysfunction: a preliminary report in 22 patients with serious neuropathic voiding disorders. J Urol. 1989;142(2 Pt 1):340–5.
3. Tanagho EA. Neural stimulation for bladder control. Semin Neurol. 1988;8(2):170–3.
4. Dijkema HE, Weil EH, Mijs PT, Janknegt RA. Neuromodulation of sacral nerves for incontinence and voiding dysfunctions. Clinical results and complications. Eur Urol. 1993;24(1):72–6.
5. Leng WW, Chancellor MB. How sacral nerve stimulation neuromodulation works. Urol Clin North Am. 2005;32(1):11–8.
6. Barboglio Romo PG, Gupta P. Peripheral and sacral neuromodulation in the treatment of neurogenic lower urinary tract dysfunction. Urol Clin North Am. 2017;44(3):453–61.

7. Gracely A, Gupta P. Pudendal neuromodulation for pelvic pain. Curr Bladder Dysfunct Rep. 2020;15:113–20.

8. Gonzalez EJ, Grill WM. Sensory pudendal nerve stimulation increases bladder capacity through sympathetic mechanisms in cyclophosphamide-induced cystitis rats. Neurourol Urodyn. 2019;38(1):135–43.

9. Ness TJ, DeWitte C, McNaught J, Clodfelder-Miller B, Su X. Spinal mechanisms of pudendal nerve stimulation-induced inhibition of bladder hypersensitivity in rats. Neurosci Lett. 2018;686:181–5.

10. Bartley J, Gilleran J, Peters K. Neuromodulation for overactive bladder. Nat Rev Urol. 2013;10(9):513–21.

11. Kalin R, Stanton MS. Current clinical issues for MRI scanning of pacemaker and defibrillator patients. Pacing Clin Electrophysiol. 2005;28(4):326–8.

12. De Wachter S, Knowles CH, Elterman DS, Kennelly MJ, Lehur PA, Matzel KE, et al. New technologies and applications in sacral neuromodulation: an update. Adv Ther. 2020;37(2):637–43.

13. Janssen PT, Kuiper SZ, Stassen LP, Bouvy ND, Breukink SO, Melenhorst J. Fecal incontinence treated by sacral neuromodulation: long-term follow-up of 325 patients. Surgery. 2017;161(4):1040–8.

14. Pope JE, Deer TR, Falowski S, Provenzano D, Hanes M, Hayek SM, et al. Multicenter retrospective study of neurostimulation with exit of therapy by explant. Neuromodulation. 2017;20(6):543–52.

15. Noblett K, Siegel S, Mangel J, Griebling TL, Sutherland SE, Bird ET, et al. Results of a prospective, multicenter study evaluating quality of life, safety, and efficacy of sacral neuromodulation at twelve months in subjects with symptoms of overactive bladder. Neurourol Urodyn. 2016;35(2):246–51.

16. Siegel S, Noblett K, Mangel J, Bennett J, Griebling TL, Sutherland SE, et al. Five-year followup results of a prospective, multicenter study of patients with overactive bladder treated with sacral neuromodulation. J Urol. 2018;199(1):229–36.

17. Hassouna MM, Siegel SW, Nyeholt AA, Elhilali MM, van Kerrebroeck PE, Das AK, et al. Sacral neuromodulation in the treatment of urgency-frequency symptoms: a multicenter study on efficacy and safety. J Urol. 2000;163(6):1849–54.

18. Schmidt RA, Jonas U, Oleson KA, Janknegt RA, Hassouna MM, Siegel SW, et al. Sacral nerve stimulation for treatment of refractory urinary urge incontinence. Sacral Nerve Stimulation Study Group. J Urol. 1999;162(2):352–7.

19. Sutherland SE, Lavers A, Carlson A, Holtz C, Kesha J, Siegel SW. Sacral nerve stimulation for voiding dysfunction: one institution's 11-year experience. Neurourol Urodyn. 2007;26(1):19–28; discussion 36.

20. Weil EH, Ruiz-Cerda JL, Eerdmans PH, Janknegt RA, Bemelmans BL, van Kerrebroeck PE. Sacral root neuromodulation in the treatment of refractory urinary urge incontinence: a prospective randomized clinical trial. Eur Urol. 2000;37(2):161–71.

21. Cottrell AM, Schneider MP, Goonewardene S, Yuan Y, Baranowski AP, Engeler DS, et al. Benefits and harms of electrical neuromodulation for chronic pelvic pain: a systematic review. Eur Urol Focus. 2020;6(3):559–71.

22. Peters KM, Carey JM, Konstandt DB. Sacral neuromodulation for the treatment of refractory interstitial cystitis: outcomes based on technique. Int Urogynecol J Pelvic Floor Dysfunct. 2003;14(4):223–8; discussion 8.

23. Marinkovic SP, Gillen LM, Marinkovic CM. Minimum 6-year outcomes for interstitial cystitis treated with sacral neuromodulation. Int Urogynecol J. 2011;22(4):407–12.

24. Peters KM, Feber KM, Bennett RC. Sacral versus pudendal nerve stimulation for voiding dysfunction: a prospective, single-blinded, randomized, crossover trial. Neurourol Urodyn. 2005;24(7):643–7.

25. Peters KM, Feber KM, Bennett RC. A prospective, single-blind, randomized crossover trial of sacral vs pudendal nerve stimulation for interstitial cystitis. BJU Int. 2007;100(4):835–9.

26. Peters KM, Killinger KA, Jaeger C, Chen C. Pilot study exploring chronic pudendal neuro-modulation as a treatment option for pain associated with pudendal neuralgia. Low Urin Tract Symptoms. 2015;7(3):138–42.
27. Peters KM, Killinger KA, Ibrahim IA, Villalba PS. The relationship between subjective and objective assessments of sacral neuromodulation effectiveness in patients with urgency-frequency. Neurourol Urodyn. 2008;27(8):775–8.
28. Peters KM, Killinger KA, Boguslawski BM, Boura JA. Chronic pudendal neuromodulation: expanding available treatment options for refractory urologic symptoms. Neurourol Urodyn. 2010;29(7):1267–71.
29. Carmel M, Lebel M, Tu LM. Pudendal nerve neuromodulation with neurophysiology guidance: a potential treatment option for refractory chronic pelvi-perineal pain. Int Urogynecol J. 2010;21(5):613–6.
30. Siegel S, Noblett K, Mangel J, Griebling TL, Sutherland SE, Bird ET, et al. Results of a prospective, randomized, multicenter study evaluating sacral neuromodulation with InterStim therapy compared to standard medical therapy at 6-months in subjects with mild symptoms of overactive bladder. Neurourol Urodyn. 2015;34(3):224–30.
31. Noblett K, Benson K, Kreder K. Detailed analysis of adverse events and surgical interventions in a large prospective trial of sacral neuromodulation therapy for overactive bladder patients. Neurourol Urodyn. 2017;36(4):1136–9.
32. Chartier-Kastler E, Le Normand L, Ruffion A, Dargent F, Braguet R, Saussine C, et al. Sacral neuromodulation with the InterStim system for intractable lower urinary tract dysfunctions (SOUNDS): results of clinical effectiveness, quality of life, patient-reported outcomes and safety in a French Multicenter Observational Study. Eur Urol Focus. 2020; https://doi.org/10.1016/j.euf.2020.06.026.
33. Peeters K, Sahai A, De Ridder D, Van Der Aa F. Long-term follow-up of sacral neuromodulation for lower urinary tract dysfunction. BJU Int. 2014;113(5):789–94.
34. Siegel S, Noblett K, Mangel J, Griebling TL, Sutherland SE, Bird ET, et al. Three-year follow-up results of a prospective, multicenter study in overactive bladder subjects treated with sacral neuromodulation. Urology. 2016;94:57–63.

Chapter 11
Botulinum Toxin for Overactive Bladder

Sophia Janes, Sara M. Lenherr, and Anne P. Cameron

Abbreviations

ACh	Acetylcholine
ASB	Asymptomatic bacteriuria
BTXA	Onabotulinum toxin A
DMSO	Dimethyl sulfoxide
GRA	Global Response Assessment
ICS	International Continence Society
NLUTD	Neurogenic lower urinary tract dysfunction
OAB	Overactive bladder
PVR	Post void residual
SNM	Sacral neuromodulation
U	Units
UTI	Urinary tract infection
UUI	Urgency urinary incontinence

S. Janes · S. M. Lenherr
Division of Urology, Department of Surgery, University of Utah Health,
Salt Lake City, UT, USA
e-mail: sophie.janes@hsc.utah.edu; sara.Lenherr@hsc.utah.edu

A. P. Cameron (✉)
Urology, University of Michigan, Ann Arbor, MI, USA
e-mail: annepell@med.umich.edu

A. P. Cameron (ed.), *Female Urinary Incontinence*,
https://doi.org/10.1007/978-3-030-84352-6_11

Introduction

Overactive bladder is discussed in detail in Chaps. 3 and 8 in this book, including risk factors, diagnosis, and conservative treatments. Briefly, the definition of overactive bladder (OAB) from the International Continence Society (ICS) is "severe urgency with or without urge urinary incontinence, usually accompanied with increased daytime frequency and nocturia, in the absence of urinary tract infection or other obvious pathology" [1]. The US Food and Drug Administration approved onabotulinum toxin A (BTXA, Allergan, Irvine, CA) in 2011 for use in neurogenic lower urinary tract dysfunction and in January 2013 for the use in OAB. BTXA is a third-line treatment for OAB, along with posterior tibial nerve stimulation and sacral neuromodulation (SNM) after conservative and pharmacologic agents have failed [2]. Because the majority of the literature available is on BTXA, rather than other formulations, this manuscript will primarily focus on the BTXA formulation unless otherwise specified. Additionally, while the subject of interest for this review is women idiopathic OAB, some evidence is only available in other patient populations and will be identified as such.

Botulinum Toxin Mechanism of Action

The botulinum neurotoxin is produced by the bacterium *Clostridium botulinum*. The lyophilized neurotoxin is reconstituted in preservative-free normal saline and injected into the detrusor muscle cystoscopically as detailed below. The primary target for the botulinum toxin is to block the presynaptic release of acetylcholine from the parasympathetic efferent nerves. However, increasing evidence suggests that afferent nerve input is also effected by BTXA [3].

When injected into the tissue, the neurotoxin is endocytosed into the presynaptic terminal via synaptic vesicle protein SV2. The toxin is then cleaved into a heavy and light chain, and the light chain binds to the SNAP25 protein complex to inhibit the release of acetylcholine (Ach) from presynaptic terminal, therefore preventing acetylcholine-mediated muscle contraction. Additionally, the BTXA neurotoxin also blocks release of other neuropeptides from vesicles such as ATP, NO, calcitonin-related peptide, and substance P [4]. ACh, NO, CRP, and substance P contribute to sensations of fullness, bladder inflammation, and detrusor muscle contractions. ACh acts on muscarinic receptors to enable detrusor contraction. Parasympathetics also release ATP and activate the P2X receptors in detrusor to induce contraction.

Neurotoxins Available Worldwide

Currently, onabotulinum toxin A (BTXA, Allergan, Irvine, CA) is the only FDA-approved toxin to treat overactive bladder in the United States. Other toxins with the identical mechanism of action have been used off-label with comparable effects, but there are no randomized controlled trials to prove equivalent therapeutic benefit. Additionally, OAB literature has a limited description of these formulations [5]. Below is a summary of these different compounds.

Dysport, Abobotulinum Toxin A *(Ipsen Biopharm Ltd., Slough, UK)*

Dysport is the other most widely available toxin available in the United States and is commonly used in pediatric NLUTD. The difference between Dysport and Botox is primarily the purification process. Dysport is purified via a column separation method, whereas Botox undergoes repeat precipitation and redissolution [5]. For NLUTD, generally speaking, there are no clinical differences identified between the two formulations, specifically Botox 300U versus Dysport 750U [6]. One single-center observational study examined the change in outcomes of Botox versus Dysport. Similar rates of reduction in daytime frequency, nocturia, incontinence, and similar duration of effect were reported. But the Dysport cohort had double the rate of symptomatic urinary retention requiring intermittent self-catheterization [7]. A separate 9-year prospective study using Dysport demonstrated similar outcomes to the standard onabotulinum toxin A. Overactive bladder symptom severity improved at similar rates, and self-catheterization rates for elevated PVR were similar in both groups (~18%). OABSS and QoL scores improved by 35% and 41%, respectively (both $p < 0.001$). Urgency incontinence abolished in 26%, and severity of incontinence decreased in 44% participants. Mean interval period between treatments was 21.3 months [8]. One single-center cohort followed 33 women with idiopathic detrusor overactivity who received repeat intradetrusor injections with 500U Dysport [9]. They used a trigone sparing method and noted a reinjection interval longer than what we typically expect for BTXA.

One study examined patients with neurogenic lower urinary tract dysfunction (NLUTD) who switched to Dysport after failing intradetrusor BTXA injections [10]. There was a significant decrease in urinary incontinence episodes, and all patients experienced a reduction in maximum detrusor pressure with 56.14% of patients deemed a treatment success. Although there is no data on this strategy in OAB, it remains to be seen if a neurotoxin switch is a possible solution to toxin resistance that can develop over time after other strategies such as dose escalation have failed [11].

Xeomin, Incobotulinum Toxin A *(Merz Pharmaceutics, Frankfurt Germany)*

Another less commonly used toxin includes Xeomin, or incobotulinum toxin A. A small cohort of elderly males with neurogenic detrusor overactivity was given Xeomin and exhibited significant improvement in daily pad use, daily incontinent episodes, daily urinary frequency, and hours in between self-catheterization [12]. More recently, some providers in the United States have started to use this product because it is more cost-effective (~$150 savings per 100U), but the efficacy has not been demonstrated in large randomized clinical trials for idiopathic OAB.

Other toxins have not been utilized in OAB or are not clinically available including *Lantox Chinese type A botulinum toxin* (Lanzhou Biological Products Institute, China), Myobloc (NeuroBlock, RimabotulinumtoxinB, Solstice Neurosciences Inc.), and Neuronox, (BONTA, Medy-Tox Inc.).

Botox Injection Techniques

Lyophilized BTXA should be reconstituted with injectable, preservative-free normal saline. No bubbling or agitation of the liquid should be performed to prevent denaturation of the protein. Lyophilized BTXA can sit at room temperature for 5 days but should be used within 5 h of reconstitution. Providers should pay careful attention to the dilution, preparation, and storage to prevent primary and secondary treatment failures.

Generally speaking, 10–30 min before injection, a 2% lidocaine is instilled in bladder with sterile technique and permitted to dwell to provide local anesthesia. A recent randomized controlled study investigated pain reduction with the addition of 10 mL 8.4% sodium bicarbonate to the standard 20 mL of 2% lidocaine before injection and found that this alkalinization protocol significantly reduced pain rating immediately following the procedure. Pain was rated (from 0 to 10) as 2.37 ± 0.31 compared to 4.44 ± 0.36 ($p < 0.01$) when the solution was not alkalinized. No differences were observed 1 h after treatment [13]. This is a very cost-effective and simple method to reduce pain without affecting complications or efficacy that deserves further attention.

Per the manufacturer and clinical trials for OAB patients, the reconstituted BTXA (100U) should be reconstituted with 10 mL sterile saline. The needle should be inserted approximately 2 mm into the detrusor, injecting in 20 sites of 0.5 mL, spaced approximately 1 cm apart and sparing the trigone.

Most providers are familiar with this 20 site template injection pattern that was utilized in the clinical trials, but there have been some basic modifications. Many providers have adjusted the dilution to decrease the number of injection sites making the procedure more easily tolerated in the office and particularly in those patients with a friable urothelium where the bleeding risk is diminished with fewer injection sites.

There is limited evidence that supports that the actual injection pattern can be variable. A single-blind randomized controlled study evaluated the efficacy and safety of different numbers of intravesical BTXA injections for OAB patients [14]. Sixty-seven patients were randomized into three different groups all with 100U BTXA diluted in 10 mL with 10 injections in the bladder body ($n = 24$), 20 injections in the bladder body ($n = 22$), and 40 injections in the bladder body ($n = 21$).

The rates of successful treatment defined as Global Response Assessment (GRA ≥ 1) were approximately 80% and were comparable between the groups at 1, 3, and 6 months after treatment with no significant difference in adverse events.

Another recent pilot study showed similar clinical efficacy in a group of OAB patients injected with three injection locations horizontally across the posterior bladder wall (2cc each injection site) [15]. This technique did not demonstrate a decline in BTXA efficacy from prior injection episodes and no increase in adverse events.

Injections in a template avoiding the trigone were standardized in the clinical trials, but many providers inject into the trigone for certain patients given the density of nervous tissue in this area. Most recently, data was presented at the International Continence Society Annual Meeting (2019) on an Allergan-funded protocol called LO-BOT demonstrating an alternate injection paradigm (Clinicaltrials.gov, NCT03052764). In this study protocol, 100U in 10 mL was administered with eight peri-trigonal and two intra-trigonal injections. When compared to prior pooled phase 3 and 4 studies, there was a lower incidence of retention requiring intermittent catheterization (6.2% vs 2.6%). They postulated that the decreased retention could be a result of the injections being more targeted to afferent trigonal nerves rather than the detrusor muscle.

Another variable for injection is depth of injection. Many parameters for adjusting injection depth are determined by the needle that is being used. Smaller gauge flexible needles will penetrate less deeply into the detrusor as compared to rigid needles. While the injection depth provided by the clinical trials was a standard 2 mm into the detrusor, the urothelium and detrusor are dynamic as the bladder fills. Some severely trabeculated bladders are predominantly type III collagen, and identifying where the neuromuscular junctions might be is a challenge. To leverage the possible efferent versus afferent effects of BTXA, some providers intentionally injection a superficial injection to cause more of a urothelial bleb. The thought is that afferent signals might be blocked in sensory urgency patients that have OAB rather than severe detrusor contractions leading to symptoms. This technique can also be used to hopefully reduce the risk of retention, but future study is required.

Other Delivery Techniques Under Investigation

While intradetrusor injection is effective and the equipment is generally widely available, there is motivation to develop other less invasive methods for delivering the neurotoxin to the bladder to reduce pain, infection, and bleeding. Direct intravesical application of BTX is not effective because of the high molecular weight of the BTXA (150 kDa) making it difficult to pass through the urothelial barrier and reach the sub-mucosal nerves. When applied into the bladder via catheter, other methods for penetrating the urothelium and attempting to get the toxin to the neuromuscular junction must be employed [16].

Liposomal formulations allow for passive diffusion of BTXA across the urothe-lial barrier, which cannot be penetrated by the large BTXA molecule alone. In patients with OAB, a double-blind RCT was done to evaluate the effectiveness of liposomal BTXA instillation versus normal saline [17]. Experimental group received intravesical instillation of Lipotoxin containing 80 mg liposomes and 200U BTXA. Total urinary frequency was monitored after 1 month. There was a signifi-cant decrease in urinary frequency in experimental group ($p = 0.0008$) and a signifi-cant decrease in urgency episodes ($p = 0.012$). There was no significant change in urinary incontinence ($p = 0.797$). Compared to intradetrusor injections, this treat-ment was not as beneficial for OAB.

Several other techniques have been trialed including intravesical thermosensitive polymer hydrogel as a vehicle for prolonged drug exposure [18], hyaluronic acid linked to phosphatidylethanolamine (HA-PE) as a carrier for large proteins, such as BTXA through the urothelium [19], disruption of urothelial barrier with 1% prot-amine sulfate or dimethyl sulfoxide (DMSO) [20], or even electromotive drug administration (EDMA) [21] or low energy shock waves [22] with varying success.

As an alternative to intravesical administration, other groups are exploring the feasibility of transvaginal injection [23]. In this feasibility study, eight female cadaver pelvises received transvaginal ultrasound-guided injection of India ink into trigone and posterior wall. Upon histologic analysis, the India ink was present within the detrusor layer suggesting feasibility and accuracy for BTXA injections. While this approach has not been replicated in a clinical practice, there might be appeal of this delivery method for some women, although the injection field is lim-ited to the trigone and posterior bladder wall.

Efficacy

Early reports on the efficacy of BTXA in OAB in small placebo-controlled random-ized trials demonstrated both clinical and urodynamic effects of the toxin in various doses [24, 25]. Symptom relief is experienced as significant changes in urgency, frequency, and urgency incontinence that can occur as early as 3 or 4 days after injection and nocturia typically improving after the first week [25, 26].

Earlier studies used the higher dose of 200 units which is the dose typically used in NGLUTD and had high rates of incomplete bladder emptying [27] but did have excellent efficacy with 75% improvement in incontinence in 72% of patients and a median duration of response of 373 days.

Contemporary large randomized controlled trials have been undertaken with phase II dose ranging studies. Dmochowski et al. [28] enrolled 313 patients (288 women) with overactive bladder and a minimum of eight urgency incontinence epi-sodes per week and were given placebo, 50 units, 100U, 150U, 200U, or 300U of BTXA. Results at 12 weeks showed that all doses of 100U or greater showed improvement over placebo for the primary outcome of reduction of weekly urgency incontinence episodes. These effects in the extension study proved to be sustained over 4 years [29]. Further analysis of the dose–response curve of various doses concluded that doses >150U did not provide demonstrable additional improvement in this outcome. The authors noted that both increases in post-void residual urine volume and use of intermittent catheterization were dose dependent and, therefore, suggested 100U as the dose in OAB that best balances benefits with safety. The urodynamic results of this same study demonstrated that all BTXA doses significantly increased bladder capacity; however, doses greater than 150 resulted in post-void residuals >200 mL [30].

Chapple et al. reported the results of a large, Phase III, multicenter, randomized, placebo-controlled, double-blind trial of injection of 100U of BTXA versus placebo for OAB in 2013 [31]. A total of 277 patients received 100U BTXA and reported a reduction in urgency incontinence episodes of 2.95 per day, compared with a reduction of 1.03 episodes in the 271 patients who received placebo ($p = 0.001$). The results for a positive response on the treatment benefit scale of "greatly improved" or "improved" were also highly significant, in that 62.8% of patients receiving BTXA reported a positive response in comparison to 26.8% of patients receiving placebo ($p = 0.001$). A similar Phase III multicenter study by Nitti et al. compared injection of 100U of BTXA to placebo in 557 patients with OAB [32]. BTXA injection resulted in a reduction of 2.65 episodes of incontinence per day compared with 0.87 for placebo ($p < 0.001$) at week 12. Treatment benefit scale responses were 60.8% positive for BTXA versus 29.2% positive for placebo ($p < 0.001$).

BTXA has been compared head to head with other standard treatments for OAB in women. The ABC double-blind randomized trial compared reduction in urgency incontinence among a group of women ($n = 241$) who either received oral solifenacin (5 mg and if needed 10 mg dose escalation) and a saline bladder injection or 100U bladder BTXA injection and daily oral placebo. These women had an average 5.0 UUI episodes per day, and in both groups the episodes were reduced by 3.4 and 3.3, respectively, ($p = 0.81$) with more dry mouth in the anticholinergic group but more retention and UTIs [33].

Another large randomized trial compared BTXA 200U to SNM in women at nine medical centers including 364 women with UUI [34]. Early results at 6 months demonstrated a slightly greater decrease in daily UUI episodes with BTXA compared to SNM (-3.9 vs -3.3; $p = 0.01$). Follow-up over 2 years showed a similar reduction in UUI in both groups with (-3.88 vs -3.50 episodes/d, 95% confidence interval [CI] $= -0.14$–0.89; $p = 0.15$), with no differences in UUI resolution, but the BTXA group had higher patient satisfaction despite a higher UTI rate with recurrent urinary tract infections (UTIs) occurring in 24% BTXA compared to 10% after SNM ($p < 0.01$), and 6% required intermittent catheterization post second injection. SNM revision and removals occurred in 3% and 9% patients, respectively [35].

BTXA has also been shown to be effective in those people who fail SNM. The assumption would be that these are more complex cases of UUI since they have already failed third-line therapy. Of the 76 patients over half stopped receiving injections over the follow-up period, but 43% of patients did report efficacy after their first injection making this a viable option in this situation [36].

Injection Complications and Other Considerations

Direct complications that are attributed to BTXA injection can be categorized as immediate and delayed. Immediate risks include pain with injection, anxiety, and bleeding. These immediate risk factors can be modified by the setting of the injection, either in the clinic or the operating room or other setting where more sedation can be administered. In the operating room, there is also more access to electrocautery for bleeding if necessary. However, many instances of bleeding can be managed with direct manual pressure of the tip of the scope against the area of bleeding.

The continuation of anticoagulation during the time of BTXA injection is contraindicated per the BTXA packaging instructions. However, using a smaller gauge needle and modification of some injection parameters (number of sites, volume of injection) generally reduces the risk of bleeding to a minimal. Additionally, keeping a patient on anticoagulation is often weighed with the risk of stopping such therapy and does help with the logistics of planning. Many providers continue anticoagulation and will perform the injection with a discussion of slightly increased risk of bleeding with the patient [37].

The delayed complications include most commonly symptomatic UTI, persistent pain, worsening urinary incontinence, constipation, and urinary retention. Management of asymptomatic bacteriuria (ASB) prior to injection of BTXA in the idiopathic OAB patient is rather controversial. According to the BTXA clinical trial design, most providers likely verify that the patient does not have a UTI by assessing symptoms and performing urinalysis at the time of injection. However, many providers across the country will inject regardless of urinalysis and give a single dose of antibiotic or empiric course along with sending a culture. This strategy has been shown to be safe in a study that compared the rate of post procedure UTI in a group of patients undergoing injection who either had a negative urinalysis (no blood, leucocyte esterase or nitrites) or a positive urine dip pre procedure. Of note none of these patients had symptoms of a UTI. There were no differences in the rate of UTI post procedure between groups [38]. Even in the presence of asymptomatic bacteriuria, the rate of hospitalization and sepsis was not different nor was the efficacy in a retrospective study of 457 injection sessions. There was an increased risk of UTI post procedure in those with ASB [39].

Immunogenicity: Timing of Other BTXA Injections

Currently, there are four major classes of FDA-approved indications for BTXA injection in the United States. In addition to urological disorders, patients can receive BTXA for movement disorders (e.g., spasticity and cervical dystonia) and dermatologic conditions (e.g., axillary hyperhidrosis) in addition to cosmetic applications. Additionally, there are many off-label indications for which providers will inject BTXA including pelvic floor tension myalgia. While the utility of BTXA should be appreciated, many patients receive these asynchronous injections from different providers and often do not inform other providers of these injections.

The concern about "asynchronous" injections is the increased risk of immunogenicity. Immunogenicity occurs because the body neutralizes or blocks the BTXA when administered, resulting in secondary treatment failures. BTXA is regarded as foreign by the host, and a potential immune response can be mounted against the antigen. The risk of this immunogenicity is increased with repeated administration in a "booster" timeline, typically 2–3 weeks apart. Whether the actual 150 kD BTXA protein or the complexing proteins stimulate the immune response is currently unknown [40]. Another theory is that failure of BTXA secondary to antibody generation is because the urinary bladder (with its urothelium) is an immunoreactive organ that is designed to be sensitized to other antigens, such as urinary tract infections [41].

To mitigate the risk of immunogenicity, the urologist should ask whether a patient has received other BTXA recently. This is especially important considering the chronicity of the conditions that BTXA treat and the nonpermanent neuromuscular junction blockade requiring repeated injections. The authors' clinical practice is to keep asynchronous injections within 1 week of each other or delay until 3 months apart. Because of this clinical paradigm, most insurance plans will not pay for repeated injections more often than 3 months. If there is a concern that treatment failure is due to neutralizing antibodies, one can do a functional assessment test injection into the temporal muscle to look for muscle response (unilateral brow injection) or assay for neutralizing antibodies against botulinum toxin [40]. However, the management of treatment failure is the same regardless of the presence of neutralizing antibodies, despite costly extra testing—transition to alternative therapies.

Distant Spread

A feared complication of BTXA injection is the distant spread of the toxin to nontarget sites. In 2009, the FDA released a black box warning discussing the symptoms, and signs of botulism then appeared following detrusor injections for cervical dystonia in cerebral palsy patients [42]. No lethal side effects have been noted, but multiple adverse effects of detrusor injections have been recorded. The most common reported side effect is muscular weakness following intradetrusor injections. In these case reports, two patients with spinal cord injuries developed muscle weakness that made transfers difficult [43], and in another report, there was transient generalized weakness in four patients with NDO [44]. Another patient with multiple sclerosis reported bilateral leg weakness after BTXA injection which was later determined to be an MS exacerbation [45]. Notably, all case reports are in patients with neurologic dysfunction, not idiopathic OAB. Distant spread of BTXA injections is a rare but serious complication of BTXA injections that requires more investigation.

Contraindications

BTXA is contraindicated in anyone who has had a prior allergic reaction to Botox or Botox cosmetics and has an active UTI or an infection at the proposed injection site. It is currently unknown how BTXA interacts with pregnant and breastfeeding individuals; however, animal studies have revealed reduced fetal body weight, decreased fetal skeletal ossification, abortions, early deliveries, and maternal death with intramuscular BTXA injections in pregnant animals (per Allergan BTXA product label). Due to the anticholinergic effects, BTXA is also not advised in patients with amyotrophic lateral sclerosis, myasthenia gravis, or Lambert Eaton syndrome; however, these conditions are not labeled as contraindication at the moment.

Conclusion

Botulinum toxin is a highly effective third-line management method for OAB, but there are many considerations to help improve outcomes. Providers should be aware of other uses of BTXA and patient use patterns. Patients should not be injected any more than every 3 months, and asynchronous injections should be clustered to help avoid immunogenicity. The methods to administer BTXA are likely to advance in the near future for patient safety and comfort.

References

1. Haylen BT, Freeman RM, Swift SE, Cosson M, Davila GW, Deprest J, et al. An International Urogynecological Association (IUGA) /International Continence Society (ICS) joint terminology and classification of the complications related directly to the insertion of prostheses (meshes, implants, tapes) & grafts in female pelvic flo. Int Urogynecol J. 2011;22(1):3–15.
2. Gormley EA, Lightner DJ, Faraday M, Vasavada SP. Diagnosis and treatment of overactive bladder (non-neurogenic) in adults: AUA/SUFU guideline amendment. J Urol [Internet]. 2015;193(5):1572–80. Available from: https://doi.org/10.1016/j.juro.2015.01.087
3. Coelho A, Cruz F, Cruz CD, Avelino A. Spread of onabotulinumtoxinA after bladder injection. Experimental study using the distribution of cleaved SNAP-25 as the marker of the toxin action. Eur Urol. 2012;61(6):1178–84.
4. Chen JL, Kuo HC. Clinical application of intravesical botulinum toxin type a for overactive bladder and interstitial cystitis. Investig Clin Urol. 2020;61:S33–42.
5. Walker TJ, Dayan SH. Comparison and overview of currently available neurotoxins. J Clin Aesthet Dermatol. 2014;7(2):31–9.
6. Stoehrer M, Wolff A, Kramer G, Steiner R, Löchner-Ernst D, Leuth D, et al. Treatment of neurogenic detrusor overactivity with botulinum toxin A: the first seven years. Urol Int. 2009;83(4):379–85.

7. Ravindra P, Jackson BL, Parkinson RJ. Botulinum toxin type A for the treatment of non-neurogenic overactive bladder: does using onabotulinumtoxinA (Botox®) or abobotulinumtoxinA (Dysport®) make a difference? BJU Int. 2013;112(1):94–9.

8. Craciun M, Irwin PP. Outcomes for intravesical abobotulinumtoxin A (Dysport) treatment in the active management of overactive bladder symptoms—a prospective study. Urology [Internet]. 2019;130:54–8. Available from: https://doi.org/10.1016/j.urology.2019.04.018

9. Abeywickrama L, Arunkalaivanan A, Quinlan M. Repeated botulinum toxin type A (Dysport®) injections for women with intractable detrusor overactivity: a prospective outcome study. Int Urogynecol J Pelvic Floor Dysfunct. 2014;25(5):601–5.

10. Bottet F, Peyronnet B, Boissier R, Reiss B, Previnaire JG, Manunta A, et al. Switch to abobotulinum toxin A may be useful in the treatment of neurogenic detrusor overactivity when intradetrusor injections of onabotulinum toxin A failed. Neurourol Urodyn. 2018;37(1):291–7.

11. Apostolidis A, Cameron AP. Neurourological management after failed Intradetrusor onabotulinumtoxinA injections. Eur Urol Focus [Internet]. 2020;6(5):814–6. Available from: https://doi.org/10.1016/j.euf.2019.10.003

12. Asafu-Adjei D, Small A, McWilliams G, Galea G, Chung D, Pak J. The intravesical injection of highly purified botulinum toxin for the treatment of neurogenic detrusor overactivity. Can Urol Assoc J. 2019;14(10):520–6.

13. Pereira e Silva R, Ponte C, Lopes F, Palma dos Reis J. Alkalinized lidocaine solution as a first-line local anesthesia protocol for intradetrusor injection of onabotulinum toxin A: results from a double-blinded randomized controlled trial. Neurourol Urodyn. 2020;39(8):2471–9.

14. Liao C-H, Chen S-F, Kuo H-C. Different number of intravesical onabotulinumtoxinA injections for patients with refractory detrusor overactivity do not affect treatment outcome: a prospective randomized comparative study. Neurourol Urodyn. 2016;35:717–33.

15. Martínez-Cuenca E, Bonillo MA, Morán E, Broseta E, Arlandis S. Onabotulinumtoxina re-injection for refractory detrusor overactivity using 3–4 injection sites: results of a pilot study. Urology. 2020;137:50–4.

16. Chen P-Y, Lee W-C, Wang H-J, Chuang YC. Therapeutic efficacy of onabotulinumtoxinA delivered using various approaches in sensory bladder disorder. Toxins (Basel). 2020;12(75):1–11.

17. Kuo HC, Liu HT, Chuang YC, Birder LA, Chancellor MB. Pilot study of liposome-encapsulated onabotulinumtoxinA for patients with overactive bladder: a single-center study. Eur Urol [Internet]. 2014;65(6):1117–24. Available from: https://doi.org/10.1016/j.eururo.2014.01.036

18. Tyagi P, Li Z, Chancellor M, De Groat WC, Yoshimura N. Sustained intravesical drug delivery using thermosensitive hydrogel. Pharm Res. 2004;21(5):832–7.

19. El Shatoury MG, DeYoung L, Turley E, Yazdani A, Dave S. Early experimental results of using a novel delivery carrier, hyaluronan-phosphatidylethanolamine (HA-PE), which may allow simple bladder instillation of botulinum toxin A as effectively as direct detrusor muscle injection. J Pediatr Urol [Internet]. 2018;14(2):172.e1–6. Available from: https://doi.org/10.1016/j.jpurol.2017.11.016

20. Petrou SP, Parker AS, Crook JE, Rogers A, Metz-Kudashick D, Thiel DD. Botulinum A toxin/dimethyl sulfoxide bladder instillations for women with refractory idiopathic detrusor overactivity: a phase 1/2 study. Mayo Clin Proc [Internet]. 2009;84(8):702–6. Available from: https://doi.org/10.4065/84.8.702

21. Ladi-Seyedian SS, Sharifi-Rad L, Kajbafzadeh AM. Intravesical electromotive botulinum toxin type "A" administration for management of urinary incontinence secondary to neuropathic detrusor overactivity in children: long-term follow-up. Urology [Internet]. 2018;114:167–74. Available from: https://doi.org/10.1016/j.urology.2017.11.039

22. Nageib M, Zahran MH, El-Hefnawy AS, Barakat N, Awadalla A, Aamer HG, et al. Low energy shock wave-delivered intravesical botulinum neurotoxin-A potentiates antioxidant genes and inhibits proinflammatory cytokines in rat model of overactive bladder. Neurourol Urodyn. 2020;39(8):2447–54.

23. Syan R, Briggs MA, Olivas JC, Srivastava S, Comiter CV, Dobberfuhl AD. Transvaginal ultrasound guided trigone and bladder injection: a cadaveric feasibility study for a novel route of intradetrusor chemodenervation. Investig Clin Urol. 2019;60(1):40–5.
24. Flynn MK, Amundsen CL, Perevich MA, Liu F, Webster GD. Outcome of a randomized, double-blind, placebo controlled trial of botulinum a toxin for refractory overactive bladder. J Urol [Internet]. 2009;181(6):2608–15. Available from: https://doi.org/10.1016/j.juro.2009.01.117
25. Sahai A, Khan MS, Dasgupta P. Efficacy of botulinum toxin-A for treating idiopathic detrusor overactivity: results from a single center, randomized, double-blind, placebo controlled trial. J Urol. 2007;177(6):2231–6.
26. Kalsi V, Apostolidis A, Gonzales G, Elneil S, Dasgupta P, Fowler CJ. Early effect on the overactive bladder symptoms following botulinum neurotoxin type a injections for detrusor overactivity. Eur Urol. 2008;54(1):181–7.
27. Brubaker L, Richter HE, Visco A, Mahajan S, Nygaard I, Braun TM, et al. Refractory idiopathic urge urinary incontinence and botulinum a injection. J Urol. 2008;180(1):217–22.
28. Dmochowski R, Chapple C, Nitti VW, Chancellor M, Everaert K, Thompson C, et al. Efficacy and safety of onabotulinumtoxina for idiopathic overactive bladder: a double-blind, placebo controlled, randomized, dose ranging trial. J Urol [Internet]. 2010;184(6):2416–22. Available from: https://doi.org/10.1016/j.juro.2010.08.021
29. Kennelly M, Dmochowski R, Schulte-Baukloh H, Ethans K, Del Popolo G, Moore C, et al. Efficacy and safety of onabotulinumtoxinA therapy are sustained over 4 years of treatment in patients with neurogenic detrusor overactivity: final results of a long-term extension study. Neurourol Urodyn. 2017;36(2):368–75.
30. Rovner E, Kennelly M, Shulte-Baukloh H, Zhou J, Haag-Molkenteller C, Dasgupta P. Urodynamic results and clinical outcomes with intradetrusor injections of onabotulinumtoxinA in a randomized, placebo-controlled dose-finding study in idiopathic overactive bladder. Neurourol Urodyn. 2011;30:556–62.
31. Chapple C, Sievert KD, Macdiarmid S, Khullar V, Radziszewski P, Nardo C, et al. OnabotulinumtoxinA 100 U significantly improves all idiopathic overactive bladder symptoms and quality of life in patients with overactive bladder and urinary incontinence: a randomised, double-blind, placebo-controlled trial. Eur Urol [Internet]. 2013;64(2):249–56. Available from: https://doi.org/10.1016/j.eururo.2013.04.001
32. Nitti VW, Dmochowski R, Herschorn S, Sand P, Thompson C, Nardo C, et al. OnabotulinumtoxinA for the treatment of patients with overactive bladder and urinary incontinence: results of a phase 3, randomized, placebo controlled trial. J Urol [Internet]. 2013;189(6):2186–93. Available from: https://doi.org/10.1016/j.juro.2012.12.022
33. Visco AG, Brubaker L, Richter HE, Nygaard I, Paraiso MFR, Menefee SA, et al. Anticholinergic therapy vs. onabotulinumtoxinA for urgency urinary incontinence. N Engl J Med. 2012;367(19):1803–13.
34. Amundsen CL, Richter HE, Menefee SA, Komesu YM, Arya LA, Gregory WT, et al. Onabotulinumtoxin a vs sacral neuromodulation on refractory urgency urinary incontinence in women: a randomized clinical trial. JAMA. 2016;316(13):1366–74.
35. Amundsen CL, Komesu YM, Chermansky C, Gregory WT, Myers DL, Honeycutt EF, et al. Two-year outcomes of sacral neuromodulation versus onabotulinumtoxinA for refractory urgency urinary incontinence: a randomized trial [figure presented]. Eur Urol [Internet]. 2018;74(1):66–73. Available from: https://doi.org/10.1016/j.eururo.2018.02.011
36. Baron M, Perrouin-Verbe MA, Lacombe S, Paret F, Le Normand L, Cornu JN. Efficacy and tolerance of botulinum toxin injections after sacral nerve stimulation failure for idiopathic overactive bladder. Neurourol Urodyn. 2020;39(3):1012–9.
37. Wells H, Luton O, Simpkin A, Bullock N, KandaSwamy G, Younis A. Intravesical injection of botulinum toxin a for treatment of overactive bladder in anticoagulated patients: is it safe? Turk J Urol. 2020;46(6):481–7.

38. Derisavifard S, Giusto LL, Zahner P, Rueb JJ, Goldman HB. Safety of intradetrusor ona-botulinumtoxinA (BTX-A) injection in the asymptomatic patient with a positive urine dip. Urology. 2020;135:38–43.
39. Aharony S, Przydacz M, Van Ba OL, Corcos J. Does asymptomatic bacteriuria increase the risk of adverse events or modify the efficacy of intradetrusor onabotulinumtoxinA injections? Neurourol Urodyn. 2020;39(1):203–10.
40. Dressler D. Clinical presentation and management of antibody-induced failure of botulinum toxin therapy. Mov Disord. 2004;19(Suppl. 8):92–100.
41. Schulte-Baukloh H, Bigalke H, Miller K, Heine G, Pape D, Lehmann J, et al. Botulinum neuro-toxin type A in urology: antibodies as a cause of therapy failure. Int J Urol. 2008;15(5):407–15.
42. Linsenmeyer TA. Use of botulinum toxin in individuals with neurogenic detrusor overactiv-ity: state of the art review. J Spinal Cord Med [Internet]. 2013;36(5):402–19. Available from: http://www.ncbi.nlm.nih.gov/pubmed/23941788
43. Wyndaele JJ, Van Dromme SA. Muscular weakness as side effect of botulinum toxin injection for neurogenic detrusor overactivity. Spinal Cord. 2002;40(11):599–600.
44. Grosse J, Kramer G, Stöhrer M. Success of repeat detrusor injections of botulinum A toxin in patients with severe neurogenic detrusor overactivity and incontinence. Eur Urol. 2005;47(5):653–9.
45. Kalsi V, Gonzales G, Popat R, Apostolidis A, Elneil S, Dasgupta P, et al. Botulinum injections for the treatment of bladder symptoms of multiple sclerosis. Ann Neurol. 2007;62(5):452–7.

Chapter 12
Augmentation Cystoplasty in the Non-neurogenic Bladder Patient

Aisha L. Siebert, Elizabeth Rourke, and Stephanie J. Kielb

Augmentation cystoplasty with bowel interposition is indicated for the treatment of low-volume, poorly compliant bladders or refractory detrusor overactivity attributed to an underlying neurologic lesion. This surgical approach can and should also be considered for a variety of non-neurologic conditions leading to bladder dysfunction refractory to medical therapies and conservative surgical interventions. Overactive bladder (OAB), interstitial cystitis (IC) or bladder pain syndrome (BPS), partial cystectomy for benign bladder lesions or fistula repair, and special circumstances resulting in decreased bladder compliance (tuberculosis, end-stage renal disease, ketamine cystitis) are discussed.

Overactive Bladder

The American Urological Association (AUA) and Society of Urodynamics, Female Pelvic Medicine & Urogenital Reconstruction (SUFU) guidelines recommend surgical bladder augmentation only for severe, refractory, complicated patients with OAB [1]. Small case series report resolution of OAB symptoms in 66–94% of patients postoperatively with higher patient reported satisfaction than serial botulinum toxin injection, with the caveat that patients progressing to bladder augmentation tend to have more severe symptoms preoperatively [2–5]. Patients demonstrate variable ability to void postoperatively, and up to 75% require clean intermittent

A. L. Siebert · S. J. Kielb (✉)
Department of Urology, Northwestern University Feinberg School of medicine, Chicago, IL, USA
e-mail: aisha.siebert@northwestern.edu; stephanie.kielb@nm.org

E. Rourke
Department of Urology, Vanderbilt University, Nashville, TN, USA

© The Author(s), under exclusive license to Springer Nature Switzerland AG 2022
A. P. Cameron (ed.), *Female Urinary Incontinence*,
https://doi.org/10.1007/978-3-030-84352-6_12

self-catheterization (CIC), and patients should be selected and counseled of this risk as part of routine preoperative assessment [6]. Grafting using porcine dermis has been described in a small number of patients, with 1 year follow-up demonstrating a 25% dry rate, overall 83% improvement rate, and no significant complications [7]; however, long-term outcomes are lacking. Augmentation cystoplasty is an invasive abdominal procedure, requiring bowel excision and re-anastomosis, and is rarely applied as fourth-line treatment for refractory OAB due to surgical risks as well as long-term need for CIC and risk of malignancy. In a select patient population, bladder augmentation can provide symptom relief, and patient satisfaction compares favorably with intra-detrusor botulinum toxin injection.

Interstitial Cystitis/Bladder Pain Syndrome

Interstitial cystitis (IC) or bladder pain syndrome (BPS) is a diagnosis of exclusion. Major surgery, including subtotal cystectomy with substitution cystoplasty, is considered sixth-line treatment for patients failing medical and endoscopic management [8]. Trigone-sparing surgery theoretically decreases the risk of urinary retention; postoperatively the majority of these patients are able to void and rarely require initiation of CIC. However, following this approach, 33% of women report persistent irritative symptoms secondary to histologically proven trigone involvement, and for this reason preoperative bladder biopsy with mapping has been recommended but not widely adopted [9]. Patient factors predictive of persistent symptoms include those reporting urethra as a primary site of pain, absence of Hunner's lesions, and patients with larger bladder capacity on cystoscopic evaluation [8]. Augmentation without bladder excision can increase bladder capacity with some reported improvement in storage symptoms including urinary frequency and nocturia, but little to no impact on bladder pain [10]. Outcomes for augmentation cystoplasty for IC/BPS include 12% Clavian Grade III complications and 29% persistent pain [11]. There may be a role for augmentation in patients with cystoscopically or urodynamically demonstrated decreased bladder capacity, but the evidence is limited. Augmentation cystoplasty alone is not indicated to address bladder pain, and subtotal cystectomy with substitution cystoplasty demonstrates variable success in addressing bladder pain.

Following Partial Cystectomy

Partial cystectomy for symptomatic benign bladder lesions may result in decreased compliance and impaired bladder function. Bladder excision has been combined with augmentation cystoplasty to preserve bladder compliance and limit impact on quality of life. Other indications for augmentation in the setting of partial cystectomy for fistula excision and trauma have been described [12, 13]. Injury to the bladder either with concomitant loss of bladder tissue or prior compromise in bladder tissue and/or compliance may require augmentation cystoplasty. Case reports have described this technique in the setting of prior irradiation, with preserved ability to void up to 7 months postoperatively [14]. Although considered a contraindication to bladder augmentation, refractory radiation cystitis can be an indication for cystectomy or subtotal cystectomy with substitution cystoplasty. The surgeon should consider the quality of tissue and negative impact on wound healing when planning to operate in an irradiated field.

Decreased Bladder Capacity

End-stage renal disease (ESRD) resulting from poor bladder compliance can result from tuberculosis, radiation complications, congenital malformations including vesicoureteral reflux and posterior urethral values, and interstitial cystitis, along with a host of neurogenic causes. When conducted as part of routine transplant evaluation, voiding cystourethrography is abnormal in up to 2.5% of patient, with <1% requiring intervention, rarely augmentation cystoplasty [15]. Of patients referred for pretransplant urodynamic evaluation for cause, upward of 70% demonstrate urologic lesions contributing to renal dysfunction and requiring intervention prior to transplantation including obstruction, reflux, or bladder dysfunction [16]. Although rare, bladder augmentation has been described either before, simultaneous to, or following renal transplantation. The transplant ureter can be anastomosed with the augmented bladder or native ureter [17]. Graft survival is excellent with 96–100% 1 year, 92% 2 year, and 77–100% at 5 years [18–20]. There is an increased risk of serious urinary tract infection (UTI) without increased risk of urosepsis and a trend toward diminished graft function [21] although some centers report stable renal function up to 4 years postoperatively [22, 23] and few no increase in incidence of graft failure when compared to transplant patients without bladder augmentations [24].

The genitourinary tract is the most common site of extrapulmonary tuberculosis manifestation, resulting in dysfunctional bladder storage. Complications arise from inflammation leading to abscess formation, strictures of the ureters and urethra, and bladder contracture often requiring surgical management and eventual renal insufficiency in severe cases. Augmentation cystoplasty increases capacity and compliance and can preserve bladder sensation [25]. Improvement in diurnal frequency to greater than 2 hours has been demonstrated with a postsurgical capacity of at least 250 ml; however, involuntary bladder contractions may persist, requiring additional medical therapies [26].

Chronic ketamine use is a rare cause bladder fibrosis, resulting in a small, contracted bladder. Small case series report a significant increase in bladder capacity with decrease in pain, urgency, frequency, and decrease in pain medication use after bladder augmentation for this indication [27].

Surgical Approach

Patients undergoing surgery for conditions failing medical and less invasive interventional management should be managed by a center specializing in these indications. Appropriate patient selection and preoperative and postoperative counseling are paramount to patient expectation setting and goals to improve postoperative quality of life. Preoperative evaluation should include urethral evaluation for competency and urinary continence, accomplished with a combination of cystoscopic evaluation, uroflowmetry or urodynamics, and assessment of ability to self-catheterize. Renal function can be negatively impacted by the underlying disease process and bladder dysfunction, so preoperative renal function evaluation and postoperative monitoring are recommended. Robotic augmentation cystoplasty has been described as a viable option by many centers, though clinical benefit over the open approach is not certain (Table 12.1). Surgeon skill and experience should dictate approach.

Ileum is the most frequently employed bowel segment for bladder augmentation; however, ileocecal, sigmoid, and stomach have been used. When using ileum, a 20–25 cm segment is harvested 15–20 cm proximal to the ileocecal valve in order to preserve micronutrient reapportion. Location and length of the segment are dictated by the corresponding vascular arcade.

Colon segment may be indicated with a history of pelvic radiation or when concomitant colon surgery such as colostomy is being performed where a bowel anastomosis could be avoided. Under these circumstances, timing of surgery as well as other factors which may impair wound healing should be carefully considered and discussed with the patient. Preoperative colonoscopy should be considered to assess candidacy for interposition in case the small bowel is deemed inappropriate for interposition at the time of surgery.

Stomach is a less frequently used source of tissue for bladder augmentation. A 10–20 cm wedge of stomach antrum or body excised along the greater curvature can be used for bladder augmentation. The flap is supplied either from the right or left gastroepiploic arteries and subsequently tunneled through transverse colon and small bowel mesentery. Gastric augments secrete less mucus and are less prone to metabolic acidosis as well as infections compared to bowel augmentation where chronic bacteriuria is common; however, hematuria-dysuria syndrome has caused gastric augments to fall out of favor.

When performing augmentation cystoplasty, the selected bowel segment is opened along the antimesenteric boarder and configured in a U, S, or W shape and anastomosed to a sagittal incision made in the native bladder dome [28]. Ureteral evaluation is indicated in patients with suspicion for multiple levels of disease. Ileal replacement of the ureter, substitution urethroplasty with buccal mucosal grafting, and ileal augmentation cystoplasty can be used individually or in combination to address multiple site of pathology [29].

Table 12.1 Application of robotic approach to augmentation cystoplasty

Reference	Journal	Outcomes	Complications	N
Robotic augmentation enterocystoplasty K. E. Al-Othman, H. A. Al-Hellow, H. M. Al-Zahrani, R. M. Seyam	Journal of Endourology 22(4):597–600 (2008)	Low postoperative narcotic requirements	Long operative time	n = 1
Robotic enterocystoplasty: technique and early outcomes J. J. Gould, J. T. Stoffel	Journal of Endourology 25(1):91–5 (2011)	Urethral continence, normal upper tract imaging	Rare ileus	n = 5
Robotic approaches to augmentation cystoplasty: ready for prime time? Prithvi Murthy, Joshua A. Cohn, Mohan S. Gundeti	Current Bladder Dysfunction Reports 9:310–7 (2014)	Faster recovery time, decreased postoperative narcotic use and adhesion formation	Expense	n = 13
Completely intracorporeal robotic-assisted laparoscopic augmentation enterocystoplasty with continent catheterizable channel Andrew S. Flum, Lee C. Zhao, Stephanie J. Kielb, Erik B. Wilson, Tung Shu, John C. Hairston	Journal of Urology 84(6):1314–8 (2014)	Faster recovery time, decreased wound/bowel complications (e.g., small bowel obstruction, ileus)	Venous thromboembolism	n = 22
Robotic-assisted laparoscopic bladder augmentation in the pediatric patient A. C. Wiestma, C. R. Estrada Jr., P. S. Cho, M. V. Hollis, R. N. Yu	Journal of Pediatric Urology 12(5):313. e1–e2 (2016)	Increased bladder capacity	Long operative time	n = 1

Augmentation Cystoplasty Techniques

AC with/without Catheterizable Channel-Open Technique

1. The patient is placed in the supine position (frog-legged for females to allow for ease of access to the urethra during the procedure) with/without kidney rest and flexion. A Foley catheter is placed on the sterile field. A midline infraumbilical incision is made and can be extended above the umbilicus as needed for adequate exposure. Once the abdomen is entered, bowel assessed, and the procedure is deemed feasible. Develop the retropubic space of Retzius and mobilize the bladder. The bladder is clam-shelled open with electrocautery extending approximately 2 cm from the bladder neck anteriorly and 2 cm from the trigone posteriorly (Fig. 12.1a). This prevents the hourglass configuration that can occur as a result of contraction along the bowel/bladder suture line.

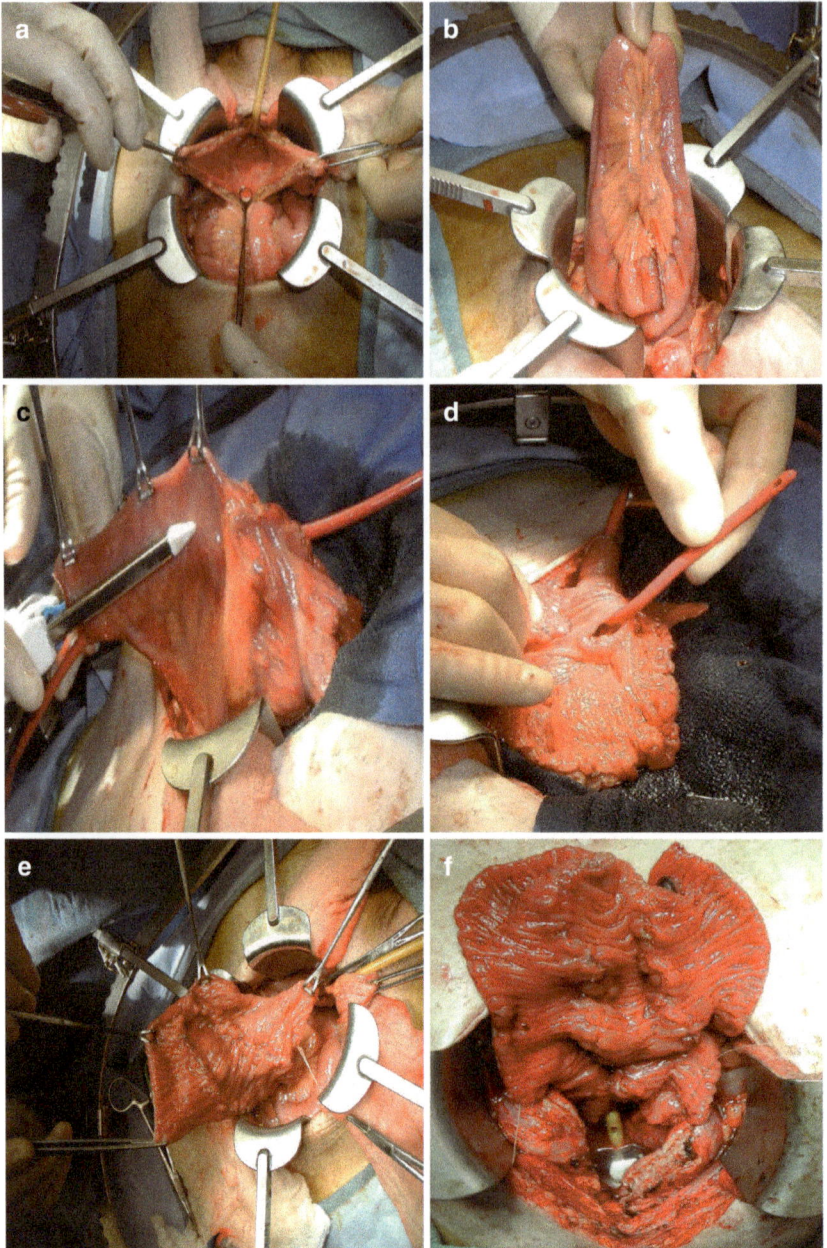

Fig. 12.1 Ileocystoplasty with continent catheterizable channel. (**a**) Bi-valved bladder both posteriorly toward trigone and anteriorly to bladder neck. (**b**) Segment length of ileum approximately 45 cm. (**c**) Creation of catheterizable channel (Mitrofanoff) over 12–14 Fr red rubber with cecal cuff. (**d**) Testing catheterizable channel to accommodate catheter. (**e**) Detubularized segment of ileum. (**f**) Anastomosis of ileal segment to bi-valved bladder. (**g**) Stoma maturation Y-V plasty. (**h**) Suprapubic catheter in augmented bladder (**i**). Twelve Fr red-rubber catheter in channel, suprapubic catheter in augment bladder, and abdominal drain. (**j**) Postoperative cystogram. (Images courtesy Melissa Kaufman MD MPH)

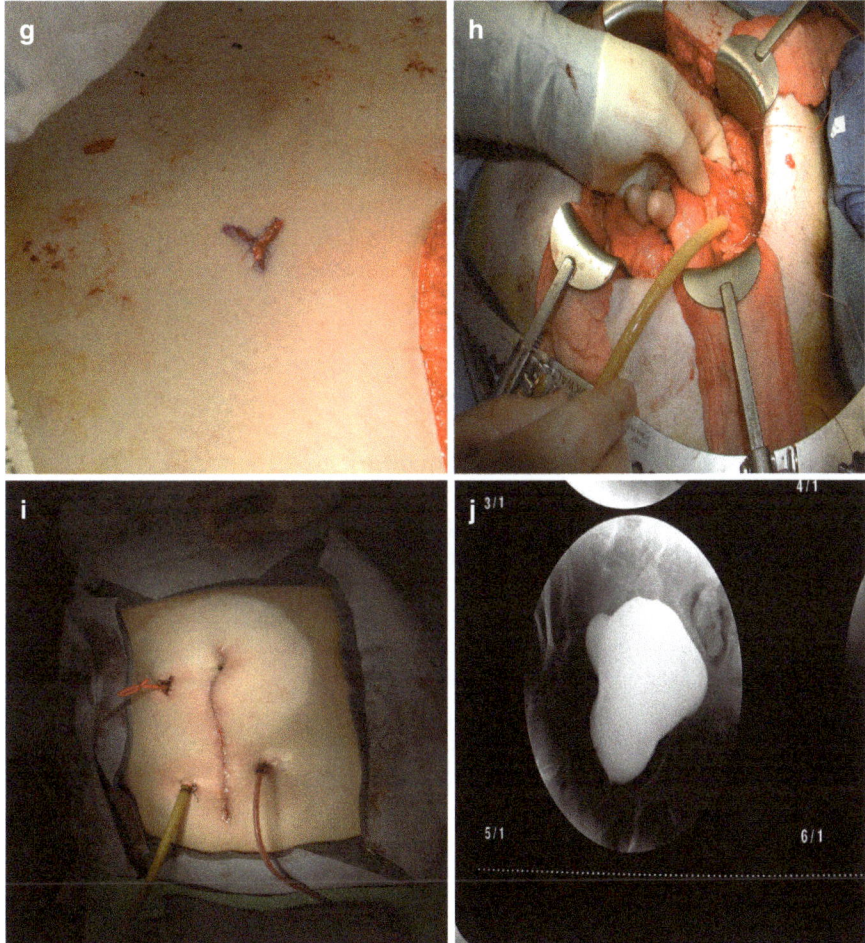

Fig. 12.1 (continued)

2. Identify the bowel segment to be used for the augment (ileum, ascending or sigmoid colon). For ileocystoplasty, utilize an approximately 25 cm segment of ileum (15–20 cm for colon) 15–20 cm from the ileocecal valve. Mark the proximal and distal ends of the segment with suture and harvest the bowel with GIA stapler. Perform bowel anastomosis oriented above the segment harvested for augmentation. Ensure all staple lines are removed from the augment segment (Fig. 12.1b). Detubularize the bowel segment on the antimesenteric border with electrocautery and approximate the backwalls of the bowel in S-shape configuration (note: straight or cup patch in a U, W, and S shape are alternative techniques for augment configuration). The mucosal edges (in the desired configuration) can be approximated with 2–0 Vicryl or 3–0 polydioxanone (PDS) (Fig. 12.1e, f). To facilitate irrigation and postoperative management, a 16–20 Fr suprapubic catheter (a Malecot catheter may also be used) is placed through the detrusor into the native bladder after completion of the posterior anastomosis (Fig. 12.1h).

Once the anterior anastomosis is complete, the bladder is irrigated/tested for leak along the suture line and bolstered as needed.

3. If a catheterizable channel is desired, this is most commonly performed with either appendix (if length is adequate) or with a portion of ileum. An appendicovesicostomy/Mitrofanoff is created by isolating the appendix from the cecum while preserving the appendiceal artery within the mesentery of the appendix and divided from the cecum. If more length is required, a portion of the cecum can be harvested with the appendix and tubularized. An additional cuff of cecum incorporated in the channel can allow for decreased risk of stomal stenosis at the skin level. Appendiceal channel length can also be augmented by removing a segment of cecum along with the appendix and tapered over the catheter with a GIA stapler (Fig. 12.1c). The appendix is then implanted into the bladder through a submucosal tunnel. It is recommended to anastomose the channel into the native bladder in the posterolateral position and not the augment patch in a location that allows for seamless passage of the catheter. The appendix can also be secured to the outer bladder wall to prevent stoma retraction. Stoma placement may vary based on length of channel and patient anatomy and is either placed in the lower abdominal wall or umbilicus (preferred). The channel should accommodate a 12–14 Fr red rubber catheter (Fig. 12.1d). If appendix is not available, a 2 cm segment of ileum, using the Yang Monti (YM) technique, can be utilized to create a channel. The selected segment is mobilized and incised transversely along the antimesenteric border and retubularized in two layers (mucosa and serosa) with 3–0/4–0 absorbable sutures along its long axis to form a long channel (typically doubles the length of the harvested segment). Retubularization is recommended around a 12–14 Fr catheter. In cases where a longer channel is needed, a double YM or spiralized YM is additional options. A double YM is created by harvesting two separate segments as described above and anastomosed end to end.

4. Stomal maturation can be performed with a Y-V, V, or U plasty incision and placed in the umbilicus or lower abdominal quadrants (Fig. 12.1g). It is ultimately most important that the location of the stoma allow for ease of catheterization. During construction, frequent testing of channel throughout this process is imperative. With a Y-V plasty, secure the apex of the V to the channel (deep dermal skin to mucosa of channel) with 3–0 Vicryl and continue to mature stoma with interrupted suture. Postoperatively, maintain a 16 Fr Foley catheter in the stoma for 3 weeks. It is imperative that the channel is secured to the posterior peritoneum/abdominal wall to ensure properly direct alignment into the bladder in order to avoid difficulties with catheterization.

5. A perivesical/intra-abdominal drain is left in place and may be removed prior to discharge if there is no concern for intrabdominal urine leak (Fig. 12.1i).

6. Postoperatively, a urethral catheter may be left in place and removed prior to patient discharge. The suprapubic catheter is irrigated daily to prevent mucous buildup and remains in place for 3 weeks postoperative with a cystogram prior to removal (Fig. 12.1j). If the cystogram demonstrates no urine extravasation, plug the suprapubic tube, and the patient will begin performing catheterization

of the channel (if present). If there are no issues with catheterization, then the suprapubic tube is removed [30, 31].

AC Laparoscopic/Robotic Technique

The adoption of robot-assisted laparoscopic techniques has evolved over the years and more recently has expanded to include minimally invasive options for complex urinary diversions including AC. The first robotic ileocystoplasty was first described by Gundeti et al. in 2008 in the pediatric neurogenic bladder setting [32]. Historically AC is approached with an open technique, and therefore robot-assisted laparoscopic total intracorporal bladder augmentation has not been well established to date with limited publications detailing safety, feasibility, and surgical technique. However, several proposed techniques are detailed below and should be considered in order to decrease morbidity and invasiveness of AC. It is imperative that patient selection is considered prior to proceeding with a robotic approach in addition to appropriate surgeon experience in robotics.

1. Patient is placed in the dorsal lithotomy position in steep Trendelenburg. A 12 mm camera port is placed 2–5 cm above the umbilicus with a Veress or Hassan technique depending on surgeon preference. Port placement is similar to robot-assisted radical cystectomy and prostatectomy with two 8 mm robot ports along the lateral border of the rectus muscle on the right and left side, an additional 8 mm robot port 2 cm above the right anterior superior iliac spine (ASIS), and a 12 mm assistant port 2 cm above the left ASIS. Each port should be placed approximately 8 cm apart. A 5 mm assistant port can be placed as needed (Fig. 12.2).

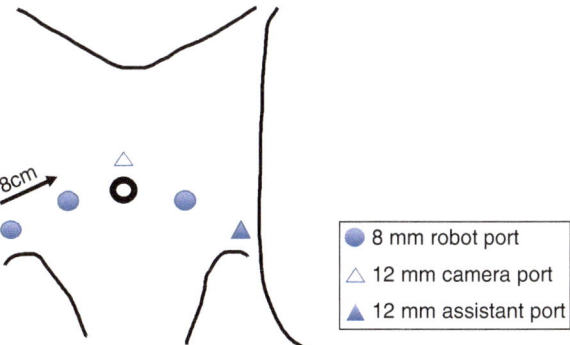

8cm

| ⬤ 8 mm robot port |
| △ 12 mm camera port |
| ▲ 12 mm assistant port |

Fig. 12.2 Port placement for robot-assisted laparoscopic ileocystoplasty. A 12 mm camera port is placed 2–5 cm above the umbilicus with assistance from a Veress needle or Hassan technique. Two 8 mm robot ports are placed along the lateral border of the rectus muscle on the right and left side, an additional 8 mm robot port placed 2 cm above the right anterior superior iliac spine (ASIS), and a 12 mm assistant port 2 cm above the left ASIS. Ports should be approximately 8 cm apart. A 5 mm assistant port can be placed as needed. (Image courtesy Melissa Kaufman MD MPH)

2. Dissection begins with a longitudinal incision along the peritoneum between the medial umbilical ligaments and access gained to the extraperitoneal space and the bladder dome exposed with a combination of blunt and cautery dissection. The bladder is distended to allow for ease of cystotomy and is bivalved in a mid-sagittal plane similarly to open technique.

3. The ileal patch is created by preserving 15 cm of ileum proximal to the ileocecal junction and 15–20 cm of distal ileum isolated. The distal end of the segment is fixed with stay sutures of the abdominal wall in order to facilitate harvesting of the ileal patch segment [33]. An endoscopic stapler is used to isolate the ileal segment, and a combination of monopolar and bipolar cautery is used to divide the mesentery. The two ileal ends are approximated for the bowel anastomosis, and the same endoscopic stapler is used again. The mesenteric window is loosely approximated and closed using 3–0 Vicryl. The staple lines are removed from the ends of the ileal augment segment and detubularized (can be assisted with the suction device to guide the direction of the incision) and configured in a U shape (or preferred configuration) with 3–0 Vicryl. (*Note: this portion can be performed extracorporally by extending the umbilical port incision.*)

4. The ileal-bladder anastomosis is performed in a similar fashion as the open technique with the posterior wall anastomosis performed first and suturing anteriorly to the bladder neck. The apex of the U should be oriented anteriorly at the bladder neck. This may be completed in a single-layer full-thickness closure with 2–0 Vicryl. The augment is tested with irrigation and buttressed as needed.

5. An abdominal drain is left in place in addition to suprapubic and urethral catheters. Abdominal drain and urethral catheter are removed prior to patient discharge and 3-week cystogram performed and suprapubic catheter removed if no complications/urine leak identified [34, 35].

Spontaneous perforation of to the augmented bladder is a serious risk with rates as high as 13% thought secondary to chronic or acute over distension and subsequent bowel wall ischemia [36–41]. The more common clinical scenario is a patient who chronically lets their bladder become overdistended or a patient who is under the influence of alcohol and allows the bladder to get overfills, and it spontaneously ruptures.

Evaluation of a suspected perforation should include computer tomography (CT) and management with either conservative management with Foley drainage, and intravenous antibiotics or surgical exploration and repair have been described. Lee et al. have proposed an algorithm for management, but due to the risk of sepsis, a low threshold for surgical exploration is recommended [42]. Patients should be counseled regarding this risk and encouraged to maintain a regular catheterization schedule.

Follow-Up

Patient undergoing augmentation cystoplasty for non-neurogenic indications require similar short-term monitoring for bowel or bladder anastomotic breakdown, fistula, and delayed return of function as well as long-term monitoring of renal function and routing screening for malignancy as indicated. This includes regular electrolytes, CBC, urinalysis, B12, and periodic ultrasound imaging. Follow-up for electrolyte disturbance and stone disease is outside of the scope of this chapter, but routine monitoring is indicated. Patients with bowel interposition as well as those who perform CIC are considered to be at an increased risk for malignancy, and hematuria should be evaluated in this patient population and not treated as a sign of infection if symptoms of such are absent.

Pregnancy after Bladder Augmentation

Multiple case reports describe uncomplicated pregnancy following bladder augmentation [43]. There is an approximately 15% risk of pyelonephritis, which compares favorably with a 20–40% incidence in pregnant women with asymptomatic bacteriuria and normal lower urinary tracts [44]. Current practice patterns mandate treatment of asymptotic bacteriuria during pregnancy, and by extension prophylactic antibiotics are sometimes employed in the setting of bowel interposition with chronic colonization. Impaired urinary drainage due to external compression from the gravid uterus is relatively uncommon (4%) as compared to ileal conduit (23%), commonly from compression of the left ureter against the sacrum [45]. C-section delivery rates are 27% similar to the general population, typically performed for obstetric indications. Patients with an augmentation cystoplasty are not at an increased risk of incontinence. Notable exceptions include those with bladder neck reconstruction or artificial urinary sphincter, in which case caesarian section delivery is indicated. Surgical approach to caesarian section must consider the position of the mesentery which draped over the uterus, is commonly displaced laterally, and can be adherent. Although uncomplicated lower segment caesarean section after bladder augmentation had been described [46], to avoid injury to the vascular supply, a high uterine incision is preferred.

Summary

Augmentation cystoplasty may be utilized for non-neurogenic conditions impacting bladder capacity, and compliance though often after other less-risky options has been exhausted. Ileum is the most commonly utilized bowel segment, and surgical approach is similar to neurologic indications. Long-term follow-up is indicated due to the risks of metabolic abnormalities, stone formation, and bladder perforation.

References

1. Lightner DJ, Gomelsky A, Souter L, et al. Diagnosis and treatment of overactive bladder (non-neurogenic) in adults: AUA/SUFU guideline amendment 2019. J Urol. 2019;202:5.
2. Kayigil Ö, Atahan Ö, Metin A. Experiences with clam ileocystoplasty. Int Urol Nephrol. 1998;30(1):45–8.
3. Andersen AV, Granlund P, Schultz A, Talseth T, Hedlund H, Frich L. Long-term experience with surgical treatment of selected patients with bladder pain syndrome/interstitial cystitis. Scand J Urol Nephrol. 2012;46(4):284–9.
4. El-Azab AS, Moeen AM. The satisfaction of patients with refractory idiopathic overactive bladder with onabotulinumtoxinA and augmentation cystoplasty. Arab J Urol. 2013;11(4):344–9.
5. Mishra NN. Clinical presentation and treatment of bladder pain syndrome/interstitial cystitis (BPS/IC) in India. Transl Androl Urol. 2015;4(5):512–23. https://doi.org/10.3978/j.issn.2223-4683.2015.10.05.
6. Sood A, Eilender B, Wong P, Atiemo H. Outcomes in patients with idiopathic overactive bladder undergoing augmentation cystoplasty in the era of onabotulinumtoxin-A and interstim. Neurourol Urodyn. 2019;38:S238–9.
7. Barrington JW, Dyer R, Bano F. Bladder augmentation using Pelvicol implant for intractable overactive bladder syndrome. Int Urogynecol J Pelvic Floor Dysfunct. 2006;17(1):50–3.
8. Hanno PM, Erickson D, Moldwin R, et al. Diagnosis and treatment of interstitial cystitis/bladder pain syndrome: AUA guideline amendment. J Urol. 2015;193:1545.
9. Nurse DE, Parry JRW, Mundy AR. Problems in the surgical treatment of interstitial cystitis. Br J Urol. 1991;68(2):153–4.
10. Zhang GK, Sidi AA, Reddy PK. Treatment of interstitial cystitis with augmentation cystoplasty. Neurourol Urodyn. 1990;9(2):222–3.
11. Downey AP, Osman NI, Park JJ, et al. Contemporary outcomes of surgery for bladder pain syndrome/interstitial cystitis. Neurourol Urodyn. 2018;37:S357.
12. Tabakov ID, Slavchev BN. Large post-hysterectomy and post-radiation vesicovaginal fistulas: repair by ileocystoplasty. J Urol. 2004;171:272–4.
13. Hsu TH, Rackley RR, Abdelmalak JB, Madjar S, Vasavada SP. Novel technique for combined repair of postirradiation vesicovaginal fistula and augmentation ileocystoplasty. Urology. 2002;59:597–9.
14. Miyamoto S, Takushima A, Harii K, Shimoi H, Nutahara K. Ileal patch graft used to repair a bladder injured during repair of an abdominal wall hernia. J Plast Surg Hand Surg. 2010;44(1):66–8.
15. Glazier DB, Whang MIS, Geffner SR, et al. Evaluation of voiding cystourethrography prior to renal transplantation. Transplantation. 1996;62(12):1762–5.
16. Theodorou C, Katsifotis C, Bocos J, Moutzouris G, Stournaras P, Kostakis A. Urodynamics prior to renal transplantation--its impact on treatment decision and final results. Scand J Urol Nephrol. 2003;37(4):335–8.
17. Power RE, O'Malley KJ, Khan MS, Murphy DM, Hickey DP. Renal transplantation in patients with an augmentation cystoplasty. BJU Int. 2000;86(1):28–31.
18. Martín MG, Castro SN, Castelo LA, Abal VC, Rodríguez JS, Novo JD. Enterocystoplasty and renal transplantation. J Urol. 2001;165(2):393–6.
19. Van Ophoven A, Oberpenning F, Hertle L. Long-term results of trigone-preserving orthotopic substitution enterocystoplasty for interstitial cystitis. J Urol. 2002;167(2 I):603–7.
20. Slagt IK, Ijzermans JN, Alamyar M, et al. Long-term outcome of kidney transplantation in patients with a urinary conduit: a case-control study. Int Urol Nephrol. 2013;45(2):405–11.

21. Pazik J, Wazna E, Lewandowski Z, et al. Factors predisposing to urinary tract infections in adult kidney allograft recipients with lower urinary tract reconstruction. Transplant Proc. 2009;41(8):3039–42.
22. Barnett MG, Bruskewitz RC, Belzer FO, Sollinger HW, Uehling DT. Ileocecocystoplasty bladder augmentation and renal transplantation. J Urol. 1987;138(4):855–8.
23. Milutinovic D, Topuzovic C, Hadzi-Djokic J. Clam ileoplasty bladder augmentation and renal transplantation. Acta Chir Iugosl. 2007;54(4):79–81.
24. Garat JM, Caffaratti J, Angerri O, Bujons A, Villavicencio H. Kidney transplants in patients with bladder augmentation: correlation and evolution. Int Urol Nephrol. 2009;41(1):1–5.
25. Singh V, Sinha RJ, Sankhwar SN, Sinha SM. Reconstructive surgery for tuberculous contracted bladder: experience of a center in northern India. Int Urol Nephrol. 2011;43(2):423–30.
26. de Figueiredo AA, Lucon AM, Srougi M. Bladder augmentation for the treatment of chronic tuberculous cystitis. Clinical and urodynamic evaluation of 25 patients after long term follow-up. Neurourol Urodyn. 2006;25(5):433–40.
27. Yee CH, Chiu PKF, Chan YS, et al. Robotic augmentation cystoplasty for contracted bladder secondary to cystitis: a 1-year outcome assessment. J Urol. 2020;203:e1017–8.
28. Morrison CD, Kielb SJ. Use of bowel in reconstructive urology: what a colorectal surgeon should know. Clin Colon Rectal Surg. 2017;30(3):207–14.
29. Singh O, Gupta SS, Arvind NK. A case of extensive genitourinary tuberculosis: combined augmentation ileo-cystoplasty, ureteric ileal replacement and buccal mucosal graft urethroplasty. Updat Surg. 2013;65(3):245–8.
30. Partin AW, Dmochowski RR, Kavoussi LR, Peters C, editors. Campbell-Walsh-Wein urology/editor-in-chief, Alan W. Partin; editors, Roger R. Dmochowski, Louis R. Kavoussi, Craig A. Peters. 12th ed. Philadelphia: Elsevier; 2020.
31. Montague DK, Gill I, Ross J, Angermeier KW, editors. Textbook of reconstructive urologic surgery. 1st ed. CRC Press; 2008.
32. Gundeti MS, Eng MK, Reynolds WS, Zagaja GP. Pediatric robotic-assisted laparoscopic augmentation ileocystoplasty and mitrofanoff appendicovesicostomy: complete intracorporeal—initial case report. Urology. 2008;72(5):1144–7.
33. Passerotti CC, Nguyen HT, Lais A, Dunning P, Harrell B, Estrada C, et al. Robot-assisted laparoscopic ileal bladder augmentation: defining techniques and potential pitfalls. J Endourol. 2008;22(2):355–60.
34. Dogra P, Regmi S, Singh P, Bora G, Saini A, Aggarwal S. Robot-assisted laparoscopic augmentation ileocystoplasty in a tubercular bladder. Urol Ann. 2014;6(2):152–5.
35. Grilo N, Chartier-Kastler E, Grande P, Crettenand F, Parra J, Phé V. Robot-assisted supratrigonal cystectomy and augmentation cystoplasty with totally intracorporeal reconstruction in neurourological patients: technique description and preliminary results. Eur Urol. 2021;79(6):858–65.
36. Metcalfe PD, Casale AJ, Kaefer MA, Misseri R, Dussinger AM, Meldrum KK, et al. Spontaneous bladder perforations: a report of 500 augmentations in children and analysis of risk. J Urol. 2006;175:1466–70; discussion 1470–1.
37. DeFoor W, Tackett L, Minevich E, Wacksman J, Sheldon C. Risk factors for spontaneous bladder perforation after augmentation cystoplasty. Urology. 2003;62:737–41.
38. Bertschy C, Bawab F, Liard A, Valioulis I, Mitrofanoff P. Enterocystoplasty complications in children. A study of 30 cases. Eur J Pediatr Surg. 2000;10:30–4.
39. Shekarriz B, Upadhyay J, Demirbilek S, Barthold JS, González R. Surgical complications of bladder augmentation: comparison between various enterocystoplasties in 133 patients. Urology. 2000;55:123–8.
40. Krishna A, Gough DC, Fishwick J, Bruce J. Ileocystoplasty in children: assessing safety and success. Eur Urol. 1995;27:62–6.
41. Rushton HG, Woodard JR, Parrott TS, Jeffs RD, Gearhart JP. Delayed bladder rupture after augmentation enterocystoplasty. J Urol. 1988;140:344–6.

42. Lee T, Kozminski DJ, Bloom DA, Wan J, Park JM. Bladder perforation after augmentation cystoplasty: determining the best management option. J Pediatr Urol. 2017;13(3):274.e1–7.
43. Norris JP, Wheeler JS, Norris DM, Rubenstein MA. Augmentation cystoplasty and ileal conduits in pregnancy. Int Urogynecol J. 1995;6(1):37–40.
44. Krieger JN. Complications and treatment of urinary tract infections during pregnancy. Urol Clin North Am. 1986;13(4):685–93.
45. Hill DE, Chantigian PM, Kramer SA. Pregnancy after augmentation cystoplasty. Surg Gynecol Obstet. 1990;170(6):485–7.
46. Shaikh A, Ahsan S, Zaidi Z. Pregnancy after augmentation cystoplasty. J Pak Med Assoc. 2006;56(10):465–7.

Chapter 13
Advanced Options for Treatment of Refractory Urgency Urinary Incontinence

Elizabeth Rourke, Alice Wang, and Melissa Kaufman

Suprapubic Catheter: Indications and Methods

Suprapubic (SP) catheter placement is considered an alternative method for management of bladder in patients with bladder underactivity and/or overflow incontinence [3]. However, SP catheter placement can also be considered after failure of third-line therapies for urgency urinary incontinence (UUI). The SP catheter is typically placed endoscopically or surgically in an infraumbilical anatomic location and cannot only avoid the complications of urethral erosion but is often more comfortable and easier to manage than a urethral catheter. Though SP catheter placement adequately drains the bladder and can improve incontinence, bladder overactivity may still be present, and an SP catheter is most often used in conjunction with pharmacotherapy and/or intradetrusor Botox and given the patent urethra may not result in continence if the woman has substantial stress incontinence.

Percutaneous Placement of SP Catheter

A percutaneous procedure can be done under local anesthetic and may be the preferred option for patients requiring emergent drainage of the bladder without options for urethral access. Prior to performing this procedure, assessment of the patient's surgical history is mandated to reveal intra-abdominal surgeries potentially resulting in disruption of the peritoneum allowing for bowel migration into the pelvis and surrounding the space of Retzius or overlying the bladder. Ultrasound at bedside

E. Rourke · A. Wang · M. Kaufman (✉)
Vanderbilt University Medical Center, Urology, Nashville, TN, USA
e-mail: Melissa.kaufman@vumc.org

© The Author(s), under exclusive license to Springer Nature Switzerland AG 2022
A. P. Cameron (ed.), *Female Urinary Incontinence*,
https://doi.org/10.1007/978-3-030-84352-6_13

can be utilized to visualize loops of bowel in the trajectory of catheter placement. If there is concern that bowel cannot be avoided without direct visualization (open approach), then the procedure should be aborted, and an alternative placement technique is considered. Interventional radiology drain placement under CT guidance is a frequently employed option with potential for subsequent upsizing to a formal catheter in the operating room or gradual upsizing in clinic. Perioperative antibiotics should be administered for skin and genitourinary bacterial coverage. At the target site approximately two fingerbreadths above the pubic symphysis in the midline, deep, and superficial local anesthetic can be applied. A 20-gauge spinal needle is advanced through the skin and into the bladder. To avoid bowel, the bladder should be fully distended, and the needle should be angled 10–15 degrees from vertical, aimed caudally and advanced until urine is aspirated. Then, a 1 cm transverse incision is made in the midline at the previously marked site two fingerbreadths above the pubic symphysis. There are various percutaneous access and dilating kits available to use, but the principle remains the same that trocar and sheath should be advanced in the same direction and depth as the needle. Once in the bladder, urine should be seen in the sheath. The inner trocar is then removed, and the sheath is kept in place. The catheter of choice is advanced through the sheath, and the balloon is inflated with sterile water. The sheath is then peeled off the catheter [4].

Endoscopic Placement of SP Catheter

For endoscopic suprapubic cystotomy placed in a retrograde fashion, the Lowsley retractor is commonly used [5]. This version of the procedure is preferable if there is urethral access and the patient has had no previous lower abdominal procedures. This technique is typically simpler in females given the shorter urethra. Proper consent is obtained, and appropriate preoperative antibiotics are given. Though this procedure is done endoscopically, general anesthesia is often utilized. The lithotomy position is preferred in both male and female patients to optimize the retractor angle. The Lowsley retractor is passed into the bladder through the urethra and aimed toward the anterior abdominal wall approximately 2 cm above the symphysis pubis. A spinal needle may be employed with cystoscopic guidance to optimize localization. The retractor is held firmly to prevent urethral trauma. A small suprapubic incision is then made through skin, subcutaneous tissue, and rectus fascia with electrocautery until the instrument is visualized. A catheter of the desired size is then attached to the Lowsley retractor and secured via a nonabsorbable suture (usually nylon or silk). The retractor is then pulled back through the bladder and exits out the urethral meatus. The suture is removed, and under direct vision, the catheter is advanced back to the bladder wall, and balloon is inflated. Direct vision placement with the Lowsley retractor prevents placement of the instrument outside the bladder and assists in avoiding potential damage of intra-abdominal viscera, which can occur during percutaneous placement [6].

Surgical Placement of SP Catheter

Surgical placement of a suprapubic catheter can be employed for patients with prior abdominal surgeries, who are at a high risk of bowel injury as well as patients with an inaccessible urethra due to urethral disruption, severe urethral stricture disease, or traumatic catheterization [7].

Proper consent is obtained, and the surgery is performed under general anesthesia. Preoperative antibiotics should be administered based on hospital and practice guidelines. The lower abdomen and genitalia are prepped with betadine or chlorhexidine. The patient is optimally positioned in dorsal lithotomy although dependent on patient anatomy this may also be performed supine. The patient can also be placed in Trendelenburg position to help relocate bowel away from the bladder. A small vertical incision (4–5 cm) is made in the midline, starting from the pubic symphysis and proceeding cephalad. Using electrocautery, dissection occurs through the subcutaneous fat and Scarpa's fascia to expose the rectus fascia. Using sharp dissection or cautery, the rectus fascia is incised in either a horizontal or vertical direction. Without dividing the muscle, retract the rectus muscle bellies to expose the underlying transversalis fascia and bladder immediately beneath. Ideally, the bladder should be full, and this can be confirmed by inserting a small-gauge needle, such as a spinal needle, attached to a syringe to aspirate urine. Once this has been confirmed, vertical stay sutures are placed with a 3-0 absorbable suture on either side of the midline of the bladder. The bladder can also be secured with Allis clamps. To avoid closure of the catheter within the incision, a separate incision can be created lateral to the incision to bring the catheter into the space for an independent tract. Using electrocautery or a scalpel, a small cystotomy is created. The catheter is then directly inserted into the cystotomy. The catheter balloons are then inflated with sterile water and pulled so that the balloon is suspended within the bladder lumen and not against the trigone or bladder neck. The cystotomy is then closed with a purse-string 3-0 absorbable suture around the site of catheter insertion. The fascia, subcutaneous tissue, and skin are closed, either independently or around the drain. The catheter can be secured with a drain stitch (silk or nylon). The SP catheter should be left in place for a minimum of 6 weeks prior to the first exchange to allow maturation of the tract and is recommended to be exchanged by the urologic surgeon initially and subsequently by nursing staff/patient.

Bladder Neck Closure Indications and Methods

Bladder outlet closure is usually reserved when other surgical interventions have failed and can be used to treat refractory incontinence. Most commonly, the refractory incontinence is due to urethral erosion from urethral catheter, severe stress incontinence, bladder neck incompetence, or difficult urethral fistulae [8]. Though bladder neck closure often has high success rates, it is to be considered a permanent and irreversible procedure and is associated with rare acute complications (such as bladder perforation) [9].

Multiple approaches for bladder neck closure are feasible, including transvaginal, transurethral, and transabdominal (retropubic), or a combination of several approaches may be required. Of note, the success of vesical neck closure requires a concomitant low-pressure urinary diversion via an SP catheter, ileovesicostomy, or augmentation cystoplasty with a continent catheterizable stoma. In a retrospective study, transvaginal and transabdominal approaches to bladder neck closure resulted in similar urethral continence rates. However, the transvaginal bladder neck closure was associated with shorter operative time, decreased length of hospitalization, and fewer short-term complications [10]. The decision to proceed with which option should depend on patient preference, functional status, and family support [11].

Transvaginal Approach

As in the transurethral approach, this approach avoids entry into the abdomen. The patient is optimally placed in the low lithotomy position. A suprapubic catheter or other form of urinary diversion should already be in place or will need to be performed at the time of bladder neck closure. The labia are retracted with a self-retaining ring retractor or sutures and a weighted speculum placed in the vagina for improved exposure. The anterior vaginal wall may be injected with saline or dilute lidocaine with epinephrine to hydrodissect the vesicovaginal space. A number 15 scalpel is used to create a wide inverted U-shape incision on the anterior vaginal wall. The apex of the U should start close to the urethral meatus and extend as proximally into the vaginal vault as possible (Fig. 13.1a). The anterior vaginal flap can be developed via retraction with Allis clamps and surgical scissors. The correct plane, revealing the underlying pubocervical fascia, should be shiny white with minimal bleeding. Once this flap has been developed, the urethra is incised circumferentially with the top edge being that of the apex of the U. The entire length of the urethra is dissected proximally to the bladder neck (Fig. 13.1b). With scissors or hemostats, the endopelvic fascia is perforated, and the bladder neck freed from the pubourethral ligaments. The urethra is transected at the level of the bladder neck and closed in multiple layers beginning with mucosa (Fig. 13.1c). The perivesical fascia is also closed. A watertight closure should be confirmed. Elevation of the closed bladder neck by fixation to the pubis is a preferred method to prevent fistula formation. A Martius flap can additionally provide an extra layer of closure and fill dead space (Fig. 13.1d). Lastly, the U-shaped vaginal flap is closed in a running fashion with a 2-0 absorbable suture, and an estrogen cream coated vaginal packing is placed in the vagina for <24 hours to assist with hemostasis [12, 13].

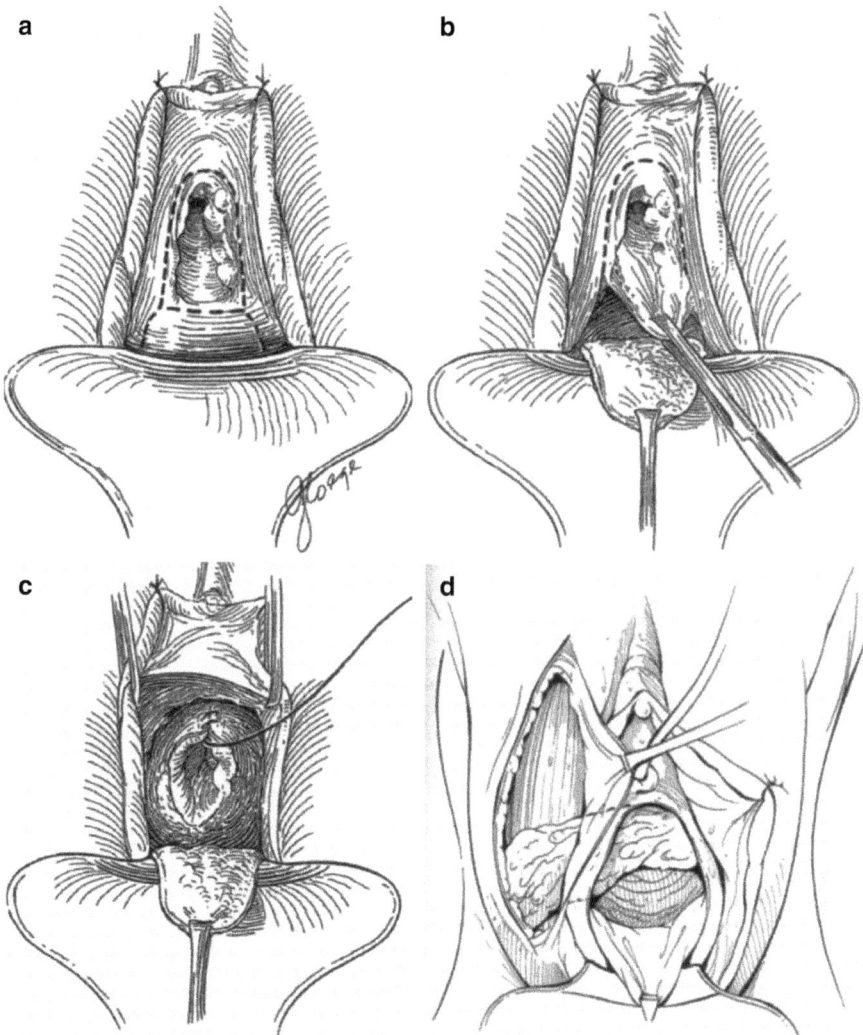

Fig. 13.1 Transvaginal bladder neck closure: (**a**) Transvaginal incision inverted U. (**b**) Development of the anterior vaginal flap and incision of bladder neck laterally. (**c**) Closure of bladder neck in a vertical running manner with a second layer closure of opposition (horizontal); repositions bladder neck behind pubic symphysis. (**d**) Martius flap to cover repair and provide additional tissue layer for prevention of fistula formation. ((**a–c**) from Raz S. Female Urology, 2nd ed. Philadelphia: WB Saunders, 1996. Copyright 1996, with permission from Springer; reprinted in Zimmern P. Vaginal Surgery for Incontinence and Prolapse) ((**d**) From Graham SD. Glenn's Urologic Surgery. Philadelphia: Lippincott-Raven, 1998 reprinted in Zimmern P. Vaginal Surgery for Incontinence and Prolapse with permission from Springer) [14]

Transurethral Approach

Similar to the transvaginal approach, adequate bladder drainage must first be obtained prior to closure of the bladder neck. The patient is placed in the low dorsal lithotomy position. A self-retaining ring retractor and/or retraction sutures are placed with a weighted vaginal speculum for adequate exposure. An elliptical incision is made around the urethra with a number 15 blade. The incision should be full thickness through the surrounding vaginal mucosa. The urethra is dissected away from the anterior vaginal wall to the bladder neck until it is completely mobilized. The endopelvic fascia is then perforated with tissue scissors. At this point, the entire length of urethra and bladder neck is mobilized. The distal urethra is then trimmed. The remaining urethra is then inverted by placing horizontal mattress sutures circumferentially around the urethra with 2–0 absorbable sutures. The bladder neck is then closed over the urethra in a purse string fashion with a similar suture. Watertight anastomoses should be confirmed with instillation of 200–300 cc of fluid into the bladder [14, 15].

Transabdominal Approach

In the transabdominal approach, drainage of the bladder is obtained during the cystotomy. Place the patient in low lithotomy position. Both the abdomen and vagina should be prepped. A Foley catheter is placed on the field. A low midline or Pfannenstiel incision is made. After entering the abdomen, the space of Retzius is dissected and developed bluntly. The endopelvic fascia is then encountered, and the dorsal venous complex is ligated with a zero absorbable suture. The urethra is dissected as widely as possible and the pubourethral ligaments transected with suture ligatures or sealing electrocautery. At this point the urethra is completely mobile and is ready to be transected. The dorsal aspect of the urethra is transected as far distally as possible. Once the foley catheter is exposed, it is divided so that it can be pulled upward to provide traction on the bladder neck. The ventral aspect of the urethra is then transected. The distal urethra is closed in two layers. The bladder is then opened anteriorly through the bladder neck. The ureteral orifices should be visualized before moving forward, and this can be done with the aid of intravenous methylene blue instillation or ureteral catheterization. The bladder neck is then transected from the proximal urethra. The bladder neck and bladder should be mobilized off the vesicovaginal space. Suprapubic catheter placement may be done at this time, or alternatively a catheterizable channel may be created. The bladder neck is now closed in two layers, ensuring inversion of the mucosal layer. Watertight closure is ensured with instillation of 200–300 cc of fluid. A peritoneal or omental flap can be used as an interposition to prevent fistula formation. Prior to abdominal closure, an abdominal drain is often placed for postoperative management [14, 15].

Urinary Diversion: Indications and Methods

Simple Cystectomy with Conduit

One of the most common and widely utilized surgical procedures for urinary diversion is an ileal conduit and was initially described by Bricker in the 1950s. Patients with refractory OAB/UUI are counseled on surgical management options, and in select cases where the patient is unable to catheterize (either per urethra or through a catheterizable channel), they should be counseled regarding simple cystectomy (supratrigonal cystectomy) and incontinent urinary diversion with a conduit. This procedure has been well developed and allows for immediate function. It is imperative to include preoperative stomal education with a wound ostomy therapist to include pouch teaching, stomal marking, and skin/stomal care, since pouching problems are a significant source of distress in patients. The bladder is removed in this procedure given the risk of pyocystis long term in a defunctionalized bladder. Given that the bladder is not completely removed during this procedure, it is contraindicated for patients with a history of bladder cancer who should receive a radical cystectomy.

As with augmentation cystoplasty, the terminal ileum is preferred for conduit diversion as it is typically mobile, small caliber lumen, and robust constant blood supply. In certain circumstances tethering of the mesentery may prevent mobilization of the ileum out of the deep pelvis, and colon may be preferred. Additionally, in patients with a history of radiation or previous bowel surgery that may have resulted in large losses of ileum, right, transverse, and descending colon can be used. If ileum is employed, it is recommended to begin following vitamin B12 levels approximately 5 years postoperatively as loss of distal ileum may result in a lack of B12 absorption [15, 16].

Simple Cystectomy with Ileal Conduit-Open Technique

1. The patient is placed in the supine position (frog-legged for females to allow for ease of access to the urethra during the procedure) with/without kidney rest and flexion. (*Note: consider placement of ureteral catheters prior to incision to allow for ease of ureteral identification/dissection.*) A Foley catheter is placed on the sterile field. A midline infraumbilical incision is made and can be extended above the umbilicus as needed for adequate exposure.
2. After gaining access to the abdomen, it is recommended to inspect the bowel at this time to ensure that segment of bowel can be harvested for the ileal conduit. Measure 15 cm from the ileocecal junction and mark the distal end with a short suture (this will identify the skin/stomal end) and then measure 15 cm of ileum and mark the proximal end with a long suture. This segment can then be packed superiorly for creation of the ileal conduit following ureteral dissection and cystectomy.
3. Ureteral dissection begins with the left ureter which can be identified crossing the iliac vessels with the sigmoid colon retracted superiomedially. A

peritonectomy is made, and the ureter is dissected free until a right-angle clamp can be passed underneath and the ureter encircled with a vessel loop to aid in further dissection. The ureter should be freed down to the level of the bladder and proximally to the kidney with care to maintain the adventitia which provides the rich blood supply to the ureter. (*Note: aggressive dissection of the ureter that results in loss of adventitia/blood supply can increase the risk of ureteral-enteric anastomotic stricture.*) A surgical clip is placed near the intramural tunnel around the ureter and transected. A 4-0 Vicryl stitch may be placed at the 12 0'clock position of the ureteral mucosa to act both as an identifying stitch and working handle to be used during the ureteral-enteric anastomosis. The same procedure is repeated on the right side; however, there is less mobilization required for a right-sided conduit as the right ureter is positioned closer to the conduit. (*Note: if ureteral catheters were placed at the beginning of the procedure these must be removed prior to clipping the ureter.*) The left ureter is tunneled between the two peritonectomies behind the sigmoid mesentery and passed to the right side.

4. With the ureters transected, the cystectomy can be performed. The space of Retzius is developed, and the bladder is mobilized by dividing the peritoneal wings bilaterally and dissecting it from the anterior fascia. The bladder can be distended with normal saline to aid in mobilization and creation of a cystotomy. Stay sutures or Allis clamps are used to assist with retraction while making an anterior cystotomy extending to the bladder neck anteriorly and the trigone posteriorly. The bladder can be removed with Bovie or sealing electrocautery device leaving only a deep muscular layer of the bladder base. Care must be taken to avoid injury to posterior structures (vagina in women and seminal vesicles and rectum in men). The remaining urothelium is fulgurated, and the bladder neck closed with 0 Vicryl.

5. The previously identified ileal segment (or colon) is brought into the surgical field. The mesentery is transilluminated in order to identify vascular arcades, and two windows are created in the mesentery with electrocautery (at both the proximal and distal ends). The sealing electrocautery is placed between the two windows, and the mesentery is divided. If there is any mesenteric bleeding, this should be ligated with 3-0 silk suture. The mesentery is cleared away from the bowel in order to accommodate the stapler. The bowel is then harvested with a GIA stapler distally and proximally (maintain stay sutures on conduit portion of bowel). The conduit is then dropped into the pelvis, and the bowel anastomosis is performed above the conduit.

6. A side-to-side anastomosis is performed (end to end is optional). The two bowel segments can be approximated along the antimesenteric border with 3-0 Vicryl sutures (removed following completion of anastomosis). The antimesenteric corners of the proximal and distal loop of bowel are excised to accommodate the GIA-75 stapler. Ensure the antimesenteric sides are facing one another before firing the staple load. The ileoileostomy is completed by offsetting longitudinal suture lines (with allis clamps or 3-0 Vicryl suture) and the enterotomy placed in the TA 60/90 stapler and fire, cut remaining stump with mayo scissors and release stapler. Oversew anastomosis with 3-0 Vicryl above the staple line. Close both the fork and the mesenteric edge with 3-0 silk or Vicryl suture.

7. The left ureter is tunneled through the sigmoid mesocolon to reach the conduit in the right pelvis. The ureteroileal anastomosis begins with ensuring both ureters are properly aligned to enter the bowel without tension and in the correct orientation. The staple line is removed from the distal end, and a Babcock clamp (one-click) is used on this end to orient the conduit in the appropriate position for anastomosis. An enterotomy is made (typically lateral edges of the proximal end of the conduit) through serosa and mucosa (may be done with cautery or scalpel/scissors). The mucosal edges of bowel are everted with 4-0 chromic to allow easier anastomosis to the ureters. The ureter is spatulated with tenotomy/Potts scissors. The anastomosis can be performed with interrupted or running sutures depending on surgeon preference with 4-0 Monocryl (or any unbraided synthetic absorbable suture). A running anastomosis uses two sutures at the apex: one place in to out on the ureter and the other in to out on the bowel and run. Before completing the anastomosis, a wire-loaded single J stent is placed. The site of implantation of the right ureter is more distal on the conduit. The ureteral stents are pulled out through the distal end of the conduit/stoma end.
8. The stoma is made by incising the skin in a circular fashion with electrocautery through skin and subcutaneous tissue down to the fascia. It is important to draw the fascia into the orthotopic midline incision with Kocher clamps during the creation of the stoma to prevent retraction during closure. The fascia is cleared of any subcutaneous fat and a cruciate incision made in the anterior rectus fascia, the rectus muscle split, and the posterior sheath and peritoneum incised. The incision should accommodate approximately two fingers to allow the conduit to pass through the fascia with ease. A Babcock clamp is passed from the skin through the fascial incision and clamped on the distal end of the conduit, including both ureteral stents and pulled through the fascia to the skin. Ensure the conduit is properly oriented on the mesentery and not on any tension. Stomal eversion can be completed several ways either including fascia to seromuscular layer or with deep serosal layer to more superficial mucosa to deep dermal layer at four points with 2-0 Vicryl and tied down one at time accentuating the rosebud formation. The stoma is matured with skin-mucosa 3-0 Vicryl or chromic suture around the edge of the stoma.
9. An abdominal drain is placed and can be removed prior to discharge which is no concern for ureteroileal urine leak. Ureteral stents can be removed in 4–6 weeks postoperatively [15, 16].

Note: stomal placement can be right or left sided if using colonic segment. A right-side colon conduit may be preferred for patients with existing colostomy/ileostomy to avoid pouching issues postoperatively.

Conclusion

Severe urgency urinary incontinence/overactive bladder can have profound effects on overall patient quality of life and should be managed in stepwise fashion (Fig. 13.2). In patients that have failed noninvasive therapies including

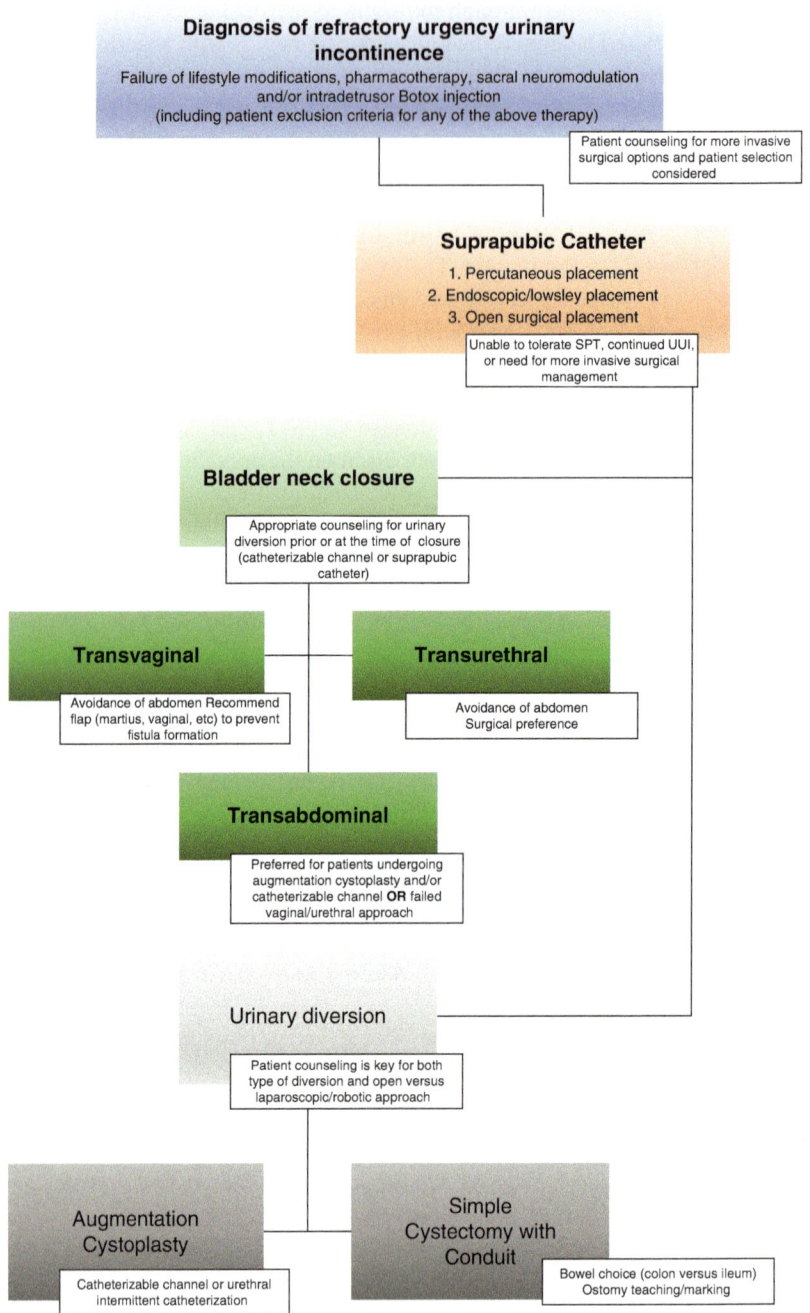

Fig. 13.2 Treatment Algorithm for Refractory Urgency Urinary Incontinence

anticholinergics/beta 3 agonist medications, intravesical injection of botox, or sacral neuromodulation, it is reasonable to offer more invasive surgical management. It is imperative that appropriate counseling occurs so that patients understand the options, complications, and impact these interventions can have on daily life. Additionally, a combination of modalities may be utilized to optimize quality of life including suprapubic catheterization (with or without intravesical Botox), bladder neck closure with urinary diversion (suprapubic catheter, catheterizable channel). In extreme cases, permanent options for urinary diversion should be considered and include augmentation cystoplasty with or without catheterizable channel and urinary diversion. The method (open versus laparoscopic/robotic) should be carefully considered by the surgeon and their appropriate skill set.

References

1. Abrams P, Cardozo L, Fall M, Griffiths D, Rosier P, Ulmsten U, et al. The standardisation of terminology of lower urinary tract function: report from the standardisation sub-committee of the International Continence Society. Neurourol Urodyn. 2002;21(2):167–78.
2. Lightner DJ, Gomelsky A, Souter L, Vasavada SP. Diagnosis and treatment of overactive bladder (non-neurogenic) in adults: AUA/SUFU guideline amendment 2019. J Urol. 2019;202(3):101097JU0000000000000309-563.
3. MacLachlan LS, Rovner ES. New treatments for incontinence. Adv Chronic Kidney Dis. 2015;22(4):279–88.
4. Jr HF. Suprapubic catheterization. In: Hinman, editor. Atlas of urologic surgery. Philadelphia, Pennsylvania: Saunders; 1998. p. 625–9.
5. Wyner LM. Easy suprapubic tube placement using a Van Buren sound. Urology. 2018;114:245.
6. Zeidman EJC. Humberto; Alarcon, Antonio; Raz, Shlomo. Suprapubic cystotomy using lowsley retractor. Urology. 1988;32(1):54–5.
7. Wolter CD, Roger. Suprapubic catheterization. In: Hashim H, AP, Dmochowski R, editors. . London: Springer; 2008. p. 128–31.
8. Boone TB, Stewart JN, Martinez LM. Additional therapies for storage and emptying failure. In: Wein AJ, Kavoussi LR, Campbell MF, editors. Campbell-Walsh-Wein urology. 12th ed. Philadelphia: Elsevier Saunders; 2012. p. 2889–904.
9. Ardelt PU, Woodhouse CR, Riedmiller H, Gerharz EW. The efferent segment in continent cutaneous urinary diversion: a comprehensive review of the literature. BJU Int. 2012;109(2):288–97.
10. Willis H, Safiano NA, Lloyd LK. Comparison of transvaginal and retropubic bladder neck closure with suprapubic catheter in women. J Urol. 2015;193(1):196–202.
11. Colli J, Lloyd LK. Bladder neck closure and suprapubic catheter placement as definitive management of neurogenic bladder. J Spinal Cord Med. 2011;34(3):273–7.
12. Rovner ES, Goudelocke CM, Gilchrist A, Lebed B. Transvaginal bladder neck closure with posterior urethral flap for devastated urethra. Urology. 2011;78(1):208–12.
13. Zimmern PE, Hadley HR, Leach GE, Raz S. Transvaginal closure of the bladder neck and placement of a suprapubic catheter for destroyed urethra after long-term indwelling catheterization. J Urol. 1985;134(3):554–7.
14. Zimmern PE, et al. In: Zimmern P, editor. Vaginal surgery for incontinence and prolapse [electronic resource]. London: Springer; 2006.

15. Smith JA Jr, Howards SS, Preminger GM, Dmochowski RR, Smith JA, Howards SS, Preminger GM, Dmochowski RR, editors. Hinman's atlas of urologic surgery. 4th ed. Philadelphia: Elsevier; 2018.
16. Dmochowski RR, Kavoussi LR, Peters CA. In: Partin AW, Partin AW, Dmochowski RR, Kavoussi LR, Peters C, editors. Campbell-Walsh-Wein urology. 12th ed. Philadelphia: Elsevier; 2020.

Part IV
Surgical Treatment for SUI

Chapter 14
Urethral Bulking Agents

Alexandra L. Tabakin and Siobhan M. Hartigan

Introduction

Urethral bulking agents (UBAs) are a minimally invasive treatment for either primary or recurrent SUI after other anti-incontinence procedures. First introduced in the early twentieth century, UBAs continue to evolve in composition, mechanism of action, and delivery method. Here we discuss indications for UBA usage, procedural aspects of injection, and historical and contemporary UBAs.

Method of Action

UBAs are used to treat stress urinary incontinence (SUI) in patients with intrinsic sphincter deficiency (ISD), a very weakened urethral closure mechanism [1]. UBAs can be injected transurethrally or through the periurethral tissue, thereby focally expanding urethral surface area and increasing pressure transmitted to the proximal urethra [2]. The bulking of the urethra improves urethral coaptation and urethral outlet resistance, preventing the leakage of urine. Injection of UBAs may also increase functional urethral length [3].

UBAs may be synthesized from biologic or synthetic materials. Biologic UBAs are comprised of decellularized membranes from either autologous, allogenic, or

A. L. Tabakin
Division of Urology, Rutgers Robert Wood Johnson Medical School,
New Brunswick, NJ, USA

S. M. Hartigan (✉)
Hunterdon Urological Associates, Flemington, NJ, USA
e-mail: smhartigan@gmail.comalliet

© The Author(s), under exclusive license to Springer Nature
Switzerland AG 2022
A. P. Cameron (ed.), *Female Urinary Incontinence*,
https://doi.org/10.1007/978-3-030-84352-6_14

xenogenic tissues [4]. Synthetic UBAs are categorized as either particulate or non-particulate. Particulate UBAs are composed of microspheres suspended in an absorbable gel carrier. As the gel is reabsorbed over time, the surrounding host tissue integrates with the remaining particles to create a bulky fibrotic capsule. Particles must be at least 80 μm in diameter to prevent migration from the original site of injection [5, 6]. Non-particulate UBAs are created from homogenous, non-absorbable gels; for these agents, the bulk is created by the thin fibrous networks that form to anchor the injected gel to the host tissue [5].

Although there are key differences in their mechanisms of action based on their composition, ideal UBAs share similar key characteristics. For a UBA to successfully support reconstruction of and augment periurethral tissue, it should be easily injectable, non-absorbable, nontoxic, and non-immunogenic. UBAs should also be acellular, nonmigratory, and induce minimal fibrosis and calcification [7, 8].

Patient Selection and Indications

UBAs are classically used in patients with SUI secondary to ISD, defined as an abdominal leak point pressure less than 60 cm H_2O on urodynamics. Ideal candidates should also lack urethral hypermobility and idiopathic detrusor contractions [9]. UBAs have been shown to be most efficacious in women with less than 2.5 episodes of SUI per day and those aged 60 years and older. The efficacy of UBAs in older women may be attributed to lower baseline activity levels as well as improvement in sphincter function through an increase in sphincter sarcomere length [10].

Although UBAs are less efficacious than the gold standard mid-urethral sling (MUS) for treating SUI with urethral hypermobility, they boast a more favorable side effect profile and have many indications [11]. UBAs can be considered in patients who are poor surgical candidates secondary to comorbidities, age, severe obesity, or inability to stop anticoagulation. UBAs can be offered to women of childbearing age who desire future pregnancies and those who want to avoid a surgery requiring general anesthesia but accept a lower rate of cure [12]. UBAs may also be utilized in cases of mild SUI, SUI with poor bladder emptying, or as an adjunct to other anti-incontinence procedures if SUI still persists [9, 12]. Contraindications to UBA injection include active urinary tract infection (UTI) or history of allergic reaction to the bulking agent of choice [12].

Procedural Aspects and Injection Techniques

UBAs can be injected under sedation or local or general anesthesia either in an office setting or the operating room [13]. To perform injections, the patient is traditionally placed in the dorsal lithotomy position. The genitals are prepped and draped in a sterile fashion. Topical anesthetics or lidocaine can be deposited transurethrally or injected within the urethral submucosa. It is recommended that practitioners administer a single dose of prophylactic antibiotics in accordance with local anti-biograms and prior patient urine cultures [14]. UBAs should be deposited into the proximal urethral mucosa near the bladder neck [15–17]. Three major methods of injection have been described.

Transurethral Injection

Transurethral injection involves the implantation of UBAs through the working channel of a cystoscope (Fig. 14.1a). The transurethral method allows the clinician to perform the injection under direct vision and select the precise location for implantation. The practitioner can also visualize urethral coaptation, potentially reducing the amount of bulking agent required. For optimal coaptation, injections should be performed at either 3 and 9 o'clock or 6 o'clock through a cystoscope [18]. Circumferential periurethral distribution and proximal urethral injection have been associated with optimal short-term success rates [19].

Periurethral Injection

Periurethral injection involves the direct placement of the UBA in the urethral mucosa in the perimeatal region (Fig. 14.1b). In comparison with the transurethral method, periurethral injection offers certain benefits including less mucosal leak-age and bleeding [20]. However, periurethral injections are associated with a higher

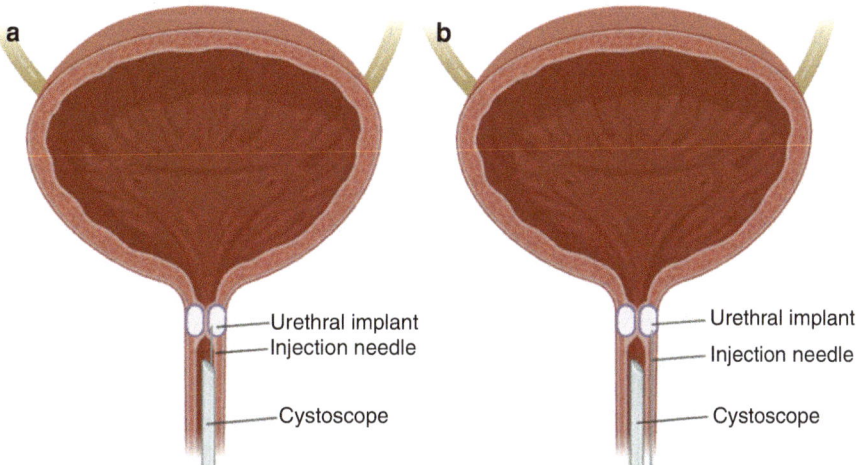

Fig. 14.1 (**a**) Technique for transurethral injection where the needle for urethral bulking agent delivery is advanced through the working channel of a cystoscope. (**b**) Technique for periurethral injection of urethral bulking agent by direct placement of the injection needle in the perimeatal region. (Created with BioRender.com)

risk of acute urinary retention, which is hypothesized to be caused by the use of higher volumes of the bulking agent, since direct visualization may not be utilized [20, 21].

Device-Guided Injection

Some UBAs are deposited through specially made dispensers. The Macroplastique™ Implantation System contains an injection device placed in the urethra to the level of the bladder neck, which is identified when urine flows through the device's central channel (Fig. 14.2a). The clinician withdraws the device 1 centimeter distally. Needles are then placed through the implantation device into the urethral mucosa at the 2, 6, and 10 o'clock positions [17].

Bulkamid™ is injected through a urethroscope containing a zero-degree lens and light cord for visualization (Fig. 14.2b). A specialized needle is inserted 1 cm into the submucosa at the 6 o'clock position. Additional injections are placed at either 2 and 10 o'clock or 3, 9, and 12 o'clock. The practitioner should visualize the formation of blebs after each submucosal injection [15].

Similarly, Urolastic™ is administered through a dispenser gun containing an applicator which is placed in the mid-urethra. Injections are then performed at the 2, 5, 7, and 10 o'clock positions for optimal urethral coaptation. If persistent leakage occurs after a cough test, additional deposits can be placed in the 3 or 9 o'clock regions [16].

Postoperative Recommendations and Findings

Practitioners should measure a PVR for all patients postoperatively [14]. Patients with PVRs greater than 100–150 ml may require a single catheterization with a 10–12 French Foley catheter. A smaller catheter is recommended as to not displace the

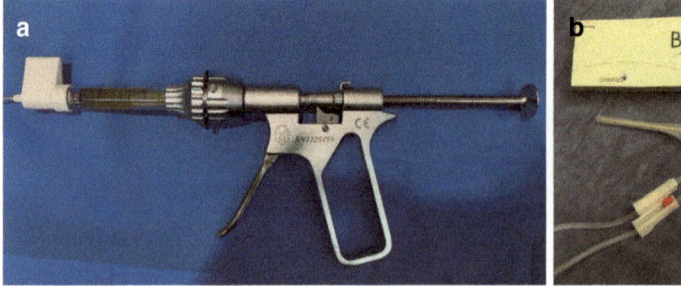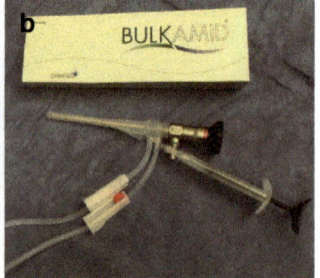

Fig. 14.2 Device-guided injection dispensers. (**a**) Macroplastique™ Implantation System contains an injection device which is placed in the urethra to the level of the bladder neck in order to optimally position the injection sites [90]. (**b**) Bulkamid™ rotatable sheath is advanced through the urethra under direct visualization, after which the clinician may perform injections [15]

recently injected bulking agent. If urinary retention persists, patients should be taught to perform clean intermittent catheterization. Patients may return to work after 24 hours if performed under general anesthesia [15, 16] or same day if done under local anesthesia. Minimal, if any, pain medication is usually required following the procedure.

Of note, bulking agents can be seen on computed tomography (CT) or magnetic resonance imaging (MRI) and can be confused with urethral masses. Some are also radiopaque (Coaptite, Durasphere) and can be mistaken for bladder stones on kidney, ureter, and bladder x-ray (KUB) (Fig. 14.3). A recent retrospective study revealed occasional misdiagnosis of periurethral bulking agents in patients with SUI [22]. In this study, urethral findings were rarely mentioned on abdominal or pelvic imaging interpretation. In the infrequent cases in which they were mentioned, greater than 60% misdiagnosed the bulking material as a genitourinary pathology such as pelvic mass or urethral diverticulum [22].

Comparison of Injection Methods

Benefits and disadvantages associated with each injection method have been described, but there is no evidence favoring one method over another in terms of clinical success rates. One study comparing transurethral ($n = 24$) to periurethral

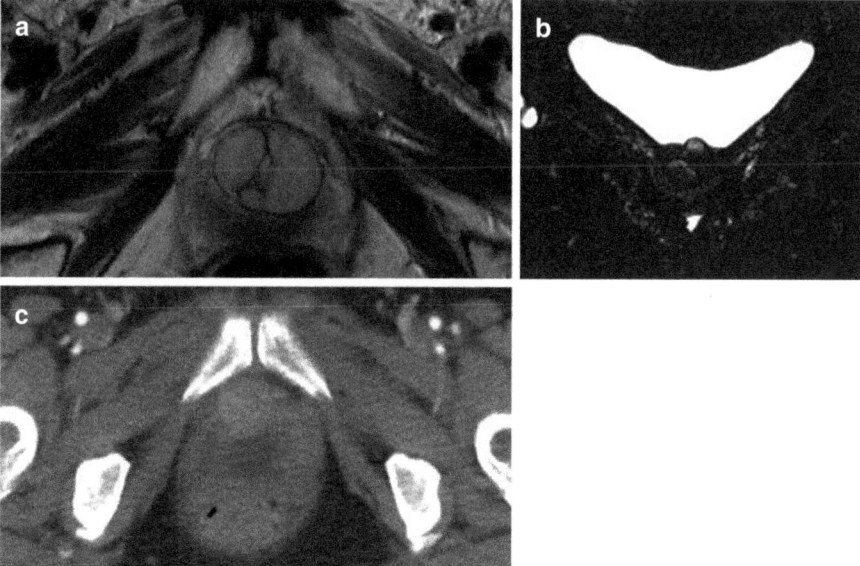

Fig. 14.3 UBAs identified on various imaging modalities can be easily misinterpreted. (**a**) Axial magnetic resonance imaging of collagen bulking agent which was correctly interpreted on radiographic read. (**b**) Coronal magnetic resonance imaging of collagen bulking agent which was radiographically interpreted as "possible urethral diverticulum." (**c**) Axial computerized tomography imaging of Macroplastique™ bulking agent which was radiographically interpreted as "increased attenuation of soft tissue". (Images **a-c** courtesy of Anne Cameron MD)

($n = 21$) collagen injection demonstrated no statistically significant difference in cure, symptomatic improvement, or complication rates after six months. However, the amount of collagen injected was lower (4.7 vs 10.1 ml) for the transurethral compared to the periurethral group, respectively [21].

These results were corroborated by an analysis of 40 women with SUI or mixed urinary incontinence (MUI) randomized to receive either periurethral or transurethral injection of dextran copolymer. There was no significant difference in dry rates or subjective mean symptomatic improvement at one, three, six, or 12 months. Primary reason for SUI (ISD vs urethral hypermobility) had no significant relationship with clinical results. Importantly, there was a significantly higher incidence of urinary retention in the periurethral group compared to the transurethral group (30% vs 5%, respectively). While there were no differences in the volume of UBA injected overall, patients in the periurethral group who experienced urinary retention had a significantly larger quantity of bulking agent deposited than those in the transurethral group (5.1 vs 3.4 ml) [20].

Summary of Urethral Bulking Agents in Women: Safety and Efficacy

Historical Agents

Historical UBAs are summarized in Table 14.1.

Table 14.1 Historical urethral bulking agents

Urethral bulking agent	Trade name(s)	Agent class	Associated complications
Sodium morrhuate	N/A	Sclerosing agent	Pulmonary embolus, cardiac arrest
Granugenol oil/Dondren	N/A	Sclerosing agent	Pulmonary embolus, urethral sloughing
Polytetrafluoroethylene	Teflon™	Microsphere particulate UBA	Particle migration, particle extrusion, periurethral abscess, urethral diverticula, granuloma formation, possible carcinogen
Autologous fat	N/A	autologous fat	Pulmonary fat embolism
Glutaraldehyde Cross-Linked (GAX) Collagen	Contigen™	Bovine collagen	Allergic reactions, pulmonary emboli, sterile abscess formation
Ethylene vinyl alcohol	Uryx™, Tegress™	Copolymer non-particulate UBA	Urethral erosions
Dextranomer with hyaluronic acid	Zuidex™, Deflux™	Microsphere particulate UBA	Sterile abscess, injection site mass, and pseudocyst formation

Sclerosing Agents

Sodium morrhuate, a sclerosing agent, was the first documented UBA. First described in 1938, Murless injected sodium morrhuate into the anterior vaginal wall to stimulate scarring of the periurethral tissue in order to prevent urethral hypermobility. While somewhat successful, some severe adverse effects ensued including pulmonary embolus and cardiac arrest [23, 24]. In 1963, Sachse injected granugenol oil, or Dondren, another sclerosing agent, into both female and male urethras. Although patients did experience some symptomatic improvement, several developed pulmonary emboli and urethral sloughing [25].

Polytetrafluoroethylene (Teflon™)

Polytetrafluoroethylene, or Teflon™, contains microparticles ranging in size from less than 50 μm to 300 μm [26]. It was used in the 1970s and 1980s with success rates as high as 75% [27] but was never approved for use in the United States due to significant complications related to particle migration to distant sites and its carcinogenic potential [23, 28]. Furthermore, there were several reports of extrusion, periurethral abscess, urethral diverticula, and granuloma formation [23, 29].

Autologous Fat

As early as 1989, several groups trialed periurethral injections of autologous fat harvested from the abdominal wall [30]. Thought to be a suitable material for a UBA for its ease of access and biocompatibility, a randomized double-blind trial comparing periurethral injections of autologous fat or saline placebo failed to demonstrate a significant difference in cure rates. One patient even experienced death secondary to pulmonary fat embolism [31], which further discouraged its usage as a UBA. The durability of autologous fat grafts is limited, as grafts lose up to 55% of volume by six months [32].

Glutaraldehyde Cross-Linked (GAX) Collagen (Contigen™)

In 1993, GAX bovine collagen in phosphate-buffered saline, marketed as Contigen™ (CR Bard, Murray Hill, New Jersey, USA), was approved by the US Food and Drug Administration (FDA) as a UBA. Initial symptomatic improvement rates ranged from 68 to 90%, usually after approximately three injections, but declined over time [33, 34]. Comprised of 95% type I collagen and 1–5% type III collagen, women undergoing Contigen injection required skin testing 30 days prior to their procedure, as it caused allergic reactions in 4% of patients due to its antigenic nature. Other adverse events included UTI, hematuria, de novo urgency, arthralgia, pulmonary emboli, and sterile abscess formation [35]. Contigen was discontinued by its manufacturer in 2011.

Ethylene Vinyl Alcohol (Uryx™, Tegress™)

Ethylene vinyl alcohol (EVA) is a copolymer suspended in dimethyl sulfoxide (DMSO), also known as Uryx™ (Genyx Medical, Inc., Aliso Viejo, CA/C.R. Bard, Murray Hill, NJ, USA) or Tegress™ (CR Bard, Murray Hill, NJ, USA). EVA was approved by the FDA in 2004 for use as a UBA. When injected and exposed to blood or extracellular fluid at body temperature, the DMSO dissolves, and the EVA forms a spongiform mass, creating the urethral bulk [36]. When compared to collagen injections, EVA injections had higher cure and symptomatic improvement rates [37]. However, it was ultimately withdrawn from the market in 2007 due to multiple adverse effects including severe urethral erosions and fistula formation [38].

Dextranomer with Hyaluronic Acid (Zuidex™, Deflux™)

Zuidex™ (Q-Med AB, Uppsala, Sweden) or Deflux™ (Oceana Therapeutics Inc., Edison, New Jersey, USA) are gels containing dextranomer microspheres suspended in hyaluronic acid. As the hyaluronic acid gel dissolves, the microspheres remain in place for four years, promoting connective tissue ingrowth. These agents are commonly used and approved for endoscopic treatment of vesicoureteral reflux in children.

A multicenter study with 142 patients with invasive-treatment naïve SUI who underwent Zuidex injections demonstrated a 77% positive response, defined as ≥50% reduction in provocation test leakage, after one year. Significant reductions were also noted for 24-hour pad-weight test and number of daily incontinence episodes. Most adverse events were transient and included urinary retention, UTI, injection site reaction, urinary urgency, vaginal discomfort, dysuria, pain, pseudocyst formation, and injection site infection [39].

A subsequent non-inferiority trial compared outcomes in patients with SUI, who were randomized to receive either midurethral injection of Zuidex ($n = 227$) or Contigen injection at the bladder neck ($n = 117$). Those who underwent Contigen injection had higher dry and positive response rates, also defined as ≥50% reduction in provocation test leakage. Although both groups had identical rates of urinary retention (28%), the Zuidex group experienced more complications, including sterile abscess, injection site mass, and pseudocyst formation [40], leading to its discontinuation as a UBA for SUI.

Contemporary UBAs

Contemporary UBAs are summarized in Table 14.2.

Table 14.2 Contemporary urethral bulking agents (Updated January 2021)

Urethral bulking agent	Trade name(s)	Composition	Mechanism of action	Particle size	Year of FDA approval
Particulate agents					
Carbon-coated zirconium	Durasphere™	Carbon-coated zirconium particles in 2.8% beta-glucan hydrogel carrier	Hydrogel degrades over times, leaving particles behind to create bulk	212 to 500 μm	1999
Calcium hydroxylapatite	Coaptite™	Calcium hydroxylapatite microspheres incarboxymethyl cellulose gel carrier		75 to 125 μm	2005
Cross-linked polydimethylsiloxane	Macroplastique™	Cross-linked polydimethylsiloxane elastomer particles in polyvinylpyrrolidone hydrogel carrier		110 μm	2006
Non-Particulate Agents					
Porcine collagen	Permacol™	Cross-linked porcine dermis	Injected collagen matrix integrates with host tissue and blood vessels	N/A	2004
Polyacrylamide hydrogel	Bulkamid™, Aquamid™	Hydrogel containing 97.5% nonpyrogenic water and 2.5% cross-linked polyacrylamide	Hydrogel invaded by macrophages and giant cells, allowing for integration with host tissue	N/A	2020
Polydimethylsiloxane	Urolastic™	Vinyl dimethyl terminated polydimethylsiloxane polymer, tetrapropoxysilane cross-linking material, and platinum divinyltetramethyl siloxane complex catalyst	Injected as a liquid which hardens and becomes encased in scar tissue	N/A	pending

Porcine Collagen (Permacol™)

Permacol™ (Covidien, Gosport, United Kingdom) is sourced from cross-linked porcine dermis. During processing, cells, DNA, and RNA are removed in such a way that allows the collagen matrix to retain its microscopic constitution [41]. The matrix resembles human dermis, allowing integration with host tissue and blood vessels. Unlike Contigen, it does not require allergy testing prior to implantation [42]. Data surrounding the efficacy of Permacol is mostly limited to one trial which randomized women with SUI to receive either injection with Permacol ($n = 25$) or Macroplastique ($n = 25$). Six weeks postinjection, Permacol patients had insignificantly higher dry rates (60% vs 41.6%). At six months, 62.5% of the Permacol patients remained dry compared with 37.5% of Macroplastique patients. Additionally, fewer Permacol patients experienced transient post-procedural urinary retention (8 vs 12%) [42].

Calcium Hydroxylapatite (Coaptite™)

Coaptite™ (Bioform Medical Inc., San Mateo, California, USA) is a synthetic UBA consisting of calcium hydroxylapatite microspheres suspended in a carboxymethyl cellulose gel carrier. Microsphere particles range in size from 75 to 125 μm [43]. The gel initially provides the bulking effect but degrades over time allowing native tissue to grow around the particles, which also eventually dissolve [43]. The volume of the Coaptite deposit decreases by approximately 40% after three months, and patients who retain more volume are more likely to have sustained symptomatic improvement [44].

The main data supporting the efficacy of Coaptite is derived from a multicenter prospective randomized control trial. In this non-inferiority study, women with SUI secondary to ISD without urethral hypermobility received injection with either Coaptite or Contigen, the gold standard at the time of publication. After one year, there was an insignificant improvement in patient success, defined as improvement of at least one Stamey grade, favoring the Coaptite group (63.4 vs 57.0%). There were also no differences in the one-year cure rate (39% vs 37%) and percentage of participants having at least 50% reduction in 24-hour pad weight (62% vs 54%) for the Coaptite and Contigen groups, respectively. Furthermore, more patients in the Coaptite group only required a single injection [43].

There were no differences between the groups in terms of most minor procedure-related adverse events, including dysuria or urinary retention, although there was a significantly lower risk of developing urge incontinence in the Coaptite group (5.7% vs 12%). Two major complications were reported in the Coaptite group, specifically vaginal wall erosion into the distal urethra and dissection of the material beneath the trigone. These serious events were attributed to injection technique and the large particle size causing pressure on host tissues [43]. Other rare side effects of Coaptite including urethral prolapse and granuloma formation requiring surgical correction have been reported [45, 46].

Carbon-Coated Zirconium (Durasphere™)

Durasphere™ (Carbon Medical Technologies, St. Paul, Minnesota, USA) contains nondegradable carbon-coated zirconium particles suspended in a dissolvable 2.8% beta-glucan hydrogel carrier. The relatively large particles range in size from 212 to 500 μm [47], which can make injection more difficult due to increased resistance [5]. It became FDA approved for use as a UBA in 1999 [48].

Durasphere was shown to have equivalent efficacy to collagen injections in a multicenter trial. The study randomized 355 women with SUI secondary to ISD to receive either Durasphere or bovine collagen. Clinicians used a significantly lower volume of Durasphere than collagen during injection (4.83 vs 6.23 ml, respectively). At one year after injection, there was no difference in pad weight or improvement in continence grade. After both one and two years, no evidence of particle migration was observed on pelvic radiographs [48]. However, after 24 months and beyond, Durasphere's objective benefits diminished [49]. With respect to adverse events, patients in the Durasphere group experienced significantly more urinary urgency and transient acute retention. Otherwise, complication profiles were similar [48]. While most adverse effects are self-limited, other serious complications including particle migration to lymph node tissue [50], periurethral abscess formation, and urethral prolapse [51] have been reported as well as visible staining/tattoo of vaginal mucosa since the product is black in color.

Durasphere has also been used in combination with Contigen. In a study comparing women who underwent combined Contigen/Durasphere injections ($n = 33$) with Contigen alone ($n = 33$), there was a significantly higher cure rate in the combined group after two weeks (72.7% vs. 39.2%). The benefits were not sustained, and dry rates after six months were equivalent between the combined and Contigen alone groups (33.3 vs 29.4%). There was no difference between groups in the need for subsequent anti-incontinence procedures [52].

Cross-Linked Polydimethylsiloxane (Macroplastique™)

Macroplastique™ (Cogentix Medical, Orangeburg, New York, USA) is a silicone polymer containing cross-linked polydimethylsiloxane elastomer particles suspended in a polyvinylpyrrolidone hydrogel carrier. After injection, the Macroplastique deposit is enveloped in a fibrin capsule, which is infiltrated with collagen. The hydrogel is absorbed and excreted by the kidneys [53]. The nondegradable particles, approximately 110 μm in size, remain in place after the gel carrier dissolves [5, 54].

The most compelling data demonstrating Macroplastique's efficacy was described in a trial of 247 women with SUI secondary to ISD who were randomized to receive transurethral injection of either Macroplastique or Contigen. At 12 months, the Macroplastique group demonstrated a significantly higher dry rate than the Contigen group (36.9% vs 24.8%). More patients in the Macroplastique cohort also improved by at least one Stamey grade (61.5% vs 48%). Both cohorts exhibited a reduction in urine loss from baseline, although there was no distinguishable difference from each other. The number and volume of injections between groups were also equivalent. Both groups had similar rates of treatment-related adverse events. The most common side effects included UTI, lower urinary tract symptoms, urinary retention, and implantation site pain. Three patients experienced urethral erosion (two in the Macroplastique group and one in the Contigen group) [54]. After two years of follow-up, 84% of patients reported continued improvement from their treatment, 67% of whom were dry. Incontinence quality of life (I-QoL) scores and mean pad weight also remained significantly improved from baseline. There were no treatment-related adverse events during the follow-up period [53].

A subsequent systematic review combining data from 958 women with SUI who underwent Macroplastique injection demonstrated short-term, mid-term, and long-term dry rates of 43%, 37%, and 36% and improvement rates of 75%, 73%, and 64%, respectively. The median reinjection rate was 30%, with 63% of those patients reporting symptomatic improvement from SUI. Adverse events were all minor, such as transient urinary retention, urge incontinence, UTI, dysuria, and hematuria [55]. However, despite an overall favorable complication profile, a number of rare and serious complications were described including extrusion secondary to suspected immune reaction, bladder neck and urethral erosion, and suburethral, vaginal, and bladder mass formation [56–60]. Several other studies have demonstrated Macroplastique's durable response with cure rates ranging from 47 to 49% after two to three years. While many patients require more than one injection, most objective improvement rates remain stable after six months. There are also sustained decreases in daily pad weight after several years of follow-up [61–63].

Macroplastique may also be useful in patients with SUI after hysterectomy. In a study of 24 cervical cancer patients who underwent radical hysterectomy with resultant SUI, Macroplastique injection was associated with a 42% dry rate and 42% improvement rate after one year. Failure was correlated with presence of ure-thral hypermobility [64].

Polyacrylamide Hydrogel (Bulkamid™, Aquamid ™)

Bulkamid™ and Aquamid™ (Contura International A/S, Soeborg, Denmark) are derived from a nondegradable hydrogel containing 97.5% nonpyrogenic water and 2.5% cross-linked polyacrylamide [7]. The viscoelastic, hydrophilic nature of poly-acrylamide hydrogel allows it to exchange water molecules, nutrients, and waste with the surrounding host tissue matrix [5]. Over several years, the hydrogel is invaded by macrophages and giant cells which are then replaced by a permanent network of thin fibers and vessels [65] to prevent migration [66].

The effects of Bulkamid have been investigated in a number of settings including SUI, mixed incontinence, and vulnerable patients. With respect to treatment for SUI and MUI, a systematic review of mostly observational studies revealed improve-ments in the number of incontinence episodes, quantity of urine leakage, and quality of life after Bulkamid injection. The overall reinjection was calculated to be 24.3%. Complications were mostly minor including pain at injection site, UTI, hematuria, and transient acute urinary retention [67]. Rare serious adverse events included abscess formation and urethral mucous membrane rupture at injection site [67–69]. The only randomized double-arm study included was a multicenter trial demonstrating the non-inferiority of polyacrylamide hydrogel to Contigen for treatment of SUI or stress-predominant MUI. After one-year postinjection, cure/improvement rates were 77.1% and 70% for the polyacrylamide hydrogel and Contigen groups, respectively. There was no difference in complication rates between cohorts, which were mostly limited to minor, transient lower urinary tract symptoms, urinary retention, and de novo incontinence. Only one serious treatment-related adverse effect, transient hematuria, was reported in the polyacrylamide hydrogel group [8]. On post hoc analysis, a 90% treatment effect rate and 38% cure rate were seen in women over age 60, compared to just a 13% cure rate for younger women [10].

In addition to improving incontinence, Bulkamid has been shown to have a positive effect on sexual activity. Leone Roberti Maggiore et al. described the effects Bulkamid injection on sexual function in 29 women with SUI. After one year of follow-up, 100% of the 23 previously sexually active patients were able to resume sexual activity after injection. These women reported less incontinence or fear of incontinence during intercourse, improvement in desire, climax, and satisfaction with their sex lives. The remaining six nonsexually active women were able to reestablish sexual activity as well [70].

Bulkamid has also been successfully utilized in a number of special populations including octogenarians and postradiation patients [71, 72]. In a group of 20 octogenarians with a mean age of 84.5 years old, Vecchioli-Scaldazza et al. found a significant reduction in urine lost with a cough stress test and number of pads needed after two years after Bulkamid injection. Quality of life scores and urodynamic parameters, including abdominal leak point pressure, mean urethral closure pressure, and urethral length also improved [72]. Krhut et al. administered Bulkamid to 46 women with a history of a gynecologic cancer with resultant SUI treated with and without pelvic radiotherapy. After injection, cure rates for the radiation group and non-radiation group were 25% and 36.4%, respectively, and no severe adverse events were reported [71]. Taken together, these findings highlight how polyacrylamide hydrogel can be a useful tool with minimal risk in vulnerable patients with incontinence.

Polydimethylsiloxane (Urolastic™)

Urolastic (Urogyn BV, Nijmegen, The Netherlands) is a synthetic compound containing vinyl dimethyl terminated polydimethylsiloxane polymer, a tetrapropoxysilane cross-linking material, and a platinum divinyltetramethyl siloxane complex catalyst. The addition of titanium dioxide radio-opacifies this bulking agent [73]. Unlike Macroplastique, the Urolastic deposit does not contain any particles and is injected as a liquid. Once the liquid hardens, it is encircled in scar tissue and does not degrade, lose volume, or migrate over time [74]. Currently, Urolastic is only approved for usage in Europe.

The efficacy and complication profile of Urolastic for treating SUI has been described in a few small series [73–77]. Zajda et al. reported on 20 women with SUI who underwent Urolastic injection, 35% of whom required a second injection. After 12 and 24 months of follow-up, 68% and 45% ·of patients remained dry, respectively. Eighty-nine percent of patients reported improved continence after 12 months which was reduced to 66% at two years [74, 77]. Minor complications occurred in 30% of patients, which included hematoma formation, urinary retention, and dyspareunia or vaginal pain requiring removal of the deposit [74]. At 24 months, four out of 18 patients included in the follow-up analysis underwent implant removal because of dyspareunia and suboptimal dryness [77]. Likewise, Futyma et al. performed Urolastic injection on 105 women with either primary or recurrent SUI. After 12 months, objective success rates, defined as negative pad and cough stress tests, were 71.4% and 59.3% in the primary and recurrent groups, respectively. The overall reinjection rate was 17%. Four out of 10 patients with urinary retention required implant excision [75]. After 24 months, those with recurrent SUI had a 22.4% cure rate, with 32.7% reporting objective success (either cure or improvement) [76].

Urolastic has also been trialed in women who are medically unfit for surgery. Kowalik et al. evaluated the effects of Urolastic periurethral injection in 20 women deemed unfit for a MUS. Five patients required a second injection due to persistent incontinence, three of which required removal of the bulking agent from the first injection. Six months postinjection, 90% of patients reported subjective symptomatic improvement, and 65% of patients had a negative cough stress test. Health-related quality of life scores improved significantly in all domains, as measured by the Urogenital Distress Inventory (UDI-6) and the Incontinence Impact Questionnaire (IIQ-7). Peri-procedural complications included hematoma formation, pain, and injection of the UBA at epithelial surface requiring excision. Reported adverse events were all managed in the outpatient setting and included urinary retention immediately after injection, bulking material exposure, and spontaneous loss of bulking material [73].

Long-term success of Urolastic appears comparable to other bulking agents. In a systematic review with follow-up between six and 24 months, objective cure rates ranged between 32.7% and 67% with a pooled rate of 57%. The pooled subjective improvement rate was 84%. A second injection was required in 16.7%–35% of study cohorts. The pooled complication rate was 36%, the most common of which was urgency, post-void residual greater than 150 ml, and exposure or erosion [78]. Ultimately up to 18% of patients may require excision of Urolastic for persistent pain, exposure, or erosion [79].

The Use of UBAs Compared with Other Anti-Incontinence Procedures

Practices for managing SUI widely vary among clinicians, as there is no accepted standardized algorithm. The 2017 American Urological Association/Society of Urodynamics, Female Pelvic Medicine, and Urogenital Reconstruction (AUA/

SUFU) Guidelines for SUI state that in index patients with SUI considering surgical treatment, clinicians may offer UBAs as well as synthetic MUS, autologous fascial pubovaginal sling, or a Burch colposuspension. The Guidelines also state that UBAs may be offered to non-index patients with ISD in addition to retropubic MUS and pubovaginal slings. No recommendations are given with respect to the order in which these treatment options should be trialed, although the discussion statement does express that UBAs should be offered to patients who want a minimally invasive procedure and acknowledges that repeat injections are common [80]. Similarly, the European Association of Urology (EAU) 2018 Guidelines on urinary incontinence state that bulking agents should be offered to women with SUI who desire a low-risk procedure and understand that they will likely require repeat injections [81].

The precise location in which UBAs should fall on the SUI surgical management decision tree is unknown. This ambiguity is likely due to a paucity of randomized prospective studies comparing UBAs to other anti-incontinence procedures [82].

In a 2015 systematic review and meta-analysis, the authors identified just three studies comparing UBAs to other anti-incontinence procedures, only two of which were randomized control trials. The analysis concluded that UBAs are associated with significantly higher objective recurrence rates for both primary and recurrent SUI when compared with other anti-incontinence procedures, which included pubovaginal slings, MUS, bladder neck suspensions, and Burch colposuspensions. UBAs were associated with less voiding dysfunction. However, the small size of this meta-analysis and numerous other limitations highlight the need for additional comparative data [82].

More recently, a trial randomized 224 women with primary SUI to receive either tension-free vaginal tape ($n = 111$) or polyacrylamide hydrogel injection ($n = 113$). After one year of follow-up, patients who underwent MUS reported higher patient satisfaction scores and higher rates of dryness as measured by a negative cough stress test compared with those who underwent polyacrylamide hydrogel injection (95% vs 66.4%, respectively). Women in both groups exhibited improved sexual function and health-related quality of life, particularly in the domains of physical and social functioning. However, MUS was associated with a higher rate of perioperative complications and reoperations [11, 83]. Therefore, it is important to counsel patients with SUI on both options, as some patients may be willing to accept the trade-off between lower cure rates with UBAs and higher complication rates associated with MUS [84]. Ultimately, more prospective data comparing UBAs to other anti-incontinence procedures evaluated in diverse patient settings are needed to clearly define the role of UBAs in managing primary and recurrent SUI.

UBAs as a Salvage Procedure After Failed MUS

There is currently no established gold standard or consensus for the ideal salvage technique after a failed MUS [66]. In a survey of the members of the International Urogynecological Association, UBAs were reported as the preferred salvage procedure in patients without urethral hypermobility [85]. Despite the proclivity of some surgeons to trial UBAs for recurrent SUI after a sling, the evidence regarding the efficacy and durability of UBAs as a salvage procedure for recurrent SUI after a failed MUS is limited to small retrospective reports and lacks high-quality evidence.

A study including 23 women who underwent salvage injection with either Macroplastique or Durasphere after a failed MUS demonstrated a cure rate of 34.8% after just 10 months, despite improved I-QoL scores and 92% perceived benefit of treatment [86]. Similarly, Dray et al. examined 73 patients with recurrent SUI after MUS placement who underwent salvage injection with either Macroplastique or collagen. After an average of 2.6 injections, 71% of patients reported symptomatic improvement, 24.7% of whom had complete resolution of SUI. Just two of 40 women with long-term follow-up information after a mean of 39.5 months reported complete resolution of SUI, although there was a significant improvement in most domains on the Michigan Incontinence Symptom Index (M-ISI) [18]. In an analysis of 17 women who underwent injection with 2 ml of Bulkamid after failed MUS, Clark et al. reported a 42% reinjection rate (occurring between 10 and 46 months after the initial injection) but a 71% perceived rate of benefit [87]. Zivanovic et al. performed a retrospective observational analysis looking at 60 patients with refractory SUI or MUI after a failed MUS who underwent injection with 1 to 3 ml of Bulkamid. After one month, 93.3% of patients were either cured or had symptomatic improvement, which slightly dropped to 88.3% and 83.6% at six and 12 months, respectively. The most common adverse event was persistent urge urinary incontinence in 20%, 16.7%, and 20% of patients after one, six, and 12 months, respectively. Other adverse events were seen in a small minority of patients and included voiding dysfunction, UTI, de novo urgency, hematuria, injection site laceration, and hematoma [66].

Only one analysis has directly compared repeat MUS ($n = 98$) with UBA using either Contigen, Coaptite, or Macroplastique ($n = 67$) as a salvage technique after failed MUS. Those who underwent UBA injection experienced a significantly higher risk of failure after one year of follow-up compared to repeat MUS patients (38.8% vs 11.2%, respectively), although there was no difference in complication rates [88].

UBAs have also been utilized as a salvage technique after MUS removal. Rodriguez et al. evaluated 70 women who underwent UBA injection with Macroplastique after excision of failed MUS. They demonstrated a 69% overall success rate, with an 83% subjective improvement rate and 78% reduction in pad usage [89]. While these studies are small, it does appear that multiple types of UBAs offer both subjective and objective symptomatic benefit to many women when used as an adjunctive salvage procedure or after MUS removal, although the benefit diminishes over time and may require reinjection.

Conclusion

UBAs are an important tool in a urologist's armamentarium for managing SUI. They are particularly useful in women who are not surgical candidates or who wish to avoid general anesthesia. Although associated with lower rates of cure than other anti-incontinence procedures, UBAs demonstrate more favorable complication profiles. More prospective randomized data is necessary to elucidate the optimal composition and long-term outcomes of UBAs.

References

1. D'Ancona C, Haylen B, Oelke M, et al. The International Continence Society (ICS) report on the terminology for adult male lower urinary tract and pelvic floor symptoms and dysfunction. Neurourol Urodyn. 2019;38(2):433–77.
2. Radley SC, Chapple CR, Lee JA. Transurethral implantation of silicone polymer for stress incontinence: evaluation of a porcine model and mechanism of action in vivo. BJU Int. 2000;85(6):646–50.
3. Wasenda EJ, Kirby AC, Lukacz ES, et al. The female continence mechanism measured by high resolution manometry: urethral bulking versus midurethral sling. Neurourol Urodyn. 2018;37(5):1809–14.
4. Davis NF, Kheradmand F, Creagh T. Injectable biomaterials for the treatment of stress urinary incontinence: their potential and pitfalls as urethral bulking agents. Int Urogynecol J. 2013;24(6):913–9.
5. Chapple C, Dmochowski R. Particulate versus non-particulate bulking agents in the treatment of stress urinary incontinence. Res Rep Urol. 2019;11:299–310.
6. Kirchin V, Page T, Keegan PE, et al. Urethral injection therapy for urinary incontinence in women. Cochrane Database Syst Rev. 2017;7:CD003881.
7. Lose G, Mouritsen L, Nielsen JB. A new bulking agent (polyacrylamide hydrogel) for treating stress urinary incontinence in women. BJU Int. 2006;98(1):100–4.
8. Sokol ER, Karram MM, Dmochowski R. Efficacy and safety of polyacrylamide hydrogel for the treatment of female stress incontinence: a randomized, prospective, multicenter North American study. J Urol. 2014;192(3):843–9.
9. Kocjancic E, Mourad S, Acar O. Complications of urethral bulking therapy for female stress urinary incontinence. Neurourol Urodyn. 2019;38(Suppl 4):S12–20.
10. Elmelund M, Sokol ER, Karram MM, et al. Patient characteristics that may influence the effect of urethral injection therapy for female stress urinary incontinence. J Urol. 2019;202(1):125–31.
11. Itkonen Freitas AM, Mentula M, Rahkola-Soisalo P, et al. Tension-free vaginal tape surgery versus polyacrylamide hydrogel injection for primary stress urinary incontinence: a randomized clinical trial. J Urol. 2020;203(2):372–8.
12. Mamut A, Carlson KV. Periurethral bulking agents for female stress urinary incontinence in Canada. Can Urol Assoc J. 2017;11(6Suppl2):S152–S4.
13. Corcos J, Collet JP, Shapiro S, et al. Multicenter randomized clinical trial comparing surgery and collagen injections for treatment of female stress urinary incontinence. Urology. 2005;65(5):898–904.
14. Li H, Westney OL. Injection of urethral bulking agents. Urol Clin North Am. 2019;46(1):1–15.
15. Bulkamid standard operating procedure: Contura; Available from: https://bulkamid.com/wp-content/uploads/2019/03/BULK_2018_041.2_SOP_12.04.18.pdf.
16. Urolastic instructions for use: Urogyn BV; Available from: https://www.urogynbv.com/wp-content/uploads/2015/09/Urolastic-IFU-EN-rev6-06OCT2014.pdf.
17. Tamanini JT, D'Ancona CA, Tadini V, et al. Macroplastique implantation system for the treatment of female stress urinary incontinence. J Urol. 2003;169(6):2229–33.
18. Dray EV, Hall M, Covalschi D, et al. Can urethral bulking agents salvage failed slings? Urology. 2019;124:78–82.
19. Hegde A, Smith AL, Aguilar VC, et al. Three-dimensional endovaginal ultrasound examination following injection of Macroplastique for stress urinary incontinence: outcomes based on location and periurethral distribution of the bulking agent. Int Urogynecol J. 2013;24(7):1151–9.

20. Schulz JA, Nager CW, Stanton SL, et al. Bulking agents for stress urinary incontinence: short-term results and complications in a randomized comparison of periurethral and transurethral injections. Int Urogynecol J Pelvic Floor Dysfunct. 2004;15(4):261–5.
21. Faerber GJ, Belville WD, Ohl DA, et al. Comparison of transurethral versus periurethral collagen injection in women with intrinsic sphincter deficiency. Tech Urol. 1998;4(3):124–7.
22. Gaines N, Gupta P, Khourdaji AS, et al. Radiographic misdiagnoses after Periurethral bulking agents. Female Pelvic Med Reconstr Surg. 2018;24(4):312–4.
23. Hussain SM, Bray R. Urethral bulking agents for female stress urinary incontinence. Neurourol Urodyn. 2019;38(3):887–92.
24. Murless BC. The injection treatment of stress incontinence. J Obstet Gynaecol Br Emp. 1938;45:67–73.
25. Sachse H. Treatment of urinary incontinence with sclerosing solutions. Indications, results, complications. Urol Int. 1963;15:225–44.
26. Taylor AK, Dielubanza E, Hairston J. Use of injectable urethral bulking agents in the management of stress urinary incontinence. Curr Bladder Dysfunct Rep. 2011;6:159(2011).
27. Politano VA. Periurethral polytetrafluoroethylene injection for urinary incontinence. J Urol. 1982;127(3):439–42.
28. Malizia AA Jr, Reiman HM, Myers RP, et al. Migration and granulomatous reaction after periurethral injection of polytef (Teflon). JAMA. 1984;251(24):3277–81.
29. Kiilholma PJ, Chancellor MB, Makinen J, et al. Complications of Teflon injection for stress urinary incontinence. Neurourol Urodyn. 1993;12(2):131–7.
30. Santiago Gonzalez de Garibay AM, Castro Morrondo J, Castillo Jimeno JM, et al. Endoscopic injection of autologous adipose tissue in the treatment of female incontinence. Arch Esp Urol. 1989;42(2):143–6.
31. Lee PE, Kung RC, Drutz HP. Periurethral autologous fat injection as treatment for female stress urinary incontinence: a randomized double-blind controlled trial. J Urol. 2001;165(1):153–8.
32. Horl HW, Feller AM, Biemer E. Technique for liposuction fat reimplantation and long-term volume evaluation by magnetic resonance imaging. Ann Plast Surg. 1991;26(3):248–58.
33. Dmochowski RR, Appell RA. Injectable agents in the treatment of stress urinary incontinence in women: where are we now? Urology. 2000;56(6 Suppl 1):32–40.
34. Winters JC, Appell R. Periurethral injection of collagen in the treatment of intrinsic sphincteric deficiency in the female patient. Urol Clin North Am. 1995;22(3):673–8.
35. Sweat SD, Lightner DJ. Complications of sterile abscess formation and pulmonary embolism following periurethral bulking agents. J Urol. 1999;161(1):93–6.
36. Mukkamala A, Latini JM, Cameron AP. Urethrocutaneous fistula after use of Tegress bulking agent: case report and review of the literature. Can Urol Assoc J. 2013;7(11-12):E833–6.
37. Dmochowski RR. Tegresstrade mark urethral implant phase III clinical experience and product uniqueness. Rev Urol. 2005;7(Suppl 1):S22–6.
38. Hurtado EA, Appell RA. Complications of Tegress injections. Int Urogynecol J Pelvic Floor Dysfunct. 2009;20(1):127; author reply 9.
39. Chapple CR, Haab F, Cervigni M, et al. An open, multicentre study of NASHA/Dx Gel (Zuidex) for the treatment of stress urinary incontinence. Eur Urol. 2005;48(3):488–94.
40. Lightner D, Rovner E, Corcos J, et al. Randomized controlled multisite trial of injected bulking agents for women with intrinsic sphincter deficiency: mid-urethral injection of Zuidex via the Implacer versus proximal urethral injection of Contigen cystoscopically. Urology. 2009;74(4):771–5.
41. Permacol(TM) Surgical implant: Medtronic; 2020. Available from: https://www.medtronic.com/covidien/en-us/products/hernia-repair/permacol-surgical-implant.html.
42. Bano F, Barrington JW, Dyer R. Comparison between porcine dermal implant (Permacol) and silicone injection (Macroplastique) for urodynamic stress incontinence. Int Urogynecol J Pelvic Floor Dysfunct. 2005;16(2):147–50; discussion 50.

43. Mayer RD, Dmochowski RR, Appell RA, et al. Multicenter prospective randomized 52-week trial of calcium hydroxylapatite versus bovine dermal collagen for treatment of stress urinary incontinence. Urology. 2007;69(5):876–80.
44. Unger CA, Barber MD, Walters MD. Ultrasound evaluation of the urethra and bladder neck before and after transurethral bulking. Female Pelvic Med Reconstr Surg. 2016;22(2): 118–22.
45. Lai HH, Hurtado EA, Appell RA. Large urethral prolapse formation after calcium hydroxylapatite (Coaptite) injection. Int Urogynecol J Pelvic Floor Dysfunct. 2008;19(9):1315–7.
46. Palma PC, Riccetto CL, Martins MH, et al. Massive prolapse of the urethral mucosa following periurethral injection of calcium hydroxylapatite for stress urinary incontinence. Int Urogynecol J Pelvic Floor Dysfunct. 2006;17(6):670–1.
47. Summary of safety and effectiveness data: Durasphere(TM) Injectable Bulking Agent: United States Food and Drug Administration; 1999. Available from: https://www.accessdata.fda.gov/cdrh_docs/pdf/P980053b.pdf.
48. Lightner D, Calvosa C, Andersen R, et al. A new injectable bulking agent for treatment of stress urinary incontinence: results of a multicenter, randomized, controlled, double-blind study of Durasphere. Urology. 2001;58(1):12–5.
49. Chrouser KL, Fick F, Goel A, et al. Carbon coated zirconium beads in beta-glucan gel and bovine glutaraldehyde cross-linked collagen injections for intrinsic sphincter deficiency: continence and satisfaction after extended followup. J Urol. 2004;171(3):1152–5.
50. Pannek J, Brands FH, Senge T. Particle migration after transurethral injection of carbon coated beads for stress urinary incontinence. J Urol. 2001;166(4):1350–3.
51. Ghoniem GM, Khater U. Urethral prolapse after durasphere injection. Int Urogynecol J Pelvic Floor Dysfunct. 2006;17(3):297–8.
52. Sokol ER, Aguilar VC, Sung VW, et al. Combined trans- and periurethral injections of bulking agents for the treatment of intrinsic sphincter deficiency. Int Urogynecol J Pelvic Floor Dysfunct. 2008;19(5):643–7.
53. Ghoniem G, Corcos J, Comiter C, et al. Durability of urethral bulking agent injection for female stress urinary incontinence: 2-year multicenter study results. J Urol. 2010;183(4):1444–9.
54. Ghoniem G, Corcos J, Comiter C, et al. Cross-linked polydimethylsiloxane injection for female stress urinary incontinence: results of a multicenter, randomized, controlled, single-blind study. J Urol. 2009;181(1):204–10.
55. Ghoniem GM, Miller CJ. A systematic review and meta-analysis of Macroplastique for treating female stress urinary incontinence. Int Urogynecol J. 2013;24(1):27–36.
56. Bennett AT, Lukacz ES. Two cases of suspected rejection of polydimethylsiloxane urethral bulking agent. Female Pelvic Med Reconstr Surg. 2017;23(3):e10–e1.
57. Kulkarni S, Davies AJ, Treurnicht K, et al. Misplaced Macroplastique injection presenting as a vaginal nodule and a bladder mass. Int J Clin Pract Suppl. 2005;(147):85–6.
58. Rodriguez D, Jaffer A, Hilmy M, et al. Bladder neck and urethral erosions after Macroplastique injections. Low Urin Tract Symptoms. 2020;13:93.
59. Thompson A, Daborn JP. A vaginal mass and ulceration 8 years following Macroplastique(R) injection. Int Urogynecol J. 2015;26(10):1547–9.
60. Wasenda EJ, Nager CW. Suburethral mass formation after injection of polydimethylsiloxane (Macroplastique(R)) urethral bulking agent. Int Urogynecol J. 2016;27(12):1935–6.
61. Serati M, Soligo M, Braga A, et al. Efficacy and safety of polydimethylsiloxane injection (Macroplastique((R))) for the treatment of female stress urinary incontinence: results of a series of 85 patients with >/=3 years of follow-up. BJU Int. 2019;123(2):353–9.
62. Tamanini JT, D'Ancona CA, Netto NR Jr. Treatment of intrinsic sphincter deficiency using the Macroplastique implantation system: two-year follow-up. J Endourol. 2004;18(9):906–11.
63. Tamanini JT, D'Ancona CA, Netto NR. Macroplastique implantation system for female stress urinary incontinence: long-term follow-up. J Endourol. 2006;20(12):1082–6.
64. Plotti F, Zullo MA, Sansone M, et al. Post radical hysterectomy urinary incontinence: a prospective study of transurethral bulking agents injection. Gynecol Oncol. 2009;112(1):90–4.

65. Christensen LH, Nielsen JB, Mouritsen L, et al. Tissue integration of polyacrylamide hydrogel: an experimental study of periurethral, perivesical, and mammary gland tissue in the pig. Dermatol Surg. 2008;34 Suppl 1:S68–77; discussion S.
66. Zivanovic I, Rautenberg O, Lobodasch K, et al. Urethral bulking for recurrent stress urinary incontinence after midurethral sling failure. Neurourol Urodyn. 2017;36(3):722–6.
67. Kasi AD, Pergialiotis V, Perrea DN, et al. Polyacrylamide hydrogel (Bulkamid(R)) for stress urinary incontinence in women: a systematic review of the literature. Int Urogynecol J. 2016;27(3):367–75.
68. Gopinath D, Smith AR, Reid FM. Periurethral abscess following polyacrylamide hydrogel (Bulkamid) for stress urinary incontinence. Int Urogynecol J. 2012;23(11):1645–8.
69. Martan A, Masata J, Svabik K, et al. Transurethral injection of polyacrylamide hydrogel (Bulkamid((R))) for the treatment of female stress or mixed urinary incontinence. Eur J Obstet Gynecol Reprod Biol. 2014;178:199–202.
70. Leone Roberti Maggiore U, Alessandri F, Medica M, et al. Periurethral injection of polyacrylamide hydrogel for the treatment of stress urinary incontinence: the impact on female sexual function. J Sex Med. 2012;9(12):3255–63.
71. Krhut J, Martan A, Jurakova M, et al. Treatment of stress urinary incontinence using polyacrylamide hydrogel in women after radiotherapy: 1-year follow-up. Int Urogynecol J. 2016;27(2):301–5.
72. Vecchioli-Scaldazza CV, Smaali C, Morosetti C, et al. Polyacrylamide hydrogel (bulkamid(R)) in female patients of 80 or more years with urinary incontinence. Int Braz J Urol. 2014;40(1):37–43.
73. Kowalik CR, Casteleijn FM, van Eijndhoven HWF, et al. Results of an innovative bulking agent in patients with stress urinary incontinence who are not optimal candidates for midurethral sling surgery. Neurourol Urodyn. 2018;37(1):339–45.
74. Zajda J, Farag F. Urolastic-a new bulking agent for the treatment of women with stress urinary incontinence: outcome of 12 months follow up. Adv Urol. 2013;2013:724082.
75. Futyma K, Miotla P, Galczynski K, et al. An open multicenter study of clinical efficacy and safety of Urolastic, an injectable implant for the treatment of stress urinary incontinence: one-year observation. Biomed Res Int. 2015;2015:851823.
76. Futyma K, Nowakowski L, Galczynski K, et al. Nonabsorbable urethral bulking agent - clinical effectiveness and late complications rates in the treatment of recurrent stress urinary incontinence after 2 years of follow-up. Eur J Obstet Gynecol Reprod Biol. 2016;207:68–72.
77. Zajda J, Farag F. Urolastic for the treatment of women with stress urinary incontinence: 24-month follow-up. Cent Eur J Urol. 2015;68(3):334–8.
78. Capobianco G, Azzena A, Saderi L, et al. Urolastic(R), a new bulking agent for treatment of stress urinary incontinence: a systematic review and meta-analysis. Int Urogynecol J. 2018;29(9):1239–47.
79. Casteleijn FM, Kowalik CR, Berends C, et al. Patients' satisfaction and safety of bulk injection therapy Urolastic for treatment of stress urinary incontinence: a cross-sectional study. Neurourol Urodyn. 2020;39(6):1753–63.
80. Kobashi KC, Albo ME, Dmochowski RR, et al. Surgical treatment of female stress urinary incontinence: AUA/SUFU guideline. J Urol. 2017;198(4):875–83.
81. Burkhard FC, Bosch, JLHR, Cruz F, Lemack GE, Nambiar AK, Thiruchelvam N, Tubaro A, Ambühl D, Bedretdinova DA, Farag F, Lombardo R, Schneider MP. Urinary incontinence 2018. Available from: https://uroweb.org/guideline/urinary-incontinence/.
82. Leone Roberti Maggiore U, Bogani G, Meschia M, et al. Urethral bulking agents versus other surgical procedures for the treatment of female stress urinary incontinence: a systematic review and meta-analysis. Eur J Obstet Gynecol Reprod Biol. 2015;189:48–54.
83. Itkonen Freitas AM, Mikkola TS, Rahkola-Soisalo P, et al. Quality of life and sexual function after TVT surgery versus Bulkamid injection for primary stress urinary incontinence: 1 year results from a randomized clinical trial. Int Urogynecol J. 2020;32:595.

84. Casteleijn FM, Enklaar RA, El Bouyahyaoui I, et al. How cure rates drive patients' preference for urethral bulking agent or mid-urethral sling surgery as therapy for stress urinary incontinence. Neurourol Urodyn. 2019;38(5):1384–91.
85. Giarenis I, Thiagamoorthy G, Zacche M, et al. Management of recurrent stress urinary incontinence after failed midurethral sling: a survey of members of the International Urogynecological Association (IUGA). Int Urogynecol J. 2015;26(9):1285–91.
86. Lee HN, Lee YS, Han JY, et al. Transurethral injection of bulking agent for treatment of failed mid-urethral sling procedures. Int Urogynecol J. 2010;21(12):1479–83.
87. Clark R, Welk B. The use of polyacrylamide hydrogel in the setting of failed female stress incontinence surgery. Can Urol Assoc J. 2018;12(4):95–7.
88. Gaddi A, Guaderrama N, Bassiouni N, et al. Repeat midurethral sling compared with urethral bulking for recurrent stress urinary incontinence. Obstet Gynecol. 2014;123(6):1207–12.
89. Rodriguez D, Carroll T, Alhalabi F, et al. Outcomes of Macroplastique injections for stress urinary incontinence after suburethral sling removal. Neurourol Urodyn. 2020;39(3):994–1001.
90. Macroplastique® Implantation System (MIS): Cogentix Medical; 2021. Available from: https://www.cogentixmedical.com/health-care-professionals/products/macroplastique/implantation-system.

Chapter 15
Burch Colposuspension

Ali Luck and Samantha Raffee

Introduction

Burch colposuspension was the "gold standard" for correcting stress urinary incontinence (SUI) from urethral hypermobility in the twentieth century until the advent of the mid-urethral sling. It was first described by John C. Burch in 1961 as he was trying to overcome challenges encountered while performing the Marshall-Marchetti-Krantz (MMK) procedure. He found that attaching the bladder neck to Cooper's ligament was more robust and better able to restore the normal anatomy of the bladder neck [1]. The predecessor to the Burch was the MMK procedure. It is the attachment of the bladder neck (urethrovesical junction) to the periosteum of the pubic symphysis which at times did not prove to be a reliable point of attachment and had the risk of developing osteitis pubis. Burch and his colleagues found similar success rates when compared to MMK. The MMK procedure has largely been replaced by the Burch colposuspension when comparative trials were performed showing similar efficacy with less morbidity [2].

Since it was first described, variations of the Burch colposuspension technique have been described. Emil A. Tanagho's publication in 1976 made modifications, helping to standardize the Burch procedure [3]. It is the most widely adopted approach used by surgeons today. Due to advent of the minimally invasive

A. Luck (✉)
Department of Women's Health, Obstetrics & Gynecology, Female Pelvic Medicine Reconstructive Surgery, Henry Ford Health Systems, Detroit, MI, USA
e-mail: Aluck1@hfhs.org

S. Raffee
Department of Urology, Female Pelvic Medicine Reconstructive Surgery, Henry Ford Health Systems, Detroit, MI, USA
e-mail: Sraffee1@hfhs.org

© The Author(s), under exclusive license to Springer Nature Switzerland AG 2022
A. P. Cameron (ed.), *Female Urinary Incontinence*,
https://doi.org/10.1007/978-3-030-84352-6_15

257

mid-urethral sling (MUS), the trend in use of Burch colposuspension has waned since 2000 [4]. In 2008, the US Food and Drug Administration (FDA) investigated the use of polypropylene synthetic mesh for MUS and pelvic organ prolapse. It was not until 2013 that the FDA declared that the multi-incision sling procedure was safe and effective for up to one year [5]. In the 5 years that lapsed as synthetic mesh was being investigated, there was confusion separating the use of synthetic mesh for MUS and prolapse portrayed in the media. The medical legal entities became involved, strategically targeting patients that had received the MUS. Patients gave pause to the most common surgical treatment for SUI. Some nations went as far as banning use of all synthetic mesh [6]. Patients were now looking for alternative non-mesh procedures to surgically correct SUI. It was also at this time that pelvic floor surgeons started to revisit the use of the Burch colposuspension procedure.

This procedure has had proven safety and efficacy for more than 20 years. It has been adapted to the laparoscopic and robotic platform. Indications for the use of the Burch include providing an alternative to synthetic mesh and an option to be used during concomitant open surgery, such as an abdominal hysterectomy.

This chapter will cover the techniques to perform the Burch procedure and explore theories on how it treats SUI, its reported safety, efficacy, and complications. The technique described will be for an open approach; however, the laparoscopic principles are the same once the retropubic space is accessed. Other chapters in this book have addressed in detail other surgical treatments and the nonsurgical treatments for SUI.

Mechanism of Action

The exact mechanism of Burch colposuspension has yet to be elucidated. Two dueling theories exist. The first suggests that the pressure transmission is better distributed along the urethra when the bladder neck is stabilized above the pelvic floor, restoring normal anatomy [7]. The second theory states that changes occurring in the urethra lead to higher urethral resistance and subsequent continence [8]. Retropubic procedures evolved out of what is now the anatomic theory, explaining the etiology of SUI set forth by Dr. Victor Bonney. In 1923, he published a paper, "On Diurnal Incontinence of Urine in Women," describing SUI and theorized that SUI occurs due to the defect in the support of the bladder neck. In this paper, it is quoted that "Incontinence appears to be due to the laxity of the front part of the pubo-cervical muscle-sheet, so that it yields under sudden pressure and allows the bladder to slip down behind the symphysis pubis and the urethra to carry downwards and forwards by wheeling round the sub-pubic angle" [9]. Bonney's work set the stage for other investigators to follow. With the radiographic innovation in the 1930s, the watch-chain cystogram was used by investigators to study the bladder neck of patients with SUI and noticed what was described as a "funneling of the bladder floor" [10]. It was deduced that funneling of the bladder neck led to weakness and ultimately, SUI. It may not necessarily be the defect in the support of the bladder by the vagina and surrounding periurethral which cause SUI but rather problems with the urethral sphincter itself.

The idea that the defect may be due to the urethral sphincter was then further investigated by Barnes (1940) and Enhorning (1960) with the use of manometry, the predecessor to video multichannel urodynamics [10, 11]. They were able to study the pressure inside the urethra and noticed how pressure was being transmitted. They noted that when intra-abdominal pressure rose, there was poor distribution of this pressure along the urethra, such as when there is a sagging of the bladder neck, and incontinence occurred. This became the basis of the pressure transmission theory.

Burch colposuspension was theorized to be effective based on this theory. The suspension sutures of the Burch colposuspension would restore the anatomy of the bladder neck, thus making the closure of the urethral sphincter more effective and allow equal distribution of the pressure along the urethra, leading to continence. The studies that looked at this concept started in the early 1980s. Hilton and Stanton studied pressure transmission ratios (PTR), examining continent and incontinent women [12]. The PTR is calculated to be the change in urethral pressure over the change in the vesical pressure expressed in percentage: $\Delta U/\Delta V \times 100\%$. During urodynamic testing, the pressure transmission in the urethra is calculated along the length of the urethra during rest and cough provocation. It was noted that continent women had greater maintenance of transmission in the proximal urethra with highest PTR in the mid-urethra with values approaching 100% or higher. It was determined that continence was an "all or none effect." This idea was supported by their findings that patients who underwent Burch colposuspension had PTR approaching 100% or greater of those whose surgeries were deemed successful [13].

Bump et al. (1988) took a closer look at the PTR and complications after SUI surgery [14]. They concluded that if the PTR were close to 100%, continence was achieved; however, if more than 100%, this could lead to greater obstruction, resulting in detrusor instability. Of note, the patient population of this early study was small and heterogeneous with regard to the type of SUI surgeries performed. This continence PTR threshold concept was further explored by Rosenzweig et al. They examined variables of the PTR contributing to incontinence, patient characteristics affecting PTR, the effects of Burch colposuspension on the PTR, and whether changes in the PTR predicted surgical success. They noted that there was not a percentage that predicted continence, but rather it was dependent on changes in preoperative and postoperative PTR. The higher the difference between preoperative and postoperative PTR, the more successful the surgery. It was also noted that some continent patients had PTR < 100%, suggesting that the Burch suspension may not have to be obstructive to be successful.

In the mid-1990s, DeLancey described the "hammock effect" tying together the anatomic theory and the pressure transmission theory [15]. The restoration of the pubocervical fascia provided the compensatory mechanism by which the urethra could be compressed, preventing abnormal transmission of abdominal pressure. DeLancey also tried to tie in the neuromuscular control of SUI. Through his cadaver work, he identified that the pubocervical fascia inserted at the arcus tendineus fascia pelvis (ATFP) which also served as the attachment of the levator muscles. During increased intra-abdominal pressure, the levator muscles are activated, pulling up on the ATFP and pubocervical fascia to facilitate coaptation of the urethra.

In the late 1990s and early 2000s, several investigators called into the possibility that the colposuspension may be effective partly due to its high urethral resistance. Klutke et al. (1999) examined UDS parameters of patients who underwent Burch, modified Pereyra, and anterior repair and then plotted it on the Abrams-Griffiths nomogram (later named the bladder outlet obstruction index, BOOI) [16]. It was noted that the mean urethral resistance was significantly higher in the Burch group between preoperative and postoperative parameters. It was noted that only 50% of the patients that were considered "cured" were in the unobstructive zone and 10% in the obstructed zone. This led them to conclude that there may be a compensatory mechanism to the Burch procedure. There may not have to be an overcorrection of the bladder neck, which can lead to voiding dysfunction, to achieve continence. This observation was also seen in the large, randomized control trial of 655 women undergoing the Burch colposuspension or autologous sling, the Stress Incontinence Surgical Treatment Efficacy Trial (SISTEr) [17]. The BOOI was higher after undergoing Burch and the autologous fascial sling. The autologous fascial sling had a higher BOOI score and likely explaining the higher number of patients with voiding dysfunction in this group.

Surgical Technique

Anatomy

Before performing the procedure, it is important to understand the vital structures in the retropubic space to prevent vascular and neurologic complications. The retropubic space is an avascular space bounded by the pubic symphysis anteriorly, laterally by the pubic rami and the pelvic muscles (obturator internus, pubococcygeus, and puborectalis) with the proximal and mid-urethra and extraperitoneal bladder inferiorly. The peritoneum/anterior abdominal wall serves as the roof of this space [18].

The vesical venous plexus is the most common site of bleeding. Pathi et al. (2009) looked at 15 unembalmed female cadavers and noted that there were interconnections of 2–5 rows of vessels within the paravaginal connective tissue that ran parallel to bladder. The vital structures that should be identified prior to the dissection into this space include the obturator neurovascular bundle, accessory (aberrant) obturator vessels, and the external iliac vessels. The obturator canal is approximately 2 cm below the superior pubic ramus at a point 6 cm lateral from the superior pubic symphysis. In cadaveric studies, the accessory obturator veins can be seen 52–70% and accessory obturator arteries in 19–34% of the time [19, 20]. Figure 15.1 illustrates the anatomy in relation to the Burch sutures.

Fig. 15.1 Retropubic anatomy and location of Burch sutures. (Reprinted from Pathi et al. [19]. With permission with minimal modification from Elselvier). (*yellow arrows*) Burch sutures at the bladder neck (PS) pubic symphysis; (OC) obturator canal; (EI) external Iliac vessels; (B) Bladder; (*) ischial spine; (*arrowhead*) spatial relationship of the right vesical venous plexus and its connecting branch to the internal iliac vein

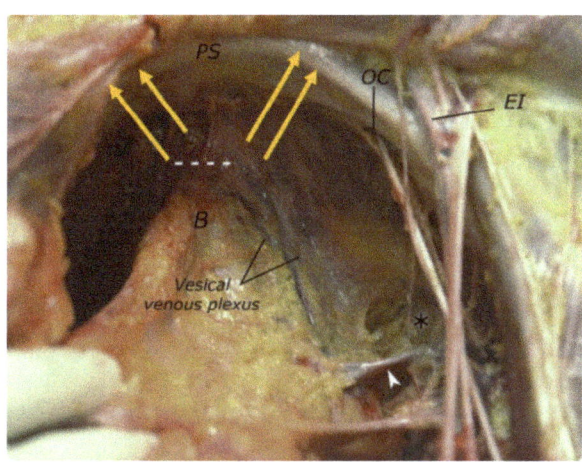

Surgical Steps

As with most pelvic floor surgeries, it is best accomplished in the supine dorsal lithotomy position. For the optimal placement of the Burch sutures, the surgeon will need one hand in the vagina to elevate the vagina and one hand in the retropubic space to place the sutures. Because of this, it is best to have the patient's lower extremities in surgical boot stirrups (Allen stirrups, Yellowfin stirrups) versus the strap stirrups (candy cane stirrups). Care should be given to avoid hyperextension and flexion at the knees and hips and abduction and internal rotation of the hips. The boot stirrups will allow easier adjustment as one has to go from the abdomen to the vagina and vice versa during the surgery. A 16 or 20 French Foley catheter with a 20 to 30 mL balloon will help delineate the bladder neck during dissection. A three-way catheter can be helpful, though not necessary to facilitate backfilling the bladder for visualization of the bladder. Saline or water mixed with methylene blue can be helpful to backfill the bladder; immediate recognition of injury to the bladder or urethra can be easily seen if entered with the Burch sutures. Preoperative antibiotics and thromboembolic prevention measures should be administered. A safety pause is performed prior to the start of surgery.

1. Access to the retroperitoneal space

    (a) The abdominal skin incision may be dictated by the concomitant surgery such as a hysterectomy. It is possible that the rectus muscle would need to be split to have better access to this area. The exposure of the retropubic space is key to have good visualization of the vital structures. If Burch colposuspension is performed in isolation, a small (6–9 cm) low transverse Pfannenstiel incision, 2 cm above the pubic rami, can be used to provide less morbid access. A Cherney or Maylard incision can be made to help with exposure of the retropubic space, if necessary. The Cherney incision, separating the rectus muscle at the tendinous insertion to the pubic symphysis, is preferred if reattaching the rectus muscle is the goal at the end of the procedure. The end of the tendinous insertion can be better approximated and serves as a sturdier anchor point versus having the sutures go through the rectus muscle itself as seen in the Maylard incision. Be cognizant of the inferior epigastric vessels while separating the rectus tendon from the pyramidalis muscle. The furthest lateral structure to identify is the obturator canal which can be 5–8 cm from the pubic symphysis. When using retractors for visualization, be cognizant of the external iliac vessels.

2. Adequate exposure of the bladder neck and pectineal ligament (Cooper's ligament)

   (a) Palpate and identify the obturator canal to prevent dissecting too laterally and injuring the neurovascular bundle when clearing the loose fatty areolar tissue off the pectineal ligament.
   (b) Start mobilizing the loose areolar tissue away from the proximal urethra and bladder neck while applying pressure to the bladder to bring it cephalad. Be methodical and gentle. Depress the tissue right behind the pubic symphysis approximately 2 cm on either side of the midline trying to find the avascular space and work laterally. Try to stay away from the midline since this is the area that is most vascular. Your gloved finger, back end of pickups or Yankauer suction can aid in this dissection.
   (c) Have the vaginal assistant start backfilling the bladder until outline of the bladder is obvious. The vaginal assistant should gently pull back on the Foley bulb to the bladder neck and place a finger on either side of the Foley bulb and catheter while elevating the anterior vaginal wall. This will help to identify how medial one can start to move the tissue away until the fibromuscular layer (endopelvic fascia) of the vagina is identified. The fibromuscular layer of the vagina should be white, almost glistening in nature. Be aware of the vesical venous plexus that are running parallel to the bladder. The goal is to clear an area approximately 2 cm from the periurethral tissue on either side so that sutures can be safely placed. Excess fat can be cleared away with the use of radiopaque sponges mounted on the end of ring forceps. If the ATFP can be identified, this should be the lateral boundary of the dissection.

3. Suture placement

   (a) In the joint report on the terminology for surgical procedures to treat stress urinary incontinence in women by the American Urogynecologic Society and the International Urogynecological Association (2020), the use of delayed absorbable or permanent sutures was advocated [21]. Non-braided sutures are preferred to avoid future sinus track formation. The authors prefer monofilament permanent sutures, 0-polypropylene. The preference for permanent sutures was standardized in the SISTEr trial [17], and permanent sutures may decrease the possibility of postoperative voiding dysfunction. If using delayed absorbable suture, tensioning of sutures should not leave space between the bladder neck and pectineal ligament. There is a theoretical risk that if the suture reabsorbs before scar formation, then the colposuspension may not be effective.

(b) With the surgeon's nondominant finger in the vagina, elevating the bladder neck, place the most distal suture at the proximal 1/3 of the urethra, 2 cm lateral to the urethra, through the fibromuscular layer of the vagina. Avoid perforation of the vaginal epithelium. Bring the suture through the ipsilateral pectineal ligament at the same level and place a tag. The second suture should be placed at the bladder neck, 2 cm lateral to the urethra in a similar fashion and brought through the ipsilateral pectineal ligament. An anatomic gross dissection study by J. Hamner et al. (2018) demonstrated a "zone of safety" 2 cm from the periurethral tissue to the ATFP at the level of the bladder neck [18].

A figure of eight should be taken through the fibromuscular layer of the vagina to decrease the risk of sutures pulling through. To avoid injury to the surgeon's finger, a stainless-steel thimble can be placed over the surgeon's finger [22]. Place the sutures on the contralateral side in a similar fashion and secure a tag until cystoscopy has been performed.

(c) Cystoscopy should be performed. Tension and tie down the sutures after cystoscopy has been performed to confirm that the sutures did not perforate the urethra and bladder. Leave a 2–3 cm suture bridge between the periurethral tissue and the pectineal ligament when tying the sutures. The goal of the procedure is to correct the hypermobility of the bladder neck and not over elevate the bladder neck leading to obstruction. Tighter is not better. Figure 15.1 shows a drawing depicting the relationship of the sutures to the surrounding vital structures in the retropubic space.

(d) When bleeding is encountered, there are several options to secure hemostasis. If bleeding occurs while placing sutures through the fibromuscular layer of the vagina, the offending suture can be tied by the abdominal surgical assistant before being brought through to the pectineal ligament. It is most likely venous bleeding from the vesical venous plexus thus applying pressure by compressing with the vaginal and abdominal hand can help. If massive bleeding is encountered and it is believed to be from the vesical venous plexus, an intentional cystotomy, for direct intravesical visualization, can be performed so that the hemostatic sutures will not compromise the bladder or ureters. A hemostatic agent should be placed in this area when concerned for bleeding. A surgical drain can be placed if a large amount bleeding was encountered and there is concern for a hematoma at the closure of the procedure.

4. Reapproximating the abdominal incision

The classical Cherney was originally described with reattachment of the muscles to its tendinous insertion at the pubic symphysis [23]. There is a lack of data on the outcomes regarding pain with or without reattachment of the muscles. The authors prefer to reattach the muscles to its tendinous insertion. The rectus muscle is grasp with a Kelly clamp and pulled toward the pubic rami. A horizontal mattress suture using a delayed absorbable or permanent suture is brought through the rectus muscle tendon sheath at the muscle end and then through the cut tendinous insertion at the pubic symphysis and secured. A similar attachment should be performed on the contralateral rectus muscle if they were split. The peritoneum should be closed if combined with an intraperitoneal procedure. The fascia and skin are closed in the usual fashion.

5. Bladder drainage

   A 16 Fr Foley catheter should be left in place at the end of the procedure with voiding trial on postoperative day one.

Surgical Outcomes

With the development of the Burch colposuspension occurring in 1961, a wealth of long-term data is available in regard to its efficacy and overall outcomes. Further, it has served as a benchmark for comparison with the development of other anti-incontinence procedures such as the pubovaginal and mid-urethral slings. A 2017 Cochrane review of open retropubic colposuspension examined 231 full-text articles, ultimately including 152 reports (55 studies) in a qualitative analysis and 142 reports (50 studies) in a quantitative analysis [2]. This review concluded that continence within the first year after treatment is approximately 85–90% while continence after 5 years drops to approximately 80% [2]. Randomized data has largely been made available from the Stress Incontinence Surgical Treatment Efficacy Trial (SISTEr), a multicenter, randomized control trial comparing Burch colposuspension and fascial sling procedures. The initial publication reported two-year patient satisfaction of 78% and 86%, for the Burch colposuspension and fascial sling, respectively [17]. This cohort was later evaluated at five years with the E-SISTEr trial reporting patient satisfaction of 73% for the Burch colposuspension and 83% for patients that had received a fascial sling [24]. Though the satisfaction rates were relatively high, the rates of success specific to stress incontinence were reported at 66% for the fascial sling and 49% for the Burch colposuspension at 2 years [17]. This lower success rate was felt to be secondary to their stricter definition of success using a composite outcome measure, as opposed to one single outcome measure. Additionally, the discrepancy between subjective and objective outcomes was drastic, pointing to the multiple factors that influence a patient's interpretation of surgical success [17]. Kupasertkul et al. reported 15-year outcomes from a single participating institution with three out of 21 patients undergoing reoperation (two Burch, one fascial sling) [25]. Alcalay et al. reported a cure of incontinence following a Burch colposuspension at 10–20 years being 69% [26].

Minimally invasive sling procedures and laparoscopic Burch colposuspension procedures provide similar success rates to open Burch colposuspension when reviewed in the 2017 Cochrane review [2]. Studies comparing the Burch colposuspension to the TVT and TOT reported similar subjective cure rates of 70–85% at 2 and 5 years [27–29]. However, a study comparing 12-year data at a single institution did identify a difference in success between TVT and Burch colposuspension with 14/127 (Burch) and 3/180 (TVT), undergoing repeat urinary incontinence surgery ($p < 0.001$) [30]. Additionally, a meta-analysis of randomized control trials comparing anti-incontinence procedures concluded that patients receiving a mid-urethral sling had significantly higher overall (82% vs 74%) and objective continence rates (79.7% vs 67.8%) than those receiving an open Burch colposuspension [31]. More data is likely needed to further elucidate if there is a difference between open and laparoscopic colposuspension at a long-term follow-up, as the longest follow-up in the Cochrane review was a small study at 5–7 years with results favoring the laparoscopic approach but not reaching significance [2]. See Table 15.1 for a summary of select study outcomes.

With lower objective cure rates, efforts have been made to understand factors associated with poor outcomes. Preoperative weight greater than 80 kg, previous bladder neck surgery, intraoperative blood loss greater than one liter, and the development of postoperative detrusor instability have been associated with decreased success [27]. Further, a retrospective evaluation of 258 patients who underwent a Burch colposuspension showed age, parity, menopausal status, use of hormone replacement therapy, previous hysterectomy, and occurrence of postoperative complications did not significantly influence the failure rate [32].

Traditionally, the Burch colposuspension has been used for patients with urethral hypermobility. Intrinsic sphincter deficiency (ISD), defined as urodynamic Valsalva leak point pressure less than 60 mm Hg, has been shown to be a risk factor for surgical failure [33]. However, Hsieh et al. showed 21/24 patients with ISD were continent on postoperative cystometry, arguing that low Valsalva leak point pressure alone, without other parameters associated with ISD (e.g., maximum urethral closure pressure less than 20 mg Hg), is not an independent risk factor for surgical failure [34].

Burch colposuspension has been used as a secondary procedure in the setting of failed anti-incontinence surgeries. A small retrospective review of 16 patients that underwent laparoscopic Burch colposuspension after a failed mid-urethral sling reported objective and subjective cure rates of 54.5% and 92.9%, respectively, at a median follow-up of 24.5 months [35]. Agur et al. noted no significant difference between Burch colposuspension and retropubic mid-urethral sling in a systematic review and meta-analysis of the management of recurrent stress urinary incontinence [36].

Complications and Adverse Events

The open Burch colposuspension, though more invasive than other anti-incontinence procedures, has not been shown to have significantly higher morbidity or complication rates [2]. Dimerci et al. described risk of bleeding secondary to dissection in the wrong plane involving paravaginal veins. Their review noted a risk of transfusion or

Table 15.1 Burch study outcomes

Study	Study design	N	Operative details	Follow-up period	Outcomes	Adverse outcomes
Burch colposuspension versus fascial sling						
Albo 2007	Multicenter randomized control trial	Sling: 326 Burch: 328	NA	24 months	SUI reported success: 66% sling, 49% Burch ($P < 0.001$) Satisfaction: 86% sling, 78% Burch ($P = 0.02$)	Serious adverse events: 13% sling, 10% Burch ($P = 0.20$) Adverse events: 63% sling, 47% Burch ($P < 0.001$) Voiding dysfunction: 14% sling, 2% Burch ($P < 0.001$)
Brubaker 2012	Prospective observational	Sling: 183 Burch: 174	NA	5 years	Overall continence: 24% Burch, 31% sling ($p = 0.05$) Satisfaction: 83% sling, 73% Burch ($p = 0.04$)	Serious adverse events: none Adverse events: 9% sling, 10% Burch 72/75 adverse events were recurrent UTI
Demirci 2001	Single institution, prospective randomized control trial	Sling: 23 Burch: 23	Operative time: 60 min sling, 54 min Burch No major intraoperative complications	12 months	Dry (symptom free): 16/17 sling, 15/17 Burch	De novo DI: one sling, one Burch Suprapubic pain: three sling, zero Burch Prolapse: zero sling, two Burch
Burch colposuspension versus TVT						
El Barky 2005	Single institution, prospective randomized control trial	Sling: 25 Burch: 25	Operative time: 57 min Burch, 20 min sling	24 months	Cure: Burch 72%, TVT 72%	De novo urgency: 12% Burch, 8% sling Retention: 12% Burch, 20% sling

Ward 2004	Multicenter, randomized control trial	Sling: 137 Burch: 108	NA	24 months	Negative 1 hour pad test: Burch 80%, TVT 81%	Repeat surgery for stress urinary incontinence: 1.8% TVT, 3.4% Burch Surgery for prolapse: 0 TVT, 4.8% Burch
Ward 2008	Multicenter, randomized control trial	Sling: 98 Burch: 79	NA	5 years	Satisfied/very satisfied: Burch 90%, TVT 91% Negative 1 hour pad test: Burch 81%, TVT 90%	Repeat surgery for stress urinary incontinence: 2.3% TVT, 3.4% Burch Surgery for prolapse: 1.8% TVT, 7.5% Burch
Burch colposuspension versus TOT						
Asicioglu 2013	Retrospective	Sling: 272 Burch: 498	Operative time: Burch 41.5 min, sling 23.7 min Estimated blood loss: Burch 119.3 cc, sling 52.7 cc	5 years	Objective cure: Burch 73.9%, sling 77.5% ($p = 0.991$) Subjective cure: Burch 76.8%, sling 81.7% ($p = 0.791$)	Urinary retention: Burch 24%, Sling 7.6% ($p = 0.001$) De novo urgency: Burch 6.7%, Sling 2.8% ($p = .169$) Long-term voiding dysfunction: Burch 5.3% ($p = 0.005$)
Sivaslioglu 2007	Prospective randomized control trial	Sling: 49 Burch: 51	Operative time: Burch 48 min, Sling 23.2 min Blood loss >100 ml: Burch 1, sling 0	24 months	Objective cure: Burch 83.8%, sling 87.5% ($p = 0.6$) Subjective cure: Burch 87%, sling 87.5% ($p = 0.9$)	De novo urge incontinence: Burch 5.8%, TOT 2% ($p = 0.3$) Post-op retention >100 cc after day 2: Burch 5.8%, TOT 2% ($p = 0.3$)

(continued)

Table 15.1 (continued)

Study	Study design	N	Operative details	Follow-up period	Outcomes	Adverse outcomes
Open Burch colposuspension versus laparoscopic Burch colposuspension						
Carey 2006	Multicenter randomized control trial	Open: 104 Lap: 96	Operative time: Open: 42 Min, Lap: 87 min ($p < 0.001$) EBL: open: 170 cc, Lap: 126 cc ($p = 0.03$)	24 months	Patient satisfaction (% score > 80): open 70%, Lap 58% ($p = 0.10$)	Frequent urinary urgency: open 10%, Lap 23% ($p = 0.40$) Frequent urge incontinence: open 10%, Lap 18% ($p = 0.21$)
Ankardal 2004	Multicenter, prospective randomized trial	Open: 120 Lap: 120	Operative time: Open 60 Min, Lap 75 min ($p < 0.0001$) -EBL: open 105 cc, Lap 35 cc ($p < 0.0001$)	12 months	Subjectively dry: open 89%, Lap 64% ($p < 0.001$) Leakage <8 g/24 hr at 48 hr: open 92%, Lap 74% ($P < 0.001$)	Urinary tract infection (within 1 month): open: 20%, Lap: 10% (NS) Wound infection: open: 3%, Lap 2% (NS) Urinary retention >5 days: open: 26%, Lap: 9% ($p = 0.002$)

hematoma being 0.02–4.8% with one surprising study showing a transfusion rate of 33% [37]. Decreased blood loss has been found using a laparoscopic approach, however, with the tradeoff of longer reported operative time [38, 39]. The most common serious adverse events reported in the SISTEr trial included incidental cystotomy (3%) and wound complications requiring surgical intervention (4%). Overall, the most common adverse event was urinary tract infection (62%), though significantly less than those that received a fascial sling (93%) [17].

An important risk that patients must be counseled on prior to any anti-incontinence procedure is postoperative voiding dysfunction. This can be difficult to quantify due to various definitions and amount of time postoperatively that these symptoms are considered. Because of this, a large range of postoperative urinary retention (0–24%) has been reported, though only 3% were reported as permanent need for self-catheterization [37]. Further, preoperative urodynamic testing was not shown to be predictive of postoperative voiding dysfunction [40].

In addition to difficulty emptying, new onset or worsening urgency, frequency, and urge urinary incontinence can occur after surgical intervention. De novo detrusor instability has been reported at 3–8% after a Burch colposuspension [41]. Of the 174 women that underwent a Burch colposuspension in the E-SISTEr trial and completed the 5-year follow-up, 29 had persistent urge urinary incontinence, and seven had de novo urge urinary incontinence [25]. This rate of de novo urge urinary incontinence was similar to that reported by Ward et al. at 5 years (4%) [42].

Burch's original article describing his colposuspension suggested a correlation with the development of vaginal prolapse postoperatively, specifically enterocele, though the numbers were small [1]. Further studies have supported this finding over the years. Wiskind et al. showed 26.7% of their cohort (131 patients) required operative correction of genital prolapse postoperatively [43]. Another study of 109 patients showed 30% required rectocele or enterocele repair during the 10–20 years follow-up period [26]. In a study comparing patients with recurrent incontinence after a Burch colposuspension to those without recurrence, it was found that incontinent patients had significantly higher postoperative cystocele and rectoceles, while the rate of enteroceles was similar (24%) [44]. When comparing Burch to synthetic mid-urethral sling procedures, similar outcomes have been noted [42].

Conclusion

Burch colposuspension is a well-studied procedure for hypermobile stress urinary incontinence proven to be safe and effective. It is a suitable primary procedure for the non-morbidly obese patient who desires an alternative to mesh. Laparoscopic adaption of the Burch is likely to decrease pain, blood loss, and quicker return to daily activity; however, more research is needed to look at its long-term safety and efficacy. As with any anti-incontinence surgery, patient should be counseled on the development of de novo urgency, frequency, and urge incontinence.

References

1. BURCH JC. Urethrovaginal fixation to Cooper's ligament for correction of stress incontinence, cystocele, and prolapse. Am J Obstet Gynecol. 1961;81:281–90.
2. Lapitan MCM, Cody JD, Mashayekhi A. Open retropubic colposuspension for urinary incontinence in women. Cochrane Database Syst Rev. 2017;7(7):CD002912.
3. Tanagho EA. Colpocystourethropexy: the way we do it. J Urol. 1976;116(6):751–3.
4. Jonsson Funk M, Levin PJ, Wu JM. Trends in the surgical management of stress urinary incontinence. Obstet Gynecol. 2012;119(4):845–51. https://doi.org/10.1097/AOG.0b013e31824b2e3e.
5. Souders CP, Eilber KS, McClelland L, Wood LN, Souders AR, Steiner V, Anger JT. The truth behind transvaginal mesh litigation: devices, timelines, and provider characteristics. Female Pelvic Med Reconstr Surg. 2018;24(1):21–25.
6. Zacche MM, Mukhopadhyay S, Giarenis I. Changing surgical trends for female stress urinary incontinence in England. Int Urogynecol J. 2019;30(2):203–9.
7. Hilton P, Stanton SL. A clinical and urodynamic assessment of the Burch colposuspension for genuine stress incontinence. Br J Obstet Gynaecol. 1983;90(10):934–9.
8. Klutke JJ, Klutke CG, Bergman J, Elia G. Urodynamics changes in voiding after anti-incontinence surgery: an insight into the mechanism of cure. Urology. 1999;54(6):1003–7.
9. Bonney V. On diurnal incontinence of urine in women. J Obset Gynaecol Br Emp. 1923;30:358–65.
10. Barnes A. A method for evaluating the stress of urinary incontinence. Am J Obstet Gynecol. 1940;40:381–90.
11. Enhorning G. Simultaneously recording of intravesical and intra-urethral pressure: a study on urethral closure in normal and stress incontinent women. Acta Chir Scand. 1961;suppl 276:1-68.
12. Hilton P, Stanton SL. Urethral pressure measurement by microtransducer: the results in symptom-free women and in those with genuine stress incontinence. Br J Obstet Gynaecol. 1983;90:919–33.
13. Hilton P, Stanton SL. A clinical and urodynamic assessment of the Burch colposuspension for genuine stress incontinence. Br J Obstet Gynaecol. 1983;90(10):934–9.
14. Bump RC, Fantl JA, Hurt WG. Dynamic urethral pressure profilometry pressure transmission ratio determinations after continence surgery: understanding the mechanism of success, failure, and complications. Obstet Gynecol. 1988;72(6):870–4.
15. DeLancey JO. The pathophysiology of stress urinary incontinence in women and its implications for surgical treatment. World J Urol. 1997;15(5):268–74.
16. Klutke JJ, Klutke CG, Bergman J, Elia G. Urodynamics changes in voiding after anti-incontinence surgery: an insight into the mechanism of cure. Urology. 1999;54(6):1003–7.
17. Albo ME, Richter HE, Brubaker L, Norton P, Kraus SR, Zimmern PE, Chai TC, Zyczynski H, Diokno AC, Tennstedt S, Nager C, Lloyd LK, FitzGerald M, Lemack GE, Johnson HW, Leng W, Mallett V, Stoddard AM, Menefee S, Varner RE, Kenton K, Moalli P, Sirls L, Dandreo KJ, Kusek JW, Nyberg LM, Steers W. Urinary Incontinence Treatment Network. Burch colposuspension versus fascial sling to reduce urinary stress incontinence. N Engl J Med. 2007;356(21):2143–55.
18. Hamner JJ, Carrick KS, Ramirez DMO, Corton MM. Gross and histologic relationships of the retropubic urethra to lateral pelvic sidewall and anterior vaginal wall in female cadavers: clinical applications to retropubic surgery. Am J Obstet Gynecol. 2018;219(6):597.e1–597.e8.
19. Pathi SD, Castellanos ME, Corton MM. Variability of the retropubic space anatomy in female cadavers. Am J Obstet Gynecol. 2009;201(5):524.e1–5.
20. Kinman CL, Agrawal A, Deveneau NE, Meriwether KV, Herring NR, Francis SL. Anatomical relationships of Burch colposuspension sutures. Female Pelvic Med Reconstr Surg. 2017;23(2):72–4.

21. Joint report on the terminology for surgical procedures to treat stress urinary incontinence in women. Developed by the Joint Writing Group of the American Urogynecologic Society and the International Urogynecological Association. Int Urogynecol J. 2020;31(3):465–78.
22. Loughlin KR. The thimble: a useful adjunct to needle suspension procedures for female stress incontinence. Urology. 2000;56(6):1050–1.
23. CHERNEY LS. Transverse low abdominal incision with detachment of the recti from the pubis: follow-up study of eight hundred cases. J Am Med Assoc. 1955;157(1):23–6.
24. Brubaker L, Richter HE, Norton PA, Albo M, Zyczynski HM, Chai TC, Zimmern P, Kraus S, Sirls L, Kusek JW, Stoddard A, Tennstedt S. Gormley EA; Urinary Incontinence Treatment Network. 5-year continence rates, satisfaction and adverse events of burch urethropexy and fascial sling surgery for urinary incontinence. J Urol. 2012;187(4):1324–30.
25. Kuprasertkul A, Christie AL, Lemack GE, Zimmern P. Long-term results of Burch and autologous sling procedures for stress urinary incontinence in E-SISTEr participants at 1 site. J Urol. 2019;202(6):1224–9.
26. Alcalay M, Monga A, Stanton SL. Burch colposuspension: a 10–20 year follow up. Br J Obstet Gynaecol. 1995;102(9):740–5. Erratum in: Br J Obstet Gynaecol 1996;103(3):290.
27. Sivaslioglu AA, Caliskan E, Dolen I, Haberal A. A randomized comparison of transobturator tape and Burch colposuspension in the treatment of female stress urinary incontinence. Int Urogynecol J Pelvic Floor Dysfunct. 2007;18(9):1015–9.
28. El-Barky E, El-Shazly A, El-Wahab OA, Kehinde EO, Al-Hunayan A, Al-Awadi KA. Tension free vaginal tape versus Burch colposuspension for treatment of female stress urinary incontinence. Int Urol Nephrol. 2005;37(2):277–81.
29. Asıcıoglu O, Gungorduk K, Besımoglu B, Ertas IE, Yıldırım G, Celebı I, Ark C, Boran B. A 5-year follow-up study comparing Burch colposuspension and transobturator tape for the surgical treatment of stress urinary incontinence. Int J Gynaecol Obstet. 2014;125(1):73–7. https://doi.org/10.1016/j.ijgo.2013.09.026. Epub 2013 Dec 14
30. Holdø B, Verelst M, Svenningsen R, Milsom I, Skjeldestad FE. Long-term clinical outcomes with the retropubic tension-free vaginal tape (TVT) procedure compared to Burch colposuspension for correcting stress urinary incontinence (SUI). Int Urogynecol J. 2017;28(11):1739–46.
31. Fusco F, Abdel-Fattah M, Chapple CR, Creta M, La Falce S, Waltregny D, Novara G. Updated systematic review and meta-analysis of the comparative data on Colposuspensions, Pubovaginal slings, and Midurethral tapes in the surgical treatment of female stress urinary incontinence. Eur Urol. 2017;72(4):567–91.
32. Sun MJ, Ng SC, Tsui KP, Chang NE, Lin KC, Chen GD. Are there any predictors for failed Burch colposuspension? Taiwan J Obstet Gynecol. 2006;45(1):33–8.
33. Koonings PP, Bergman A, Ballard CA. Low urethral pressure and stress urinary incontinence in women: risk factor for failed retropubic surgical procedure. Urology. 1990;36(3):245–8.
34. Hsieh GC, Klutke JJ, Kobak WH. Low valsalva leak-point pressure and success of retropubic urethropexy. Int Urogynecol J Pelvic Floor Dysfunct. 2001;12(1):46–50.
35. De Cuyper EM, Ismail R, Maher CF. Laparoscopic Burch colposuspension after failed suburethral tape procedures: a retrospective audit. Int Urogynecol J Pelvic Floor Dysfunct. 2008;19(5):681–5.
36. Agur W, Riad M, Secco S, Litman H, Madhuvrata P, Novara G, Abdel-Fattah M. Surgical treatment of recurrent stress urinary incontinence in women: a systematic review and meta-analysis of randomised controlled trials. Eur Urol. 2013;64(2):323–36.
37. Demirci F, Petri E. Perioperative complications of Burch colposuspension. Int Urogynecol J Pelvic Floor Dysfunct. 2000;11(3):170–5.
38. Carey MP, Goh JT, Rosamilia A, Cornish A, Gordon I, Hawthorne G, Maher CF, Dwyer PL, Moran P, Gilmour DT. Laparoscopic versus open Burch colposuspension: a randomised controlled trial. BJOG. 2006;113(9):999–1006.
39. Ankardal M, Ekerydh A, Crafoord K, Milsom I, Stjerndahl JH, Engh ME. A randomised trial comparing open Burch colposuspension using sutures with laparoscopic colposuspension using mesh and staples in women with stress urinary incontinence. BJOG. 2004;111(9):974–81.

40. Lemack GE, Krauss S, Litman H, FitzGerald MP, Chai T, Nager C, Sirls L, Zyczynski H, Baker J, Lloyd K. Steers WD; Urinary Incontinence Treatment Network. Normal preoperative urodynamic testing does not predict voiding dysfunction after Burch colposuspension versus pubovaginal sling. J Urol. 2008;180(5):2076–80.
41. Sohlberg EM, Elliott CS. Burch Colposuspension. Urol Clin North Am. 2019;46(1):53–9.
42. Ward KL. Hilton P; UK and Ireland TVT Trial Group. Tension-free vaginal tape versus colposuspension for primary urodynamic stress incontinence: 5-year follow up. BJOG. 2008;115(2):226–33.
43. Wiskind AK, Creighton SM, Stanton SL. The incidence of genital prolapse after the Burch colposuspension. Am J Obstet Gynecol. 1992;167(2):399–404; discussion 404-5.
44. Kjølhede P. Genital prolapse in women treated successfully and unsuccessfully by the Burch colposuspension. Acta Obstet Gynecol Scand. 1998 Apr;77(4):444–50.

Chapter 16
The Innovation of Midurethral Slings: Where We've Been and Where We Are Today

Suzette E. Sutherland and Ellen C. Thompson

Introduction

The innovation leading to the development of mid-urethral slings (MUS) revolutionized our thinking about, and subsequent treatment for, female stress urinary incontinence (SUI). Today the mid-urethral sling is the most widely studied and performed surgical treatment for female stress urinary incontinence, with almost 20 years of outcome data available in the medical literature and with over ten million cases worldwide (IUGA global). The risk/benefit ratio has been reported as one of the safest and most efficacious surgical treatments for female stress urinary incontinence to date, such that the American Urogynecologic Society (AUGS) and the Society of Urodynamics, Female Pelvic Medicine and Urogenital Reconstruction (SUFU), the American Urological Association (AUA), the European Association of Urology (EAU) and European Urogynecological Association (EUGA), and the International Urogynecological Association (IUGA) have all published position statements declaring the mid-urethral sling the standard of care for the surgical treatment for female stress urinary incontinence [4, 5, 14, 51, 52].

Although uncommon, severe complications have occurred and have received widespread amplification through widely publicized litigation and social media. With respect to polypropylene MUS for SUI, the FDA in 2013 clearly stated "the safety and effectiveness of multi-incision slings is well established in clinical trials"

S. E. Sutherland (✉)
Female Urology/Urogynecology, UW Medicine Pelvic Health Center, Seattle, WA, USA

Department of Urology, University of Washington School of Medicine, Seattle, WA, USA

E. C. Thompson
Department of Urology, University of Minnesota School of Medicine,
Minneapolis, MN, USA

© The Author(s), under exclusive license to Springer Nature Switzerland AG 2022
A. P. Cameron (ed.), *Female Urinary Incontinence*,
https://doi.org/10.1007/978-3-030-84352-6_16

273

[35]. With ongoing efforts of vocal anti-mesh groups, unsubstantiated notions of implanted mesh leading to autoimmune diseases [15] and cancer [15, 16, 61, 62], it is not inconceivable that the MUS could one day no longer be available. Unfortunately, the elimination of MUS could essentially put women at a greater surgical safety risk by denying them a highly effective, yet minimally invasive procedure for SUI, forcing them to seek more invasive surgical alternatives.

This chapter hopes to present the rationale for the appropriate ongoing use of the mid-urethral sling and the innovative evolution from the initial retropubic transvaginal tape (TVT) device—to the transobturator tape (TOT) version—to the single-incision sling (SIS) and to provide evidence-based support through contemporary comparative data that describes the performance of current generation slings as they compare to other traditional incontinence procedures, all with their associated risks, benefits, and outcomes when performed by trained surgeons.

Stress Urinary Incontinence: Historical Pearls

To understand the truly innovative conceptual thinking that led to the development of the mid-urethral sling, it proves helpful to take a step back and review the historical theories throughout the twentieth century concerning the pathophysiological mechanisms of SUI that subsequently led to the development of prior anti-incontinence procedures. Advances in understanding of the pathophysiology of urinary incontinence have gone hand in hand with advances in technology and surgical treatment of SUI. For generations, SUI has presented both conceptual and therapeutic challenges to physicians [54]. Topics of study concerning the potential etiologies for SUI have included intrabdominal pressure changes during Valsalva-related physical maneuvers, loss of support through weakening pelvic floor muscles and ligamentous structures, changes in intrinsic urinary sphincter properties resulting in urethral coaptation deficiency, complex voiding neurophysiological factors leading to urethral sphincter denervation, and of course including the myriad interrelationships among these (See Table 16.1).

Very early surgical techniques focused on reinforcing urethral sphincter strength by encircling the urethra with gracilis or pyramidal muscle or through fascial flaps [95]. In the early 1900s, improvements in cystoscopy allowed Kelly to visualize and describe the structure of the internal and external urinary sphincters, noting a compromised internal sphincter with subsequent bladder neck funneling in patients with SUI [55]. He developed the Kelly plication technique [9], which reinforced the proximal urethra-bladder neck support by creating a narrow posterior urethra-vesical angle through midline plication of peri-urethral and

Table 16.1 Summary: innovation leading to SUI treatment designs

Year	Innovation	SUI treatment
1900s	Sphincter muscle defect	Muscle "sling" Urethral wrap with gracilis or pyramidalis muscle
1910s	Internal sphincter defect leading to BN funneling	Kelly Plication Peri-urethral/pubocervical fascia midline plication at prox urethra/BN
1920s–1930s	Increased urethro-vesical angle below pubis with valsalva	Kelly Plication PVS – Fascia Lata
1940s	*Pelvic Floor Muscle Support*	Kegel Exercises
1940s–1960s	*Pressure Transmission Theory*	Retropubic Urethropexy Stabilize prox urethra/BN in retropubic position
		PVS – Rectus Fascia MMK Burch
1960s–1970s	Minimally invasive techniques	Retropubic Needle Suspensions
	Still stabilizing prox urethra/BN complex	Pereyra Stamey Raz
1980s	*Concept of ISD* due to sphincter denervation;	UHM = Kelly, Burch
	Dichotomy of SUI theory UHM vs ISD	ISD = PVS
1990s	*Hammock Theory* Integration of muscle, fascia and neurological component	PVS – Rectus Fascia "Gold Standard" Addressing both UHM and IDS
1990s	*Integral Theory* Ligamentous and Muscular support drive function	MUS dynamic "kinking" at midurethra
		TVT (RPS) in US 1996
2000s	Improve safety of MUS by avoiding the retropubic space	TOT in US 2001 SIS in US 2006
2008, 2011	FDA – safety notifications transvaginal mesh for SUI and POP	MUS PVS
2014, updated 2016 and 2017	*Societal Position Statements* in support of mesh MUS AUGS/SUFU/AUA EAU/EUGA	Support RPS and TOT "Gold Standard"
	IUGA Global Statement	Data on SIS still too immature
2017	*SUFU/AUA guidelines for SUI*	For Index Patient MUS
		PVS – good option, especially for more complex patients, but with increased risk
2018	*EAU guidelines for SUI*	MUS is first-line
		PVS if MUS can not be done

pubocervical fascia. In spite of its fairly high failure rate of up to 30% at 1 year [46], the Kelly plication was utilized for many decades [95]. In the 1920s–1930s, Bonney continued this focus on the proximal urethra, noting a loss of peri-urethral support and increased urethra-vesicle angle that allowed the bladder to drop below the pubis during Valsalva-related activities in patients with SUI [23]. Kegel, in the 1940s–1950s, brought a new focus on the pelvic floor musculature, which had a lasting impact on pelvic floor physical rehabilitation, and today remains a mainstay of nonsurgical treatment for urinary incontinence, as well as many other pelvic floor disorders [54]. In the 1960s Enhoerning focused on pressure transmission to the bladder and urethra during events of physical stress, seeming to validate surgical techniques that attempted to preserve an intra-abdominal position of the proximal urethra in order to prevent urinary leakage [30, 31]. Procedures like the fascial pubovaginal sling (fascia lata,1933; rectus fascia,1942 [2]) and the retropubic urethropexies (Marshall-Marchetti-Krantz (MMK),1949 [71]; Burch colposuspension,1961 [12]) relied upon an understanding of continence through stabilization of the proximal urethra in a retropubic position [107] and were all in common use during this time. Less invasive urethropexy options were tried (Pereyra [86], Stamey needle suspension [100, 101], Raz urethropexy [89] and Raz four-corner suspension [90]), but did not hold up well over time and were aborted. A Cochran review evaluating needle suspension urethropexies again noted an almost 30% failure rate at just 1 year [46].

In the 1980s, denervation injury to the urethral sphincter mechanism was further described and termed intrinsic sphincter deficiency (ISD) [107], thereby dichotomizing the etiological theories about SUI: anatomical (lack of support leading to urethral hypermobility) versus functional (denervation injury leading to ISD). This further led to a treatment dichotomy with the use of the Kelly plication and Burch colposuspension for patients with urethral hypermobility and the pubovaginal sling (autologous rectus fascial PVS, as described by Blaivas [10]) for those with concomitant ISD [72–74]. DeLancey's "Hammock Theory" in the 1990s described the importance of all components together—muscular, fascial and neurological—for maintaining continence [25, 26]. This further supported the use of the pubovaginal sling (PVS) for SUI as it was able to address both urethral hypermobility and concurrent ISD [13] and was therefore considered the "gold standard" for surgical treatment of SUI in the mid-to-late 1990s.

And then came the integral theory, by Petros and Ulmsten [87], and the innovation that led to the mid-urethral sling.

Integral Theory

While early surgical approaches relied upon an understanding of continence through stabilization of the proximal urethra/bladder neck complex in a retropubic position [107], integral theory, a musculoelastic theory, posited by Petros and Ulmsten in 1990, identified an anatomic area about the mid-urethra referred to as the pubourethral ligament (PUL). Rather than stabilizing the entire urethra, this PUL serves to supports the mid-urethra during moments of increased Valsalva-related activity, thereby acting as a fulcrum around which the proximal urethra rotates. This allows for dynamic "kinking" at the mid-urethra and thereby eliminates unwanted urine leakage related to physical stress maneuvers, or specifically SUI (see Figs. 16.1 and 16.2) [87].

Fig. 16.1 Sling Placement: Location matters for mechanism of action (MOA)

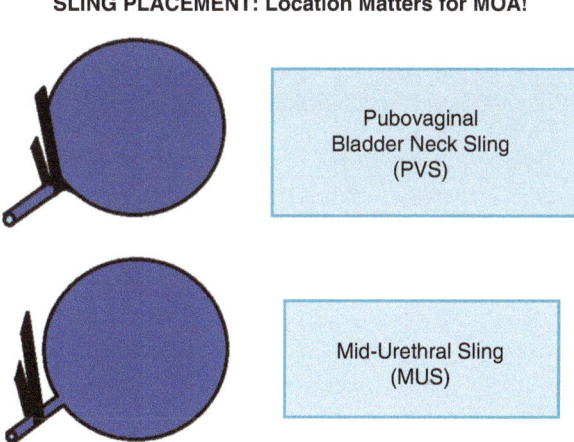

Fig. 16.2 Integral theory Ligamentous (PUL) stabilization of the mid-urethra during Valsalva leading to dynamic urethral kinking and maintenance of continence. Mechanism of action for the mid-urethral slings (MUS)

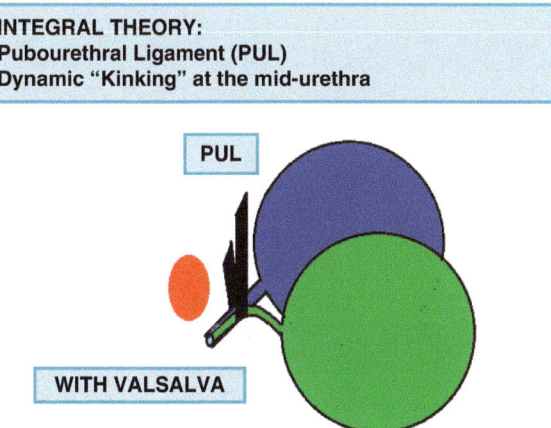

Evolution of the Mid-Urethral Sling

This focus on the mid-urethra, rather than the proximal urethra/bladder neck complex, challenged the traditional way of thinking about female SUI—and how to treat it—and provided the inspiration and innovation that gave us the first surgical synthetic mid-urethral sling, the tension-free vaginal tape procedure (TVT) [103]. Acting as a "pseudo-pubovaginal ligament," the synthetic mesh mid-urethral sling was meant to restore or reinforce the sub-urethral vaginal hammock and the para-urethral connective tissue at the level of the mid-urethra. Tissue ingrowth into the sling—using the visual analogy of ivy growing on latticework—secures the sling in position during healing, thereby providing a backboard of support for the urethra during times of physical stress. This mechanism understandably works optimally in patients with urethral hypermobility.

The initial approach to the mid-urethral sling drew from the prior experience surgeons had in the retropubic (RP) space. This retropubic TVT formed a U-shaped sling under and along the lateral aspects of the urethra, with mesh arms extending up through the retropubic (RP) space, traversing directly behind the pubic bone, and exiting through two small stab incisions in the suprapubic region of the lower anterior abdominal wall (see Fig. 16.3). With the aid of trocars, this retropubic mid-urethral sling (RPS) was placed starting in the vagina through a small midline incision under the urethra (bottom-up approach). Later technique developments allowed for placement of the mid-urethral sling with passage of the trocars starting at the abdomen and moving down to the vagina (top-down approach). Either way, focus on the mid-urethra lent itself to a more anatomically accessible and therefore less invasive target for anti-incontinence surgery through a transvaginal approach.

Efficacy of the synthetic RPS has been well established with long-term data extending out to almost 20 years [81]. Although infrequent, there are serious complications associated with the blind retropubic trocar and mesh passage. These include bladder perforation which if not recognized can lead to retained mesh in the bladder with subsequent urinary tract infections and bladder stones, bowel injury,

Fig. 16.3 Evolution of mid-urethral slings. RPS Retropubic sling, TOT Transobturator tape, SIS Single-incision sling

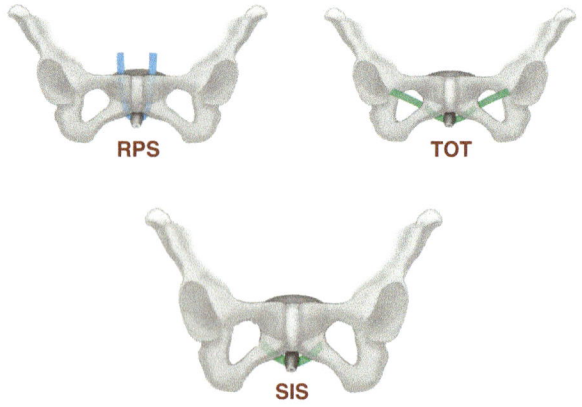

major vessel injury, bleeding, and even death. This provided the inspiration for the development of a second generation sling, the transobturator tape (TOT), by Delorme in 2001 (see Fig. 16.3) [28]. The TOT served to place the mesh sling in the same mid-urethral position as the RPS, but without traversing the retropubic space. This was accomplished by passage of helical trocars through the obturator foramen and around the inferior pubic rami bilaterally, staying superior and medial in the obturator space to avoid the obturator nerve/artery/vein complex which is located in the superior-lateral aspect of the obturator foramen. By staying out of the retropubic space, these serious complications are theoretically avoided. With the transobturator approach—developed as an outside-in (obturator to vagina) or inside-out (vagina to obturator) approach [27]—more groin pain and mesh-related dyspareunia were initially seen. Recognizing the location of the adductor longus tendon and keeping it out of the trocar trajectory by proper high lithotomy position of the legs served to improve the incidence of postoperative groin pain. Furthermore, ensuring an adequate depth and angle of dissection below the vaginal epithelium behind the inferior pubic rami toward the 2 and 10 o'clock positions eliminates buttonholing or scything of the vaginal epithelium (with risk of future mesh extrusion) and mesh arm banding out to the vaginal side wall that could potentially lead to dyspareunia.

With proper surgical technique and allowing for the learning curve associated with tensioning differences between the RP and TOT approaches, these two midurethral slings have repeatedly noted comparable efficacy in contemporary randomized control trials [8, 19, 24, 37, 43, 59, 66, 91, 97, 104, 109].

Further innovation led to the development of a third generation mid-urethral sling, the single-incision sling (SIS), first introduced in 2006 (see Fig. 16.3) [76]. The incentive here was to avoid both RP and TO spaces and their inherent potential complications based on their respective designs and trocar passage. The truly novel aspect of the contemporary SIS is the anchoring tip that allows for a more reliable mechanism to secure the mesh in place during the healing tissue ingrowth process. The anchor is placed perpendicularly into the obturator internus muscle, in the same area as the TOT, without traversing the entire obturator foramen and thigh, thereby avoiding bleeding, bruising, hematoma formation, and pain in the thigh. Other advantages are a much smaller overall "mesh burden" left behind in the body, narrower trocar requiring less dissection through a single 1–2 cm sub-urethral incision, less bleeding and postoperative discomfort, and a quicker return to work and all normal activities, including vigorous exercise. Most commonly performed with a combination of local anesthesia and IV sedation, the SIS procedure has successfully transitioned to an office procedure utilizing only local anesthesia in some centers across the United States.

The first SIS, the TVT Secur (Gynecare® [76]), launched at the International Urogynecological Association (IUGA) meeting in 2006, experienced unacceptably high failure rates due to two main issues: (1) an ineffective "anchoring" system based on a simple Vicryl pledget and (2) nonadherence to tighter tensioning techniques as compared to the predecessor RPS and TOT. With respect to proper tensioning, the importance of respecting the "learning curve" has been noted when transitioning from an RP approach to a TOT and then from either of these to the SIS [57, 98, 99]. The SIS needs to be placed flat and snug against the mid-urethra with no spacing. The early TVT Secur failures were widely publicized, along with a very high medium-term failure rate of 70% at 4.5 years, and the product was subsequently removed from the market in 2012 [20, 21]. This unfortunately gave the SIS concept a bad name from the start. But further study of contemporary SIS devices with improved anchoring technology and adherence to proper SIS-specific tensioning techniques has noted vastly improved results with comparable efficacy to both RP and TOT, yet with minimal complications [79].

Contemporary Comparative Data for SUI Surgical Treatments

As previously mentioned, the PVS was considered the "gold standard" for surgical treatment of SUI in the 1990s. With the addition of the mid-urethral sling to the SUI armamentarium, this position of the PVS has been challenged. In 2017 the American Urological Association (AUA) and Society of Urodynamics, Female Pelvic Medicine and Urogenital Reconstruction (SUFU) published guidelines for the surgical treatment of SUI in the index patient and stated the following procedures should be considered: mid-urethral sling (synthetic), autologous fascia pubovaginal sling, Burch colposuspension, and urethral bulking agents [64] (see Fig. 16.4).

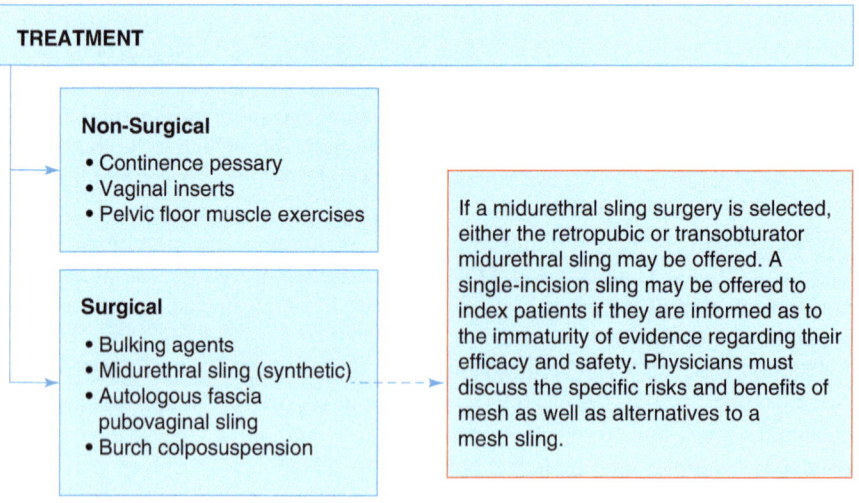

Fig. 16.4 2017 AUA/SUFU Guidelines for the treatment of female stress urinary incontinence (SUI). (Reprint permission granted by the AUA; Kobashi KC, et al. J Urol [64])

The success rate of any SUI surgical treatment is dependent on the definition of success. Unfortunately, there is a great amount of variability within the literature when it comes to the definition of success, which complicates adequate comparisons between treatments and studies [7]. Furthermore, comparisons in success need to be discussed in relationship to durability, which often is not easily identifiable. The duration of most studies dealing with surgical intervention for SUI is just 1 year, rarely beyond 3–5 years. For an invasive surgical procedure, this interval—especially 1 year—is inadequate for proper counseling of patients concerning the anticipated durability of the intervention and likelihood of requiring repeat surgical intervention.

Comparable Efficacy: Burch, Pubovaginal Slings, Mid-Urethral Sling

Although comparative trials have noted similar efficacy between Burch, PVS, and MUS at 1 year [6, 37, 43, 49, 65, 75], duration of cure has not been consistently appreciated with Burch or PVS to the same degree as has been seen with MUS. A 2017 Cochrane review of various trials involving Burch colposuspension noted an overall 1-year success rate of 85–90% but a 5-year success of only 70% [65]. The SISTer Trial (Stress Incontinence Surgical Treatment Efficacy Trial), a well-designed RCT by the Urinary Incontinence Treatment Network (UITN), compared Burch and PVS at 2 and 5 years. Here the stress-specific continence rates, as strictly defined using composite scores that included both objective and subjective measures of success (a negative cough stress test, no subjective reports of SUI, and no retreatment of any kind) noted superior efficacy for the PVS compared to the Burch, but the overall decline in efficacy over time was quite notable for both: stress-specific continence rates for PVS versus Burch at 2 years were 66% and 49%, respectively, and at 5 years, only 31% and 24%, respectively [1, 11]. Another RCT including short 10 cm autologous fascial PVS on a string (Prolene suture) versus long 21 cm autologous fascial PVS (allowing for more scarification in the retropubic space) again noted poor longevity with 5-year recurrence of subjective SUI at 49% and 57%, respectively, as defined by the Urogenital Distress Inventory Short Form Questionnaire (UDI-6) [60].

Compared to MUS, Burch is notably inferior with respect to long-term efficacy and safety [43, 82]. PVS, however, has demonstrated comparable efficacy with MUS in some studies up to 5 years. In a recent meta-analysis involving a large number of patients (n = 15,855) with long-term follow-up (at least 60 months), the superiority of MUS over both PVS and Burch was confirmed when evaluating for both efficacy and safety [43]. Although efficacy was deemed similar between MUS and PVS at 5 years, longer-term (>5 year) comparative data is still lacking.

Comparable Efficacy: Mid-urethral Slings (Retropubic, Transobturator, Single-Incision Slings)

The "full length" slings, RPS and TOT, have been studied extensively since the late 1990s and early 2000s, respectively. The longest published study to date is Nilsson with 17 year follow-up describing the original TVT and noting objective and subjective success of 91% and 87%, respectively [81]. A recent systematic review and meta-analysis on RPS and TOT noted excellent long-term efficacy as well [67]. Furthermore, RCTs comparing RPS and TOT exist abound, with most noting similar efficacy [8, 19, 24, 43, 59, 66, 91, 97, 104, 109]. A meta-analysis of 55 comparative trials between RPS and TOT noted similar objective and subjective cure rates, some out to 5 years: objective success RPS 87% and TOT 86%; subjective success RPS 71–97% and TOT 62–98% [37]. The TOMUS trial (Trial of Mid-urethral Slings), in its extended analysis, noted only a slight trend toward enhanced durability with the RPS as compared to TOT at 5 years [59]. In the case of significant concomitant ISD, however, the RPS does seem to fair better than TOT, with retreatment at 3 years required in only 1.4% of RPS versus 20% of TOT [38, 94]. Overall, slightly higher longer-term rates of SUI cure have been noted with RPS compared to TOT but at the cost of higher intraoperative complications and postoperative voiding dysfunction [43].

By comparison, SIS arrived on the scene much later. A relatively recent 2017 Cochrane review noted insufficient long-term data in the published literature to adequately compare SIS to the more traditional "full length" slings, the RPS and TOT [80]. Comparable short-term (12–24 month) efficacy and safety of the SIS was demonstrated, compared to RPS and TOT, which was unaffected by age, BMI, or obstetrical history [3, 42, 78, 79, 85]. In 2014, a meta-analysis of RCTs evaluating efficacy and safety of SIS (excluding TVT-Secure) compared to "full-length" slings (RPS and TOT) noted no significant differences in objective cure (88% vs 90%), subjective cure (83% vs 90%), impact on QoL, or sexual function with a mean of 18 months follow-up [79]. But longer-term data was still lacking. Accordingly, the 2017 AUA/SUFU Guidelines panel statement on surgical treatment for SUI reflected the recommendation that longer-term data were necessary before a stronger statement regarding the use of SIS could be made [64].

More recently, however, there are a number of large RCTs, comparative trials, and systematic reviews with meta-analyses to support these initial findings of relative comparable efficacy and safety for the SIS compared to RPS and TOT [3, 41, 69, 70, 105]. An FDA-mandated 522 post-market approval study comparing SIS to TOT noted comparable composite success (objective and subjective) at 3 years of 90.4% and 88.9%, respectively [105]. A large RCT between SIS and TOT noted similar results at 3 years with objective and subjective cure at 89% and 86% for SIS and 88% and 87% for TOT, respectively; no differences were seen between years 1, 2, or 3 [93]. Very low risk of complications overall was seen, yet with significantly less postoperative pain with SIS. Similarly 3- and 5-year subjective and objective cure rates of 83% and 88% and 85% and 80% for SIS have been reported [69, 70]. And even more recently, a 10-year retrospective review of 60 patients with SIS noted no deterioration of efficacy over time—comparing 2 years to 10 years—with objective and subjective cure rates of 86% and 88%, respectively [41].

Assessing short- and long-term (6–36 months) impact of SIS (Solyx) versus TOT (Obtryx II) on sexual function, significant improvements in the Pelvic Organ Prolapse/Urinary Incontinence/Sexual Function Questionnaire (PISQ-12) scores were seen by both groups, owing to the elimination of SUI. Moreover, exceedingly rare de novo dyspareunia was noted out to 36 months (SIS 1/141; TOT 0/140, $p = 1.00$) [106]. A meta-analysis of randomized control trials of various mid-urethral slings indicated single-incision slings were associated with significantly greater improvement in sexual function (PISQ-12) and lower postoperative pain when compared to traditional mid-urethral slings [33].

Mesh Complications

Due to their proven long-term efficacy, synthetic mid-urethral slings are the most commonly adopted surgical procedure worldwide for female SUI. A recent 2017 Cochrane review of MUS noted "Midurethral sling operations have been the most extensively researched surgical treatment for SUI in women and have a good safety profile. Irrespective of the routes traversed, they are highly effective in the short and medium term, and accruing evidence demonstrates their effectiveness in the long term" [37]. However, there has still been much controversy over the use of synthetic mesh in the vagina, primarily due to the concerns about mesh-related complications: mesh exposure (through the vaginal wall), mesh erosion (into a neighboring organ), infections and poor healing, dyspareunia, and pain. But despite these concerns, the real risk of serious complications following mesh surgery for incontinence is reportedly very low. As noted in a population-based Scottish review conducted over 20 years (1997–2016), there were comparatively less immediate and long-term (5 years) complications with mesh mid-urethral slings as compared to all other non-mesh anti-incontinence procedures [77]. Specifically, with respect to the retropubic mesh mid-urethral sling, equal efficacy to non-mesh alternatives was seen (up to 5 years), but the relative risk of immediate complications with the RPS was 50% lower than all other non-mesh procedures. At this point, there are over 20 years of data describing the safety and efficacy of MUS. When comparing the three approaches, the RPS is associated with more postoperative obstruction and voiding dysfunction, including de novo urgency and urge incontinence requiring subsequent intervention [58]. Due to the RP approach, major vascular or visceral injuries, bladder or urethral perforations, and suprapubic pain have been described, while the TOT approach has seen more groin and thigh complications, including bleeding and pain [37, 102]. By comparison, SIS has seen less intraoperative injuries, postoperative and long-term pain, and higher sexual function scores when compared to the full RPS and TOT approach [33, 36, 79, 92, 96, 108].

What has been seen over time is the decrease in both intraoperative and postoperative complications associated with MUS as products evolved and improved, and providers gained more surgical experience and a better understanding about patient-related factors that may increase the risk of potential complications.

Initial reports of mesh-related complications and reoperation rates most often involved mesh extrusion through the vaginal epithelium. The reoperations dealt with excision of the exposed mesh, which most often was a very small area, and could be managed in the office or outpatient surgery setting, since the sling is so readily accessible from the introitus. In small (<1 cm) asymptomatic cases, local vaginal estrogen and/or no treatment-observation can be utilized in women who are not sexually active [48]. There have been more serious cases requiring extensive sling revision due to intraoperative surgical mishaps and poor healing, but these are uncommon. Very early reports of mesh complications were notably higher than with contemporary slings, with mesh exposure through the vaginal wall making up the vast majority of all mesh-related complications. That being said, the mesh exposure rate is still very low at <5%, with most managed via simple excision or expectant management in the otherwise asymptomatic patient [48, 68]. Likewise, reoperation rates overall are very low. According to a recent population-based retrospective review of >90,000 women receiving mid-urethral slings from 2006 to 2015 in England, the overall reoperation rate at 9 years for sling removal (partial or total) or recurrent SUI was very low at 6.9%; for sling removal only, 3.3%; and for recurrent SUI only, 4.5% [47].

To summarize, the current evidence points to the superiority of MUS over Burch and PVS for the treatment of SUI in patients with urethral hypermobility when evaluating for both long-term (>5 year) efficacy and safety. Although comparable efficacy between MUS and PVS has been demonstrated at 5 years, longer-term data describing further durability of PVS is lacking. And compared to MUS, PVS is associated with significantly more postoperative voiding dysfunction, along with the additional morbidity of the rectus fascial harvest.

With the mechanism of action at the bladder neck, the PVS is eloquently designed to address more difficult ISD-related SUI [10]. The Burch, with its comparatively inferior efficacy and greater morbidity associated with the open abdominal approach, may be recommended during salvage situations or perhaps when other open procedures are already required [88].

For all three types of MUS, similar efficacy is noted between RPS, TOT, and SIS out to 5 years. And with all three, both surgery-related and mesh-related complications are low. The RPS is noted to have a slightly higher success rate over time but at a cost of more intraoperative complications (bladder and vaginal perforations) and postoperative pain and voiding dysfunction. With TOT, more groin pain, vaginal mesh exposure, and mesh-related dyspareunia have been seen; much less so with SIS.

What About Urethral Bulking Agents?

With their mechanism of action at the bladder neck causing coaptation and increased resistance, urethral bulking agents have traditionally been used to treat ISD-associated SUI [63]. They are traditionally office-based cystoscopic procedures with very low morbidity, which adds to their appeal [18].

A new bulking agent, Bulkamid® (polyacrylamide hydrogel), was introduced into the US market in January 2020 but has already experienced widespread use in Europe since 2006, with good long-term results when compared to other available urethral bulking agents [84]. Its novelty and thus-far perceived advantage over the other urethral bulking agents is that it is completely non-reabsorbable, thereby providing relatively sustainable results. In spite of the enhanced durability noted, it still seems to provide better outcomes when used for mild-to-moderate SUI patients, which is similar to the other urethral bulking agents [29]. But although complete clinical success defined as dry rate has been low, up to 80% of patients report a partial response, which was deemed satisfactory. And this comes with a very low risk of associated adverse events that would require subsequent surgical intervention. With this in mind, the question has been posed to the viability of Bulkamid® challenging MUS's position as the primary treatment of choice for SUI in the index patient, especially for those who want to avoid the use of mesh. However, when compared to MUS in a recent head-to-head randomized control trial for primary SUI, the superiority of MUS with respect to efficacy at 1 year was significantly notable, both objectively and subjectively: negative cough stress test and pad test, TVT 95% versus Bulkamid® 66%; patient satisfaction, TVT 95% versus Bulkamid® 60%. These outcomes include the 53% of Bulkamid® patients who received a second injection procedure because of unsatisfactory initial results. With respect to adverse events requiring subsequent surgical intervention with the use of Bulkamid®, there were none reported, although there are many who would consider unsatisfactory results requiring repeat surgery a "complication." In the TVT group, few mesh-related complications requiring surgical intervention were seen. As clear superiority of the TVT versus Bulkamid® with respect to cure rates and patient satisfaction was established, the conclusion was that "Tension-free vaginal tape should be offered as first line treatment in women who expect to be completely cured by the initial treatment and are willing to accept the complication risks" [50]. For those women who would be satisfied with accepting lower efficacy in order to avoid the use of mesh, Bulkamid® is a good minimally invasive option.

Current Guidelines for SUI and the Worldwide Standard

The most recent 2017 AUA/SUFU Guidelines for the surgical treatment of SUI recommends considering the following surgical options for the index patient: mid-urethral sling (synthetic), autologous fascia pubovaginal sling, Burch colposuspension, and urethral bulking agents (Strong Recommendation; Evidence Level: Grade A). Concerning synthetic mid-urethral slings, the "full-length" RPS and TOT slings are specifically recommended (Moderate Recommendation; Evidence Level: Grade A), with the caveat for single-incision slings that the patient be "…informed as to the immaturity of evidence regarding their efficacy and safety" (Conditional Recommendation; Evidence Level: Grade B) (see Fig. 16.4) [64].

Now in 2021, good quality long-term data does exist, including the results from the FDA-mandated 522 studies noting equal efficacy and enhanced safety of the SIS compared to TOT at 3+ years [105].

Of particular importance, national and international professional and academic societies dealing with urogynecological procedures have all published formal position statements endorsing the overall safety and efficacy of MUS. The American Urogynecologic Society (AUGS) and Society of Urodynamics, Female Pelvic Medicine, and Urogenital Reconstruction (SUFU) open their joint position statement with "The purpose of this position statement…is to support the use of the midurethral sling in the surgical management of stress urinary incontinence." They go on to conclude "The polypropylene mesh midurethral sling is the recognized worldwide standard of care for the surgical treatment of stress urinary incontinence. The procedure is safe, effective, and has improved the quality of life for millions of women" (AUGS/SUFU). Further support for this statement is noted by endorsements from the American College of Obstetricians and Gynecologists (ACOG), the Society of Gynecologic Surgeons (SGS), the International Urogynecological Association (IUGA), the National Association for Continence (NAFC), and the American Association of Gynecologic Laparoscopists (AAGL). Similarly acknowledging the favorable risk/benefit profile and advocating for the MUS, the American Urological Association (AUA) position statement formally declares "It is the AUA's opinion that any restriction of the use of synthetic polypropylene mesh suburethral slings would be a disservice to women who choose surgical correction of SUI" [5].

In Europe, the European Commission Scientific Committee on Emerging and Newly Identified Health Risks (SCENIHR) concluded "synthetic sling SUI surgery is an accepted procedure with proven efficacy and safety in the majority of patients with moderate to severe SUI, when used by an experienced and appropriately trained surgeon. Therefore, the SCENIHR supports continuing synthetic sling use for SUI, but emphasized the importance of appropriately trained surgeons and detailed counseling of patients about the associated risk/benefits. …There is robust evidence to support the use of MUS from over 2,000 publications, making this treatment the most extensively reviewed and evaluated procedure for female SUI now in use" [32].

Concurrent with this statement, the European Association of Urology (EAU) and European Urogynecological Association (EUGA) consensus guidelines (revised 2017) also recognize the far-reaching positive impact mid-urethral slings have had on the quality of life of women throughout Europe and recommended it as the preferred surgery for uncomplicated SUI while recommending PVS for those patients in whom MUS cannot be considered [14]. Even in the setting of recurrent SUI after synthetic MUS (which was only 6% at 5 years), a nationwide Danish study from 1998 to 2007 evaluated 5,820 MUS and noted the retreatment procedure of choice was most often a repeat MUS (45.5%), reflecting the perceived ease and safety profile of the procedure with traditionally excellent long-term efficacy [39, 40].

And in its global position statement endorsed by 53 international urogynecological societies, the International Urogynecological Association (IUGA) further acknowledges the equal efficacy of the polypropylene MUS compared to traditional surgeries but with clinically meaningful advantages of shorter operative and hospital admission times, fewer surgical complications, and a quicker return to normal activities. It is precisely this very favorable risk/benefit ratio that "resulted in MUS becoming the operation of choice in Europe, Asia, South America, South Africa, Australasia and North America for treatment of SUI with several million procedures performed worldwide" (IUGA 2014 global position statement).

Conclusion

Despite the controversy surrounding the use of mesh in the vagina, it is important to recognize that synthetic mid-urethral slings are still the mainstay surgical treatment for female SUI associated with a predominance of urethral hypermobility. Since the introduction of MUS, the number of surgeries for stress urinary incontinence has significantly increased worldwide [45, 56, 83]. In the United States, an estimated 27% increase in the rate of surgeries from 2000 to 2009 was noted, which was attributed to the wide adoption of MUS as a less invasive, yet equally effective (if not more effective) treatment for SUI compared to other traditional surgical alternatives (Burch, PVS, urethral bulking agents) [53]. MUS is the most widely studied anti-incontinence procedure to date, with the highest long-term (>5 years and up to 17 years) efficacy and the lowest rate of short-, medium-, and long-term complications, mild and serious [37, 50]. Due to this, they have been deemed the "Gold Standard" surgical treatment for SUI (AUA/SUFU) (AUGS/SUFU) (EAU/EUGA) (IUGA) (IUGA global) [22].

Today, in 2021, the synthetic mid-urethral sling is still the most commonly performed procedure worldwide to treat female SUI. Despite all the controversy and medicolegal consequences surrounding the use of vaginal mesh, most physicians have continued to provide MUS for their patients as the primary surgical choice for

SUI. Even shortly after the 2011 FDA [34] safety notification on the use of transvaginal mesh, 99% of American Urogynecologic Society (AUGS) members who treat SUI still reported using MUS [17]. This was true for our international colleagues too, as noted through a survey of the International Urogynecological Association (IUGA) members describing the MUS as the preferred method of treatment for SUI, regardless of prior treatments, concomitant surgeries, or preoperative examination findings [44]. This is because most physicians practice evidence-based medicine, as they strive to provide the best possible care for their patients. And with this in mind, adequately trained providers know when and how to use MUSs appropriately and safely to achieve those best results.

References

1. Albo ME, Richter HE, Brubaker L, et al. Burch colposuspension versus fascial sling to reduce urinary stress incontinence. N Engl J Med. 2007;356:2143.
2. Aldridge AH. Transplantation of fascia for relief of urinary stress incontinence. Am J Obstet Gynecol. 1942;44(3):398–411.
3. Alexandridis V, Rudnicki M, Jakobsson U, Teleman P. Adjustable mini-sling compared with conventional mid-urethral slings in women with urinary incontinence: a 3-year follow-up of a randomized controlled trial. Int Urogynecol J. 2019;30(9):1465–73.
4. American Urogynecologic Society (AUGS) and the Society for Urodynamics and FPMRS (SUFU). Position statement: mesh mid-urethral slings for stress urinary incontinence. https://sufuorg.com/docs/guidelines/augs-sufu-mus-position-statement.aspx . Adopted 2014; Last revised 2017. Accessed March 2021.
5. American Urological Association. AUA position statement on the use of vaginal mesh for the surgical treatment of stress urinary incontinence (SUI). https://www.auanet.org/guidelines/guidelines/use-of-vaginal-mesh-for-the-surgical-treatment-of-stress-urinary-incontinence . Adopted 2011; Last revised 2019. Accessed March 2021.
6. Bai SW, Sohn WH, Chung DJ, et al. Comparison of the efficacy of Burch colposuspension, pubovaginal sling, and tension-free vaginal tape for stress urinary incontinence. Int J Gynaecol Obstet. 2005;91:246.
7. Bakali E, Buckley BS, Hilton P, et al. Treatment of recurrent stress urinary incontinence after failed minimally invasive synthetic suburethral tape surgery in women. Cochrane Database Syst Rev. 2013;2:CD009407.
8. Ballester M, Bui C, Frobert JL, et al. Four-year functional results of the suburethral sling procedure for stress urinary incontinence: a French prospective randomized multicenter study comparing the retropubic and transobturator routes. World J Urol. 2012;30(1):117–22.
9. Barnett RM. The modern Kelly plication. Obstet Gynecol. 1969;34(5):667–9.
10. Blaivas JG, Jacobs BZ. Pubovaginal fascial sling for the treatment of complicated stress urinary incontinence. J Urol. 1991;145(6):1214–8.
11. Brubaker L, Richter HE, Norton PA, et al. Five year continence rates, satisfaction and adverse events of burch urethropexy and fascial sling surgery for urinary incontinence. J Urol. 2012;187(4):1324–30.
12. Burch JC. Urethrovaginal fixation to Cooper's ligament for correction of stress incontinence, cystocele, and prolapse. Am J Obstet Gynecol. 1961;81:281–90.
13. Chaikin DC, Rosenthal J, Blaivas JG. Pubovaginal fascial sling for all types of stress urinary incontinence: long-term analysis. J Urol. 1998;160:1312.
14. Chapple CR, Cruz F, Deffieux X, et al. Consensus statement of the European Urology Association and the European Urogynaecological Association on the use of implanted

materials for treating pelvic organ prolapse and stress urinary incontinence. Eur Urol. 2017;72(3):424–31.

15. Chughtai B, Sedrakyan A, Mao J, et al. Is vaginal mesh a stimulus of autoimmune disease? Am J Obstet Gynecol. 2017a;216(5):495.

16. Chughtai B, Sedrakyan A, Mao J, et al. Challenging the Myth: transvaginal mesh is not associated with carcinogenesis. J Urol. 2017b;198(4):884–9.

17. Clemons JL, Weinstein M, Guess MK, et al. Impact of the 2011 FDA transvaginal mesh safety update on AUGS members' use of synthetic mesh and biologic grafts in pelvic reconstructive surgery. Female Pelvic Med Reconstr Surg. 2013;19(4):191–8.

18. Corcos J, Collet JP, Shapiro S, et al. Multicenter randomized clinical trial comparing surgery and collagen injections for treatment of female stress urinary incontinence. Urology. 2005;65:898.

19. Costantini E, Kocjancic E, Lazzeri M, et al. Long-term efficacy of the trans-obturator and retropubic mid-urethral slings for stress urinary incontinence: update from a randomized clinical trial. World J Urol. 2016;34(4):585–93.

20. Cornu JN, Sebe P, Peyrat L, et al. Midterm propective evaluation of TVT-Secur reveals high failure rate. Eur Urol. 2010;58(1):157–61.

21. Cornu JN, Lizee D, Sebe P, et al. TVT SECUR single-incision sling after 5 years of follow-up: the promises made and the promises broken. Eur Urol. 2012;62(4):737–8.

22. Cox A, Hershorn S, Lee L. Surgical management of female SUI: Is there a gold standard? Nat Rev Urol. 2013;10(2):78–89.

23. Cundiff GW. The pathophysiology of stress urinary incontinence: a historical perspective. Rev Urol. 2004;6 Suppl 3(Suppl 3):S10–8.

24. Deffieux X, Daher N, Mansoor A, et al. Transobturator TVT-O versus retropubic TVT: results of a multicenter randomized controlled trial of 24 months follow-up. Int Urogynecol J. 2010;21:1337.

25. DeLancey JO. Stress urinary incontinence: where are we now, where should we go? Am J Obstet Gynecol. 1996;175(2):311–9.

26. DeLancey JO, Trowbridge ER, Miller JM, et al. Stress urinary incontinence: relative importance of urethral support and urethral closure pressure. J Urol. 2008;179:2286.

27. de Leval J. Novel surgical technique for the treatment of female stress urinary incontinence: transobturator vaginal tape insideout. Eur Urol. 2003;44(6):724–30.

28. Delorme E. Transobturator urethral suspension: mini-invasive procedure in the treatment of stress urinary incontinence in women. Prog Urol. 2001;11(6):1306–13.

29. Elmelund M, Sokol ER, Karra MM, et al. Patient characteristics that may influence the effect of urethral injection therapy for female stress urinary incontinence. J Urol. 2019;202:125–31.

30. Enhoerning G. Simulateous recording of intravesical and intra-urethral pressure. A study on urethral closure in normal and stress incontinent women. Acta Chir Scand Suppl. 1961;Suppl 276:1–68.

31. Enhoerning G, Miller ER, Hinman F Jr. Urethral closure studied with cineroentgenography and simultaneous bladder-urethra pressure recording. Surg Gynecol Obstet. 1964;118:507–16.

32. European Commission Scientific Committee on Emerging and Newly Identified Health Risks. Opinion on the safety of surgical meshes used in urogynecological surgery. 2015. Available at: http://ec.europa.eu/health/scientific_committees/emerging/Opinions/index_en.htm.

33. Fan Y, Huang Z, Yu D. Incontinence-specific quality of life measures used in trials of sling procedures for female stress urinary incontinence: a meta-analysis. Int Urol Nephrol. 2015;47(8):1277–95.

34. FDA, FDA safety communication: UPDATE on serious complications associated with transvaginal placement of surgical mesh for pelvic organ prolapse. 2011. http://wayback.archive-it.org/7993/20170722150848/https://www.fda.gov/MedicalDevices/Safety/AlertsandNotices/ucm262435.htm.

35. FDA, Considerations about surgical mesh for SUI. 2013. http://www.fda.gov/MedicalDevices/ProductsandMedicalProcedures/ImplantsandProsthetics/UroGynSurgicalMesh/ucm345219.htm.

36. Foote A. Randomized prospective study comparing Monarc and Miniarc suburethral slings. J Obstet Gynaecol Res. 2015;41:127.
37. Ford AA, Rogerson L, Cody JD, et al. Mid-urethral sling operations for stress urinary incontinence in women. Cochrane Database Syst Rev. 2017;7(7):CD006375.
38. Ford AA, Ogah JA. Retropubic or transobturator mid-urethral slings for intrinsic sphincter deficiency-related stress urinary incontinence in women: a systematic review and meta-analysis. Int Urogynecol J. 2016;27(1):19–28.
39. Foss Hansen M, Lose G, Schioler Kesmodel U, Gradel KO. Reoperation for urinary incontinence: a nationwide cohort study, 1998-2007. Am J Obstet Gynecol. 2016a;214(2):263.e1.
40. Foss Hansen M, Lose G, Schioler Kesmodel U, Gradel KO. Repeat surgery after failed midurethral slings: a nationwide cohort study, 1998-2007. Int Urogynecol J. 2016b;27:1013–19.
41. Frigerio M, Milani R, Barba M, et al. Single-incision slings for the treatment of stress urinary incontinence: efficacy and adverse effects at 10-year follow-up. Int Urogynecol J. 2021;32(1):187–91. https://doi.org/10.1007/s00192-020-04499-8. Epub 2020 Sep 9
42. Frigerio M, Regini C, Manodoro S, et al. Mini-sling efficacy in obese versus non-obese patients for treatment of stress urinary incontinence. Minerva Ginecol. 2017;69(6):533–7.
43. Fusco F, Abdel-Fattah M, Chapple CR, et al. Updated systematic review and meta-analysis of the comparative data on Colposuspensions, Pubovaginal slings, and Midurethral tapes in the surgical treatment of female stress urinary incontinence. Eur Urol. 2017;72(4):567–91.
44. Ghoniem G, Hammett J. Female pelvic medicine and reconstructive surgery practice patterns: IUGA member survey. Int Urogynecol J. 2015;26(10):1489–94.
45. Gibson W, Wagg A. Are older women more likely to receive surgical treatment for stress urinary incontinence since the introduction of the mid-urethral sling? An examination of Hospital Episode Statistics data. BJOG. 2016;123:1386–92.
46. Glazener CM, Cooper K. Bladder neck needle suspension for urinary incontinence in women. Cochrane Database Syst Rev. 2004;2:CD003636.
47. Gurol-Urganci I, Geary RS, Mamza JB, et al. Long-term rate of mesh sling removal following Midurethral mesh sling insertion among women with stress urinary incontinence. JAMA. 2018;320(16):1659–69.
48. Illiano E, Giannitsas K, Li Marzi V, et al. No treatment required for asymptomatic vaginal mesh exposure. Urol Int. 2019:1–5.
49. Mari I, Jemma H, Wallace Sheila A, et al. Surgical interventions for women with stress urinary incontinence: systematic review and network meta-analysis of randomised controlled trials. BMJ. 2019;365:l1842.
50. Itkonen Freitas AM, Mentula M, Rahkola-Soisalo P, et al. Tension-free vaginal tape surgery versus polyacrylamide hydrogel injection for primary stress urinary incontinence: a randomized clinical trial. J Urol. 2020;203(2):372–8.
51. IUGA. Position statement on mid-urethral slings for stress urinary incontinence. http://www.iuga.org/?page=mus&hSearchTerms=%22midurethral+and+slings%22.
52. IUGA. Statement in support of midurethral slings for stress urinary incontinence – on behalf of the International Urogynecological Community. http://www.iuga.org/urogynglobal.com
53. Jonsson Funk M, Levin PJ, Wu JM. Trends in the surgical management of stress urinary incontinence. Obstet Gynecol. 2012;119(4):845–51.
54. Kegel AH. The physiologic treatment of poor tone and function of the genital muscles and of urinary stress incontinence. West J Surg Obstet Gynecol. 1949;57(11):527–35.
55. Kelly HA, Dumm WM. Urinary incontinence in women, without manifest injury to the bladder. 1914. Int Urogynecol J Pelvic Floor Dysfunct. 1998;9(3):158–64.
56. Keltie K, Elneil S, Monga A, et al. Complications following vaginal mesh procedures for stress urinary incontinence: an 8 year study of 92,246 women. Sci Rep. 2017;7:12015.
57. Kennelly MJ, Moore R, Nguyen JN, et al. Prospective evaluation of a single incision sling for stress urinary incontinence. J Urol. 2010;184(2):604–9.
58. Kenton K, Richter H, Litman H, et al. Risk factors associated with urge incontinence after continence surgery. J Urol. 2009;182:2805.

59. Kenton K, Stoddard AM, Zyczynski H, et al. 5-year longitudinal followup after retropubic and transobturator mid urethral slings. J Urol. 2015;193:203.
60. Khan ZA, Manbiar A, Morley R, et al. Long-term follow-up of a multicenter randomized controlled trial comparing tension-free vaginal tape, xenograft and autologous fascial slings for the treatment of stress urinary incontinence in women. BJU Int. 2015;115(6):968–77.
61. King AB, Zampini A, Vasavada S, et al. Is there an association between polypropylene midurethral slings and malignancy? Urology. 2014;84(4):789–92.
62. King AB, Goldman HB. Current controversies regarding oncologic risk associated with polypropylene midurethral slings. Curr Urol Rep. 2014;15(11):453.
63. Klarskov N, Lose G. Urethral injection therapy: what is the mechanism of action? Neurourol Urogy. 2008;27:789.
64. Kobashi KC, Albo ME, Dmochowski RR, et al. Surgical treatment of female stress urinary incontinence: AUA/SUFU guideline. J Urol. 2017;198(4):875–83. https://www.auanet.org/guidelines/guidelines/stress-urinary-incontinence-(sui)-guideline
65. Lapitan MCM, Cody JD, Mashayekhi A. Open retropubic colposuspension for urinary incontinence in women. Cochrane Database Syst Rev. 2017;2017:1–235.
66. Laurikainen E, Valpas A, Aukee P, et al. Five-year results of a randomized trial comparing retropubic and transobturator midurethral slings for stress incontinence. Eur Urol. 2014;65:1109.
67. Leone Roberti Maggiore U, Finazzi Agro E, Soligo M, et al. Long-term outcomes of TOT and TVT procedures for the treatment of female stress urinary incontinence: a systematic review and meta-analysis. Int Urogynecol J. 2017;28(8):1119–30.
68. Linder B, El-Nashar SA, Carranza Leon DA, Trabuco E. Predictors of vaginal mesh exposure after midurethral sling placement: a case-control study. Int Urogynecol J. 2016;27(9):1321–6.
69. Lo TS, Chua S, Kao CC, et al. Five-year outcome of MiniArc single-incision sling used in the treatment of primary urodynamic stress incontinenc. J Minim Invasive Gynecol. 2018a;25(1):116–23.
70. Lo TS, Chua S, Tan YL, et al. Ultrasonography and clinical outcomes following anti-incontinence procedures (Monarc vs MiniArc): a 3-year post-operative review. PLoS One. 2018b;13(12):e0207375.
71. Marshall VF, Marchetti AA, Krantz KE. The correction of stress incontinence by simple vesicourethral suspension. Surg Gynecol Obstet. 1949;88(4):509–18.
72. McGuire EJ, Lytton B. Pubovaginal sling procedure for cure of stress incontinence. J Urol. 1978;119:82–4.
73. McGuire EJ, Cespedes RD, O'Connell HE. Leak-point pressures. Urol Clin North Am. 1996;23(2):253–62.
74. McGuire EJ. Pathophysiology of stress urinary incontinence. Rev Urol. 2004;6 Suppl 5:S11.
75. Mock S, Angelle J, Reynolds WS, et al. Contemporary comparison between retropubic midurethral sling and autologous pubovaginal sling for stress urinary incontinence after the FDA advisory notification. Urology. 2015;85(2):321–5.
76. Molden SM, Lucente VR. New minimally invasive slings: TVT secur. Curr Urol Rep. 2008;9(5):358–61.
77. Morling JR, McAllister DA, Agur W, et al. Adverse events after first, single, mesh and non-mesh surgical procedures for stress urinary incontinence and pelvic organ prolapse in Scotland, 1997-2016: a population-based cohort study. Lancet. 2017;389(10069):629–40.
78. Mostafa A, Agur W, Abdel-All M, et al. Multicenter prospective randomized study of single-incision mini-sling vs tension-free vaginal tape-obturator in management of female stress urinary incontinence: a minimum of 1-year follow-up. Urology. 2013;82:552.
79. Mostafa A, Lim CP, Hopper L, Madhuvrata P, Abdel-Fattah M. Single-incision mini-slings versus standard midurethral slings in surgical management of female stress urinary incontinence: an updated systematic review and meta-analysis of effectiveness and complications. Eur Urol. 2014;65(2):402–27.

80. Nambiar A, Cody JD, Jeffery ST, Aluko P. Single-incision sling operations for urinary incontinence in women. Cochrane Database Syst Rev. 2017;7(7):CD008709.
81. Nilsson CG, Palva K, Aarnio R, et al. Seventeen years' follow up of the tension-free vaginal tape procedure for female stress urinary incontinence. Int Urogynecol J. 2013;24:1265.
82. Novara G, Artibani W, Barber M, et al. Updated systematic review and meta-analysis of the comparative data on colposuspensions, pubovaginal slings, and midurethral tapes in the surgical treatment of female stress urinary incontinence. Eur Urol. 2010;58(2):218–38.
83. Oliphant SS, Wang L, Bunker CH, et al. Trends in stress urinary incontinence inpatient procedures in the United States, 1979-2004. Am J Obstet Gynecol. 2009;200:521.
84. Pai A, Al-Singary W. Durability, safety and efficacy of polyacrylamide hydrogel (Bulkamid(®)) in the management of stress and mixed urinary incontinence: three year follow up outcomes. Cent European J Urol. 2015;68(4):428–33.
85. Palmieri S, Frigerio M, Spelzini F, et al. Risk factors for stress urinary incontinence recurrence after single-incision sling. NeurourolUrodyn. 2018;37(5):1711–6.
86. Pereyra AJ. A simplified surgical procedure for the correction of stress incontinence in women. West J Surg Obstet Gynecol. 1959;67(4):223–6.
87. Petros PE, Ulmsten UI. An integral theory of female urinary incontinence. Experimental and clinical considerations. Acta Obstet Gynecol Scand Suppl. 1990;153:7–31.
88. Rashid TG, De Ridder D, Van der Aa F. The role of bladder neck suspension in the era of miurethral sling surgery. World J Urol. 2015;33:1235–41.
89. Raz S. Modified bladder neck suspension for female stress incontinence. Urology. 1981;17(1):82–5.
90. Raz S, Klutke CG, Golomb J. Four-corner bladder and urethral suspension for moderate cystocele. J Urol. 1989;142(3):712–5.
91. Richter HE, Albo ME, Zyczynski HM, et al. Retropubic versus transobturator midurethral slings for stress incontinence. N Engl J Med. 2010;362:2066.
92. Schellart RP, Oude Rengerink K, Van der Aa F, et al. A randomized comparison of a single-incision midurethral sling and a transobturator midurethral sling in women with stress urinary incontinence: results of 12-mo follow-up. Eur Urol. 2014;66:1179.
93. Schellert RP, Zwolsman SE, Lucot JP, et al. A randomized, nonblinded extention study of single-incision versus transobturator midurethral sling in women with stress urinary incontinence. Int Urogynecol J. 2018;29:37–44.
94. Schierlitz L, Dwyer PL, Rosamilia A, et al. Three-year follow-up of tension-free vaginal tape compared with transobturator tape in women with stress urinary incontinence and intrinsic sphincter deficiency. Obstet Gynecol. 2012;119:321.
95. Schreiner G, Beltran R, Lockwood G, Takacs EB. A timeline of female stress urinary incontinence: how technology defined theory and advanced treatment. NeurourolUrodyn. 2020;39(6):1862–7.
96. Schweitzer KJ, Milani AL, Van Eijndhoven HW, et al. Postoperative pain after adjustable single-incision or transobturator sling for incontinence: a randomized controlled trial. Obstet Gynecol. 2015;125:27.
97. Shirvan MK, Rahimi HR, Darabi Mahboub MR, et al. Tension-free vaginal tape versus transobturator tape for treatment of stress urinary incontinence: a comparative randomized clinical trial study. Urol Sci. 2014;25:54.
98. Spelzini F, Frigerio M, Regini C, et al. Learning curve for the single-incision suburethral sling procedure for female stress urinary incontinence. Int J Gynaecol Obstet. 2017;139(3):363–7.
99. Spelzini F, Cesana MC, Verri D, et al. Three-dimensional ultrasound assessment and middle term efficacy of a single-incision sling. Int Urogynecol J. 2013;24(8):1391–7.
100. Stamey TA. Endoscopic suspension of the vesical neck for urinary incontinence. Obstet Gynecol Surv. 1973;28(10):762–4.

101. Stamey TA. Endoscopic suspension of the vesical neck for urinary incontinence in females. Report on 203 consecutive patients. Ann Surg. 1980;192:465.
102. Sun X, Yang Q, Sun F, et al. Comparison between the retropubic and transobturator approaches in the treatment of female stress urinary incontinence: a systematic review and meta-analysis of effectiveness and complications. Int Braz J Urol. 2015;41:220.
103. Ulmsten U, Henriksson L, Johnson P, Varhos G. An ambulatory surgical procedure under local anesthesia for treatment of female urinary incontinence. Int Urogynecol J Pelvic Floor Dysfunct. 1996;7(2):81–5.
104. Wadie BS, Elhefnawy AS. TVT versus TOT, 2-year prospective randomized study. World J Urol. 2013;31:645.
105. White AB, Kahn B, Gonzalez R, et al. Prospective study of a single-incision sling versus transobturator sling in women with stress urinary incontinence: 3-year results. Am J Obtet Gynecol. 2020;223(4):545.e1–545.e11. https://doi.org/10.1016/j.ajog.2020.03.008. Epub 2020 Mar 14
106. White AB, Anger JT, Eilber K, et al. Female sexual function following sling surgery: a prospective parallel multi-center study of the Solyx single incision sling system versus the Obtryx II sling system (FDA-mandated 522 results at 36 months). J Urol. 2021:101097JU0000000000001830. https://doi.org/10.1097/JU.0000000000001830. Online ahead of print.
107. Whiteside J, Walters M. Pathophysiology of stress urinary incontinence. In: Urogynecology and Reconstructive pelvic surgery. 4th ed; 2015. p. 215–23.
108. Zhang P, Fan B, Zhang P, et al. Meta-analysis of female stress urinary incontinence treatments with adjustable single-incision mini-slings and transobturator tension-free vaginal tape surgeries. BMC Urol. 2015;15:64.
109. Zhu L, Lang J, Hai N, et al. Comparing vaginal tape and transobturator tape for the treatment of mild and moderate stress incontinence. A prospective randomized controlled study. Int J Gynecol Obstet. 2007;99:14.

Chapter 17
Autologous Fascial Sling

Annah Vollstedt and Priya Padmanabhan

Historical Perspective

The technique of pubovaginal sling was first described by German surgeons in the early twentieth century. In 1910, Goebel described treating incontinence in children by rotating of the pyramidalis muscles such that their insertion to the pubic bone was conserved, but the ends were joined together below the bladder neck and urethra [1]. In 1914, Frangenheim modified Goebel's procedure by incorporating the aponeurosis of the abdominal rectus muscles to the sling of the pyramidalis muscles [2]. Shortly thereafter, Stoeckel was the first to describe the abdominal and vaginal approach for placing a pubovaginal fascial sling [3]. Adopting these earlier techniques, McGuire was the first to describe a modern version of the pubovaginal sling (PVS) in the 1970s, using a strip of rectus fascia that remained attached laterally on one side [4]. The contemporary technique of harvesting a free graft from the rectus fascia, developed by Blaivas and Jacobs in 1991, allowed for the ability to tension the PVS [5].

Since approval in 1998, synthetic mesh mid-urethral slings replaced the fascial sling and needle suspension as the most commonly performed procedure for stress urinary incontinence (SUI) [6]. However, after the Food and Drug Administration Public Health Notification in 2001 and 2008 regarding transvaginal mesh for pelvic organ prolapse, there has been a decrease in the use of synthetic mesh slings for the treatment of SUI and an increase in placement of autologous fascial slings [7].

A. Vollstedt · P. Padmanabhan (✉)
Beaumont Hospital, Department of Urology, Royal Oak, MI, USA
e-mail: priya.padamanabhan@beaumont.edu

© The Author(s), under exclusive license to Springer Nature
Switzerland AG 2022
A. P. Cameron (ed.), *Female Urinary Incontinence*,
https://doi.org/10.1007/978-3-030-84352-6_17

Indications

The basic mechanism of the pubovaginal sling is to correct urethral hypermobility and modify the pressure transmission caused by an increase in intraabdominal pressure [8]. In addition to urethral hypermobility, the pubovaginal sling is indicated for the treatment of intrinsic urethral sphincter deficiency (ISD). ISD was once a strict urodynamic diagnosis of an abdominal leak point pressure of less than 60 mm H_2O [9] and/or a maximal urethral closure pressure of less than 20 cm H_2O [10]. Though still clinically relevant, the definition of ISD has now evolved to an imprecise subjective diagnosis. The International Continence Society now defines ISD as a "very weakened urethral closure mechanism" [11].

Other indications for PVS include recurrent stress urinary incontinence (SUI) after failed mid-urethral sling, SUI or insensate incontinence related to neurological diseases, tissue interposition after repair of urethral fistulae or diverticulum, or urethral reconstruction after traumatic loss of the proximal urethra from erosion of synthetic material or prolonged in-dwelling catheterization. Other causes of urethral damage in which an autologous fascial sling may serve an important role in reconstruction are protracted obstetric delivery, aggressive transurethral resection, or disruption of the bladder neck, pelvic trauma, tumors, and radiation [12].

Urethral Mechanics

Female SUI is due to urethral hypermobility and/or ISD. Once thought to be two separate components, urethral hypermobility and ISD are now recognized as two points on a continuum [13]. It is thought that the loss of structural urethral support results in descent of the bladder neck and urethra, thus causing urethral hypermobility. In the normally supported bladder neck and proximal urethra, increased intraabdominal pressure is transmitted equally to both the bladder and urethra. When this support is lost, intraabdominal pressure is then transmitted unequally to the bladder and urethra. During increased intraabdominal pressure with "stress maneuvers," such as occurs with coughing, sneezing, and laughing, the posterior wall of the urethra slides away from the anterior wall, causing the bladder neck to open (Fig. 17.1). This transmission of uneven pressure combined with opening of the bladder neck allows for SUI to occur [13]. The normal urethra remains closed despite stress maneuvers. In the case of ISD, there is an intrinsic defect in the urethra itself, regardless of anatomic position, such that the urethra is unable to coapt and remain closed to store urine in the bladder [12].

The concepts of urethral hypermobility and ISD are important in understanding the mechanism of action of the PVS. With the PVS positioned at the bladder neck, the goal is to provide compression of the proximal urethra during stress maneuvers such that there is adequate coaptation of the urethra leading to continence [12]. When there is increased intraabdominal pressure, the sling is pulled anteriorly, increasing bladder outlet resistance through rotating the bladder base posteroinferiorly and kinking the posterior meatus, which leads to decreased urine leakage (Fig. 17.2) [14].

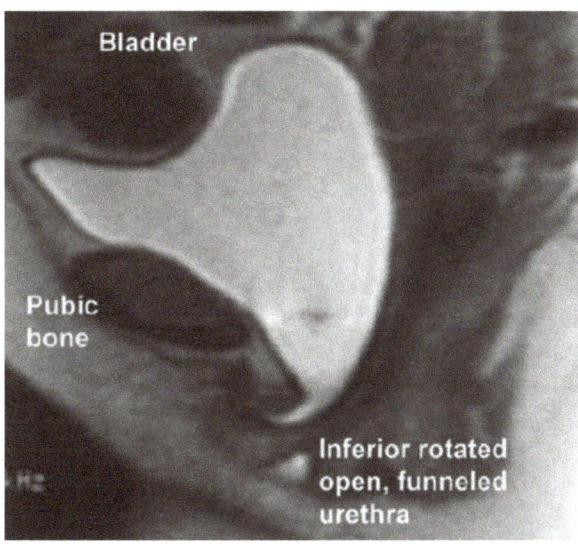

Fig. 17.1 Sagittal T2-weighted MRI during abdominal straining in a patient with stress urinary incontinence. Abdominal straining is causing downward rotational descent of the urethra, as well as funneling of the bladder neck. This leads to an open urethra with subsequent leakage. (With permission from Atlas of Vaginal Reconstructive Surgery, Raz, 2015, Springer Figure 2.7b)

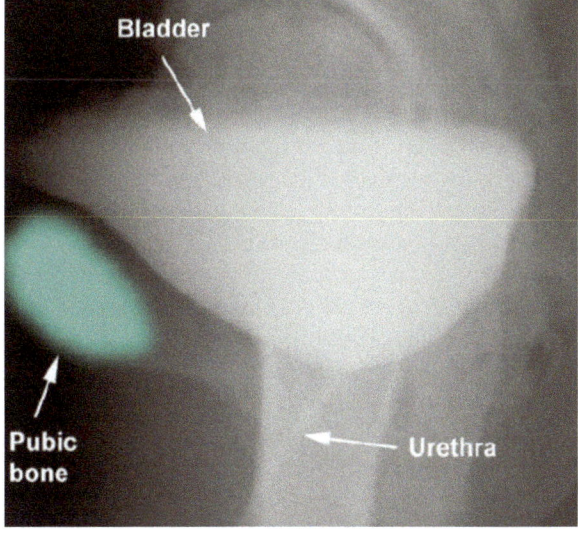

Fig. 17.2 Lateral cystogram in patient after sling placement. This sling is preventing the downward rotation and funneling of the urethra. The sling is allowing proper transmission of abdominal pressure during straining. (With permission from Atlas of Vaginal Reconstructive Surgery, Raz, Springer, 2015, Figure 2.8)

Preoperative Evaluation

The preoperative evaluation consists of a thorough history and physical exam. Specifically, the surgeon should ask about voiding symptoms, including the presence of urinary leakage with stress maneuvers, such as coughing, sneezing, and laughing. The presence of preoperative storage symptoms needs to be noted, such as urinary frequency, urgency, and urinary urgency incontinence. The patient should be counseled that these storage symptoms may not improve after the procedure and may even worsen. It should be noted that one-third of patients will have persistent urgency urinary incontinence (UUI), and about 10% of patients will develop de novo UUI [15]. A complete surgical history, including all abdominal and vaginal procedures, needs to be collected. Prior radiation also needs to be noted as this may affect the quality of the bladder and vaginal tissue and degree of ISD.

Physical examination should include a complete abdominal examination noting prior surgical scars, as well as a pelvic examination. The presence or absence of urethral hypermobility should be noted. This can be performed by either a formal Q-tip test or gross visualization. A cough stress test should be performed, noting the presence of leakage and the relative fullness of the bladder. In addition, the quality of the vaginal tissues, presence of pelvic organ prolapse, or evidence of any mesh exposures that may have been previously placed should be noted. It is important to assess for prolapse of the anterior vaginal compartment, as this may be a future cause of urethral obstruction and may need to be corrected at the time of the sling placement.

A postvoid residual should be obtained. However, per the 2017 American Urological Association (AUA)/Society of Urodynamics, Female Pelvic Medicine & Urogenital Reconstruction (SUFU), routine preoperative urodynamic studies (UDS) are not recommended for the "index patient," defined as the otherwise healthy female who is considering surgical therapy for the correction of pure stress and/or stress-predominant mixed urinary incontinence (MUI) who has not undergone previous SUI surgery [16]. In the more complex patient, UDS may be considered, especially when impaired detrusor contractility or obstruction is suspected. UDS may also detect preoperative detrusor overactivity (DO). Often, an autologous fascial sling is used to treat recurrent SUI. In these patients, preoperative UDS is commonly used. Likewise, routine preoperative cystoscopy is not recommended for the index patient unless there is a concern for a urinary tract abnormality [16].

A urine culture should be obtained prior to surgery, and the surgery should be postponed if there is an untreated infection.

The surgery may be performed under general anesthesia or spinal anesthesia. A first- or second-generation cephalosporin is the preferred antibiotic regimen and should be given 60 minutes before the incision. Per the 2019 AUA Best Practice Statement, Urologic Procedures, and Antimicrobial Prophylaxis, vaginal procedures should consider additional anaerobic coverage, which is most often afforded by the use of a second-generation cephalosporin, such as cefoxitin [17]. Additional anaerobic coverage provided by metronidazole and an antifungal may also be considered for vaginal cases, particularly for high-risk patients [17].

Operative Technique

Patient Positioning

Before induction of anesthesia, sequential compression devices (SCDs) should be placed on the lower extremities. The patient is then placed in the dorsal lithotomy position. The patient's vagina and abdomen as far cephalad as the umbilicus are prepped. The authors prefer to use a weighted Scherbak vaginal speculum for retraction of the posterior vaginal wall. A 16 French catheter is placed for bladder drainage. Moderate Trendelenburg (head down) position is helpful for visualization of and access to the anterior vaginal wall. The surgeon may use a vaginal ring retraction (such as a disposable Lone Star® retractor) for labial retraction. Alternatively, the labia majora can be sutured laterally to the inner thigh with a silk suture.

Rectus Fascia Graft Harvest

A 5- to 7-cm Pfannenstiel incision is made approximately two-fingerbreadth cephalad to the pubic bone. This incision is dissected down to the level of the rectus fascia (Fig. 17.3a). A self-training retractor, such as the Alexis® Wound Protector, can be used to help with visualization and retraction of the subcutaneous tissues. The borders of an 8 cm long by 2 cm wide strip of rectus fascia are marked with either a marking pen or electrocautery. An Allis clamp is used on the lateral aspect of the graft to help free the fascia from the underlying rectus muscle using electrocautery. Once free, the graft is set aside on the back table in normal saline. The fascia is then reapproximated with a #1 polydioxanone (PDS) suture on a CTX-tapered needle, either in a running or interrupted fashion.

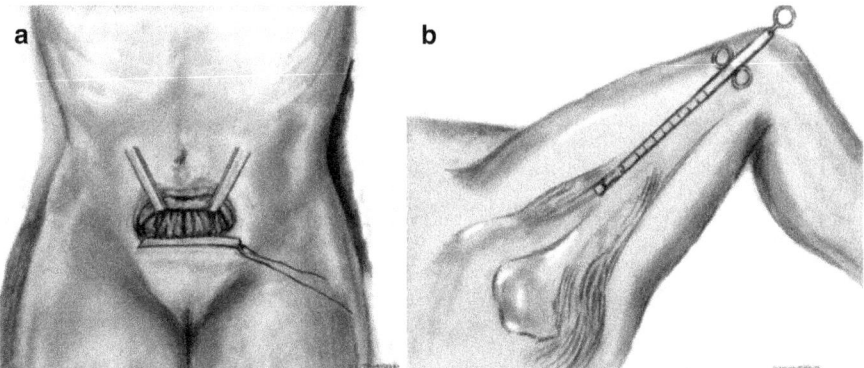

Fig. 17.3 (**a**) Rectus fascia harvest. (**b**) Fascial lata harvest. (Dmochowski et al. [12])

Any excess fat is then removed from the graft. A running whip stitch with a #1 PDS suture on a CTX-tapered needle is placed on each end of the graft for later placement and tensioning. Care is taken to leave even ends to the whip stitch. The whip stitch is tied down, and the sutures are left long.

Vaginal Dissection

Hydrodissection of the anterior vaginal wall is performed with either injectable saline or local anesthetic with or without epinephrine. Using a 15 blade, an inverted-U incision or a midline vertical incision is made along the anterior wall with the most distal portion of the incision approximately 2 cm proximal to the urethral meatus (Fig. 17.4). An Allis clamp below the meatus is helpful for countertraction and marking the most distal aspect of the incision. The most proximal aspect of the incision should be at the level of the bladder neck, which can be determined by palpating the Foley catheter balloon. The vaginal epithelial flap is dissected free from the underlying periurethral and pubocervical fascia using sharp dissection with Metzenbaum scissors. The vaginal flaps are dissected sharply until the tip of the scissors palpates the ischiopubic rami. At this point, with the scissors aiming upward and toward the ipsilateral shoulder, the endopelvic fascia is then perforated immediately under the ischiopubic ramus at the superior margin of the dissection (Fig. 17.5). Prior to perforation, always confirm the bladder is completely decompressed to avoid bladder injury. After perforation in the superolateral direction, the scissors are opened widely to aid in dissection. The scissors are left slightly open and removed from the wound. The index finger is then used to complete further blunt dissection (Fig. 17.6). This dissection leads to a connection between the infrapubic and retropubic spaces. The bladder may be palpated medially; however, care should be taken to avoid aggressive mobilization medially to avoid a bladder injury.

Fig. 17.4 Inverted U incision along the anterior wall of the vagina. (Dmochowski et al. [12])

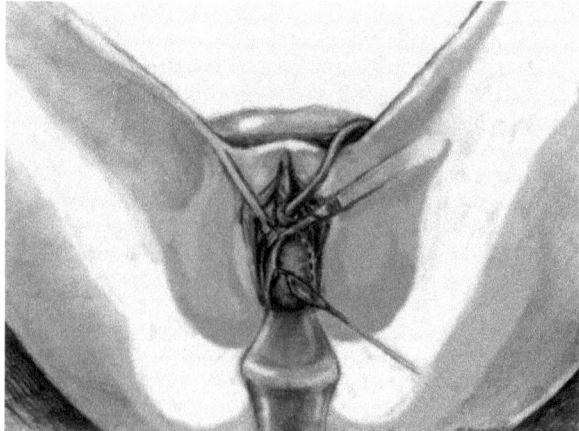

Fig. 17.5 Perforation of
endopelvic fascia.
(Dmochowski et al. [12])

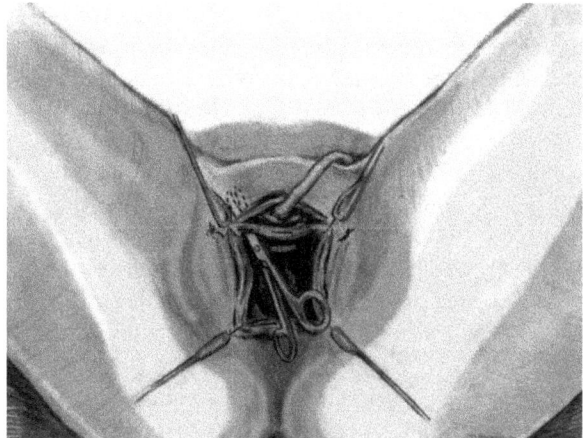

Fig. 17.6 Blunt dissection
of the retropubic space.
(Dmochowski et al. [12])

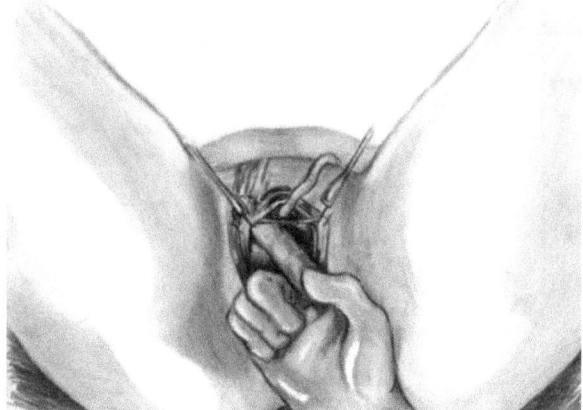

Sling Placement and Fixation

It is important to again confirm that the bladder is completely drained prior to sling placement. For placement of the sling, the authors prefer to use 15-degree Stamey needles. Other surgeons have used large clamps such as a Tonsil clamp or the double-pronged ligature carrier (i.e. Raz needle passer). Through the previously made Pfannenstiel incision, the Stamey needle is passed from behind the pubic bone (Fig. 17.7). The index finger is placed into the vaginal incision on the ipsilateral side so that the tip of the needle is palpated. The vaginally placed finger guides the Stamey needle through the space of Retzius and out the ipsilateral endopelvic fascial opening created with perforation and blunt dissection. It is important when passing the needles that no tissue should be palpable between the needle and the vaginal finger. If a thicker layer is felt between the finger and the needle, it may be the bladder. In this case, further careful dissection is needed to avoid injury to the bladder.

After passage of the needles, rigid cystoscopy is performed with the 30- and 70-degree lens. The urethra should be inspected with a short-beaked sheath. The authors find this step to be nonoptional to avoid a delayed recognition of a bladder injury. The 2010 AUA Update on the Surgical Management of Incontinence states that intraoperative cystourethroscopy is considered standard of care [15]. If a bladder injury is seen, the needle is removed and repassed with the bladder decompressed. The Foley is replaced once Stamey needles are in place, and confirmation cystoscopy has been performed. The ends of the graft suture are placed through the eye of the needle, and the needle is pulled up through the abdominal incision. The needles are removed and the ends of the suture are brought out through the abdominal incision and tagged with hemostat clamps. The sling length should be long enough to allow it to penetrate into the retropubic space (Fig. 17.8). The midpoint of the graft is approximated to the proximal third of the urethra with two simple 4–0 polyglactin (Vicryl ®) sutures.

Fig. 17.7 The Stamey needle is passed behind the pubic bone and brought out lateral to the bladder and urethra through the vaginal incision. (Dmochowski et al. [12])

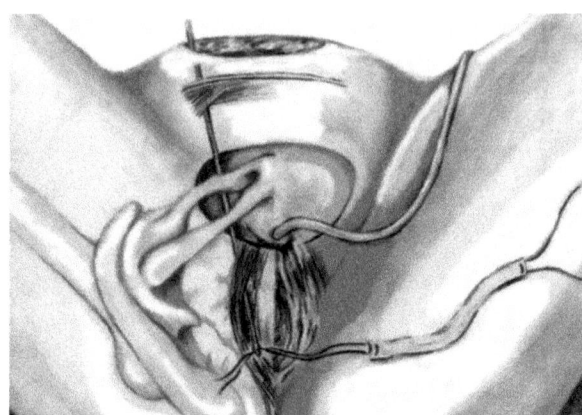

Fig. 17.8 Sagittal view of the fascial sling in place, located in the retropubic space, positioned at the bladder neck. (Dmochowski et al. [12])

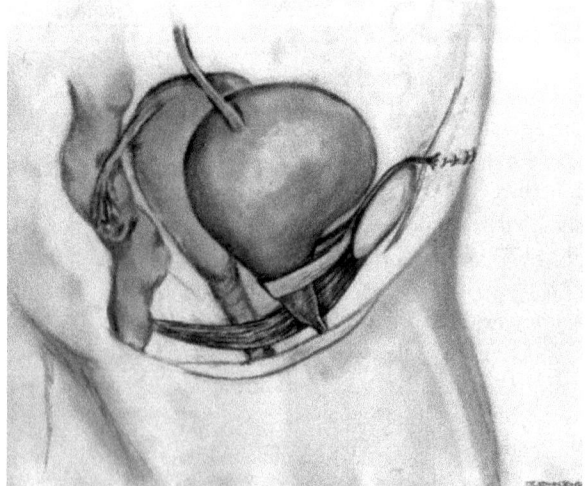

It is the authors' practice to close the vaginal incision and remove the weighted speculum prior to sling tensioning to eliminate factors that may affect final tensioning. The vaginal incision is irrigated and inspected for hemostasis. The vaginal incision is then closed with a running 2.0 polyglactin (Vicryl®) suture.

The PDS sutures are tied down above the rectus fascia. Concurrent rigid cystoscopy with a 30-degree lens has been described to simultaneously watch for adequate coaptation of the proximal urethra. It is our practice to perform tensioning with only the Foley catheter in place (Fig. 17.9). There should be approximately a two-fingerbreadth width between the rectus fascia and the suture knots. Lastly, the sutures are tied together in the center above the rectus fascia with the ability to place one or two fingers between the knot and the fascia. However, the amount of tension may vary based on the patient's anatomy, urethral mobility, and goal to purposefully cause urinary retention or close the bladder outlet. It should be noted that there are no standardized techniques for determining appropriate tensioning of the sling.

In certain situations, it may be desirable to completely close the bladder outlet with an occlusive fascial sling, such as that for refractory SUI, urethral erosion, and incompetent bladder outlet. Concomitant continent cutaneous bladder augmentation or placement of a suprapubic tube is typically performed. Occlusive fascial sling may be preferable to bladder neck closure so that emergent access to the bladder is still permitted. Excessive tensioning should be avoided to prevent urethral erosion or damage.

After irrigation, the abdominal wound is irrigated and hemostasis is achieved. The wound is closed in several layers to decrease the risk of a seroma formation. A Foley catheter is left for drainage, and a vaginal packing is placed.

Fascia Lata Considerations

Harvest of fascial lata (Fig. 17.10) may be preferred over rectus fascial if the patient is obese or has had multiple prior abdominal surgeries, particularly abdominoplasty or hernia repairs. Some surgeons may elect to perform fascia lata harvest primarily.

Fig. 17.9 Tensioning and tying of the sling. (Dmochowski et al. [12])

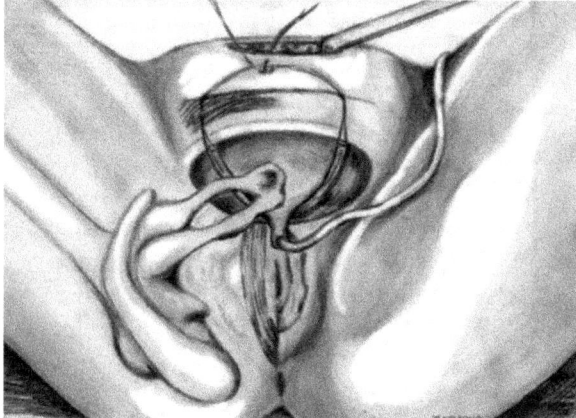

Fig. 17.10 The tensor fascia lata and the gluteal muscle form a tendinous extension to the tibia called the iliotibial band, which inserts to the lateral aspect of the tibial bone. This band is well-defined in most patients. (Permission from Atlas of Vaginal Reconstructive Surgery, Raz, Spring, 2015, Figure 2.66)

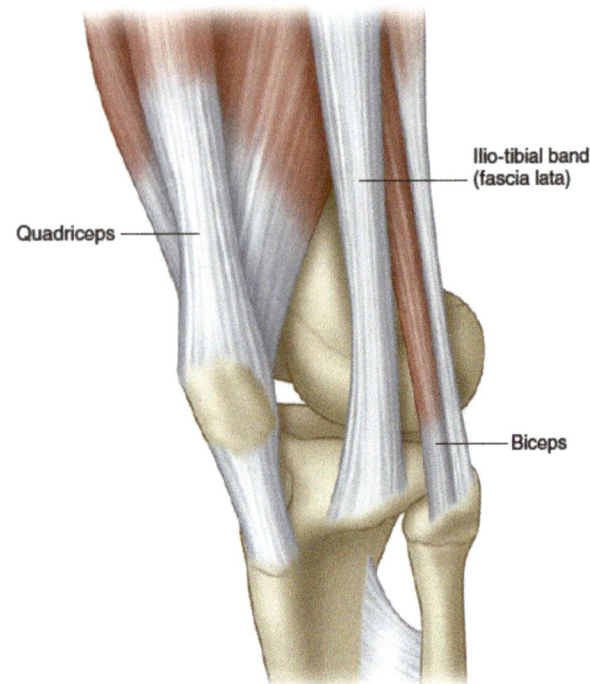

If fascia lata is to be harvested, the lower extremity of interest is internally rotated at the hip. The anterolateral aspect of the patient's thigh is prepped and draped from the greater trochanter to the distal patella. The SCD is placed below the patella on the harvest site. The greater trochanter and the lateral femoral condyle of the femur, which denote the proximal and distal attachments of the fascia lata, are palpated and marked with a marking pen. A 3-cm longitudinal incision is marked starting just above the patella over the iliotibial band. Dissection is carried down to the level of the fascia lata. Two parallel incisions are made longitudinally in the fascia lata, 2-cm apart, perpendicular to the skin incision in the direction of the fascial fibers. The undersurface of the fascia is dissected off the muscle as far as possible. The two parallel incisions are then connected to the one free end of the graft. A 2–0 permanent monofilament suture is placed in a horizontal mattress at the free end of the graft. A malleable retractor is placed just under the planned fascial graft to free it from the underlying muscle. The Crawford stripper can then be used starting at the free end of the graft, extending proximally [18] (Fig. 17.3b).

If a Crawford stripper is not available, a 6 cm × 2 cm fascia lata graft may be harvested "free-hand" via a 4-cm incision made longitudinally, starting three-fingerbreadth cephalad to the patella. A measuring tape cut to 6 cm can be helpful in marking out the borders of the graft with electrocautery at 1-cm intervals.

After irrigation and meticulous hemostasis, the wound is closed in three layers without closing the fascia. Once the skin of the thigh is closed, a compressive wrap is placed. The compression dressing should remain in place for at least 8 hours or until the morning of postoperative day one. Early ambulation should be encouraged [19].

Postoperative Care

On postoperative day one, the vaginal packing is removed and a trial of void may be performed. The patient may be discharged after confirmation of bladder emptying with a postvoid. If there are high postvoid residuals, then the catheter is placed again and the trial of void is repeated in 5 days as an outpatient or patient can be taught self-catheterization. Patients should be instructed to avoid lifting anything greater than 10 pounds for 3 months. Nothing should be placed intravaginally for 8 weeks. Sexual activity may be resumed after 8 weeks, after physical examination by the surgeon.

Outcomes and Complications

Cure/Improvement Rates

McGuire's original studies on the autologous pubovaginal sling showed an improvement in SUI in 50 of his 52 patients. Later, Blaivas et al. reported an 82% success rate [4] [5]. In more recent studies, cure rates vary based on the definition used, from 31% to 100% [12, 20]. The challenge is the lack of direct correlation between objective and subjective measures of improvement or cure after incontinence procedures [21]. From the AUA 2010 review on surgical management of SUI, estimated cure/dry rates associated with autologous fascial sling without prolapse surgery ranged between 90% at 12–23 months and 82% at 48 months or longer [15]. Though several other retrospective and cohort studies have been published, Table 17.1 summarizes outcome data based on available randomized control trials.

The Stress Incontinence Surgical Treatment Efficacy Trial (SISTEr), published in 2012, randomized 655 patients to either an autologous fascial sling or a Burch colposuspension. Primary outcomes were overall urinary incontinence (including self-reported symptoms, pad weight tests, and further medical or surgical treatment for urinary incontinence) and stress-specific measures (including self-reported symptoms, and negative stress test) over a 24-month postoperative period. The autologous fascial sling showed superior results for overall urinary incontinence (47% vs. 38%, $p = 0.01$), as well as stress-specific incontinence (66% vs. 49%, $p < 0.001$) [22]. However, the Burch colposuspension group had lower rates of urinary tract infection (32% vs. 48%) and postoperative voiding dysfunction (2% vs. 14%, $p < 0.001$). All subsequent surgical procedures performed to reduce voiding

Table 17.1 Summary of outcomes of randomized control trials involving fascial slings

Study	Assessment of outcome	Follow-up time	Design	Number of pts	% Reaching outcome
			Study design and results		
Albo, 2007 [22] (SISTEr trial)	Pad weight, stress test, voiding diary	24 months	Rectus PVS	326	66%
			BC	329	49%
Wadie, 2005 [26]	Stress test, complete dryness with no usage of pads	9 months	Rectus PVS	15	92%
			TVT	17	92.9%
Al-Azzawi, 2014 [60]	Patient-perceived dryness, stress test, Qmax >15 mL/sec	1 year	Rectus PVS	40	98%
			TOT	40	95%
Basok, 2008 [61]	Pad test, patient questionnaire	12 months	Cadaveric fascial lata	67	79%
			Intravaginal slingplasty	72	70.8%
Khan, 2015 [62]	Patient reported "completely dry" or "improved"	10 years	Autologous PVS	61	75.4%
			Xenograft PVS	38	73%
			TVT	63	58%
Bai, 2005 [63]	Patient-report of absence of SUI, stress test	12 months	Rectus PVS	28	92.8%
			TVT	31	87%
			BC	33	87.8%
Tcherniakovsky, 2009 [64]	UDS, stress test	12 months	Rectus PVS	20	95%
			TOT	21	90.5%
Culligan, 2003 [65]	Stress test, pad weight	73 months	PVS	17	100%
			BC	19	82%
Amaro, 2009[a] [66]	Complete dryness, no usage of pads	44 months	Rectus PVS	21	57%
			TVT	20	65%
Guerrero, 2010 [67]	Patient-reported complete dryness or improvement	12 months	Rectus PVS	79	90%
			TVT	72	93%
			Allograft PVS	50	61%
Sharifiaghdas, 2008[a] [68]	Stress test	40 months	Rectus PVS	36	83%
			TVT	25	80%
Sharifiaghdas, 2017 [69]	Stress test	10.5 years	Rectus PVS	36	84%
			TVT	25	81.5%
Sharma, 2020 [70]	ICIQ scores	6 months	Rectus PVS	15	100%
			TOT	15	100%
Kuprasertkul, 2019 [71]	Reoperation-free survival	15.1 years	Rectus PVS	15	90%
			BC	14	80.8%

[a]Results of PVS inferior to comparator

TVT tension-free vaginal tape, *PVS* pubovaginal sling, *BC* Burch colposuspension, *TOT* transobturator tape, *SUI* stress urinary incontinence, *UDS* urodynamics, *ICIQ* International Consultation on Incontinence Questionnaire

symptoms or improve urinary retention were performed exclusively in the PVS group, in which 19 patients underwent a total of 20 procedures [22]. The 5-year results of the Extended-SISTEr study showed that women who underwent fascial sling continued to have higher satisfaction despite increased incidence of voiding dysfunction [23].

A 2017 Cochrane review showed a significantly greater improvement in patient-reported SUI symptoms, both within and after 1 year, with autologous fascia. There was no evidence of a difference in perioperative complications or postoperative morbidity between autologous fascia and other materials [24]. However, the studies were small and had short-term follow-up, particularly related to mesh-related complications. In addition, the studies did not stratify outcomes based on preoperative severity of SUI.

A large cohort study compared three-year outcomes in 79 fascial sling patients (performed by a urologist) to 163 synthetic mesh mid-urethral sling patients (performed by a gynecologist). The synthetic mesh group showed relatively higher success than the autologous fascial sling group for any urinary incontinence, severe incontinence, and stress-specific incontinence. There was no difference in the complications; however, the fascial group had a higher incidence of urinary retention requiring clean intermittent catheterization, urethrolysis, or prolonged suprapubic tube use [25]. In a randomized trial of 53 patients, there was no difference in the cure rate between an autologous fascial group and the tension-free vaginal tape group [26].

Voiding Dysfunction/Urgency/Retention

Postoperative voiding dysfunction is the most important complication after autologous fascial sling placement. Voiding dysfunction can present with a range of symptoms, ranging from the development of de novo urgency to frank urinary retention.

The rate of de novo urge incontinence is estimated between 3% and 20%, and the rate of postoperative urge incontinence is between 8% and 25% [15, 18, 27]. The AUA 2010 meta-analysis reported that in patients with preoperative urgency urinary incontinence (UUI), 33% have continued UUI despite resolution of their SUI [15].

Voiding dysfunction has been reported at a higher rate in autologous fascial sling compared to both Burch colposuspension and synthetic mesh mid-urethral sling. The SISTEr trial reported voiding dysfunction in 14% of the fascial sling group versus 2% in the Burch colposuspension group ($p < 0.001$) [22]. In another study by Athanasopoulos et al., of over 260 patients undergoing fascial sling, 10% reported postoperative voiding dysfunction [27]. Most had resolution of their voiding dysfunction by 2 months, but five patients (overall 1.9%) required urethrolysis [27].

Detrusor overactivity and impaired detrusor contractility (underactive bladder) are factors that may also exacerbate iatrogenic outlet obstruction from a fascial sling. Although postoperative urgency and UUI are strongly related to failure, studies have not shown consensus on the preoperative risk factors prior to fascial sling. Prior studies have suggested that a postvoid residual urine volume greater than 100 mL or a Qmax less than or equal to 20 mL/second may lead to a higher risk of needing prolonged clean intermittent catheterization, though these urodynamic factors did not reach statistical significance [28]. Likewise, Nager et al. analyzed the pre- and postoperative urodynamic data in patients enrolled in the SISTEr trial and found the presence of detrusor overactivity and the level of Valsalva leak point pressure were not predictive of postoperative voiding dysfunction or risk of surgical revision in those undergoing a fascial sling [29].

Postoperative retention is defined as lasting longer than 1 month or requiring intervention. The rate of postoperative retention is less common than postoperative urgency or UUI, and is estimated to be 8% without concomitant prolapse treatment and 5% in those with concomitant prolapse treatment [15]. The risk of iatrogenic obstruction is most likely a function of intraoperative technique. When the sling is overly tensioned, there is excessive elevation of the bladder neck toward to pubic bone, causing "hypersuspension" or overcorrection of the urethrovesical angle [12].

Proper tensioning of the sling is the most complex portion of the procedure, and techniques vary between surgeons. In a recent study by Preece et al., postoperative voiding dysfunction was predicated by the lax sling height when the knotted suture is tented above the rectus fascia. The authors showed that a lax sling height of less than 40 mm was associated with a higher risk of postoperative retention and the need for intermittent self-catheterization and urethrolysis [30].

The most important clinical factor is the temporal relationship between the sling placement and the presentation of the voiding symptoms. Physical examination can reveal an abnormal urethral angle or a nonmobile urethra. A postvoid residual should be recorded, although there is no consensus regarding a specific cut-off for a "normal" value. Cystoscopy may be useful to rule out bladder pathology, sling erosion, and a hypersuspended urethra. Videourodynamics may also be helpful in assessing for obstruction, detrusor overactivity, or detrusor underactivity. However, it has also been shown that when voiding symptoms or urinary retention is the primary indication for intervention after sling placement, urodynamic findings are not predictive of outcomes after intervention to relieve obstruction [31].

There is no consensus regarding the management of postoperative voiding dysfunction. Transient urinary retention is common, and most patients return to spontaneous voiding within the first 10 days [32]. For this reason, if postvoid residuals remain high or patient develops new or worsening urgency or UUI, the authors prefer to manage with timed voiding, double voiding, biofeedback, pelvic floor muscle training, antimuscarinics, and clean intermittent catheterization for 3 months prior to consideration of a urethrolysis.

Surgical management of obstruction after a fascial sling involves complete urethrolysis via a retropubic, transvaginal, or suprameatal approach with success rates ranging from 45% to 100% [12]. Persistent or recurrent obstruction, detrusor overactivity, impaired detrusor contractility, or learned voiding dysfunction may contribute to the failure of urethrolysis [12]. However, the most common reason is an incomplete dissection and lysis of the urethra. In one small study of 24 patients undergoing repeat urethrolysis, surgeons performed an "aggressive" urethrolysis by either a transvaginal or retropubic approach in all 24 cases. The authors reported that 22 of the 24 patients had resolution of their urinary retention. However, UUI only completely resolved in 12% of cases. The authors conclude that it is reasonable to consider a repeat urethrolysis after the first failure or when the extent of the initial urethrolysis is unknown [33]. Understandably, the patient may be concerned about the risk of recurrent SUI after urethrolysis; however, this rate is reported to be relatively low, ranging from 0% to 34% [12] [33].

Erosion and Extrusion

In contrast to synthetic mesh materials, urethral erosion and vaginal extrusion after autologous fascia pubovaginal sling are extremely rare. Leach et al. showed an urethral erosion rate of 0.003% and a vaginal extrusion rate of 0.0001% in patients undergoing autologous and allograft sling [34]. Causes of erosion of autologous fascial sling are typically due to perioperative technique, including incorrect technique in sling passage, position of the sling, excessive tensioning, or traumatic catheterization in the immediate postoperative period. Management would consist of excision of the eroded portion of the sling and closure of the urethra [35].

Other Complications

Overall perioperative urinary tract infection rates range from 11% to 48% [15, 22]. Bladder injury rate from improper retropubic needle passage has been shown to be 4% [15]. Wound complication rate is reported to be 8% [15]. In a 2015 meta-analysis comparing synthetic mid-urethral slings (MUS) to autologous fascial sling, MUS had a higher rate of erosion, pelvic pain, and de novo overactive bladder syndrome, while autologous fascial sling showed an increase risk of wound infection [36]. In a recent systematic review and meta-analysis comparing different procedures for SUI, autologous fascial sling was shown to result in lower rates of wound infection, bladder or vaginal perforation, and bowel injury compared to Burch colposuspension [37].

Autologous Fascial Sling after Synthetic Mesh Sling

The autologous fascial sling can be considered as a treatment option for patients with recurrent or persistent SUI after a synthetic mid-urethral sling procedure. Petrou et al. published a retrospective study of 21 patients with at least 36 months of follow-up of autologous fascial sling after failed MUS. About three-quarters of the patients reported improvement, reporting they were completely dry or only slightly incontinent. Overall, 86% stated they would recommend the procedure to others [38]. Likewise, Milose et al. showed that in 16 patients with pure SUI who underwent autologous fascial sling as a salvage procedure after prior failed sling procedure, 70% reported cured SUI [39].

A secondary analysis of the SISTEr and the Trial of Midurethral Slings (TOMUS) trials showed autologous fascial sling patients had retreatment rate of 5%, compared to Burch colposuspension at 10%, transobturator MUS at 6%, and retropubic MUS at 4%. The majority of these patients underwent an autologous fascial sling as their salvage procedure [40].

There is no consensus regarding how the prior mid-urethral sling mesh is removed, and timing of the removal in relation to placement of the fascial sling affects clinical outcomes [39]. Some surgeons prefer to excise the mesh sling and place the fascial sling in one operation, and others choose to stage the procedures. In a recent prospective study, Parker et al. compared autologous sling as primary treatment to autologous sling as secondary treatment following failed mid-urethral sling. Reasons for failure of mid-urethral sling included recurrent SUI, sling extrusion, or obstruction. At a median follow-up time of 15 months, both groups showed significant improvement in the number of pads used and in the patients' scoring of the validated questionnaires. There was no difference in complication rates. Urinary retention was more common in patients who had prior MUS (8.5%) compared to the primary autologous fascia group (3.1%). Patients who had prior MUS in the study tended to continue to need additional incontinence procedures after the salvage autologous fascial sling (13.6%), compared to those who had the autologous sling as their primary treatment (3.5%) [41].

Autologous fascial sling is not the only option for treating recurrent SUI after mid-urethral sling. Some surgeons may prefer to perform a repeat mid-urethral sling. Aberger et al. retrospectively compared outcomes of 224 patients who failed prior MUS and subsequently underwent either synthetic retropubic mid-urethral sling (153 patients or 68.3%) or autologous rectus fascia sling (ARFS) (71 patients or 31.6%). The median follow-up in the study was 29 (minimum of 12) months. At a median follow-up of 29 months, the overall cure rate was 61.4% in the mid-urethral sling group and 66.1% in the ARFS group with no statistically significant difference [42].

Rectus Fascia Versus Fascia Lata

Many urologists prefer to harvest rectus fascia over fascia lata based on their familiarity with the abdominal anatomy. In addition, many feel the incision is less conspicuous compared to the incision needed on the lateral aspect of the leg for fascia lata harvest. Advantages of fascia lata harvest include the potential benefit of decreased postoperative pain, lower risk of seroma and incisional hernia, and perhaps a stronger graft. One study found that fascia lata had a tension strength four-times greater than rectus fascia and its thought that the longitudinal fibers of the fascia lata may be more supportive than the horizontally oriented fibers of rectus fascia [43, 44]. In addition, harvest of fascia lata may be easier in patients with an extensive abdominal surgical history. Disadvantages of fascia lata harvest include the need to reposition and the morbidity of second incisional site.

A recent retrospective study compared the outcomes of 21 fascia lata patients to 84 rectus fascia patients. Operative time was similar between the two groups. The only statistically significant difference between the two groups was a lower estimated blood loss in the fascia lata group. The fascia lata group also had a shorter length of stay, fewer wound complications, and fewer Clavien grade 2 or greater complications, but these different perioperative outcomes did not reach statistical significance. Dry rates at 1 month, 1 year, and last follow-up were similar between the two groups [45].

Autologous Graft Compared to Allograft Materials

The use of allograft (tissue taken from another human) has become increasingly popular in an effort to decrease operative time, morbidity, pain, and hospital stay. Unlike allograft materials, autologous materials offer complete biocompatibility. Histological examination of autologous fascial slings has shown extensive fibroblast infiltration and neovascularization with minimal inflammatory reaction [46].

It has been shown that the processing of allograft cadaveric tissue may compromise the integrity of the graft and may be associated with a higher long-term failure rate. The specifics in processing technique can also make a difference in the tissue integrity. Tissue freezing, as opposed to solvent dehydration, leads to ice crystal formation that can lead to disruption of the collagen matrix, which weakens the tissue [47]. Failure rates for frozen or freeze-dried grafts range from 6.0% to 38% [12]. For this reason, solvent-dehydrated allograft has predominated.

When utilizing allograft material, the surgeon must consider the increased risk of transmission of infectious disease, given the transferring of DNA and protein material. Theoretically, infections caused by prions are possible, and allograft-associated transmission of human immunodeficiency virus may occur in one in eight million cases [48–50]. Also notable, the preoperative discussion must include the fact that tissue from a human will be used. This is important for patients who may have specific religious or moral objections to implanting tissue from another human.

Researchers have assessed the outcomes of pubovaginal sling with autologous fascia versus cadaveric allograft fascia. The literature is mixed. Some researchers have reported equally high success rates and no difference in complications, concluding that allograft may be used to reduce operative time and morbidity [51, 52]. Other authors have shown that allograft may be associated with inferior outcomes, recurrent symptoms, and a higher reoperative rate [53–56]. Larger, randomized, prospective studies with long-term follow-up comparing success rates of autologous versus solvent-dehydrated cadaveric allograft fascia lata are needed. Table 17.2 outlines the advantages and disadvantages of allograft versus autologous graft.

Table 17.2 Allograft versus Autologous Graft

	Allograft	Autologous Graft
Advantages	Smaller suprapubic incision Reduced operative time Decreased operative pain	Complete biocompatibility Minimum tissue reaction
Disadvantages	Increased cost Less tensile strength Risk of transmitting infectious diseases, such HIV and prion diseases	Increased operative time Need to reposition patient[a] Risk of suprapubic seroma[b] Risk of suprapubic incisional hernia[b]

[a]Specific to fascia lata harvest
[b]Specific to rectus fascia harvest

Autologous Fascia Use for Transobturator Slings

There has been some interest in using autologous fascia as the material for a transobturator sling. In one study from Egypt, a sling fashioned with autologous fascia in the middle and polypropylene arms laterally was placed in a transobturator route. Subjective cure rate at 1 year was 90.5%, and objective cure defined by a negative cough stress test was 93% [57]. In a more recent study from 2020, a similar sling was placed after treatment of urethral diverticulum in two patients and showed that both patients had no SUI at 6 months postoperatively [58]. Perhaps the largest study is by Cubuk et al., in which 36 patients underwent the autologous fascia transobturator sling and were compared to 81 traditional transobturator slings. The authors showed no difference in subjective or objective cure rates between the two sling types at 12 months [59]. Larger, randomized trials with longer follow-up are needed to further evaluate the use of autologous fascia for a transobturator sling.

References

1. Zacharin RF. Abdominoperineal urethral suspension in the management of recurrent stress incontinence of urine- a 15-year experience. Obstet Gynecol. 1983;62(5):644–54.
2. Frangenheim P. Zur operativen Behandlung der Inkontinenz der männlichen Harnröhre. Verh Dtsch Ges Chir. 1914;43:149–56.
3. Stoeckel W. Über die Verwendung der Musculi pyramidales bei der operativen Behandlung der Incontinentia urinae. Zentralbl Gynak. 1917;41:11–9.
4. McGuire EJ, Lytton B. Pubovaginal sling procedure for stress incontinence. J Urol. 1978;119(1):82–4.
5. Blaivas JG, Jacobs BZ. Pubovaginal fascial sling for the treatment of complicated stress urinary incontinence. J Urol. 1991;145(6):1214–8.
6. Geller EJ, Wu JM. Changing trends in surgery for stress urinary incontinence. Curr Opin Obstet Gynecol. 2013;25(5):404–9.
7. Rac G, et al. Stress urinary incontinence surgery trends in academic female pelvic medicine and reconstructive surgery urology practice in the setting of the food and drug administration public health notifications. Neurourol Urodyn. 2017;36(4):1155–60.

8. Blaivas JG, Olsson CA. Stress incontinence: classification and surgical approach. J Urol. 1988;139(4):727–31.
9. Wan J, et al. Stress leak point pressure: a diagnostic tool for incontinent children. J Urol. 1993;150(2 Pt 2):700–2.
10. McGuire EJ. Urodynamic findings in patients after failure of stress incontinence operations. Prog Clin Biol Res. 1981;78:351–60.
11. D'Ancona CD, Haylen B, Oelke M, Herschorn S, Abranches-Monteiro L, Arnold EP, Goldman HB, Hamid R, Homma Y, Marcelissen T, Rademakers K, Schizas A, Singla A, Soto I, Tse V, de Wachter S. An International Continence Society (ICS) report on the terminology for adult male lower urinary tract and pelvic floor symptoms and dysfunction. Neurourol Urodyn. 2019.
12. Dmochowski RR, Padmanabhan P, Scarpero HM. Slings: autologous, biologic, synthetic, and midurethral. In: Kavoussi LR, Wein AJ, Novick AC, editors. Campbell-Walsh urology. 10th ed. Philadelphia: Elsevier-Saunders; 2012. p. 2115–67.
13. Chapple CR, Milson I. Urinary incontinence and pelvic prolapse: epidemiology and patho-physiology. In: Wein A, editor. Campbell-Walsh urology. Philadelpia: Elsevier; 2012.
14. Plagakis S, Tse V. The autologous pubovaginal fascial sling: an update in 2019. Low Urin Tract Symptoms. 2020;12(1):2–7.
15. Dmochowski RR, et al. Update of AUA guideline on the surgical management of female stress urinary incontinence. J Urol. 2010;183(5):1906–14.
16. Kobashi KC, et al. Surgical treatment of female stress urinary incontinence: AUA/SUFU guideline. J Urol. 2017;198(4):875–83.
17. Lightner DJ, et al. Best practice statement on urologic procedures and antimicrobial prophy-laxis. J Urol. 2020;203(2):351–6.
18. Blaivas JG, et al. Surgery for stress urinary incontinence: autologous fascial Sling. Urol Clin North Am. 2019;46(1):41–52.
19. Dwyer NT, et al. Fascia lata sling. In: Raz LVRS, editor. Female urology. W.B. Saunders; 2008. p. 406–14.
20. Mahdy A, Ghoniem GM. Autologous rectus fascia sling for treatment of stress urinary incon-tinence in women: a review of the literature. Neurourol Urodyn. 2019;38 Suppl 4:S51–8.
21. Padmanabhan P, Nitti VW. Female stress urinary incontinence: how do patient and physician perspectives correlate in assessment of outcomes? Curr Opin Urol. 2006;16(4):212–8.
22. Albo ME, et al. Burch colposuspension versus fascial sling to reduce urinary stress inconti-nence. N Engl J Med. 2007;356(21):2143–55.
23. Brubaker L, et al. 5-year continence rates, satisfaction and adverse events of burch urethropexy and fascial sling surgery for urinary incontinence. J Urol. 2012;187(4):1324–30.
24. Rehman H, et al. Traditional suburethral sling operations for urinary incontinence in women. Cochrane Database Syst Rev. 2017;7(7):Cd001754.
25. Trabuco EC, et al. Medium-term comparison of continence rates after rectus fascia or midure-thral sling placement. Am J Obstet Gynecol. 2009;200(3):300.e1–6.
26. Wadie BS, Edwan A, Nabeeh AM. Autologous fascial sling vs polypropylene tape at short-term followup: a prospective randomized study. J Urol. 2005;174(3):990–3.
27. Athanasopoulos A, Gyftopoulos K, McGuire EJ. Efficacy and preoperative prognostic factors of autologous fascia rectus sling for treatment of female stress urinary incontinence. Urology. 2011;78(5):1034–8.
28. Mitsui T, et al. Clinical and urodynamic outcomes of pubovaginal sling procedure with autolo-gous rectus fascia for stress urinary incontinence. Int J Urol. 2007;14(12):1076–9.
29. Nager CW, et al. Urodynamic measures do not predict stress continence outcomes after sur-gery for stress urinary incontinence in selected women. J Urol. 2008;179(4):1470–4.
30. Preece PD, et al. Optimising the tension of an autologous fascia pubovaginal sling to minimize retentive complications. Neurourol Urodyn. 2019;38(5):1409–16.
31. Aponte MM, et al. Urodynamics for clinically suspected obstruction after anti-incontinence surgery in women. J Urol. 2013;190(2):598–602.

32. Cross CA, Cespedes RD, McGuire EJ. Our experience with pubovaginal slings in patients with stress urinary incontinence. J Urol. 1998;159(4):1195–8.

33. Scarpero HM, Dmochowski RR, Nitti VW. Repeat urethrolysis after failed urethrolysis for iatrogenic obstruction. J Urol. 2003;169(3):1013–6.

34. Leach GE, et al. Female Stress Urinary Incontinence Clinical Guidelines Panel summary report on surgical management of female stress urinary incontinence. The American Urological Association. J Urol. 1997;158(3 Pt 1):875–80.

35. Blaivas JG, Sandhu J. Urethral reconstruction after erosion of slings in women. Curr Opin Urol. 2004;14(6):335–8.

36. Blaivas JG, et al. Safety considerations for synthetic sling surgery. Nat Rev Urol. 2015;12(9):481–509.

37. Schimpf MO, et al. Sling surgery for stress urinary incontinence in women: a systematic review and metaanalysis. Am J Obstet Gynecol. 2014;211(1):71.e1–71.e27.

38. Petrou SP, et al. Salvage autologous fascial sling after failed synthetic midurethral sling: greater than 3-year outcomes. Int J Urol. 2016;23(2):178–81.

39. Milose JC, et al. Success of autologous pubovaginal sling after failed synthetic mid urethral sling. J Urol. 2015;193(3):916–20.

40. Zimmern PE, et al. Management of recurrent stress urinary incontinence after burch and sling procedures. Neurourol Urodyn. 2016;35(3):344–8.

41. Parker WP, Gomelsky A, Padmanabhan P. Autologous fascia pubovaginal slings after prior synthetic anti-incontinence procedures for recurrent incontinence: a multi-institutional prospective comparative analysis to de novo autologous slings assessing objective and subjective cure. Neurourol Urodyn. 2016;35(5):604–8.

42. Aberger M, Gomelsky A, Padmanabhan P. Comparison of retropubic synthetic mid-urethral slings to fascia pubovaginal slings following failed sling surgery. Neurourol Urodyn. 2016;35(7):851–4.

43. Govier FE, et al. Pubovaginal slings using fascia lata for the treatment of intrinsic sphincter deficiency. J Urol. 1997;157(1):117–21.

44. Choe JM, et al. Autologous, cadaveric, and synthetic materials used in sling surgery: comparative biomechanical analysis. Urology. 2001;58(3):482–6.

45. Peng M, et al. Rectus fascia versus fascia lata for autologous fascial pubovaginal sling: a single-center comparison of perioperative and functional outcomes. Female Pelvic Med Reconstr Surg. 2020;26(8):493–7.

46. Woodruff AJ, et al. Histologic comparison of pubovaginal sling graft materials: a comparative study. Urology. 2008;72(1):85–9.

47. Lemer ML, Chaikin DC, Blaivas JG. Tissue strength analysis of autologous and cadaveric allografts for the pubovaginal sling. Neurourol Urodyn. 1999;18(5):497–503.

48. Buck BE, Malinin TI. Human bone and tissue allografts. Preparation and safety. Clin Orthop Relat Res. 1994;303:8–17.

49. Wilson TS, Lemack GE, Zimmern PE. Management of intrinsic sphincteric deficiency in women. J Urol. 2003;169(5):1662–9.

50. Bayrak Ö, et al. Pubovaginal sling materials and their outcomes. Turk J Urol. 2014;40(4):233–9.

51. Flynn BJ, Yap WT. Pubovaginal sling using allograft fascia lata versus autograft fascia for all types of stress urinary incontinence: 2-year minimum followup. J Urol. 2002;167(2 Pt 1):608–12.

52. Elliott DS, Boone TB. Is fascia lata allograft material trustworthy for pubovaginal sling repair? Urology. 2000;56(5):772–6.

53. Dora CD, et al. Time dependent variations in biomechanical properties of cadaveric fascia, porcine dermis, porcine small intestine submucosa, polypropylene mesh and autologous fascia in the rabbit model: implications for sling surgery. J Urol. 2004;171(5):1970–3.

54. McBride AW, et al. Comparison of long-term outcomes of autologous fascia lata slings with suspend Tutoplast fascia lata allograft slings for stress incontinence. Am J Obstet Gynecol. 2005;192(5):1677–81.

55. Simsiman AJ, et al. Suburethral sling materials: best outcome with autologous tissue. Am J Obstet Gynecol. 2005;193(6):2112–6.
56. Soergel TM, Shott S, Heit M. Poor surgical outcomes after fascia lata allograft slings. Int Urogynecol J Pelvic Floor Dysfunct. 2001;12(4):247–53.
57. El-Gamal O, et al. Use of autologous rectus fascia in a new transobturator hybrid sling for treatment of female stress urinary incontinence: a pilot study. Scand J Urol. 2013;47(1):57–62.
58. Ito WE, et al. Hybrid Sling for the treatment of concomitant female urethral complex diverticula and stress urinary incontinence. Res Rep Urol. 2020;12:247–53.
59. Cubuk A, et al. Modified autologous transobturator tape surgery – a prospective comparison with transobturator tape surgery. Urology. 2020.
60. Al-Azzawi IS. The first Iraqi experience with the rectus fascia sling and transobturator tape for female stress incontinence: a randomised trial. Arab J Urol. 2014;12(3):204–8.
61. Basok EK, et al. Cadaveric fascia lata versus intravaginal slingplasty for the pubovaginal sling: surgical outcome, overall success and patient satisfaction rates. Urol Int. 2008;80(1):46–51.
62. Khan ZA, et al. Long-term follow-up of a multicentre randomised controlled trial comparing tension-free vaginal tape, xenograft and autologous fascial slings for the treatment of stress urinary incontinence in women. BJU Int. 2015;115(6):968–77.
63. Bai SW, et al. Comparison of the efficacy of Burch colposuspension, pubovaginal sling, and tension-free vaginal tape for stress urinary incontinence. Int J Gynaecol Obstet. 2005;91(3):246–51.
64. Tcherniakovsky M, et al. Comparative results of two techniques to treat stress urinary incontinence: synthetic transobturator and aponeurotic slings. Int Urogynecol J Pelvic Floor Dysfunct. 2009;20(8):961–6.
65. Culligan PJ, Goldberg RP, Sand PK. A randomized controlled trial comparing a modified Burch procedure and a suburethral sling: long-term follow-up. Int Urogynecol J Pelvic Floor Dysfunct. 2003;14(4):229–33. discussion 233
66. Amaro JL, et al. Clinical and quality-of-life outcomes after autologous fascial sling and tension-free vaginal tape: a prospective randomized trial. Int Braz J Urol. 2009;35(1):60–6. discussion 66-7
67. Guerrero KL, et al. A randomised controlled trial comparing TVT, Pelvicol and autologous fascial slings for the treatment of stress urinary incontinence in women. BJOG. 2010;117(12):1493–502.
68. Sharifiaghdas F, Mortazavi N. Tension-free vaginal tape and autologous rectus fascia pubovaginal sling for the treatment of urinary stress incontinence: a medium-term follow-up. Med Princ Pract. 2008;17(3):209–14.
69. Sharifiaghdas F, et al. Long-term results of tension-free vaginal tape and pubovaginal sling in the treatment of stress urinary incontinence in female patients. Clin Exp Obstet Gynecol. 2017;44(1):44–7.
70. Sharma JB, et al. A comparative study of autologous rectus fascia pubovaginal sling surgery and synthetic transobturator vaginal tape procedure in treatment of women with urodynamic stress urinary incontinence. Eur J Obstet Gynecol Reprod Biol. 2020;252:349–54.
71. Kuprasertkul A, et al. Long-term results of burch and autologous aling procedures for stress urinary incontinence in E-SISTEr participants at 1 site. J Urol. 2019;202(6):1224–9.

Chapter 18
Managing Complications After Surgical Treatment of Stress Urinary Incontinence

Alyssa K. Gracely

Introduction

As the population ages, the yearly incidence of stress urinary incontinence (SUI) is reported at approximately 4–10% [1], with some studies reporting a yearly incidence in mid-life and older women of up to 14.9% [2]. With the steady increase in SUI prevalence, it is imperative not only to understand the management of SUI, but the potential complications that may arise with each treatment option. The increased success rates associated with surgical treatment of SUI compared to their less-invasive counterparts are balanced by a potentially higher complication rate. Surgical treatment options for SUI include retropubic suspensions, transvaginal needle suspensions, pubovaginal slings, and synthetic midurethral slings (MUS). While many complications are shared between all surgical options, a few complications are procedure-specific. This chapter will discuss the complications that can arise after surgical treatment of SUI, with a specific focus on complications associated with the "gold standard" MUS, as this has attracted significant media and regulatory attention. While prior chapters have focused on the importance of the preoperative evaluation of SUI, surgical decision-making, surgical technique, and intraoperative complications, this chapter focuses specifically on postoperative complications and their respective management.

A. K. Gracely (✉)
Chesapeake Urology Associates, Salisbury, MD, USA
e-mail: agracely@chesuro.com

© The Author(s), under exclusive license to Springer Nature Switzerland AG 2022
A. P. Cameron (ed.), *Female Urinary Incontinence*,
https://doi.org/10.1007/978-3-030-84352-6_18

Evaluation and Diagnosis

When patients present with new voiding symptoms in the postoperative period after surgical treatment for SUI, a thorough evaluation is warranted. This begins with an understanding of their preoperative voiding habits. The change in pre- and postoperative symptoms, as well as the timing of onset of symptoms can provide insight into the etiology of their new voiding complaints and help guide treatment. When available, review of preoperative urodynamics (UDS) can be useful to identify factors that are associated with postoperative urinary retention including: detrusor underactivity, Valsalva voiding, or preoperative obstruction [3, 4]. In one recent study, women with detrusor underactivity or Valsalva voiding on UDS were more likely to have postoperative urinary retention after sling procedure compared to their counterparts. Furthermore, an elevated preoperative postvoid residual and decreased preoperative maximum urinary flow rate were associated with increased risk of postoperative urinary retention [5]. In the setting of a new patient referral, a review of operative notes can prove helpful as this can often reveal unambiguous descriptions of complications or improper technique.

After obtaining a thorough history with a timeline of presenting symptoms in relation to the surgical intervention, a urinalysis and postvoid residual should be performed. When infection is present, culture-guided treatment should be offered and symptoms reassessed. Physical exam to evaluate for urethral mobility, angulation, and mesh exposure should be performed. In the setting of new onset irritative symptoms, recurrent urinary tract infections (UTIs), or hematuria, in-office cystourethroscopy should be performed to evaluate for mesh erosion into urethra or bladder. When body habitus or concomitant pelvic organ prolapse makes a pelvic exam difficult, concomitant vaginoscopy at the time of cystourethroscopy can prove helpful to evaluate for vaginal mesh exposure. If in-office examination or cystourethroscopy is not possible due to patient discomfort, habitus, or preference, it is reasonable to perform an exam under anesthesia and cystoscopy in the operating room. Depending on index of suspicion and patient counseling, one can then proceed with the indicated surgical intervention at the time of the exam under anesthesia, or plan to return in a staged fashion.

Additional diagnostic procedures may be warranted based on exam findings and patient symptoms. In select cases, UDS may prove useful, especially in women with persistent voiding symptoms and normal post void residuals or those with complex surgical history such as multiple prior sling procedures or revisions. In these instances, the addition of fluoroscopy (video urodynamics) or a separate voiding cystourethrogram can aid in identifying the location of anatomic obstruction, but is not always necessary [6] (Fig. 18.1).

The diagnosis of obstruction on UDS in women can be challenging, with no true cutoffs for pressure and flow rates existing [7]. Recently, urodynamic parameters to diagnose bladder outlet obstruction after SUI procedures have been defined, with the most common pressure-flow voiding pattern among women with voiding dysfunction after MUS placement being a normal pressure and poor flow [6, 8]. In

Fig. 18.1 Fluoroscopic images during the voiding phase of a urodynamic study capture evidence of obstruction at the midurethra in a woman with a history of urinary retention after midurethral sling

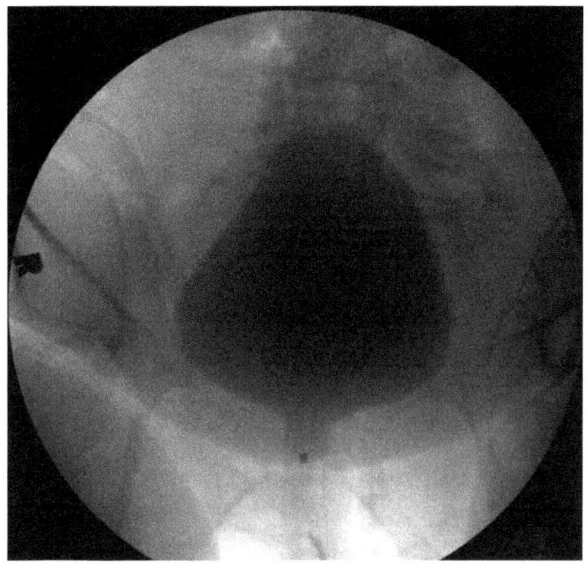

instances of new onset urinary retention or incomplete emptying after surgical intervention for SUI, clinical suspicion alone is likely sufficient to proceed with intervention. Occasionally, further imaging studies, such as ultrasonography (US), computed tomography (CT), or magnetic resonance imaging (MRI), may be indicated to identify hematomas or abscesses. Calcification identified in the lower urinary tract should raise suspicion of underlying mesh erosion. MRI can prove useful to identify mesh in patients presenting with pain or wound complications concerning for infected mesh (Fig. 18.2). Translabial or endovaginal US is another useful tool to identify mesh location, especially in patients presenting without prior operative records where it is unknown whether mesh was placed, or who have already had prior revision surgeries (Fig. 18.3).

Bladder Outlet Obstruction

Perhaps the most common complication, the exact incidence of bladder outlet obstruction after incontinence surgery is unknown, though it has been estimated to range from 2% to 25% [9–12]. It should be noted that this is likely underreported as women who undergo surgical intervention for SUI may be less likely to report voiding difficulties due to satisfaction over resolution of their incontinence, and those who do frequently seek treatment from a physician other than their original surgeon [13].

Symptoms of bladder outlet obstruction vary and include: immediate and complete urinary retention, spontaneous micturition with elevated postvoid residuals,

Fig. 18.2 An MRI in a woman with a history of transobturator midurethral sling who presented with a draining sinus in her right groin. This image captures an elongated abscess between the urethra and anterior vaginal wall at the site of the prior mesh sling which gives rise to a sinus tract extending through the right obturator externus and right gracilis muscle to the skin in the right inguinal crease

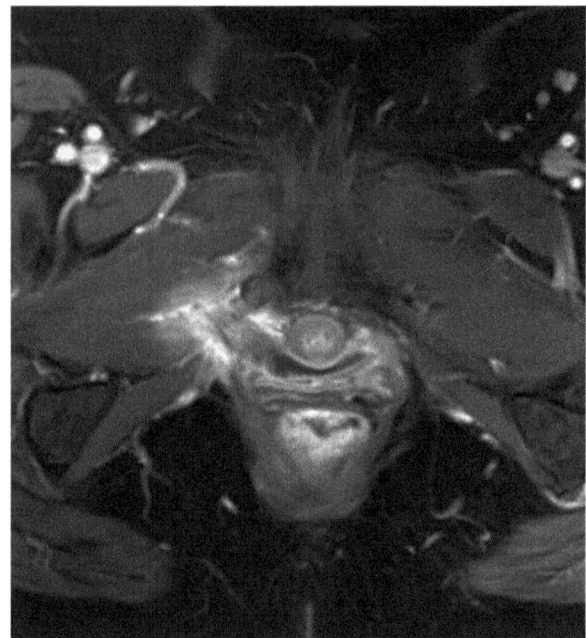

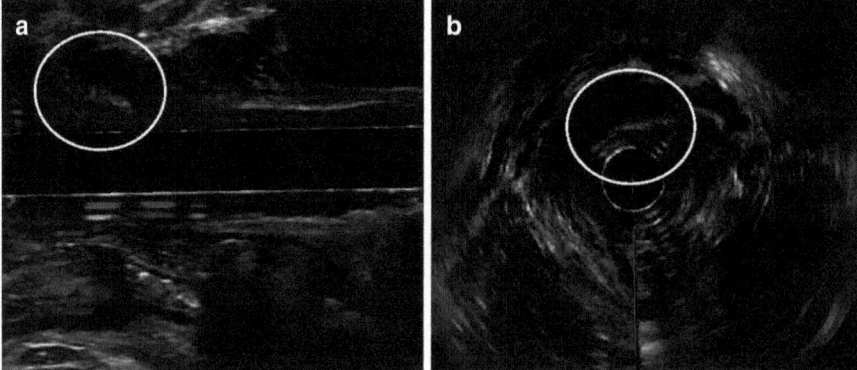

Fig. 18.3 Endovaginal ultrasound of a woman presenting with a history of transobturator midurethral sling with a draining sinus in her right groin with the mesh. The mesh can be visualized within the white circles on the (**a**) sagittal and (**b**) coronal ultrasound images

need to strain or perform positional voiding, increased or new storage symptoms, or an increased frequency of urinary tract infections.

Immediate postoperative urinary retention can occur after any surgical procedure for the treatment of SUI. Acute urinary retention is reported in 41% of women who underwent transvaginal needle suspension [14], up to 27% of women who underwent retropubic suspension [15], 5–20% of patients who underwent pubovaginal sling [16, 17], and 2.5–25% after midurethral synthetic sling [18–21]. Risk factors for postoperative urinary retention following MUS have been proposed to include: older age, concomitant surgery, vaginal vault prolapse, low preoperative urinary flow rate, and low detrusor contractility [22].

The diagnosis of acute urinary retention is relatively straightforward and is most commonly made after a failed trial of void in the recovery room, though the definition of what constitutes a successful void trial is by no means standardized. Occasionally, however, patients will undergo a successful void trial in the recovery room and present in a delayed fashion, as was reported in 3.4% of 59,556 women undergoing midurethral sling placement by Punjani et al. [21]. This presentation can be relatively straightforward with complete inability to void, weak stream, straining, or positional voiding, or may be subtler, such as new onset urinary urgency, frequency, or urgency incontinence. It is important for the physician to have a high index of suspicion of retention in patients who present in the immediate postoperative period with acute onset new voiding symptoms, as retention can be present in the absence of complete inability to void.

There is lack of consensus among urologists and urogynecologists as to the appropriate management strategy for postoperative bladder outlet obstruction following surgical intervention for SUI [23]. Acute urinary retention will frequently resolve with conservative management over time and may not always require surgical intervention. It is estimated that urinary retention will persist for longer than 4 weeks in 5% of patients undergoing retropubic and transvaginal suspensions, and 8% of sling procedures, with pubovaginal slings being associated with a higher rate of retention than MUS [10]. More recently, the average incidence of postoperative retention after MUS requiring surgery to relieve outlet obstruction has been reported at only 1–2% [24]. Furthermore, normal spontaneous voiding is reported to resume in 81–87.5% of women who required temporary intermittent catheterization for acute postoperative urinary retention following MUS [25, 26]. However, many obstructed women who are eventually able to void without a catheter continue to report significant voiding dysfunction after the initial period of retention [23, 27]. This combined with evidence suggesting that postoperative urinary retention within 30 days of MUS may be associated with future mesh problems requiring surgical intervention may prompt some to advocate for earlier surgical intervention [21]. Some studies suggest that earlier intervention for iatrogenic obstruction may be associated with better outcomes [28]. However, it is unknown whether early surgical intervention for postoperative urinary retention following SUI surgery decreases the risk of subsequent complications, and the optimal timing of reoperation is unclear.

As such, treatment of postoperative bladder outlet obstruction following SUI surgery is determined by a host of factors including patient symptoms severity and bother, temporal relationship of symptoms in relation to surgery, and procedure type. Given the increased risk of urinary retention following pubovaginal sling, many providers will elect to place a suprapubic catheter at the time of index surgery, especially in patient with a complicated history of prior MUS placement or complications requiring revision or removal. This is generally kept in place until normal emptying resumes in 1–4 weeks. Alternatively, many surgeons elect to have all patients routinely taught to perform clean intermittent catheterization (CIC) after pubovaginal sling placement and to perform postvoid catheterization until residuals have decreased below a certain threshold. Aside from these prophylactic measures, in the setting of acute postoperative urinary retention following SUI surgery, urinary drainage may be accomplished via CIC or an indwelling urethral foley catheter when the patient is unable to perform CIC. In many cases, postoperative bladder outlet obstruction will resolve after a few days of catheterization, making this conservative measure the often-preferred initial treatment choice [26, 29, 30].

When postoperative bladder outlet obstruction is not resolved with catheterization, surgical intervention is the mainstay for treatment. Urethral dilatation, often with associated downward pressure to "loosen a sling," has been reported to improve voiding dysfunction in greater than 80% of patients with bladder outlet obstruction after surgery for SUI [31, 32]. Despite this reported success, this procedure is often not well tolerated and can cause considerable damage to the urethra itself and the surrounding tissue, is associated with future mesh erosion into the urethra, and, as such, is not recommended for the treatment of iatrogenic bladder outlet obstruction [13]. Surgical options for the management of iatrogenic bladder outlet obstruction include sling mobilization, sling incision, and urethrolysis.

In patients who present with acute urinary retention immediately following a sling procedure, sling loosening or mobilization may be the most appropriate treatment option. This has been reported to successfully resolve postoperative urinary retention in 87–100% of cases without compromising continence (Table 18.1) [25, 31, 33–38]. In general, this is easiest and best performed within the first 2 weeks following surgery [25] but has been reported as being feasible up to 21 days after the primary operation [37]. While this can be performed in select patients in an office setting [33], most often sling loosening or mobilization is performed under anesthesia in the operating room. Under local or general anesthetic, the vaginal incision is opened and the sling is identified. Adequate exposure is key, and the use of self-retaining retractors such as the Lone Star retractor or handheld retractors can prove helpful. If the surgeon continues to have difficulty identifying the sling, a cystoscope or urethral sound can be placed into the urethra with gentle upward traction to help expose the sling. Once the sling is identified, a right-angle clamp or hemostat can then be positioned behind the sling and downward traction applied to

Table 18.1 Sling mobilization success and continence rates

Authors and ref. no	N	Resolution of retention	Continent
Moksnes et al. [25]	136	89.7%	92.6%
Price et al. [31]	33	87.8%	100%
Klutke et al. [32]	17	100%	94.1%
Chang et al. [34]	5	80%	100%
Rautenberg et al. [35]	61	96.7%	95.1%
Nguyen [36]	10	100%	100%
Glavind [37]	5	100%	100%
Glavind and Shim [38]	17	100%	94%

displace the sling approximately 1 cm to relieve obstruction. If difficulty is encountered passing an instrument behind the sling initially, a suture can be placed at the midpoint of the sling to aid in sling manipulation [34].

Sling incision is also reported with similar efficacy, especially in patients presenting more than 3 weeks out from their index operation. It should be noted, however, that sling incision is associated with a higher rate of SUI recurrence than mobilization, with rates of recurrent SUI generally reported at around 14–28% [25, 39–41], with one study reporting recurrent SUI in as many as 60% of patients who underwent sling incision [42]. In general, recurrent SUI is less likely to occur when interventions are performed more than 180 days after the initial anti-incontinence procedure [13]. Various techniques have been described, including: midline sling incision, lateral sling incision, and bilateral sling incision as well as excision of the suburethral portion of the sling. When sling incision is performed shortly after the index operation or by the index surgeon, a midline incision of the vaginal epithelium is appropriate. In instances where sling incision is occurring in a delayed fashion, or by a surgeon other than the one who placed the index sling, it may be prudent to proceed with an inverted U incision to optimize exposure and minimize risk of subsequent mesh extrusion or incisional breakdown. Obtaining the previous operative report can again prove useful to determine what type of sling was placed as this may aid in identification of the sling. In cases of simple iatrogenic obstruction, once the sling is isolated, incision at the midline is usually adequate to relieve the obstruction without formal urethrolysis for both pubovaginal and midurethral slings [39, 40, 43]. Frequently, after the sling is incised, a distinct retraction of the sling material and release of the tethered urethra is noted. In instances of a more complicated presentation such as concomitant pain or mesh extrusion, it is prudent to remove the suburethral portion of the sling, and we advocate excising the sling to the right and left of midline to prevent subsequent sling exposure or erosion. This can be performed by incising the sling laterally to avoid injury to the urethra and then gently dissecting the sling off of the periurethral fascia laterally on each side until the pubic bone is reached at which time each arm of the sling can be transected. When synthetic sling material is excised, it should be sent to pathology, and patients should be informed of how to either obtain the sling material or pathology results for their records when requested. For patients with solely iatrogenic obstruction, complete sling excision with aggressive resection and counter incisions is not recommended due to increased risk of incontinence.

When bladder outlet obstruction is present after retropubic or transvaginal needle suspensions, in circumstances where the sling is not identifiable, or after failed sling incision, a formal urethrolysis may be warranted. This technique can be performed transvaginally or via a retropubic approach with cure rates reported from 63% to 93% and recurrent SUI of around 13–18% [3, 44–49]. The goal of urethrolysis is to restore mobility to the urethra, bladder neck, and anterior vaginal wall.

Retropubic urethrolysis has been well described by Webster and Kreder [48]. A low midline or Pfannenstiel incision is made, and access to the retropubic space of Retzius is achieved. All retropubic adhesions are sharply excised, with any visible suspension sutures or slings being incised. The dissection may need to extend laterally to the ischial tuberosities, which create a paravaginal defect. In the original description of the procedure, a formal paravaginal repair was then commonly performed by reapproximating the paravaginal fascia to the arcus tendineus fascia pelvis.

More commonly now, urethrolysis is performed transvaginally and has been described extensively in the literature [44, 50, 51]. The most common technique involves making an inverted U-incision on the anterior vaginal wall with the apex at the midurethra and the base at the bladder neck. Once the vaginal flap has been developed, dissection is performed sharply medial-to-lateral along the periurethral fascia toward the endopelvic fascia. The endopelvic fascia is then perforated sharply into the retropubic space. Further dissection is performed to mobilize the urethra from the underside of the pubic symphysis using both blunt and sharp dissection.

Suprameatal urethrolysis has also been described by Petrou et al. [52] whereby a semilunar, inverted U-incision is made 1 cm above the urethral meatus from 3 o' clock to 9'o clock. The perineal membrane is incised in the midline, and dissection is carried out sharply in the plane just above the urethra, thereby releasing the urethra, bladder neck, and bladder from the pubic bone and pelvic attachments. Using blunt dissection, the retropubic space can be entered ventral to the bladder, thereby disrupting the obstructing fibrous attachments with a medial-to-lateral sweeping motion. When present, the obstructing pubovaginal sling or suspension sutures can be identified and divided from this approach. The potential benefit of this approach is that the lateral endopelvic fascia remains preserved, which may improve urethral support and minimize recurrent SUI. However, the reported success rate of suprameatal urethrolysis is lower than transvaginal and retropubic urethrolysis with relief of obstructive symptoms reported at about 65% [52].

It is debated whether tissue interposition should be performed to mitigate risk of recurrent obstruction and in general is reserved for particular circumstances such as prior failed urethrolysis. This can be performed using omentum in the case of retropubic urethrolysis [53], or via interposition of a Martius labial fat pad graft after transvaginal urethrolysis [54].

Chronic Irritative Symptoms

Irritative (storage) symptoms such as frequency, urgency, and urge urinary incontinence [UUI] may occur after SUI surgery, either as persistent or de novo symptoms. Patients should be counseled to expect some worsening of irritative symptoms in the initial postoperative period, and that these symptoms are likely to persist for up to 4 weeks. When acute postoperative irritative symptoms occur, it is important to confirm that the patient is emptying well and to rule out infection. In these patients, a short course of anticholinergics or beta-3 agonist may be initiated during the acute recovery period.

Patients with preexisting irritative symptoms are more likely to have continued symptoms postoperatively. In one large review, persistent postoperative urgency was present in 36–66% of women who underwent retropubic suspension, 54% of those who underwent transvaginal suspension, and 34–46% of women who underwent sling procedures. This was compared to women without preoperative urgency, where de novo urgency occurred in 8–16% of those with retropubic suspensions, 3–10% of those with transvaginal suspensions, and 3–11% of those with slings [10]. Some studies report resolution of irritative symptoms after MUS in patients with mixed urinary incontinence (MUI). Segal et al. noted resolution of preoperative urgency and frequency of 57.3%, resolution of preoperative urge urinary incontinence of 63%, and cessation of anticholinergic medication in 57.7% of women who underwent MUS for MUI [55]. Zyczynski et al. found that most women with MUI reported improvement in overactive bladder symptoms 1 year after surgical treatment of SUI with 56.6% reporting improvement after pubovaginal sling, 67.9% reporting improvement after retropubic suspension, and 65–70% reporting improvement after MUS. This improvement was noted to decline to 36.5–54.1% at 5 years [56]. Despite these findings, most studies suggest that women with a predominant urge component of their MUI will have worse outcomes after surgery [17, 57–59], making it imperative to appropriately diagnose and counsel patients prior to surgical intervention so that expectations are well-managed. Surprisingly, in one study comparing retropubic suspension and pubovaginal slings, 92% of women with MUI expected their urgency, frequency, and nocturia to improve despite counseling efforts to the contrary [60]. This highlights the importance of detailed and perhaps repeated counseling with use of decision aids to appropriately set expectations in women with MUI prior to surgical intervention for SUI, and underscores how persistence of any irritative symptom can deleteriously affect a patient's perception of success. While there are no firm predictors for resolution of irritative symptoms after surgery for SUI, increased age, increased time from index surgery [17, 56], and increased number of prior incontinence procedures [55] appear to be associated with a higher rate of postoperative irritative voiding symptoms.

When irritative symptoms persist after the initial recovery period following surgery for SUI, the first step is to rule out bladder outlet obstruction and erosion. Among patients with persistent incontinence, or those who have had multiple anti-incontinence procedures, UDS may prove particularly useful in their evaluation. In the absence of obstruction or erosion, irritative voiding symptoms may be managed with any of the available treatment options in the arsenal for the management of overactive bladder including: behavioral modification, pelvic floor physical therapy, anticholinergics, beta-3 agonists, neuromodulation, or intradetrusor injection of onabotulinum toxin.

Infection

Urinary tract infection (UTI) is a common complication after SUI surgery, with estimates of postoperative UTIs occurring in 4.5–46.7% of patients, depending on the length of postoperative surveillance and the diagnostic criteria used [61–68]. Risk factors for postoperative UTI include: a history of recurrent UTIs [63, 66, 69], longer operative times [70], age older than 65 years [71], body mass index greater than 40 [71], and most notably, elevated postvoid residual [63, 72] and postoperative catheterization [66, 73]. As many as 80% of postoperative UTIs are attributed to indwelling urinary catheters [74], with one meta-analysis reporting UTI rate between 4.3% and 32% among patients who underwent MUS and required bladder catheterization postoperatively [75]. Despite this elevated risk, good antibiotic stewardship is essential to contain the emergence of superbugs. Antibiotic prophylaxis for women who require catheterization after SUI surgery remained controversial. While several studies support the use of prophylactic antibiotics in this population [76, 77], other studies fail to find benefit. Based on the best available evidence, postoperative oral antibiotics do not appear to be effective at reducing UTI rates in women after midurethral sling who require bladder catheterization compared to placebo [75]. When patients present with acute UTI symptoms in the first few months after surgery, it is important to evaluate for urinary retention and to obtain a urine culture. If the culture is positive, treating with appropriate antibiotics is warranted. Empiric treatment of irritative voiding symptoms after surgery for SUI in the absence of a culture should be limited when possible as irritative symptoms may increase in the immediate postoperative period in the absence of infection. In the setting of recurrent UTIs after incontinence surgery in the absence of incomplete emptying of the bladder, cystoscopy should be performed to rule out suture or mesh erosion.

Wound infections are a less common complication, with an incidence of 0.1–16%, depending on the incontinence surgery performed [67, 68, 78–80]. In one study of 30,723 women in the state of Washington who underwent SUI surgery before and after the introduction of the MUS, wound infection rates were reported at 0.1% in the MUS era compared to 0.4% prior to the introduction of the MUS [80]. Wound infections are reported more often following pubovaginal sling when compared to the less-invasive MUS, with one study reporting wound infection in 7.7% of patients who underwent pubovaginal sling [68] compared to 0.4% after TVT [81]. Risk factors for surgical site infection are similar to those of any other surgical procedure and include: obesity, diabetes, smoking status, and reoperation. Strategies such as preoperative antibiotics, changing gloves when transitioning from the vaginal to the abdominal surgical field, and wound irrigation have been shown to reduce postsurgical infections [82, 83].

Pelvic abscesses are rare but have been reported in the setting of infected hematoma after MUS placement. In one case series of two infected hematomas following MUS, both were successfully managed with ultrasound-guided aspiration and intravenous broad-spectrum antibiotics. Neither case required operative intervention or mesh removal, and continence was preserved [84].

Pain

Postoperative pain and neuropathy are recognized risks of SUI surgery. The mechanism of pain can be related to the involvement of pelvic muscles and/or nerves in the trajectory of the suture or sling, sling tension, infection, or erosion. The true incidence of postoperative pain following SUI surgery is difficult to assess in part due to the use of heterogeneous terms to define pain and pain location. The use of diagrams to establish location of pain has been shown to be helpful when evaluating new onset pain after incontinence surgery [85]. When patients present with pain out of proportion to examination, especially with concomitant irritative voiding symptoms or recurrent UTIs, cystourethroscopy should be considered to rule out mesh erosion [86]. The incidence of groin pain following midurethral sling has been reported between 1.3% and 32% [85, 87–91]. Using a strict definition of pain, a secondary analysis of the Trial of Midurethral slings demonstrated that surgical pain after midurethral sling surgery was completely resolved in approximately 70% of patients by 2 weeks and 90% by 6 weeks, with the odds of pain resolution increasing by 12% each day up to 6 weeks after surgery. By week six, only 5.4% and 3.4% of patients in the transobturator and retropubic groups, respectively, were using medication for pain related to their operation [92]. It should also be noted that patient satisfaction with the procedure seems largely unrelated to postoperative pain [85, 92]. When conservative pain management fails, vaginal suburethral MUS removal can lead to pain relief in 60–80% of women [93–96]. Among 52 women who underwent suburethral MUS removal, only 31% required a secondary procedure to remove the sling arms in the setting of persistent pain, and of those who underwent complete mesh removal, 56% had unchanged or worse pain [93]. There is some controversy as to whether a limited vaginal MUS removal will be adequate to relieve pain or if a more extensive removal is required, with no specific determinants of who might benefit from a partial versus complete mesh excision in individuals who present with pain after MUS [93, 97]. The morbidity associated with complete mesh excision is not insignificant, and patients should be thoroughly counseled as to these risks before proceeding, including the risk of persistent pain. Our practice is to remain conservative and endorse a staged approach, excepting unique situations where there is concern that mesh infection is the source of pain.

The obturator nerve can be at risk with the placement of MUS, specifically via transobturator approach. Cadaveric studies have demonstrated the proximity of transobturator MUS to branches of the obturator nerve of around 20 mm [98]. Obturator nerve injury is likely caused by placing the sling too laterally. This may be prevented by making sure the patient's legs are correctly positioned to avoid excessive flexion and provide sufficient abduction. Symptoms may include medial thigh or groin pain, weakness with leg adduction, and sensory loss in the medial thigh. While the incidence of thigh pain has been reported around 5% after transobturator MUS [88], true obturator nerve injury is a much less often at 0.7–0.9/1000 MUS placements [99]. The key to managing obturator nerve injury is early diagnosis which can usually be made based on clinical findings alone. Decline of symptoms by infiltration of local anesthetic to the area can be used to confirm the diagnosis and provide short-term pain management [100, 101]. There is insufficient literature to determine the optimal treatment of an obturator nerve injury. Spontaneous recovery generally occurs with conservative therapy; however, if a patient has significant neurological symptoms or if symptoms persist beyond 6 weeks, surgical intervention including complete removal of the involved mesh arm is recommended [101, 102]. While primary nerve repair or grafting would be unexpected following obturator nerve injury after transobturator MUS, a neurosurgery consultation is prudent in the setting of significant neurologic symptoms.

The anatomy of the ilioinguinal nerve makes it vulnerable to entrapment near its exit from the superficial inguinal ring, where it lies almost directly superior to the pubic tubercle. Entrapment or injury of the ilioinguinal nerve can occur at the time of suprapubic transverse incisions, needle, or trocar passage. Ilioinguinal nerve entrapment can result in pain starting in the suprapubic region with radiation to the medial groin, mons, labia majora, and inner thigh and may be exacerbated with ambulation. Passage of needles and trocars closer to the midline and adjacent to the pubic bone should reduce the risk of ilioinguinal nerve injury. This complication has been reported after needle suspension in up to 8–16% of patients [103–105] as well as after tension-free vaginal tape placement [106]. The diagnosis can be confirmed and managed in the short term with an ilioinguinal nerve block. Symptoms can resolve with conservative management including ilioinguinal nerve block, physical therapy, and the aid of a walker without need for suture or mesh removal. However, if pain persists for more than 6 weeks or conservative measures are inadequate, surgical intervention for suture or mesh removal may be required [104].

Vaginal Mesh Exposure and Extrusion

Synthetic mesh midurethral slings provide a reliable and efficacious long-term treatment for stress urinary incontinence. As such, polypropylene mesh midurethral slings are supported as being the "standard of care for the surgical treatment of SUI" by the Society of Urodynamics, Female Pelvic Medicine and Urogenital Reconstruction (SUFU) as well as the American Urogynecologic Society (AUGS) [107]. Despite the level A evidence behind the use of synthetic mesh midurethral slings, the use of transvaginal mesh for SUI is not without risk. One of the more common and unique complications is that of mesh exposure. The Food and Drug Administration performed a systematic review of all published literature from 1996 to 2011 and reported that the rate of mesh exposure and extrusion through the vagina is 2% at 1 year following surgery [108]. To better aid in the discussion of unique mesh complications, the International Urogynecologic Association and the International Continence Society published joint classification to standardize the terminology of complications related to surgical mesh [109]. The term "exposure"

Fig. 18.4 Mesh extrusion at the right vaginal fornix is noted here on exam with the aid of a half speculum and two Allis clamps in the operating room. (Image courtesy Anne Cameron MD)

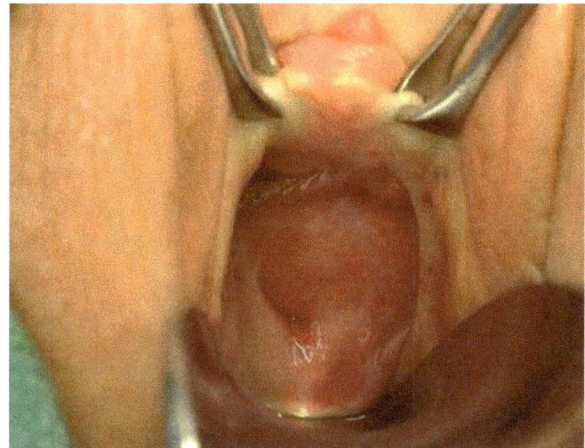

will be used to describe vaginal mesh identified visually or by palpation at the surgical incision site while "extrusion" describes the passage of mesh out of a body structure or tissue, and can include the delayed process of mesh gradually passing through the vaginal wall (Fig. 18.4).

As previously stated, the rate of mesh exposure or extrusion occurs in approximately 2% of sling placements, with a range of 0–8.1% reported in the literature [108, 110, 111]. The reported rate is for type 1 large-pore monofilament polypropylene mesh, which is the current standard for synthetic slings. Older slings such as the Obtape and Uratape have been known to have a higher rate of exposure and extrusion, as they were made of different mesh material which was not as porous, did not allow for adequate tissue ingrowth, and had higher infection rates [112]. Risk factors that may predispose to mesh exposure and extrusion include patients with diabetes, active smokers, and deficient nutritional status, as well as surgeon experience [113–116]. Possible causes of mesh exposure or extrusion are errors during sling placement, inadequate vaginal incision closure, vaginal incision breakdown, subclinical infection, impaired wound healing, or mesh contraction.

The clinical presentation of mesh exposure or extrusion may be quite variable. It is not uncommon for patients to be asymptomatic on presentation and to be diagnosed based on exam alone. Partner pain during intercourse may also be the first indication of sling exposure [117]. Other symptoms may include vaginal bleeding or discharge, dyspareunia, recurrent infections, or palpable mesh on self-exam [112, 118].

When mesh exposure or extrusion is suspected, pelvic examination should be performed with a half speculum. The exposed mesh may present as visible or palpable mesh through the vaginal tissue or as an area of granulation tissue. The course of the sling should be visually inspected and palpated. Vaginoscopy may be used as an adjunct to the exam if a high suspicion exists with inability to thoroughly examine the course of the sling due to patient discomfort or habitus. If there is concern for concomitant mesh erosion, cystourethroscopy may also be performed. When patients present with concern for mesh erosion or exposure having had their index surgery performed by another surgeon, it is valuable to obtain the operative report to guide in evaluation and treatment. The type of sling placed may also influence the location of delayed mesh exposure, with the transobturator approach often noted to expose at the fornix due to trocar trajectory. Postoperative mesh exposure is more likely to occur with transobturator slings [1.3%] compared with retropubic slings [0.7%] [119].

Upon identifying mesh exposure or extrusion, treatment will depend on a number of factors including: patient symptoms and degree of bother, the time frame between index surgery and mesh exposure/extrusion, the size and location of the exposure, and the quality of her vaginal tissue. Conservative management with observation and topical estrogen cream application for 6–12 weeks is reasonable in the asymptomatic or minimally symptomatic woman with a small exposure of less than 0.5 cm and may be successful in up to 40% of patients [96, 120]. Office-based mesh trimming may be considered for the appropriately selected patient with a small, easily visible region of exposed mesh. This treatment option is challenging however, due to patient discomfort and lack of exposure which can result in difficulty visualizing the mesh. Women should be counseled that the success rate of in-office mesh trimming is low, and that most patients will eventually require further exploration and excision in the operating room [120].

For larger mesh exposures, especially those presenting with early wound separation within the first 6 weeks after index surgery, local vaginal flaps can be created at the exposure site and advanced to close over the exposed mesh. This treatment option is appealing as it preserves continence. The literature evaluating success of vaginal flap closure reports mixed success rates of 36–100% [121–123], though it should be noted that time from index surgery to exposure is quite variable in these studies and include vaginal flap closure of mesh extrusions as well as exposures. It is our experience that for early mesh exposure at the surgical incision, vaginal flap closure is the preferred first-line treatment.

If conservative measures fail, or for larger or more delayed mesh extrusions, partial mesh excision should be offered. The decision on how much mesh to remove will depend in part on the location and size of the exposure, and it should be noted that incontinence rates after excision seem to increase with additional lengths of mesh removed. In one recent study evaluating incontinence rates after partial mesh excision [defined as removing only the part of the sling exposed] versus complete mesh excision [defined as removing the entire suburethral portion out to bilateral pubic rami], recurrent SUI was seen in 7% of patients with partial excision versus 59% of those who had removal of the entire suburethral component [124]. In the setting of simple mesh exposure or extrusion, total mesh excision is rarely indicated and however may be considered when infection or severe pelvic pain is present. Patients should be counseled about the risks and benefits of total sling excision, including the risk of persistent pain as well as recurrent stress urinary incontinence.

Urinary Tract Erosion

Mesh or suture erosion into the urinary tract is a rare complication of surgical management of SUI. First reported in 2001 [125], there has been an increase in mesh erosion over time with a current incidence rate of 0.02–5.4% [10, 126]. Risk factors of urinary tract erosion include: unrecognized trocar perforation into the bladder at time of sling placement, dissection too close to the urethra with thinning and devascularization of the tissue, urethral dilation post sling, excessive tensioning, or unrecognized direct urethral injury. Patient may present with irritative or obstructive voiding symptoms, recurrent UTIs, or hematuria. As previously noted, a high index of suspicion is necessary when evaluating these patients, and cystourethroscopy should be performed. Sutures or slings that have eroded into the urinary tract may act as a nidus for stone formation (Fig. 18.5).

Endoscopic management is a reasonable first-line treatment option for both erosions into the bladder or urethra. Endoscopic treatment can be performed with either a laser or endoscopic excision using an electrode loop or endoscopic scissors. In one systematic review of endoscopic management of mesh erosions in 198 patients, the initial success rate with laser excision was 67% compared to 80% with loop or scissor excision. Many patients subsequently underwent repeat endoscopic removal with only 2–7% requiring subsequent open surgical removal for a final success rate of 92–98%. Complication rates were 24% and 28% in the laser and endoscopic

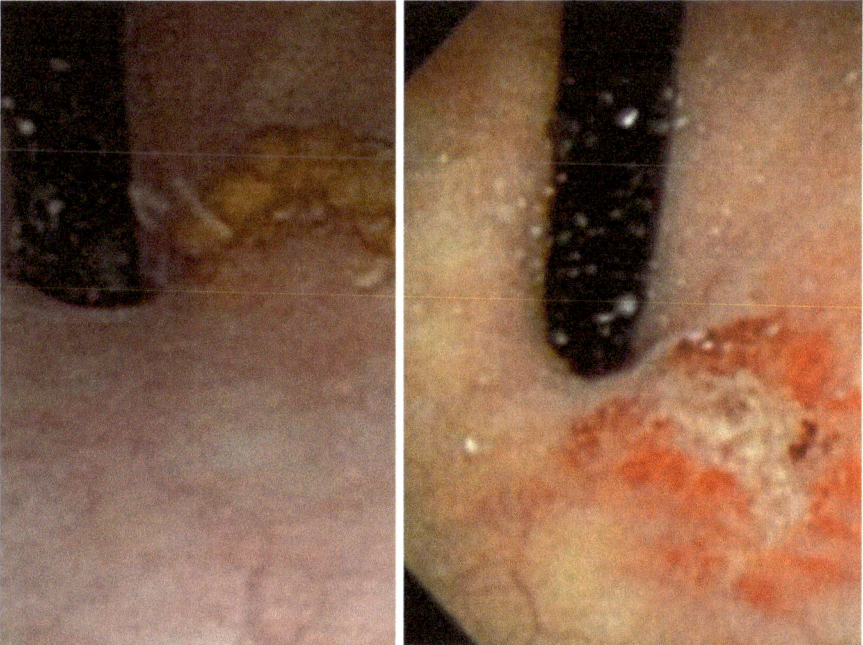

Fig. 18.5 Flexible cystourethroscopy evaluation of a mesh sling eroded at the bladder neck before and after laser treatment of the stone encrusting the mesh. (Image courtesy Anne Cameron MD)

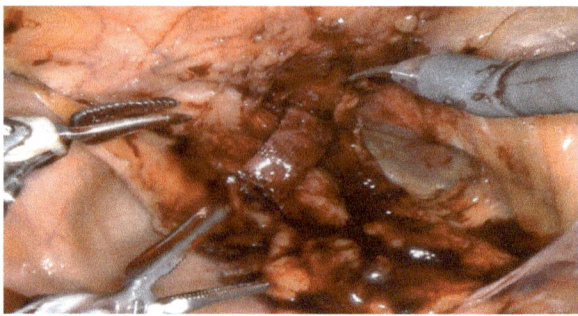

Fig. 18.6 Robotic-assisted laparoscopic cystotomy for the removal of a transvaginal tape mesh arm eroded into the bladder

groups, respectively, with 21% experiencing recurrent SUI. It should be noted that three vesicovaginal fistulas occurred in the group that utilized an electrode loop or scissors for treatment [127].

When endoscopic removal is unsuccessful, surgical removal of the eroded mesh should be performed. This can be done via a transvaginal approach in the setting of urethral or bladder neck erosion, or via suprapubic cystotomy in instances of erosion of the mesh arms into the bladder. Cystotomy via laparoscopic or robotic approach is a reasonable alternative for mesh erosion into the bladder, and has been successfully described in a number of case series without major complication [128, 129] (Fig. 18.6).

Sexual Dysfunction

Sexual dysfunction is reported in 42–56% of women with urinary incontinence [130]. Vaginal innervation may be concentrated on the anterior vagina and may be affected by surgery for SUI [131, 132]. It is postulated that disruption of the innervation of the anterior vaginal wall may be involved in the development of dyspareunia [133]. Cayan et al. found that in women undergoing surgery for SUI, sexual function decreased more in women who underwent Burch colposuspension compared to vaginal sling, particularly in arousal, lubrication, and orgasm scores [134]. Mazouni and colleagues reported that 25.6% of women experience some deterioration in sexual function after TVT placement [135]. Conversely, a number of studies have reported improvement in sexual function after surgical treatment of SUI [130, 136, 137]. Further prospective studies are required to discern the impact of surgical treatment of SUI on sexual function.

Conclusions

Complications following surgical treatment of stress urinary incontinence are not uncommon. It is important to perform a complete history and physical exam before proceeding with treatment so that the most appropriate surgical procedure for an individual can be selected. Shared decision-making, where patients understand a range of treatment options as well as their success and complication rates, will aid in fostering trust and patient satisfaction should complications arise. Physicians should have a high index of suspicion for complications when patients present with new voiding or storage symptoms, retention, recurrent urinary tract infections, or pain following surgical treatment for SUI. When a complication is suspected, a thorough history and physical exam should be performed, with additional diagnostic tests such as cystourethroscopy or urodynamics utilized when prudent. The choice of treatment option for each complication should involve an assessment of patient bother and should include a discussion of the risk of recurrent SUI or failure to relieve symptoms, especially in regard to pelvic pain as this is likely multifactorial in nature and can be difficult to treat.

References

1. Milsom IAD, Lapitan MC, Nelson R, Sillen U, Thom D. Epidemiology of urinary (UI) and faecal (FI) incontinence and pelvic organ prolapse (POP). Committee 1. International Continence Society; 2009.
2. Legendre G, Fritel X, Panjo H, Zins M, Ringa V. Incidence and remission of stress, urge, and mixed urinary incontinence in midlife and older women: a longitudinal cohort study. Neurourol Urodyn [Internet]. 2020;39(2):650–7. Available from: https://onlinelibrary.wiley.com/doi/abs/10.1002/nau.24237.
3. Tse V, Chan L. Outlet obstruction after sling surgery. BJU Int [Internet]. 2011;108:24–8. Available from: http://doi.wiley.com/10.1111/j.1464-410X.2011.10712.x.
4. Nitti VW, Tu LM, Gitlin J. Diagnosing bladder outlet obstruction in women. J Urol [Internet]. 1999;161(5):1535–40. Available from: http://www.ncbi.nlm.nih.gov/pubmed/10210391.
5. Gracely A, Major N, Zheng Y, Silverii H, Lim C, Rittenberg L, et al. Do urodynamics predict urinary retention after sling placement in the complex patient: the value of reproducing symptoms on urodynamics. Int Urogynecol J [Internet]. 2021;32(1):81–6. Available from: http://link.springer.com/10.1007/s00192-020-04623-8.
6. Rodrigues P, Hering F, Dias EC. Female obstruction after incontinence surgery may present different urodynamic patterns. Int Urogynecol J [Internet]. 2013;24(2):331–6. Available from: http://link.springer.com/10.1007/s00192-012-1869-x.
7. Brucker BM, Shah S, Mitchell S, Fong E, Nitti MD, Kelly CE, et al. Comparison of urodynamic findings in women with anatomical versus functional bladder outlet obstruction. Female Pelvic Med Reconstr Surg [Internet]. 2013;19(1):46–50. Available from: http://journals.lww.com/01436319-201301000-00010.
8. Gammie A, Kirschner-Hermanns R, Rademakers K. Evaluation of obstructed voiding in the female. Curr Opin Urol [Internet]. 2015;1. Available from: http://journals.lww.com/00042307-900000000-99465.
9. Welk B, Al-Hothi H, Winick-Ng J. Removal or revision of vaginal mesh used for the treatment of stress urinary incontinence. JAMA Surg [Internet]. 2015;150(12):1167. Available from: http://archsurg.jamanetwork.com/article.aspx?doi=10.1001/jamasurg.2015.2590.
10. Leach GE, Dmochowski RR, Appell R, Blaivas JG, Hadley HR, Luber KM, et al. Female stress urinary incontinence clinical guidelines panel summary report on surgical management of female stress urinary incontinence. J Urol [Internet]. 1997;875–80. Available from: http://journals.lww.com/00005392-199709000-00054.
11. Dmochowski RR, Blaivas JM, Gormley EA, Juma S, Karram MM, Lightner DJ, et al. Update of AUA guideline on the surgical management of female stress urinary incontinence. J Urol

[Internet]. 2010;183(5):1906–14. Available from: http://www.jurology.com/doi/10.1016/j.juro.2010.02.2369.

12. Plagakis S, Tse V. The autologous pubovaginal fascial sling: an update in 2019. LUTS Low Urin Tract Symptoms [Internet]. 2020;12(1):2–7. Available from: https://onlinelibrary.wiley.com/doi/abs/10.1111/luts.12281.

13. Malacarne DR, Nitti VW. Post-sling urinary retention in women. Curr Urol Rep [Internet]. 2016 27;17(11):83. Available from: http://link.springer.com/10.1007/s11934-016-0639-6.

14. Kelly M, Zimmern, Philippe E, Leach G. Complications of bladder neck suspension procedures. Urol Clin N Am. 1991;18(2):339.

15. Parnell JP, Marshall VF, Vaughan ED. Management of recurrent urinary stress incontinence by the Marshall-Marchetti-Krantz vesicourethropexy. J Urol [Internet]. 1984;132(5):912–914. Available from: http://www.jurology.com/doi/10.1016/S0022-5347%2817%2949943-5.

16. Athanasopoulos A, Gyftopoulos K, McGuire EJ. Efficacy and preoperative prognostic factors of autologous fascia rectus sling for treatment of female stress urinary incontinence. Urology [Internet]. 2011;78(5):1034–1038. Available from: https://linkinghub.elsevier.com/retrieve/pii/S0090429511021923.

17. Chaikin DC, Rosenthal J, Blaivas JG. Pubovaginal fascial sling for all types of stress urinary incontinence: long-term analysis. J Urol [Internet]. 1998;160(4):1312–6. Available from: http://www.ncbi.nlm.nih.gov/pubmed/9751343.

18. Levin I, Groutz A, Gold R, Pauzner D, Lessing JB, Gordon D. Surgical complications and medium-term outcome results of tension-free vaginal tape: a prospective study of 313 consecutive patients. Neurourol Urodyn [Internet]. 2004;23(1):7–9. Available from: http://doi.wiley.com/10.1002/nau.10164.

19. Karram M. Complications and untoward effects of the tension-free vaginal tape procedure. Obstet Gynecol [Internet]. 2003;101(5):929–932. Available from: http://linkinghub.elsevier.com/retrieve/pii/S0029784403001224.

20. de Tayrac R, Deffieux X, Droupy S, Chauveaud-Lambling A, Calvanèse-Benamour L, Fernandez H. RETRACTED: a prospective randomized trial comparing tension-free vaginal tape and transobturator suburethral tape for surgical treatment of stress urinary incontinence. Am J Obstet Gynecol [Internet]. 2004;190(3):602–608. Available from: https://linkinghub.elsevier.com/retrieve/pii/S0002937803019380.

21. Punjani N, Winick-Ng J, Welk B. Postoperative urinary retention and urinary tract infections predict midurethral sling mesh complications. Urology [Internet]. 2017;99:42–48. Available from: https://linkinghub.elsevier.com/retrieve/pii/S0090429516307324.

22. Takacs P, Medina CA. Tension-free vaginal tape: poor intraoperative cough test as a predictor of postoperative urinary retention. Int Urogynecol J [Internet]. 2007;18(12):1445–1447. Available from: http://link.springer.com/10.1007/s00192-007-0364-2.

23. Hashim H, Terry T. Management of recurrent stress urinary incontinence and urinary retention following midurethral sling insertion in women. Ann R Coll Surg Engl [Internet]. 2012;94(7):517–522. Available from: https://publishing.rcseng.ac.uk/doi/10.1308/003588412X13373405385610.

24. Jonsson Funk M, Siddiqui NY, Pate V, Amundsen CL, Wu JM. Sling revision/removal for mesh erosion and urinary retention: long-term risk and predictors. Am J Obstet Gynecol [Internet]. 2013;208(1):73.e1–7. Available from: https://linkinghub.elsevier.com/retrieve/pii/S0002937812010782.

25. Moksnes LR, Svenningsen R, Schiøtz HA, Moe K, Staff AC, Kulseng-Hanssen S. Sling mobilization in the management of urinary retention after mid-urethral sling surgery. Neurourol Urodyn [Internet]. 2017;36(4):1091–6. Available from: http://www.ncbi.nlm.nih.gov/pubmed/27241330.

26. Hong B, Park S, Kim HS, Choo M. Factors predictive of urinary retention after a tension-free vaginal tape procedure for female stress urinary incontinence. J Urol [Internet]. 2003;170(3):852–6. Available from: http://www.ncbi.nlm.nih.gov/pubmed/12913715.

27. Çetinel B, Tarcan T. Management of complications after tension-free midurethral slings. Korean J Urol [Internet]. 2013;54(10):651. Available from: https://icurology.org/DOIx. php?id=10.4111/kju.2013.54.10.651.

28. Abraham N, Makovey I, King A, Goldman HB, Vasavada S. The effect of time to release of an obstructing synthetic mid-urethral sling on repeat surgery for stress urinary incontinence. Neurourol Urodyn [Internet]. 2017;36(2):349–353. Available from: http://doi.wiley. com/10.1002/nau.22927.

29. Shukla A, Paul SK, Nishtar A, Bibby J. Factors predictive of voiding problems following insertion of tension-free vaginal tape. Int J Gynecol Obstet [Internet]. 2007;96(2):122–126. Available from: http://doi.wiley.com/10.1016/j.ijgo.2006.10.013.

30. Bailey C, Matharu G. Conservative management as an initial approach for post-operative voiding dysfunction. Eur J Obstet Gynecol Reprod Biol [Internet]. 2012;160(1):106–109. Available from: https://linkinghub.elsevier.com/retrieve/pii/S0301211511005409.

31. Price N, Slack A, Khong S-Y, Currie I, Jackson S. The benefit of early mobilisation of tension-free vaginal tape in the treatment of post-operative voiding dysfunction. Int Urogynecol J [Internet]. 2009;20(7):855–858. Available from: http://link.springer.com/10.1007/s00192-009-0858-1.

32. Klutke C, Siegel S, Carlin B, Paszkiewicz E, Kirkemo A, Klutke J. Urinary retention after tension-free vaginal tape procedure: incidence and treatment. Urology [Internet]. 2001;58(5):697–701. Available from: http://www.ncbi.nlm.nih.gov/pubmed/11711343.

33. Greiman A, Kielb S. Revisions of mid Urethral slings can be accomplished in the office. J Urol [Internet]. 2012;188(1):190–193. Available from: http://www.jurology.com/doi/10.1016/j.juro.2012.02.2560.

34. Chang W-C, Sheu B-C, Huang S-C, Wu M-T, Hsu W-C, Chou L-Y, et al. Postoperative transvaginal tape mobilization in preventing voiding difficulty after tension-free vaginal tape procedures. Int Urogynecol J [Internet]. 2010;21(2):229–33. Available from: http://www.ncbi.nlm.nih.gov/pubmed/19834633.

35. Rautenberg O, Kociszewski J, Welter J, Kuszka A, Eberhard J, Viereck V. Ultrasound and early tape mobilization--a practical solution for treating postoperative voiding dysfunction. Neurourol Urodyn [Internet]. 2014;33(7):1147–51. Available from: http://www.ncbi.nlm.nih.gov/pubmed/23818418.

36. Nguyen JN. Tape mobilization for urinary retention after tension-free vaginal tape procedures. Urology [Internet]. 2005;66(3):523–6. Available from: http://www.ncbi.nlm.nih.gov/pubmed/16140070.

37. Glavind K, Glavind E. Treatment of prolonged voiding dysfunction after tension-free vaginal tape procedure. Acta Obstet Gynecol Scand [Internet]. 2007;86(3):357–60. Available from: http://www.ncbi.nlm.nih.gov/pubmed/17364313.

38. Glavind K, Shim S. Incidence and treatment of postoperative voiding dysfunction after the tension-free vaginal tape procedure. Int Urogynecol J [Internet]. 2015;26(11):1657–60. Available from: http://www.ncbi.nlm.nih.gov/pubmed/26068102.

39. Moore CK, Goldman HB. Simple sling incision for the treatment of iatrogenic bladder outlet obstruction. Int Urogynecol J [Internet]. 2013;24(12):2145–2146. Available from: http://link.springer.com/10.1007/s00192-013-2241-5.

40. Wu S-Y, Kuo H-C. Long-term outcomes of anti-incontinence surgery and subsequent transvaginal sling incision for urethral obstruction. Int Urogynecol J [Internet]. 2019;30(5):761–766. Available from: http://link.springer.com/10.1007/s00192-018-3733-0.

41. Yoost T, Rames R, Lebed B, Bhavsar R, Rovner E. Predicting for postoperative incontinence following sling incision. Int Urogynecol J [Internet]. 2011;22(6):665–669. Available from: http://link.springer.com/10.1007/s00192-010-1339-2.

42. Viereck V, Rautenberg O, Kociszewski J, Grothey S, Welter J, Eberhard J. Midurethral sling incision: indications and outcomes. Int Urogynecol J [Internet]. 2013;24(4):645–653. Available from: http://link.springer.com/10.1007/s00192-012-1895-8.

43. Nitti VW, Carlson K V, Blaivas JG, Dmochowski RR. Early results of pubovaginal sling lysis by midline sling incision. Urology [Internet]. 2002;59(1):47–51. Available from: https://linkinghub.elsevier.com/retrieve/pii/S009042950101559X.
44. Foster HE, McGuire EJ. Management of urethral obstruction with transvaginal urethrolysis. J Urol [Internet]. 1993;150(5 Part 1):1448–51. Available from: http://www.jurology.com/doi/10.1016/S0022-5347%2817%2935805-6.
45. Nitti VW, Raz S. Obstruction following anti-incontinence procedures: diagnosis and treatment with transvaginal urethrolysis. J Urol [Internet]. 1994;152(1):93–98. Available from: http://www.jurology.com/doi/10.1016/S0022-5347%2817%2932825-2.
46. Anger JT, Amundsen CL, Webster GD. Obstruction after Burch colposuspension: a return to retropubic urethrolysis. Int Urogynecol J [Internet]. 2006;17(5):455–459. Available from: http://link.springer.com/10.1007/s00192-005-0037-y.
47. Petrou SP, Young PR. Rate of recurrent stress urinary incontinence after retropubic urethrolysis. J Urol [Internet]. 2002;613–5. Available from: http://journals.lww.com/00005392-200202000-00035.
48. Webster GD, Kreder KJ. Voiding dysfunction following cystourethropexy: its evaluation and management. J Urol [Internet]. 1990;144(3):670–673. Available from: http://www.jurology.com/doi/10.1016/S0022-5347%2817%2939550-2.
49. Starkman JS, Duffy JW, Wolter CE, Kaufman MR, Scarpero HM, Dmochowski RR. The evolution of obstruction induced overactive bladder symptoms following urethrolysis for female bladder outlet obstruction. J Urol [Internet]. 2008;179(3):1018–1023. Available from: http://www.jurology.com/doi/10.1016/j.juro.2007.10.051.
50. Cross CA, Cespedes RD, English SF, McGuire EJ. Transvaginal urethrolysis for urethral obstruction after anti-incontinence surgery. J Urol [Internet]. 1998;159(4):1199–201. Available from: http://www.ncbi.nlm.nih.gov/pubmed/9507832.
51. Zimmern PE, Hadley HR, Leach GE, Raz S. Female urethral obstruction after Marshall-Marchetti-Krantz operation. J Urol [Internet]. 1987;138(3):517–520. Available from: http://www.jurology.com/doi/10.1016/S0022-5347%2817%2943244-7.
52. Petrou SP, Brown JA, Blaivas JG. Suprameatal transvaginal urethrolysis. J Urol [Internet]. 1999;161(4):1268–71. Available from: http://www.ncbi.nlm.nih.gov/pubmed/10081883.
53. Carr LK, Webster GD. Voiding dysfunction following incontinence surgery: diagnosis and treatment with retropubic or vaginal urethrolysis. J Urol [Internet]. 1997;157(3):821–3. Available from: http://www.ncbi.nlm.nih.gov/pubmed/9072576.
54. Carey JM, Chon JK, Leach GE. Urethrolysis with martius labial fat pad graft for iatrogenic bladder outlet obstruction. Urology [Internet]. 2003;61(4):21–25. Available from: https://linkinghub.elsevier.com/retrieve/pii/S0090429503001171.
55. Segal JL, Vassallo B, Kleeman S, Silva WA, Karram MM. Prevalence of persistent and de novo overactive bladder symptoms after the tension-free vaginal tape. Obstet Gynecol [Internet]. 2004;104(6):1263–9. Available from: http://www.ncbi.nlm.nih.gov/pubmed/15572487.
56. Zyczynski HM, Albo ME, Goldman HB, Wai CY, Sirls LT, Brubaker L, et al. Change in overactive bladder symptoms after surgery for stress urinary incontinence in women. Obstet Gynecol [Internet]. 2015;126(2):423–30. Available from: http://www.ncbi.nlm.nih.gov/pubmed/26241434.
57. Chou EC-L, Flisser AJ, Panagopoulos G, Blaivas JG. Effective treatment for mixed urinary incontinence with a pubovaginal sling. J Urol [Internet]. 2003;170(2 Pt 1):494–7. Available from: http://www.ncbi.nlm.nih.gov/pubmed/12853807.
58. Stoffel JT, Smith JJ, Crivellaro S, Bresette JF. Mixed incontinence: does preoperative urodynamic detrusor overactivity affect postoperative quality of life after pubovaginal sling? Int Braz J Urol [Internet]. 2008;34(6):765–771. Available from: http://www.scielo.br/scielo.php?script=sci_arttext&pid=S1677-55382008000600012&lng=en&tlng=en.
59. Kulseng-Hanssen S, Husby H, Schiotz HA. The tension free vaginal tape operation for women with mixed incontinence: do preoperative variables predict the outcome? Neurourol Urodyn [Internet]. 2007;26(1):115–21; discussion 122. Available from: http://www.ncbi.nlm.nih.gov/pubmed/16894616.

60. Mallett VT, Brubaker L, Stoddard AM, Borello-France D, Tennstedt S, Hall L, et al. The expectations of patients who undergo surgery for stress incontinence. Am J Obstet Gynecol [Internet]. 2008;198(3):308.e1–6. Available from: http://www.ncbi.nlm.nih.gov/pubmed/18313452.

61. Debodinance P, Delporte P, Engrand JB, Boulogne M. Complications of urinary incontinence surgery: 800 procedures. J Gynecol Obstet Biol Reprod (Paris) [Internet]. 2002;31(7):649–62. Available from: http://www.ncbi.nlm.nih.gov/pubmed/12457137.

62. Anger JT, Litwin MS, Wang Q, Pashos CL, Rodríguez LV. Complications of sling surgery among female Medicare beneficiaries. Obstet Gynecol [Internet]. 2007;109(3):707–14. Available from: http://www.ncbi.nlm.nih.gov/pubmed/17329524.

63. Nygaard I, Brubaker L, Chai TC, Markland AD, Menefee SA, Sirls L, et al. Risk factors for urinary tract infection following incontinence surgery. Int Urogynecol J [Internet]. 2011;22(10):1255–65. Available from: http://www.ncbi.nlm.nih.gov/pubmed/21560012.

64. Brubaker L, Norton PA, Albo ME, Chai TC, Dandreo KJ, Lloyd KL, et al. Adverse events over two years after retropubic or transobturator midurethral sling surgery: findings from the Trial of Midurethral Slings (TOMUS) study. Am J Obstet Gynecol [Internet]. 2011;205(5):498. e1–6. Available from: http://www.ncbi.nlm.nih.gov/pubmed/21925636.

65. Schimpf MO, Rahn DD, Wheeler TL, Patel M, White AB, Orejuela FJ, et al. Sling surgery for stress urinary incontinence in women: a systematic review and metaanalysis. Am J Obstet Gynecol [Internet]. 2014;211(1):71.e1–27. Available from: http://www.ncbi.nlm.nih.gov/pubmed/24487005.

66. Varasteh Kia M, Long JB, Chen CCG. Urinary tract infection after midurethral sling. Female Pelvic Med Reconstr Surg [Internet]. 2021;27(1):e191–5. Available from: http://www.ncbi.nlm.nih.gov/pubmed/32427625.

67. Lee RA, Symmonds RE, Goldstein RA. Surgical complications and results of modified Marshall-Marchetti-Krantz procedure for urinary incontinence. Obstet Gynecol [Internet]. 1979;53(4):447–50. Available from: http://www.ncbi.nlm.nih.gov/pubmed/440646.

68. Chan PT, Fournier C, Corcos J. Short-term complications of pubovaginal sling procedure for genuine stress incontinence in women. Urology [Internet]. 2000;55(2):207–11. Available from: http://www.ncbi.nlm.nih.gov/pubmed/10688080.

69. Sutkin G, Alperin M, Meyn L, Wiesenfeld HC, Ellison R, Zyczynski HM. Symptomatic urinary tract infections after surgery for prolapse and/or incontinence. Int Urogynecol J [Internet]. 2010;21(8):955–61. Available from: http://www.ncbi.nlm.nih.gov/pubmed/20354678.

70. Gehrich AP, Lustik MB, Mehr AA, Patzwald JR. Risk of postoperative urinary tract infections following midurethral sling operations in women undergoing hysterectomy. Int Urogynecol J [Internet]. 2016;27(3):483–90. Available from: http://www.ncbi.nlm.nih.gov/pubmed/26467938.

71. Vigil HR, Mallick R, Nitti VW, Lavallée LT, Breau RH, Hickling DR. Risk factors for urinary tract infection following mid urethral sling Surgery. J Urol [Internet]. 2017;197(5):1268–73. Available from: http://www.ncbi.nlm.nih.gov/pubmed/28034608.

72. Doganay M, Cavkaytar S, Kokanali MK, Ozer I, Aksakal OS, Erkaya S. Risk factors for postoperative urinary tract infection following midurethral sling procedures. Eur J Obstet Gynecol Reprod Biol [Internet]. 2017;211:74–7. Available from: http://www.ncbi.nlm.nih.gov/pubmed/28192735.

73. Dieter AA, Amundsen CL, Edenfield AL, Kawasaki A, Levin PJ, Visco AG, et al. Oral antibiotics to prevent postoperative urinary tract infection: a randomized controlled trial. Obstet Gynecol [Internet]. 2014;123(1):96–103. Available from: http://www.ncbi.nlm.nih.gov/pubmed/24463669.

74. Sedor J, Mulholland SG. Hospital-acquired urinary tract infections associated with the indwelling catheter. Urol Clin N Am [Internet]. 1999;26(4):821–8. Available from: http://www.ncbi.nlm.nih.gov/pubmed/10584622.

75. Sanaee MS, Hutcheon JA, Larouche M, Brown HL, Lee T, Geoffrion R. Urinary tract infection prevention after midurethral slings in pelvic floor reconstructive surgery: a systematic

review and meta-analysis. Acta Obstet Gynecol Scand [Internet]. 2019;98(12):1514–22. Available from: http://www.ncbi.nlm.nih.gov/pubmed/31112286.

76. Marschall J, Carpenter CR, Fowler S, Trautner BW, CDC Prevention Epicenters Program. Antibiotic prophylaxis for urinary tract infections after removal of urinary catheter: meta-analysis. BMJ [Internet]. 2013;346:f3147. Available from: http://www.ncbi.nlm.nih.gov/pubmed/23757735.

77. Sutkin G, Lowder JL, Smith KJ. Prophylactic antibiotics to prevent urinary tract infection during clean intermittent self-catheterization (CISC) for management of voiding dysfunction after prolapse and incontinence surgery: a decision analysis. Int Urogynecol J Pelvic Floor Dysfunct [Internet]. 2009;20(8):933–8. Available from: http://www.ncbi.nlm.nih.gov/pubmed/19582384.

78. KIRBY RS, Whiteway JE. Assessment of the results of stamey bladder neck suspension. Br J Urol [Internet]. 1989;63(1):21–23. Available from: http://doi.wiley.com/10.1111/j.1464-410X.1989.tb05117.x.

79. Morgan JE. The suprapubic approach to primary stress urinary incontinence. Am J Obstet Gynecol [Internet]. 1973;115(3):316–20. Available from: http://www.ncbi.nlm.nih.gov/pubmed/4682824.

80. Stewart LE, Eston MA, Symons RG, Fialkow MF, Kirby AC. Stress urinary incontinence surgery in Washington state before and after introduction of the mesh midurethral sling. Female Pelvic Med Reconstr Surg [Internet]. 2019;25(5):358–61. Available from: http://www.ncbi.nlm.nih.gov/pubmed/29894326.

81. Abouassaly R, Steinberg JR, Lemieux M, Marois C, Gilchrist LI, Bourque J-L, et al. Complications of tension-free vaginal tape surgery: a multi-institutional review. BJU Int [Internet]. 2004;94(1):110–3. Available from: http://www.ncbi.nlm.nih.gov/pubmed/15217442.

82. Vij SC, Kartha G, Krishnamurthi V, Ponziano M, Goldman HB. Simple operating room bundle reduces superficial surgical site infections after major urologic surgery. Urology [Internet]. 2018;112:66–8. Available from: http://www.ncbi.nlm.nih.gov/pubmed/29122621.

83. Harris JA, Sammarco AG, Swenson CW, Uppal S, Kamdar N, Campbell D, et al. Are perioperative bundles associated with reduced postoperative morbidity in women undergoing benign hysterectomy? Retrospective cohort analysis of 16,286 cases in Michigan. Am J Obstet Gynecol [Internet]. 2017;216(5):502.e1–11. Available from: http://www.ncbi.nlm.nih.gov/pubmed/28082214.

84. Neuman M. Infected hematoma following tension-free vaginal tape implantation. J Urol. 2002;168(6):2549.

85. Cadish LA, Hacker MR, Modest AM, Rogers KJ, Dessie S, Elkadry EA. Characterization of pain after inside-out transobturator midurethral sling. Female Pelvic Med Reconstr Surg [Internet]. 2014;20(2):99–103. Available from: http://www.ncbi.nlm.nih.gov/pubmed/24566214.

86. Hilton P, Mohammed KA, Ward K. Postural perineal pain associated with perforation of the lower urinary tract due to insertion of a tension-free vaginal tape. BJOG [Internet]. 2003;110(1):79–82. Available from: http://www.ncbi.nlm.nih.gov/pubmed/12504943.

87. Laurikainen E, Valpas A, Kivelä A, Kalliola T, Rinne K, Takala T, et al. Retropubic compared with transobturator tape placement in treatment of urinary incontinence: a randomized controlled trial. Obstet Gynecol [Internet]. 2007;109(1):4–11. Available from: http://www.ncbi.nlm.nih.gov/pubmed/17197581.

88. Meschia M, Bertozzi R, Pifarotti P, Baccichet R, Bernasconi F, Guercio E, et al. Peri-operative morbidity and early results of a randomised trial comparing TVT and TVT-O. Int Urogynecol J Pelvic Floor Dysfunct [Internet]. 2007;18(11):1257–61. Available from: http://www.ncbi.nlm.nih.gov/pubmed/17345002.

89. de Leval J. Novel surgical technique for the treatment of female stress urinary incontinence: transobturator vaginal tape inside-out. Eur Urol [Internet]. 2003;44(6):724–30. Available from: http://www.ncbi.nlm.nih.gov/pubmed/14644127.

90. Neuman M, Sosnovski V, Goralnik S, Diker B, Bornstein J. Comparison of two inside-out transobturator suburethral sling techniques for stress incontinence: early postoperative thigh pain and 3-year outcomes. Int J Urol [Internet]. 2012;19(12):1103–7. Available from: http://www.ncbi.nlm.nih.gov/pubmed/22882761.

91. Giberti C, Gallo F, Cortese P, Schenone M. Transobturator tape for treatment of female stress urinary incontinence: objective and subjective results after a mean follow-up of two years. Urology [Internet]. 2007;69(4):703–7. Available from: http://www.ncbi.nlm.nih.gov/pubmed/17445655.

92. Thomas TN, Siff LN, Jelovsek JE, Barber M. Surgical pain after transobturator and retropubic midurethral sling placement. Obstet Gynecol [Internet]. 2017;130(1):118–25. Available from: http://www.ncbi.nlm.nih.gov/pubmed/28594776.

93. Fuentes JL, Finsterbusch C, Christie AL, Zimmern PE. Mesh sling arm removal for persistent pain after an initial vaginal suburethral mesh sling removal procedure. Female Pelvic Med Reconstr Surg [Internet]. 2020. Available from: http://www.ncbi.nlm.nih.gov/pubmed/33208654.

94. Hou JC, Alhalabi F, Lemack GE, Zimmern PE. Outcome of transvaginal mesh and tape removed for pain only. J Urol [Internet]. 2014;192(3):856–60. Available from: http://www.ncbi.nlm.nih.gov/pubmed/24735934.

95. Ismail S, Chartier-Kastler E, Reus C, Cohen J, Seisen T, Phé V. Functional outcomes of synthetic tape and mesh revision surgeries: a monocentric experience. Int Urogynecol J [Internet]. 2019;30(5):805–13. Available from: http://www.ncbi.nlm.nih.gov/pubmed/30069725.

96. Tijdink MM, Vierhout ME, Heesakkers JP, Withagen MIJ. Surgical management of mesh-related complications after prior pelvic floor reconstructive surgery with mesh. Int Urogynecol J [Internet]. 2011;22(11):1395–1404. Available from: http://link.springer.com/10.1007/s00192-011-1476-2.

97. Wolff GF, Winters JC, Krlin RM. Mesh excision: is total mesh excision necessary? Curr Urol Rep [Internet]. 2016;17(4):34. Available from: http://www.ncbi.nlm.nih.gov/pubmed/26905696.

98. Shah NM, Jackson LA, Phelan JN, Corton MM. Medial thigh anatomy in female cadavers: clinical applications to the transobturator midurethral sling. Female Pelvic Med Reconstr Surg [Internet]. 2020;26(9):531–5. Available from: http://www.ncbi.nlm.nih.gov/pubmed/30045054.

99. Kuuva N, Nilsson CG. A nationwide analysis of complications associated with the tension-free vaginal tape (TVT) procedure. Acta Obstet Gynecol Scand [Internet]. 2002;81(1):72–77. Available from: http://doi.wiley.com/10.1034/j.1600-0412.2002.810113.x.

100. Corona R, De Cicco C, Schonman R, Verguts J, Ussia A, Koninckx PR. Tension-free vaginal tapes and pelvic nerve neuropathy. J Minim Invasive Gynecol [Internet]. 15(3):262–7. Available from: http://www.ncbi.nlm.nih.gov/pubmed/18439494.

101. Aydogmus S, Kelekci S, Aydogmus H, Ekmekci E, Secil Y, Ture S. Obturator nerve injury: an infrequent complication of TOT procedure. Case Rep Obstet Gynecol [Internet]. 2014;2014:290382. Available from: http://www.ncbi.nlm.nih.gov/pubmed/25343052.

102. Lee SH, Jung JH, Chung WS, Park YY, Yoon H. Obturator nerve injury complicating a tension-free vaginal tape. BJU Int [Internet]. 2003;92(Suppl 3):e12. Available from: http://www.ncbi.nlm.nih.gov/pubmed/19125469.

103. Monga M, Ghoniem GM. Ilioinguinal nerve entrapment following needle bladder suspension procedures. Urology [Internet]. 1994;44(3):447–50. Available from: http://www.ncbi.nlm.nih.gov/pubmed/8073565.

104. Miyazaki F, Shook G. Ilioinguinal nerve entrapment during needle suspension for stress incontinence. Obstet Gynecol [Internet]. 1992;80(2):246–8. Available from: http://www.ncbi.nlm.nih.gov/pubmed/1635738.

105. Kelly MJ, Zimmern PE, Leach GE. Complications of bladder neck suspension procedures. Urol Clin N Am [Internet]. 1991;18(2):339–8. Available from: http://www.ncbi.nlm.nih.gov/pubmed/2017815.

106. Geis K, Dietl J. Ilioinguinal nerve entrapment after Tension-free Vaginal Tape (TVT) Procedure. Int Urogynecol J [Internet]. 2002;13(2):136–138. Available from: http://link.springer.com/10.1007/s001920200029.

107. Nager C, Tulikangas P, Miller D, Rovner E, Goldman H. Position statement on mesh midurethral slings for stress urinary incontinence. Female Pelvic Med Reconstr Surg [Internet]. 2014;20(3):123–125. Available from: http://journals.lww.com/01436319-201405000-00001.

108. Devices CF, Health R. Urogynecologic surgical mesh implants-considerations about surgical mesh for SUI. [Internet]. Available from: http://www.fda.gov/MedicalDevices/ProductsandMedicalProcedures/ImplantsandProsthetics/UroGynSurgicalMesh/ucm345219.htm.

109. Haylen BT, Freeman RM, Swift SE, Cosson M, Davila GW, Deprest J, et al. An International Urogynecological Association (IUGA)/International Continence Society (ICS) joint terminology and classification of the complications related directly to the insertion of prostheses (meshes, implants, tapes) and grafts in female pelvic flo. Neurourol Urodyn [Internet]. 2011;30(1):2–12. Available from: http://www.ncbi.nlm.nih.gov/pubmed/21181958.

110. Clemons JL, Weinstein M, Guess MK, Alperin M, Moalli P, Gregory WT, et al. Impact of the 2011 FDA transvaginal mesh safety update on AUGS members' use of synthetic mesh and biologic grafts in pelvic reconstructive surgery. Female Pelvic Med Reconstr Surg [Internet]. 19(4):191–8. Available from: http://www.ncbi.nlm.nih.gov/pubmed/23797515.

111. Osborn DJ, Dmochowski RR, Harris CJ, Danford JJ, Kaufman MR, Mock S, et al. Analysis of patient and technical factors associated with midurethral sling mesh exposure and perforation. Int J Urol [Internet]. 2014;21(11):1167–70. Available from: http://www.ncbi.nlm.nih.gov/pubmed/25039945.

112. Giusto LL, Zahner PM, Goldman HB. Management of the exposed or perforated midurethral sling. Urol Clin N Am [Internet]. 2019;46(1):31–40. Available from: http://www.ncbi.nlm.nih.gov/pubmed/30466700.

113. Linder BJ, El-Nashar SA, Carranza Leon DA, Trabuco EC. Predictors of vaginal mesh exposure after midurethral sling placement: a case-control study. Int Urogynecol J [Internet]. 2016;27(9):1321–6. Available from: http://www.ncbi.nlm.nih.gov/pubmed/26811112.

114. Kokanalı MK, Cavkaytar S, Kokanalı D, Aksakal O, Doganay M. A comperative study for short-term surgical outcomes of midurethral sling procedures in obese and non-obese women with stress urinary incontinence. J Obstet Gynaecol [Internet]. 2016;36(8):1080–5. Available from: http://www.ncbi.nlm.nih.gov/pubmed/27759469.

115. Velemir L, Amblard J, Jacquetin B, Fatton B. Urethral erosion after suburethral synthetic slings: risk factors, diagnosis, and functional outcome after surgical management. Int Urogynecol J Pelvic Floor Dysfunct [Internet]. 2008;19(7):999–1006. Available from: http://www.ncbi.nlm.nih.gov/pubmed/18202812.

116. Withagen MI, Vierhout ME, Hendriks JC, Kluivers KB, Milani AL. Risk factors for exposure, pain, and dyspareunia after tension-free vaginal mesh procedure. Obstet Gynecol [Internet]. 2011;118(3):629–36. Available from: http://www.ncbi.nlm.nih.gov/pubmed/21860293.

117. Petri E, Ashok K. Partner dyspareunia--a report of six cases. Int Urogynecol J [Internet]. 2012;23(1):127–9. Available from: http://www.ncbi.nlm.nih.gov/pubmed/21800200.

118. Bergersen A, Hinkel C, Funk J, Twiss CO. Management of vaginal mesh exposure: a systematic review. Arab J Urol [Internet]. 2019;17(1):40–8. Available from: http://www.ncbi.nlm.nih.gov/pubmed/31258942.

119. Richter HE, Albo ME, Zyczynski HM, Kenton K, Norton PA, Sirls LT, et al. Retropubic versus transobturator midurethral slings for stress incontinence. N Engl J Med [Internet]. 2010;362(22):2066–76. Available from: http://www.ncbi.nlm.nih.gov/pubmed/20479459.

120. Abbott S, Unger CA, Evans JM, Jallad K, Mishra K, Karram MM, et al. Evaluation and management of complications from synthetic mesh after pelvic reconstructive surgery: a multi-center study. Am J Obstet Gynecol [Internet]. 2014;210(2):163.e1–8. Available from: http://www.ncbi.nlm.nih.gov/pubmed/24126300.

121. Giri SK, Sil D, Narasimhulu G, Flood HD, Skehan M, Drumm J. Management of vaginal extrusion after tension-free vaginal tape procedure for urodynamic stress incontinence. Urology [Internet]. 2007;69(6):1077–80. Available from: http://www.ncbi.nlm.nih.gov/pubmed/17572190.

122. Kim SY, Park JY, Kim HK, Park CH, Kim SJ, Sung GT, et al. Vaginal mucosal flap as a sling preservation for the treatment of vaginal exposure of mesh. Korean J Urol [Internet]. 2010;51(6):416–9. Available from: http://www.ncbi.nlm.nih.gov/pubmed/20577609.

123. Karmakar D, Dwyer PL, Nikpoor P. Mid-urethral sling revision for mesh exposure-long-term outcomes of two surgical techniques from a comparative clinical retrospective cohort study. BJOG [Internet]. 2020;127(8):1027–33. Available from: http://www.ncbi.nlm.nih.gov/pubmed/32107882.

124. Jambusaria LH, Heft J, Reynolds WS, Dmochowski R, Biller DH. Incontinence rates after midurethral sling revision for vaginal exposure or pain. Am J Obstet Gynecol [Internet]. 2016;215(6):764.e1–5. Available from: http://www.ncbi.nlm.nih.gov/pubmed/27448731.

125. Koelbl H, Stoerer S, Seliger G, Wolters M. Transurethral penetration of a tension-free vaginal tape. BJOG [Internet]. 2001;108(7):763–5. Available from: http://www.ncbi.nlm.nih.gov/pubmed/11467707.

126. Novara G, Galfano A, Boscolo-Berto R, Secco S, Cavalleri S, Ficarra V, et al. Complication rates of tension-free midurethral slings in the treatment of female stress urinary incontinence: a systematic review and meta-analysis of randomized controlled trials comparing tension-free midurethral tapes to other surgical procedures and d. Eur Urol [Internet]. 2008;53(2):288–308. Available from: http://www.ncbi.nlm.nih.gov/pubmed/18031923.

127. Karim SS, Pietropaolo A, Skolarikos A, Aboumarzouk O, Kallidonis P, Tailly T, et al. Role of endoscopic management in synthetic sling/mesh erosion following previous incontinence surgery: a systematic review from European Association of Urologists Young Academic Urologists (YAU) and Uro-technology (ESUT) groups. Int Urogynecol J [Internet]. 2020;31(1):45–53. Available from: http://www.ncbi.nlm.nih.gov/pubmed/31468095.

128. Misrai V, Rouprêt M, Xylinas E, Cour F, Vaessen C, Haertig A, et al. Surgical resection for suburethral sling complications after treatment for stress urinary incontinence. J Urol [Internet]. 2009;181(5):2198–202; discussion 2203. Available from: http://www.ncbi.nlm.nih.gov/pubmed/19296973.

129. Macedo FIB, O'Connor J, Mittal VK, Hurley P. Robotic removal of eroded vaginal mesh into the bladder. Int J Urol [Internet]. 2013;20(11):1144–6. Available from: http://www.ncbi.nlm.nih.gov/pubmed/23600850.

130. Thiagamoorthy G, Srikrishna S, Cardozo L. Sexual function after urinary incontinence surgery. Maturitas [Internet]. 2015;81(2):243–7. Available from: http://www.ncbi.nlm.nih.gov/pubmed/25899565.

131. Hilliges M, Falconer C, Ekman-Ordeberg G, Johansson O. Innervation of the human vaginal mucosa as revealed by PGP 9.5 immunohistochemistry. Acta Anat (Basel) [Internet]. 1995;153(2):119–26. Available from: http://www.ncbi.nlm.nih.gov/pubmed/8560964.

132. Zivkovic F, Tamussino K, Ralph G, Schied G, Auer-Grumbach M. Long-term effects of vaginal dissection on the innervation of the striated urethral sphincter. Obstet Gynecol [Internet]. 1996;87(2):257–60. Available from: http://www.ncbi.nlm.nih.gov/pubmed/8559535.

133. Lemack GE, Zimmern PE. Sexual function after vaginal surgery for stress incontinence: results of a mailed questionnaire. Urology [Internet]. 2000;56(2):223–227. Available from: https://linkinghub.elsevier.com/retrieve/pii/S0090429500006269.

134. Cayan F, Dilek S, Akbay E, Cayan S. Sexual function after surgery for stress urinary incontinence: vaginal sling versus Burch colposuspension. Arch Gynecol Obstet [Internet]. 2008;277(1):31–6. Available from: http://www.ncbi.nlm.nih.gov/pubmed/17653739.

135. Mazouni C, Karsenty G, Bretelle F, Bladou F, Gamerre M, Serment G. Urinary complications and sexual function after the tension-free vaginal tape procedure. Acta Obstet Gynecol Scand [Internet]. 2004;83(10):955–961. Available from: http://doi.wiley.com/10.1111/j.0001-634.2004.00524.x.

136. Zyczynski HM, Rickey L, Dyer KY, Wilson T, Stoddard AM, Gormley EA, et al. Sexual activity and function in women more than 2 years after midurethral sling placement. Am J Obstet Gynecol [Internet]. 2012;207(5):421.e1–6. Available from: http://www.ncbi.nlm.nih.gov/pubmed/22840975.

137. Glavind K, Tetsche MS. Sexual function in women before and after suburethral sling operation for stress urinary incontinence: a retrospective questionnaire study. Acta Obstet Gynecol Scand [Internet]. 2004;83(10):965–968. Available from: http://doi.wiley.com/10.1111/j.0001-6349.2004.00555.x.

Chapter 19
Failure of Treatment of Stress Urinary Incontinence

Caroline Dowling and Sandra Elmer

Failed Sling Pathophysiology and Treatment

When a sling fails, it is a devastating moment for the patient and also the surgeon. Expectations for success and normalisation of function are high. Setting of expectations is often inadequate pre-operatively [1].

The analysis of sling failure is also now coloured by the regulatory and practice changes that have occurred in the wake of the Food and Drug Administration (FDA) warning in 2011 and subsequent litigation around synthetic materials or mesh, in the management of Stress Urinary Incontinence (SUI). Local professional bodies [2] continue to include synthetic mid-urethral slings (MUS) for primary SUI in their algorithms, but clinical practice and the regulatory bodies [3] have moved away from the use of the mesh MUS, particularly the transobturator route and repeating a synthetic sling in the event of failure.

The analysis of failure of slings to treat SUI is hampered by a lack of quality systematic data and the incomplete understanding of how slings fundamentally work. It is recognised that successful surgery for SUI is associated with increased urethral resistance based on urodynamic parameters such as Q_{max}, bladder outlet

C. Dowling (✉)
Eastern Health, Department of Urology, Box Hill, VIC, Australia

Monash University, Eastern Health Clinical School, Level 2, Box Hill, VIC, Australia

Epworth Healthcare, Richmond, VIC, Australia
e-mail: caroline@urologyworks.com

S. Elmer
Epworth Healthcare, Richmond, VIC, Australia

Department of Urology, Royal Melbourne Hospital, Parkville, VIC, Australia

Department of Urology, Austin Health, Heidelberg, VIC, Australia

343

obstructive index (BOOI), increased pDet and increased post void residual (PVR), suggesting that success relies on the creation of obstructive voiding [4].

Recent advances in the research field of urethral function [5] are an important reminder that the understanding of the mechanism of a sling is incomplete. Historically, the emphasis has been on the interplay of correction of urethral hypermobility and intrinsic sphincter deficiency (ISD) with more focus on the mobility of the urethra as the key mechanism. This becomes a challenge in the recurrent case where the hypermobility has been corrected.

Definition of Failure

Failure can be defined as either the persistence of SUI subjectively or objectively post-operatively, the recurrence of SUI (rSUI) where patient was dry for 6 weeks or more, the emergence of urge incontinence (de novo overactive bladder or OAB) or complications including obstruction and voiding dysfunction and those specific to synthetic materials, exposure, erosion and pain [6–8].

Escobar [9] in a comprehensive recent review of urodynamics in the assessment of failure includes both rSUI, new or worsening OAB and de novo voiding dysfunction or bladder outflow obstruction (BOO) as the three definitions of failure. For the purposes of this chapter, we will address rSUI (including persistent) and de novo OAB. Voiding dysfunction, pain and mesh-specific complications have been dealt with in Chap. 18.

Whether failure or recurrence is being reported needs to be examined when looking at outcomes of secondary procedures, and failure is considered when occurring prior to 12 months post-operatively and recurrence beyond this time [6]. The rate of failure at 5-year follow-up is highly variable and has been reported to lie between 8% and 57% [7], and more than 50% of patients who were retreated in the Stress Incontinence Surgical Treatment Efficacy Trial (SISTeR) and transobturator MUS (TOMUS) trials were retreated within the first year [10]. A figure of around 15% seems useful and reflective. It is important to also remember that very few patients who have recurrent urinary incontinence have actual isolated rSUI on presentation [11].

Patients lose faith in their surgeon in the event of failure, particularly if there is a perception of inadequate evaluation. This may impact the figures around the frequency of failure [12].

Pathophysiology of Failure

The causes of failure in terms of rSUI are incompletely understood, but most failures to treat SUI have elements of persistent intrinsic sphincter deficiency (ISD), urethral hypermobility and mixed symptoms. Previous anti-incontinence surgery itself is an independent risk factor for failure [13].

There are published risk factors for sling failure. Stav [14] demonstrated that there is an increased risk in patients with a body mass index (BMI) >25, those with mixed symptoms pre-operatively, those who have had previous surgery for SUI, those who are diabetics and those with the presence of ISD pre-operatively. Stav found that concomitant surgery for pelvic organ prolapse (POP) was associated with a lesser risk of failure, but most other studies see concomitant surgery as an increased risk [14]. A 2013 systematic review by Pradhan [15] on the efficacy of the MUS in the treatment of recurrent SUI showed that risk factors for recurrent or persistent urinary incontinence after surgical treatment include age, obesity, medical comorbidities (e.g. diabetes mellitus), previous high-grade incontinence, mixed urinary incontinence and previous failed surgery.

Richter demonstrated in a study of over 600 women that prior SUI surgery, maximum Q tip excursion and severity by pad weight were all independent risk factors for failure [16]. This large randomised study of transobturator MUS versus retropubic MUS (TOMUS study) corroborates the Stav finding of mixed symptoms as risks for failure and additionally notes the presence of increased pad weight, age and increased severity scores on pre-operative assessment [16, 17].

The position of the sling relative to the urethral length has been shown to influence the risk of failure. Bogusiewicz showed in a study on a transobturator-based sling that more proximal placement was associated with a higher rate of failure [18]. The relationship to the symphysis has also been examined with ultrasound showing a benefit in one study of closer placement of the TVT to the symphysis [19]. Several further studies have attempted to correlate ultrasound findings post sling such as dynamic compression, which if absent may indicate loosening, distances from sling to urethra and sling to pubis, with clinical outcomes, but have largely been inconclusive, and the techniques are evolving and their current applications are best studied and used in experienced centres [20].

The Ghoniem review examined the mechanics of Autologous Fascial Sling (AFS) in management of SUI with videourodynamics and showed the AFS is required to compress the urethra during activity [21]. Hence, its position along the urethra and the tension is relevant with overtension also more relevant than lack of tension.

Management of Failure

The management of rSUI, regardless of material, should proceed stepwise through a careful evaluation of the history with emphasis on the onset, severity (subjective pad use) and characterisation of current symptoms and the difference to the pre-operative symptoms, and determine if the correct type of incontinence was treated in the first instance. The degree of bother is very important. The type of surgery, approach, synthetic implant used, preferably with the original operation report in hand, and the pre-operative urodynamics, if present, should be reassessed. Bladder diaries and standardised questionnaires (e.g. International Consultation on Incontinence Questionnaire (ICIQ)) are recommended [7].

Examination of the patient should include assessment of urethral mobility (though standardisation of this is not established), presence and degree of POP, objective evidence of SUI on cough stress test, presence of Genitourinary Syndrome of Menopause (GSM), attention to the unique issues of MUS including extrusion, erosion and pain, and the assessment of any neurological symptoms. The patients should be examined with a comfortably full bladder, and an objective assessment of SUI with cough and Valsalva made. A comprehensive discussion of the methods of assessing patient's post failure is provided in excellent reviews by Escobar [9] and Fontenot [22]. The use of validated tools for these assessments is key for reproducibility.

Whilst mandatory pre-operative urodynamics in SUI surgery are a point of controversy as neatly summarised in the review by Clarke [23], the importance of their existence becomes obvious in the event of failure. The ability to review pre-operative urodynamics suddenly becomes highly relevant. Failure is associated with a lower abdominal leak point pressure on urodynamics as demonstrated by several authors, and the failure to recognise this prior to primary surgery inherently increases the risk of a poor outcome [24]. A continuing search for urodynamic predictors of success or failure continues, and a recent publication on the utility of the bladder volume at first leakage as a predictor of poor outcome demonstrates this [25]. The specifics of the urodynamics study are well detailed by Escobar and Brucker [9] but should include a subtracted study assessing for the SUI itself and an assessment for ISD but also the presence of detrusor overactivity and the impact on voiding. Urodynamics after failed surgery are recommended by the National Institute for Health and Care Excellence (NICE) guidelines [26].

Investigations should include as a minimum the assessment of the PVR and a mid-stream urine (MSU) analysis for microscopy and culture. The addition of flexible cystoscopy or cystoscopy with a 70-degree lens to adequately inspect the bladder neck particularly in the case of previous MUS [6, 27] depends then on the complexity, concerns about the possibility of presence of perforation of mesh into bladder, the findings of the PVR and the patient's motivation for further surgery [28]. Imaging to look at MUS position relative to the mid urethra to guide if there is sling misplacement and raise the option of a repeat sling [29] is supported by international guidelines [26, 30]. The surgeon should then be able to make judgements about the possible reasons for failure based on these assessments and undertake shared decision making with the patient as to the best way forward. This is done with the understanding of incomplete evidence to guide this decision making and rapid changes in local guidelines and regulatory arrangements around synthetic slings in particular. The recent publication in the Cochrane Database [31] reaches the sobering conclusion that despite the vast numbers of MUS placed, there is an absence of any evidence comparing the management alternatives in the event of failure and that "clinicians must largely rely on expert opinion and personal experience" [31].

De Novo OAB

De novo OAB occurs in approximately 9% of patients post sling surgery and has not been systematically demonstrated to occur more frequently in one sling approach versus another [32]. De novo OAB is a troubling symptom associated with lower quality-of-life scores post-operatively [33]. The mechanism for de novo OAB in the absence of obstruction, infection and mesh exposure is poorly understood but an interruption to the autonomic innervation as a result of surgical dissection has been postulated. There is no doubt held by surgeons who place slings that this symptom is associated with a high rate of patient dissatisfaction. There are identifiable risk factors that should be considered such as age, previous surgery for SUI, increased parity and caesarean section delivery and previous anticholinergic therapy that increase the risk of post-operative OAB [34].

The management of de novo OAB should proceed stepwise through a careful evaluation as outlined previously with particular attention to the timing of symptoms to determine that they are de novo and not pre-existing, and that important causal pathologies such as hormonal status, neurological pathologies, urinary tract infection, stones and pelvic organ prolapse. The history and examination should be focussed on these conditions.

All patients should have urinalysis and an assessment of their PVR. In the event of an uncomplicated picture after these and the clinical assessment, it is reasonable to trial first- and second-line therapy for OAB as one would in an index case as there is an expected high rate of spontaneous resolution [34].

Cystoscopy and urodynamics should be used in those cases where BOO, foreign body/mesh perforation into bladder, previously unrecognised neurology, is suspected. Urodynamics should proceed with fluoroscopy when BOO is suspected and attention to slowing the fill in the case of suspected detrusor overactivity.

Treatment of de novo OAB post sling with second-line anticholinergic medications has been studied and shown to be effective [35]. Beta-3 medication has not been systematically studied or shown to be as effective but is safe to be trialled with the same caveats that would be applied in the index case. Third-line therapy post sling for de novo OAB is also hampered by a paucity of data, in the case of Onabotulinum Toxin A. Miotla [36] compared 53 idiopathic and 49 post MUS treated with 100 units of Onabotulinum Toxin A and demonstrated similar outcomes in terms of success. There were 4 patients who required intermittent self-catheterisation for incomplete bladder emptying that was symptomatic, and of these, 3 were in the sling group; however, these are too smaller numbers to draw firm conclusions. Sacral neuromodulation has been less well studied, but it was shown that a trial was more likely to be successful in younger patients (under 65 years old) and within 4 years of sling placement [37].

The Treatment of the Failed Sling with Recurrent SUI

Conservative and Medical Therapy

In the event of rSUI, treatment should begin with discussion of conservative measures such as weight loss, pelvic floor exercises, continence pessaries and oestrogen replacement. The evidence for this is largely extrapolated from the treatment of primary SUI and is not well studied in the context of failure. The Society of

Obstetrics and Gynaecology of Canada recommends conservative measures as first-line management in recurrent SUI [38]. There is however no consensus on the role of physiotherapy after failed surgery, and this area needs further research. Some experts have expressed it is unfair to ask women to do this again, whilst other expert opinions state it should be revisited [7], and there is some evidence in mild cases of rSUI that it is effective [15]. Conservative measures, however, are not as effective as surgery and should be mainly considered in women who decline, or are otherwise not candidates for, surgery or have very mild symptoms.

Duloxetine has been approved in Europe for the treatment of SUI and has been shown to be effective for SUI in women [39], but the associated harms in its side effects, particularly gastrointestinal and psychiatric, are reported to outweigh the benefits [40]. The NICE guidelines recommend that Duloxetine should not be used as a first-line treatment or routinely offered as a second-line treatment for SUI, given that pelvic floor muscle training is more effective and less costly than Duloxetine and that surgery is more cost effective than Duloxetine [26, 28]. The use of off-label imipramine to increase sphincter tone has been discouraged due to its cardiac side effects [22].

Surgical Management of Recurrent SUI

The decision to undertake repeat surgery for rSUI must be shared between patient and surgeon and well counselled. The results from repeat surgery are universally lesser than for primary surgery [13, 41]. The balance of risks of the repeat surgery versus benefits should be carefully considered. The use of a repeat synthetic MUS has fallen out of favour, despite outperforming urethral bulking agents (UBA) and sling manipulation, due to the increasing realisation of the risks of the use of synthetic materials, particularly repetitively, and the magnitude of litigation since the FDA warnings. The advent of newer materials for UBA has made this a more appealing and low-risk choice for management. The AFS in a 2015 review [42] found to have a 79.3% pooled success rate and was the first choice of surgeons for failures in the TOMUS trial [10].

Studies of management options in rSUI from 2014 showed then that most urogynaecologists would choose a second MUS, and urologists will in 27% of cases recommend an AFS [28]. Urogynaecologists studied favoured repeat retropubic MUS and urethral bulking agents (UBA) as their preferred option for salvage after a failed MUS in 81.5% and 48.6% of respondents. This pattern of practice has changed with the issues around the use of transvaginal synthetic mesh for both POP and SUI management, but that has not yet been well documented aside from an established reduction in the use of synthetic mesh materials [43, 44].

Factors that may influence surgical decision making in rSUI include the presence or absence of urethral hypermobility after the primary procedure, the mean urethral closure pressure (MUCP) and the position of the original sling in the case of a primary MUS [28]. In considering a repeat MUS, synthetic material would not be recommended if the urethral mucosa is breached during dissection (including intentionally such as for diverticulum or fistula repair) or after excision of an eroded synthetic sling [27]. Certain other high-risk groups are now identified where synthetics are best avoided including complex pelvic pain and/or dyspareunia, chronic steroid therapy, previous irradiation or extensive tissue fibrosis and scarring.

It is notable that NICE guidelines in the United Kingdom [26] recommend that women referred for management of a failed anti-incontinence procedure are managed in a tertiary centre by a multidisciplinary team, and this would be consistent with best practice. Ultimately, it is a shared decision and influenced by factors centred around acceptance of a synthetic material and willingness to undertake a major procedure [45]. There is a recognised trade-off between efficacy and morbidity [46].

The surgical options for failed sling management are presented in approximate order of utility with caveats to particular situations for each intervention. Assessment of all of the interventional options is limited by poor-quality studies dominated by case series, short follow-up, heterogeneous populations and historical procedures and devices.

1. *Autologous Fascial Sling (AFS)*
2. *Bulking Agents*
3. *Repeat mid-urethral synthetic sling including adjustable sling*
4. *Colposuspension – laparoscopic or open*
5. *Sling plication and manipulation*
6. *Bladder Neck Suspension techniques*
7. *Spiral or obstructing AFS*
8. *Adjustable Continence Therapy (ACT)*
9. *Stem Cell Treatment*
10. *Artificial Urinary Sphincter*

Autologous Fascial Sling (AFS)

Welk and Herschorn published the first series in 2012 of 33 patients using the AFS post failed MUS. They demonstrated a significant reduction in pad use and good patient satisfaction using a 13×2 cm sling. Publications from 2015 onwards acknowledge the shift in practice due to the controversies surrounding the use of synthetic materials for the management of SUI and POP [29]. There has been a shift towards the AFS as the preferred salvage procedure [21].

The analysis of the AFS as both a primary and secondary treatment for SUI is limited by the varying surgical methods presented in the literature. A large study of 288 women undergoing a McGuire type [47] AFS examined 59 patients within the cohort who had a prior MUS, including 25 who had MUS complications of exposure or obstruction requiring sling lysis. The study showed equivalent subjective and objective outcomes for primary and secondary AFS (59.9% versus 62.4% objective and 66.1% versus 69% subjective cure rates). There were more retention and repeat surgery in the case of the secondary AFS [48].

Milose [49] studied 66 patients having a secondary AFS and showed only a 37.7% objective cure rate but a 69.7% subjective cure. A smaller study by Petrou retrospectively demonstrated that of 21 cases of AFS post sling, 52.4% were dry, and importantly, there was no statistically significant impact of excision of the prior sling [50]. The risk of more serious complications with a larger procedure such as AFS needs to be incorporated into pre-operative counselling with a risk of VTE 0.3% [51].

AFS as compared with retropubic MUS (RP MUS) has been studied in a retrospective series of 224 patients where one-third had an AFS and two-thirds had RP MUS with a patient choice-driven methodology [52]. The primary procedures were all slings, and two-thirds were synthetic MUS. The outcomes for both AFS and MUS secondarily were equivalent at a median follow-up of 29 months, and 61.4% in the synthetic group and 66.1% in the AFS group were described as cured with no significant difference statistically. Six patients in the synthetic group needed a third procedure, an AFS. It is not articulated how many patients overall had a total of two synthetic slings and whether this was a factor in outcome or the development of later mesh-specific complications.

A study published nearly 10 years ago in 2011 that looked at current practice amongst urogynaecologists in the UK in the management of recurrent or persistent SUI post sling showed that 51% would consider an AFS after 2 failed procedures [28]. At the time, it was stated in a review article that the AFS was "unlikely to remain a commonly performed procedure for recurrent SUI after failed MUS" [53]. This is unlikely to be the case in contemporary practice.

The decision to place an AFS at the time of mesh excision or subsequently depends on the presence or absence of SUI at the time of mesh excision and is favoured if there is extensive peri-urethral dissection or when questionable tissue quality is present. The reason for mesh excision also informs the choice. Patients need to be involved in decision making as to a concomitant or staged approach [21], and there are only small series with wide-ranging variables as to the cause for mesh excision published; hence, we are only informed by expert opinion.

Consideration of important clinical and urodynamic factors like incomplete emptying or detrusor underactivity needs to be taken into account when choosing an AFS for management of rSUI given the obstructive nature of slings and the likelihood of worsening emptying further [54]. This coupled with the longer length of surgery and recovery and risk of needing clean intermittent catheterisation (CIC) post-operatively [51] make urethral bulking a legitimate choice for many patients.

Modifications of the traditional McGuire [47] technique are evolving in a bid to make the AFS less morbid and more analogous to its synthetic counterpart. Twenty-six per cent of the patients in Malde's small case series who had a 6 × 1 cm sling via a 3 cm suprapubic incision were for treatment of rSUI [55]. Eighty per cent in the rSUI group of ten cases reported improvement overall, and this was not markedly different to the primary group (82%). Of the entire cohort of 38, de novo OAB occurred in 3, 2 of whom were in the rSUI group. Further modifications including standardised tensioning will improve the outcomes from AFS in the management of primary and rSUI. Recently, Australian data were presented, indicating that post-operative voiding dysfunction can be predicted by the lax sling height when the knotted suture is tented above the rectus fascia. The study concluded that a lax sling height of less than 40 mm was associated with a higher risk of post-operative urinary retention and the need for intermittent self-catheterisation and urethrolysis [56].

Bulking Agents

The assessment of the efficacy of UBA is made difficult by the relatively recent advent of newer agents and their FDA approval. Data on all agents are limited with small single series studies dominating the literature. The agents currently most widely available include carbon-coated zirconium (Durasphere®); calcium hydroxyl apatite (Coaptite®); polydimethylsiloxane elastomer (Macroplastique®) and poly-acrylamide hydrogel (PAHG, Bulkamid®). The latest product, PDMS-U (Urolastic®), is a silicone gel that polymerises when injected.

The optimal UBA will be biocompatible, durable, non-migratory and hypoal-lergenic, whilst evoking healing with minimal scarring. With this in mind, PAHG has the greatest utility. In the rSUI population in an observational study of 60 women including around a third with mixed symptoms or ISD, PAHG treatment was associated with an 83.6% rate of cure or improved at 12 months as defined by a negative cough stress test or pad weigh less than 2 gm [57]. Durability is always the question with UBA. The longest follow-up for PAHG in a primary population is two-year follow-up, which demonstrated a sustained response [58]. Long-term evidence is available and demonstrates durable efficacy. Data suggest that 80% of patients cured or improved at 7 years when Bulkamid® was used as first-line treatment for SUI [59]. Three-year follow-up data from a UK study demonstrated 82% cure/significant improvement at 3 months, results that were maintained at final follow-up [60].

Older agents such as silicone-based Macroplastique® have a risk of exposure with resultant stone formation, recurrent urinary tract infection and difficulty removing the agent that is rarely captured in the short-term literature [61]. Macroplastique® as a salvage agent had a published cure rate of around 35% at less than one-year follow-up in small series (23 women), but 77% of patients were said to be satisfied with the result [62]. In the series by Dray [11], 71% of patients experienced a positive response to either Macroplastique® or collagen which was durable to a mean of 35 months. Interestingly, more than 50% of the cohort had a BMI greater than 30, and more than half the cohorts were followed to 40 months. Only 12.3% of patients went on to further surgery with the majority undertaking an AFS. Similar results were achieved in a retrospective review of Macroplastique® with a second injection often required to achieve subjective improvement of 83% with a mean follow-up of 46.4 months in a population that had their sling removed prior to injection, which refutes the theory that the presence of the sling supports the injectable and improves its efficacy, but this has not been systematically studied [63]. Collagen (glutaralde-hyde-treated bovine collagen) was withdrawn worldwide in 2011 due to its tendency to be reabsorbed and lead to recurrence of symptoms [64]. Durasphere® has been studied post sling in 74 patients with a success rate of 40% [65].

Comparison of UBA (67 patients) versus repeat MUS (165) in a retrospective cohort study showed a failure rate of 38.8% in the UBA group versus 11.2% in the MUS group [66]. Accepting the limitations of the study design, a balanced discussion needs to take place with patients as to the accepted risks of repeat sling versus slightly lowered efficacy in the UBA group, again rationalising the complex relationship of the efficacy/morbidity trade-off [46].

Based on these overall poor outcomes, Kavanagh in 2017 [66] suggested UBA should not be used except in the elderly or where there was contraindication to a further sling. As with the comments on the demise of the AFS, this no longer likely mirrors contemporary practice, and American Urological Association (AUA) guidelines recommend UBA as an option which offers the patient lesser recovery time and less invasive surgery but that patients should be counselled over the success rates and risk of repeat treatment [27].

Repeat Mid-urethral Synthetic Sling Including Using an Adjustable Sling

The vogue for repeat MUS is diminishing with time. Several studies were published in previous years, and the large landmark series by Stav [41] with 1100 patients, 77 of which were repeat slings, demonstrated the superiority of the retropubic (RP) approach in repeat surgery over the transobturator (TO) route. The same group published the improved outcome for the RP route in the treatment of ISD, often a causal event in failed initial treatment [67]. This was corroborated in a retrospective study of 637 patients with ISD, which showed that a secondary TO MUS was associated with a 12 times increased risk of failure [6].

In the event of a second MUS, inherently a high-risk situation for rSUI, the TO route cannot be recommended [40, 68, 69]. A review examining some 10 retrospective series showed widely varying success (40–100% success) and much lesser efficacy than primary treatment and supports the recommendation of the RP route in repeat management [7]. The 2017 Cochrane Review found that RP MUS lowers the risk of reoperation in ISD in the primary case [70].

Contrary to this, Abdel-Fattah in a sub-analysis of a larger TO sling study with 9-year follow-up looked at 46 patients who had a TO sling as a secondary procedure and found on PGI-I the outcome compared favourably with the primary cohort with 62% success on this criterion. However, the study showed high rates of groin pain and erosion in the small cohort and was limited by numbers and only 63% of the group having the full 9 years of follow-up available [71].

The presence of unmanaged urethral hypermobility makes sense in predicting those who may benefit from a second sling-based procedure, whether that be synthetic or AFS. It is suggested that the more severe groups post sling failure are managed with AFS, but this will likely involve a trade off with voiding function and a higher complication rate and longer recovery and therefore needs clear counselling [7]. Women who were followed for an 11-year period after repeat MUS post a failed

Burch or MUS had a subjective cure rate of 67% and an objective cure rate of 65% with satisfactory quality-of-life scores and a 78% perception of success on a PGI-I [72].

Owing to the fine line between overtensioning a sling and undertreating SUI, the concept of an adjustable sling has held appeal. However, these slings have not gained widespread use in either primary or recurrent incontinence. Their use has been reported in the recurrent case in a retrospective series in 102 women and a mean follow-up over 2 years [73]. A validated severity index for incontinence was used to evaluate the outcome, and 87.2% achieved satisfaction. This seems high compared with non-adjustable sling literature but with small numbers, retrospective design and a need for delayed sling adjustment in almost 14%, this technique requires further evaluation before being adopted mainstream. The European Guidelines of 2018 recommend these slings are only used in a trial setting [30].

The role of mesh removal prior to the secondary MUS surgery should be considered in the context of the individual case. If there is no complication related to the synthetic mesh material, there is no indication for its removal at the time of rSUI surgery and no direction from the literature in this regard [68]. Two series where removal was undertaken prior to second sling showed comparable outcomes for the secondary sling, but there is insufficient literature to be certain if this is required and should be a consideration on a case-by-case basis and in the context of any complications such as mesh exposure [46, 74]. Given the rates are similar when compared with a repeat MUS without removal, it is hard to justify removal of the primary sling in absence of specific mesh complications.

At this point, it is relevant to give pause and consider the three main options for surgical management of rSUI, the AFS, UBA and MUS, which are the most likely procedures to be offered [22, 27]. It is evident that these procedures are very different to one another, and decision making for patients and clinicians alike is difficult. The use of scientific infographics (Fig. 19.1) for decision making in clinical practice may assist with this process and allow patients to understand visually the considerations of their recovery time, their other co-morbidities, the presence of ISD, the original procedure undertaken and whether they are willing to have mesh again or for the first time, the presence of complicating issues such as radiation, fistula or excessive scarring, previous abdominal surgery and OAB and if they are needing to consider a tight sling and permanent clean intermittent catheterisation (CIC). Clear indications for AFS over a repeat synthetic MUS include pain, mesh erosion or fistula [13]. Surgeons are more likely to recommend a repeat MUS but women are more likely to exclude the procedure which already failed from their list of options, by numbers alone this is more likely to be a MUS [75].

Colposuspension: Laparoscopic or Open

The literature on the use of colposuspension techniques for salvage is sufficiently sparse that the approach is excluded from major guidelines [27]. A study of 16 women with recurrent SUI described a 55% objective and 93% subjective sure rate

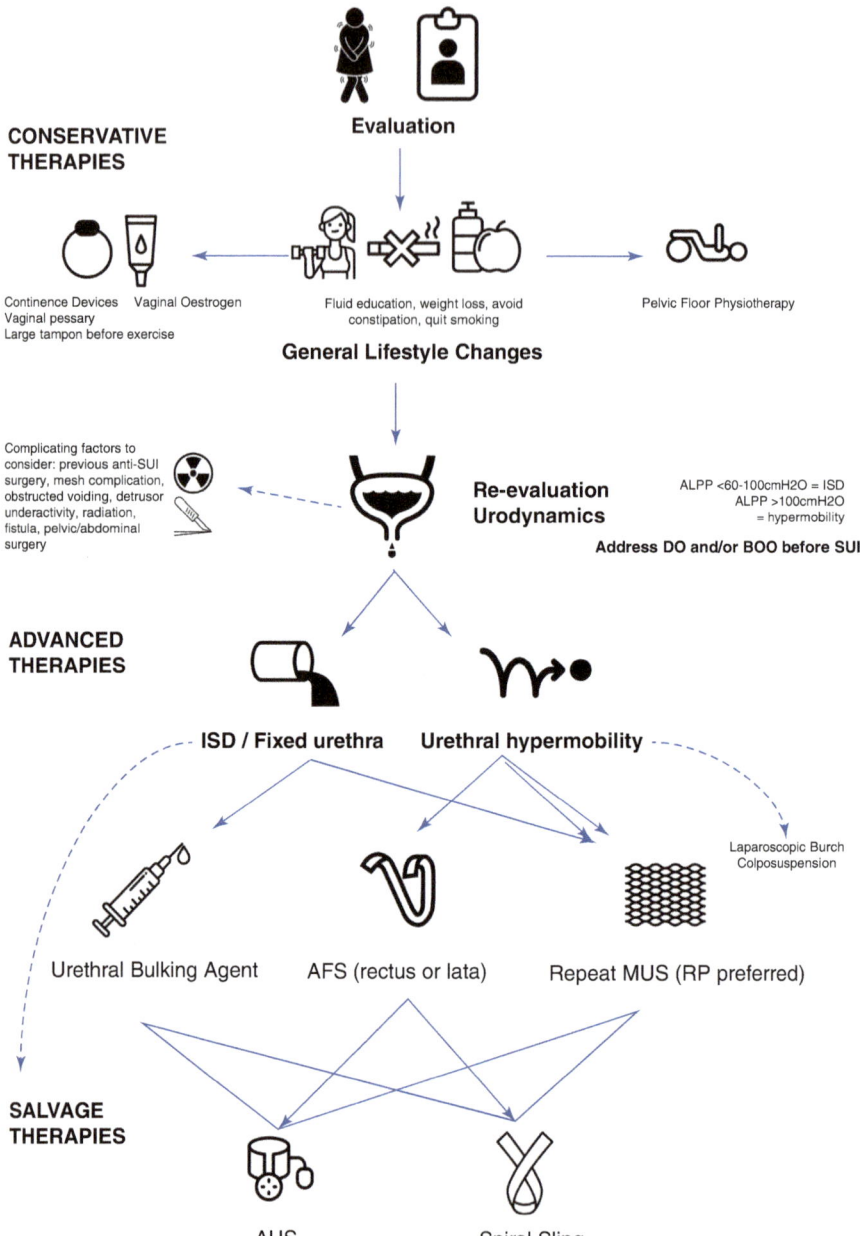

CONSERVATIVE THERAPIES

Continence Devices   Vaginal Oestrogen
Vaginal pessary
Large tampon before exercise

Evaluation

Fluid education, weight loss, avoid
constipation, quit smoking

General Lifestyle Changes

Pelvic Floor Physiotherapy

Complicating factors to
consider: previous anti-SUI
surgery, mesh complication,
obstructed voiding, detrusor
underactivity, radiation,
fistula, pelvic/abdominal
surgery

**Re-evaluation
Urodynamics**

ALPP <60-100cmH2O = ISD
ALPP >100cmH2O
= hypermobility

Address DO and/or BOO before SUI

ADVANCED THERAPIES

ISD / Fixed urethra   Urethral hypermobility

Laparoscopic Burch
Colposuspension

Urethral Bulking Agent   AFS (rectus or lata)   Repeat MUS (RP preferred)

SALVAGE THERAPIES

AUS   Spiral Sling

Fig. 19.1 Failed sling and recurrent stress incontinence

after open colposuspension with the initial failed procedure poorly defined [76]. Giarenis in 2011 published open colposuspension after failed MUS and demonstrated an objective cure rate of 77% and subjective rate of 85% [40]. The pooled analysis in the Nikolopoulos review showed an objective cure rate of 76% [42]. The open Burch colposuspension is invasive, increases the risk of POP and does not adequately address ISD. Laparoscopic and robotic Burch colposuspension for their minimally invasive approach hold appeal in the presence of ongoing hypermobility and where concomitant POP surgery by that same approach is being performed.

Sling Plication and Manipulation

Small case series have studied the outcome of either plication [77], adjustable techniques using polypropylene [78] or tape shortening [79], but all are limited by their numbers. Five small retrospective series were pooled for an overall success rate of 61% [80] with a higher success rate in the RP group compared with TOT. The lack of data and ongoing publications in this area lead these authors to the same conclusion as Kavanagh [7] who states that sling plication cannot be recommended for failure.

Despite this, the technique continues to be practiced and reported on with a small case series published in 2019 with 36 patients [81], with approximately ¾ RP and ¼ TO and a short duration prior to plication of 6.8 weeks. Success was seen in 76%, and this was statistically significantly predominant in the RP group ($p = 0.034$) and a short follow-up of less than 2 years. A cautious individualised approach would be advised with this option for treatment.

Bladder Neck Suspension Techniques

Bladder neck suspension (BNS) via the vaginal, retropubic or needle approach has been a procedure long practiced but not widely continued. In the era of increasing concerns around synthetic materials, however, a device-free technique to suspend the bladder neck and improve continence during activity has appeal. Using a traditional anterior vaginal wall plication was historically employed but has been shown to have a high failure rate for SUI and has been therefore abandoned [82]. Rashid et al. [29] conclude that BNS may have a role in concomitant anterior vaginal wall prolapse repair, in whom a MUS is contraindicated or in the presence of persistent hypermobility with persistent or rSUI but the technique has been superseded by the MUS and is inferior to AFS or UBA as a salvage technique based on world-wide practice.

Spiral or Obstructing Slings

Spiral and obstructing slings have been used over many years for salvage surgery. The particular subset of patients who fail an initial sling and have a non-mobile or pipe stem urethra pose a challenge for surgical management as it is difficult to achieve urethral compression in the face of fibrosis, denervation and disruption of the peri-urethral fascia. There is also a role for compression of the urethra in a deliberately obstructive way in female patients with neurological conditions who are on CIC and continue to leak urethrally despite good bladder pressure management. The spiral or obstructing sling fashioned from autologous tissue or in some instances synthetic material offers a legitimate alternative to the artificial sphincter or formal bladder neck closure and continent diversion.

In the salvage neurologically intact case, a spiral sling should be considered in patients with low Abdominal Leak Point Pressures (ALPP) <60 cmH$_2$o who are willing and able to CIC. Patients with higher ALPP can be considered where there is concern continence will not be achieved without compression.

Topical vaginal oestrogen as an adjunct peri-operatively should be considered. The pre-operative assessment of patients should otherwise proceed according to the previous recommendations with particular attention to the urodynamic findings of relevance, the ALPP and bladder pressure in the case of a neuropath and the inclusion of EMG and fluoroscopy in these complex cases [83]. This latter case is at risk of upper tract deterioration in the event of unchecked bladder pressure in combination with outflow obstruction produced deliberately by the sling, which will also exacerbate any incontinence driven by detrusor overactivity.

Technical aspects of the procedure include careful attention to urethrolysis prior to sling placement to allow for greatest compression and the sling can be placed with the cross over dorsally or ventrally, relative to the urethra. Sling measurements vary and also depend on if synthetic or autologous material is used. Synthetic materials of 16 × 1 cm were used in one study [84]. In their technique, the urethra was mobilised, and the sling passed dorsally and crossed ventrally and then held with an Allis clamp to prevent over tensioning around the urethra during subsequent passage of the retropubic sling arms. Safe passage dorsally is assisted by close proximity to the periosteum to avoid injuring the urethra or the dorsal venous complex and careful dissection with a small curved Satinsky clamp is advised to achieve this part of the procedure. In reality, many of these cases have had several surgeries and, analogous to the bladder neck artificial urinary sphincter, may require a modified open or laparoscopic or robotic-assisted approach to ensure there is not perforation of other structures and to allow the sling to be placed accurately. There is a high rate of urethral and bladder neck iatrogenic entry during dissection in all series cited.

In the series by Rodriguez, 21 cases had a synthetic sling and 5 an autologous sling and three had their sling placed laterally after cross over (both limbs on one side). Patients had a mean of 3.5 procedures at presentation, 7 pads daily and 90% had an ALPP <60 cmH$_2$O. One of the lateral synthetic slings failed and 5 of the bilateral synthetic slings. Two from each of those failed groups required bulking. None of the autologous cases failed. Mean pad use decreased to 0.9 per day and the mean follow-up period was 15 months. This group was able to maintain spontaneous voiding whilst correcting ISD in all but three cases who required CIC (all from the synthetic group). There was a low rate of de novo OAB [75]. Technically, the authors advise that the tension in the sling arms is critical to keep this low and then rely on the wrap for effect, and the low tension then maintains the voiding capacity.

Similar results were found in 28 women studied with a mean follow-up of 26 months and a polypropylene mesh wrap with a dorsally based cross over with a "cure" of SUI in 71.4% of patients [85].

The original series on spiral slings by Raz and colleagues [86] for urethral incompetence in neurological disease or congenital conditions or iatrogenic injury in multiple failed incontinence surgeries described the spiral sling using a 15×1 cm polypropylene mesh with a soft polyglactin zero suture on each end. Their results are similar for the 40 of the 47 patients followed up at 12 months, 68% success if the 7 lost to follow-up are considered failures. Forty-five per cent reported wearing no pads. Of the 40 patients studied, 3 required subsequent bladder neck closure and continent diversion. Overall, there were no other patients who required CIC.

The mechanism for such a high success rate and maintenance of spontaneous voiding is unclear but postulated to be about supporting the mid urethra and circumferentially coapting with increased abdominal pressure [39]. It would be valuable to know the longer-term outcomes in these patients in terms of voiding function, de novo OAB and mesh-specific complications beyond 12 months and also the management of the mesh in situ prior to placing a wrap of mesh, if that is the chosen material. The number and nature of the neurological conditions in this series were also not specified. Our own contemporary management of such cases has been a conventionally placed AFS that is tightened at the time of placement against a 22F cystoscope sheath held in the urethra in a horizontal plane. A similar technique in patients with incontinence post vesicovaginal fistula repair, often with significant vaginal fibrosis as a result, is described using tightening against a Valsalva with a bladder filled with dye [87]. This was undertaken in 40 cases and a fascia lata harvested graft used. Only one patient required ongoing CIC post-operatively. This study was limited by follow-up and design. The use of the spiral sling has not been systematically evaluated in the irradiated population.

Adjustable Continence (ACTs)

This device which functions like an adjustable implantable bluking agent has never gained traction as an option and there are limited studies in it use in primary or secondary SUI treatment. A cohort with 58% of patients with a failed sling and a 52% dry rate using pad weigh of <2 gm as the definition. Eighty per cent of patients improved with lesser results with increasing severity of incontinence [88].

Kocjancic [89] published a study of 57 women all with failed previous surgery and ISD including 22 of women who had a failed previous sling. There was follow-up to 5 years and a reduction in pad use from 5.6 to 1.6 per day. Complications are mild in 28% and more serious in 5%, and there is a device explanation rate of 18%. Freton compared the outcomes of the ACT® device to the AUS AMS 800 in the treatment of SUI due to ISD in women. Results were in favour of the AUS with respect to decrease in USP SUI subscore (-7.6 vs. -3.2), number of pads per 24 h (-4.6 vs. -2.3), PGII scale (PGII = 1: 61.1% vs. 12%) and cure rate (71.4% vs. 21.7%). The authors concluded that the AUS implantation was associated with better functional outcomes than the ACT®, but with a higher intra-operative complications rate, longer operative time and a longer stay (Freton, 2018 #147).

A literature review of studies on ACT was published in 2013 [90] and reports a wide variety of results in 8 heterogeneous studies with the conclusion that the technique is relevant to the failed treatment group with ISD for whom an artificial urinary sphincter would be inappropriate. This group may also have contraindications to a spiral sling due to previous surgeries.

Stem Cell Therapy

Several publications exist and further work is in progress on the use of adipose and muscle derived stem cell-based treatments [91–93]. Mitterberger used the technique in 20 women with ISD and at 2 years 89% of women were cured. There are few publications that address stem cells in the secondary or failure case, and recent guidelines recommend they are only used in a trial setting [27].

Artificial Urinary Sphincter (Indications and Methods)

Introduction

Treatment options for recurrent or persistent SUI after previous SUI surgery include conservative management and/or surgical management. AFS, UBA and repeat MUS are the favoured options in most countries. The artificial urinary sphincter (AUS) AMS 800 (Boston Scientific™; Inc. USA) is an alternative surgical option; however, in the USA, this is not commonly used as it is not FDA approved [94] and is typically considered a "last-resort" by most international guidelines. In contrast to this, AUS is recommended in the French guidelines as the standard of care for female patients with stress urinary incontinence due to ISD [95].

In current practice, the AUS is predominantly used in male patients with post-prostatectomy incontinence, although it was originally designed mostly for women. Evidence supporting the use of AUS in female patients is scarce and of poor quality, comprising only retrospective case series. The AUS cuff is typically implanted at the bladder neck level using an abdominal approach, although there have been descriptions of a vaginal approach which was quickly abandoned, likely due to poor results. Implantation of the AUS is challenging and inherently morbid. In the mid-1990s, the AUS was not approved by the FDA, and as a result, the use of the AUS in treating female SUI has been mostly in Europe, especially France, using an open approach. The recent rise of the minimally invasive approach, as well as technological device refinements, has helped to overcome the technical complexity and lower morbidity of AUS implantation in women and there may be an increasing role for the AUS in the future [96]. Future high level of evidence studies is needed to help better define the role of AUS in the management of female patients with SUI resulting from ISD.

Indications for AUS in Women

Whilst MUS placement is recognised as the gold-standard surgical treatment for female patients with SUI resulting from urethral hypermobility, the management is less clear in women with ISD-related SUI [97]. ISD is understood to be the incomplete coaptation of the urethral lumen due to decreased outlet resistant and is usually seen in patients who have failed previous anti-incontinence surgical procedures or patients with neurogenic SUI [96]. There is, however, no universally accepted definition of SUI due to ISD. Clinical criteria described by Cour et al. include demonstrable SUI on cough stress test with lack of urethral mobility, a negative Marshall/Bonney test (leakage with the urethra fixed in place), a low maximum urethral closure pressure on urodynamics or a "fixed urethra" on examination [95], in combination with other clinical criteria that reinforce the clinical suspicion of ISD (failure of a first anti-incontinence procedure, high SUI scores, constant leakage for any daily activity and/or leakage with abdominal straining) [97].

The AMS 800 has three main components attached to each other: the inflatable cuff (surrounding the bladder neck), the hydraulic pump (placed in the labia majora) and the pressure-regulating balloon (PRB) (placed in the prevesical space). In the normal resting mode during the storage phase of the bladder cycle, the cuff is full of water, circumferentially compressing the bladder neck and increasing outlet resistance. During the voiding phase, the cuff decompresses, the bladder neck opens and the outlet resistance is lowered. The AUS theoretically restores both normal storage and voiding function. AUS can be considered in the treatment of female SUI when there is suspected ISD, i.e., patients with rSUI or persistent SUI after previous anti-incontinence procedures [97], neurogenic SUI (usually due to spinal cord injury, spina bifida, cauda equina syndrome or pelvic trauma) [98] and given the AUS is potentially less obstructive, it may be a useful option in female patients with severe detrusor underactivity [97].

The optimal timing for AUS implantation is controversial. Although ISD is the major indication for AUS implantation, not all women with this indication immediately undergo this procedure, and it is rarely used as a primary surgical intervention for female SUI, except in some neurogenic patients [99]. Chartier-Kastler et al. raised that conundrum that the AUS implantation success rate decreases with the number of previous surgical intervention, and that for this reason, they recommend that AUS implantation be considered after failure of at least one but a maximum of two previous interventions, rather than as a last resort after failure of all previous surgical options [99].

Outcomes

The level of evidence supporting the use of AUS in female patients is very low and of poor quality. Recently, a number of systematic reviews have been performed to assess the utility of offering AUS to treat women with SUI. Rue evaluated the short- to long-term AUS performance and safety outcomes in non-neurogenic adult females with severe SUI. No studies were randomised or prospective. From the 12 articles included in their review, they found that the reported zero pad rates ranged from 42% to 86%, revision rates from 6% to 44% and mechanical failure rates from 2% to 41%. They found that procedure serious adverse event rates ranged from 2% to 54%, and rates of serious adverse device effects such as explanation ranged from 2% to 27% [100].

In another systematic review performed under the auspices of the International Continence Society and following the PRISMA statement and Cochrane Handbook recommendations, Peyronnet found that surgical approach, surgical volume and experience most likely influence peri-operative morbidity and device survival. Complete continence ranged from 61.1% to 100%. The post-operative complications rates varied widely and ranged from 16.7% to 33.3% in robotic series and from 4.1% to 75% in open series. In the laparoscopic and robotic series, erosion and explanation rates ranged from 0% to 8.1% and 0% to 22.2%, respectively, with median follow-up periods of 37.5 months and 18.9 months. The two largest series of open AUS implantations reported the lowest rates of device explanation (7% and 12.8%) and mechanical failures (13.6% and 15.5%) [97, 101, 102]. More recent, larger, robot-assisted series have shown further improved outcomes with erosion and major post-operative complication rates as low as 2.1% and 4.1%, respectively, and at last follow-up, 81.6% were fully continent, 12.2% had improved continence and 6.1% had unchanged incontinence [103].

Future high level of evidence studies is needed to help better define the role of AUS in the management of female patients with SUI resulting from ISD.

Surgical Technique

Since the launch of the first AUS (AMS 721) by American Medical Systems (Boston Scientific, Minnetonka, MN, USA) over 3 decades ago, the device has undergone many modifications, resulting in the current AMS 800 model, which is implanted in women in a relatively small number of centres worldwide [99]. The implantation of the AMS 800 can be performed using one of two approaches: the retropubic [104] or the transvaginal [105] approach. The transvaginal approach was quickly abandoned as it was associated with a relatively high morbidity and infection rate [99]. The location of the placement of the inflatable cuff may vary depending on the aetiology of incontinence; however, most commonly patients undergo bladder neck placement. And whilst AUS implantation was originally described using an open technique, recent rise of minimally invasive approaches has helped to overcome the technical complexity and lower morbidity [97].

Pre-operative Considerations

When deciding on AUS implantation, the patient should be able to weigh the long-term success rate and the quality of life (QoL) improvement against the not insignificant complications risk and potential need for future revisions. AUS implantation depends on the motivation level of the patient and because the AMS 800 device should be manipulated by the patients herself at each void, it is crucial that she is accurately informed about the device before the operation [99]. Evaluate the patient's manual dexterity and mental status to assess the patient's ability to use the control pump before proceeding with AUS placement. Thorough work-up with history, examination and urodynamics should be performed, and voiding diaries, pad tests and incontinence questionnaires may also be useful. Cystoscopy should be performed to evaluate the health of the urethral tissues and exclude strictures or mesh erosion (which will require intervention and resolution before AUS implantation). A sterile pre-operative urine culture is mandatory, and peri-operative antibiotics should include coverage from skin and urinary tract pathogens to avoid colonisation of the implant. Appropriate deep venous thrombosis (DVT) prophylaxis should be prescribed.

Robot-Assisted AMS 800 Bladder Neck Implantation

Implantation of an AUS via laparoscopy with or without robotic assistance in women presents the following advantages: parietal sparing, better visualisation and a limited time of exposure to the device before implantation in order to reduce the risks of infection [106]. Skin is shaved to include the infraumbilical abdomen, genitalia and perineum, and per instructions from the manufacturer, it is recommended that the patient's skin be scrubbed with a povidone-iodine soap for 10 minutes before surgical prep (for iodine allergy, a chlorhexidine scrub can be performed).

Bladder Neck Dissection

In the technique described by Peyronnet et al. [103], the patient is positioned in 23° Trendelenburg, with arms placed along her body and held in arm rests and lower limbs in low lithotomy. A 14Fr Foley catheter is introduced and the bladder drained. Four 8 mm robotic ports are placed (camera port at umbilicus, one in the right flank, and two at the lateral edge of the right and left rectus abdominis muscles) and an additional 12 mm assistant port in the left flank. The four-arm Da Vince Si/Xi robot is placed in the right-sided docking position. Three robotic instruments are used: a bipolar Prograsp forceps (left arm), scissors (internal right arm) and basic Prograsp forceps (external right arm). The three components of the AMS 800 are prepared as per the manufacturers' guidelines.

The bladder is filled with 100–300 ml of saline to identify its boundaries, and the bladder is then dropped from the anterior abdominal wall. Retzius space is dissected and then the bladder neck and endopelvic fascia are developed, taking care to identify the bladder neck accurately. The assistant places a finger in lateral vaginal fornix and pushes it upward and laterally. With blunt dissection of the bladder neck onto the assistant's finger, the peri-vesical fascia is entered and the shiny white plane of the vagina appears (the "bald plane"), where the dissection of the bladder neck has to be carried out. Once the dissection reaches the median line, the other side of the bladder neck is dissected until the two dissected spaces are joined. The assistant confirms that the vaginal wall is intact, and the bladder is filled with methylene blue to verify the integrity of the bladder neck [103].

A posterior approach to the bladder neck and vesicovaginal space has also been described by Gondran-Tellier et al. [59], whereby the plane between the bladder and the vagina is dissected, with the aid of a vaginal valve, posteriorly past the bladder neck and then laterally to the endopelvic fascia. Once the posterior dissection has been completed, the surgeon approaches the dissection anteriorly, opening the space of Retzius and then exposing the right and left endopelvic fascia and identifying the bladder neck. Careful passage from the posterior plane to the anterior plane is performed with Maryland bipolar forceps.

AMS-800 Placement

Once the bladder neck is circumferentially dissected, the circumference is measure using a measuring tape introduced through the 12 mm port. The inflatable cuff is then introduced through the same 12 mm post and positioned around the bladder neck, taking care to handle the cuff gently and avoid any damage. A 61–70 cmH$_2$O PRB is implanted in the prevesical space via a 3 cm suprapubic incision and filled with water. The tubing from the cuff is grasped and externalised through the same suprapubic incision. The peritoneum is closed with a barbed suture, and the port sites are closed and infiltrated with local anaesthetic. The hydraulic pump is implanted in one of the labia majora by creating a subcutaneous passage starting from the suprapubic incision. The tubing from the cuff, PRB and pump is connected through the suprapubic incision, which is then closed and the device is deactivated [103]. The patient is monitored overnight with the Foley catheter in situ, and trial of void is performed the following morning. A short course of broad-spectrum oral antibiotics after discharge is used by many expert surgeons, although this is not recommended by AUA guidelines.

Conclusion

Overall, there are little systematic data to guide decision making in the management of recurrent or persistent SUI. There is diminishing enthusiasm for sling manipulation and second mesh slings with the majority of patients now likely to be offered UBA or AFS depending on their comorbidities and degree of leakage. In the presence of ISD, the AUA guidelines recommend consideration of either repeat MUS, AFS or UBA [27]. There may be unique situations where a female AUS is implanted or a spiral or obstructing sling considered. There is a clear need for ongoing follow-up and research in the field of failure to better navigate the journey for these patients.

Acknowledgements The authors wish to acknowledge the invaluable assistance of Tina Lam, Monash University and Cassandra Khoo, Auckland University of Technology, in the preparation of the graphic design elements of Fig. 19.1. The authors also wish to acknowledge the patience of their own families and thank them for their support whilst they completed the work for this important publication.

References

1. Wai CY, Curto TM, Zyczynski HM, Stoddard AM, Burgio KL, Brubaker L, et al. Patient satisfaction after midurethral sling surgery for stress urinary incontinence. Obstet Gynecol. 2013;121(5):1009–16.
2. Treatment options for stress urinary incontinence. Information for consumers. Patient resource. https://www.safetyandqualitygovau/sites/default/files/2020–11/treatment_options_for_stress_urinary_incontinence_sui_-_transvaginal_tv_mesh_-_information_for_consumers_patient_resourcepdf.
3. TGA information for medical practitioners on pending up-classification of surgical mesh devices. https://www.tgagovau/information-medical-practitioners-pending-classification-surgical-mesh-devices.
4. Liu HH, Kuo HC. Durability of retropubic suburethral sling procedure and predictors for successful treatment outcome in women with stress urinary incontinence. Urology. 2019;131:83–8.
5. Khayyami Y, Klarskov N, Lose G. The promise of urethral pressure reflectometry: an update. Int Urogynecol J. 2016;27(10):1449–58.
6. Smith AR, Artibani W, Drake MJ. Managing unsatisfactory outcome after mid-urethral tape insertion. Neurourol Urodyn. 2011;30(5):771–4.
7. Kavanagh A, Sanaee M, Carlson KV, Bailly GG. Management of patients with stress urinary incontinence after failed midurethral sling. Can Urol Assoc J. 2017;11(6Suppl2):S143–S6.
8. Gormley EA. Evaluation and management of the patient with a failed midurethral synthetic sling. Can Urol Assoc J. 2012;6(5 Suppl 2):S123–S4.
9. Escobar C, Brucker B. Urodynamics for the "failed" midurethral sling. Curr Bladder Dysfunct Rep. 2020;15(4):245–58.
10. Zimmern PE, Gormley EA, Stoddard AM, Lukacz ES, Sirls L, Brubaker L, et al. Management of recurrent stress urinary incontinence after burch and sling procedures. Neurourol Urodyn. 2016;35(3):344–8.
11. Dray EV, Hall M, Covalschi D, Cameron AP. Can urethral bulking agents salvage failed slings? Urology. 2019;124:78–82.
12. Rodrigues P, Hering F, D'Imperio M, Campagnari JC. One hundred cases of SUI treatment that failed: a prospective observational study on the behavior of patients after surgical failure. Int Braz J Urol. 2014;40(6):790–801.
13. MacLachlan LS, Rovner ES. Management of failed stress urinary incontinence surgery. Curr Urol Rep. 2014;15(8):429.
14. Stav K, Dwyer PL, Rosamilia A, Schierlitz L, Lim YN, Lee J. Risk factors of treatment failure of midurethral sling procedures for women with urinary stress incontinence. Int Urogynecol J. 2010;21(2):149–55.
15. Pradhan A, Jain P, Latthe PM. Effectiveness of midurethral slings in recurrent stress urinary incontinence: a systematic review and meta-analysis. Int Urogynecol J. 2012;23(7):831–41.
16. Richter HE, Litman HJ, Lukacz ES, Sirls LT, Rickey L, Norton P, et al. Demographic and clinical predictors of treatment failure one year after midurethral sling surgery. Obstet Gynecol. 2011;117(4):913–21.
17. Richter HE, Albo ME, Zyczynski HM, Kenton K, Norton PA, Sirls LT, et al. Retropubic versus transobturator midurethral slings for stress incontinence. N Engl J Med. 2010;362(22):2066–76.
18. Bogusiewicz M, Monist M, Galczynski K, Wozniak M, Wieczorek AP, Rechberger T. Both the middle and distal sections of the urethra may be regarded as optimal targets for 'outside-in' transobturator tape placement. World J Urol. 2014;32(6):1605–11.
19. Pedraszewski P, Wlazlak E, Wlazlak W, Krzycka M, Pajak P, Surkont G. The role of TVT position in relation to the pubic symphysis in eliminating the symptoms of stress urinary incontinence and urethral funneling. J Ultrason. 2019;19(78):207–11.
20. Chan L, Tse V. Pelvic floor ultrasound in the diagnosis of sling complications. World J Urol. 2018;36(5):753–9.

21. Mahdy A, Ghoniem GM. Autologous rectus fascia sling for treatment of stress urinary incontinence in women: a review of the literature. Neurourol Urodyn. 2019;38(Suppl 4):S51–S8.
22. Fontenot PA, Padmanabhan P. Management of recurrent stress urinary incontinence after failed mid-urethral sling placement. Curr Bladder Dysfunct Rep. 2018;13(3):93–100.
23. Clarke A Do urodynamic findings influence the approach to mid-urethral sling surgery for stress urinary incontinence? Br J Nurs. 2018;27(11):600–5.
24. Nager CW, Sirls L, Litman HJ, Richter H, Nygaard I, Chai T, et al. Baseline urodynamic predictors of treatment failure 1 year after mid urethral sling surgery. J Urol. 2011;186(2):597–603.
25. Hill B, Fletcher S, Blume J, Adam R, Ward R. Volume at first leak is associated with sling failure among women with stress urinary incontinence. Female Pelvic Med Reconstr Surg. 2019;25(4):294–7.
26. NICE guidelines urinary-incontinence-and-pelvic-organ-prolapse-in-women-management-pdf-66141657205189.pdf.
27. Kobashi KC, Albo ME, Dmochowski RR, Ginsberg DA, Goldman HB, Gomelsky A, et al. Surgical treatment of female stress urinary incontinence: AUA/SUFU guideline. J Urol. 2017;198(4):875–83.
28. Giarenis I, Thiagamoorthy G, Zacche M, Robinson D, Cardozo L. Management of recurrent stress urinary incontinence after failed midurethral sling: a survey of members of the International Urogynecological Association (IUGA). Int Urogynecol J. 2015;26(9):1285–91.
29. Rashid TG, De Ridder D, Van der Aa F. The role of bladder neck suspension in the era of mid-urethral sling surgery. World J Urol. 2015;33(9):1235–41.
30. Lucas MG, Bosch RJ, Burkhard FC, Cruz F, Madden TB, Nambiar AK, et al. EAU guidelines on surgical treatment of urinary incontinence. Eur Urol. 2012;62(6):1118–29.
31. Bakali E, Johnson E, Buckley BS, Hilton P, Walker B, Tincello DG. Interventions for treating recurrent stress urinary incontinence after failed minimally invasive synthetic midurethral tape surgery in women. Cochrane Database Syst Rev. 2019;9:CD009407.
32. Pergialiotis V, Mudiaga Z, Perrea DN, Doumouchtsis SK. De novo overactive bladder following midurethral sling procedures: a systematic review of the literature and meta-analysis. Int Urogynecol J. 2017;28(11):1631–8.
33. Sajadi KP, Vasavada SP. Overactive bladder after sling surgery. Curr Urol Rep. 2010;11(6):366–71.
34. Marcelissen T, Van Kerrebroeck P. Overactive bladder symptoms after midurethral sling surgery in women: risk factors and management. Neurourol Urodyn. 2018;37(1):83–8.
35. Serati M, Braga A, Sorice P, Siesto G, Salvatore S, Ghezzi F. Solifenacin in women with de novo overactive bladder after tension-free obturator vaginal tape--is it effective? J Urol. 2014;191(5):1322–6.
36. Miotla P, Futyma K, Cartwright R, Bogusiewicz M, Skorupska K, Markut-Miotla E, et al. Effectiveness of botulinum toxin injection in the treatment of de novo OAB symptoms following midurethral sling surgery. Int Urogynecol J. 2016;27(3):393–8.
37. Sherman ND, Jamison MG, Webster GD, Amundsen CL. Sacral neuromodulation for the treatment of refractory urinary urge incontinence after stress incontinence surgery. Am J Obstet Gynecol. 2005;193(6):2083–7.
38. Lovatsis D, Easton W, Wilkie D. No. 248-guidelines for the evaluation and treatment of recurrent urinary incontinence following pelvic floor surgery. J Obstet Gynaecol Can. 2017;39(9):e309–e14.
39. Nadeau G, Herschorn S. Management of recurrent stress incontinence following a sling. Curr Urol Rep. 2014;15(8):427.
40. Giarenis I, Cardozo L. Management of stress urinary incontinence following a failed midurethral tape. Curr Bladder Dysfunct Rep. 2011;6(2):67–9.
41. Stav K, Dwyer PL, Rosamilia A, Schierlitz L, Lim YN, Chao F, et al. Repeat synthetic mid urethral sling procedure for women with recurrent stress urinary incontinence. J Urol. 2010;183(1):241–6.
42. Nikolopoulos KI, Betschart C, Doumouchtsis SK. The surgical management of recurrent stress urinary incontinence: a systematic review. Acta Obstet Gynecol Scand. 2015;94(6):568–76.

43. Rac G, Younger A, Clemens JQ, Kobashi K, Khan A, Nitti V, et al. Stress urinary incontinence surgery trends in academic female pelvic medicine and reconstructive surgery urology practice in the setting of the food and drug administration public health notifications. Neurourol Urodyn. 2017;36(4):1155–60.
44. Hansen MF, Lose G, Kesmodel US, Gradel KO. Repeat surgery after failed midurethral slings: a nationwide cohort study, 1998-2007. Int Urogynecol J. 2016;27(7):1013–9.
45. Plagakis S, Tse V. The autologous pubovaginal fascial sling: an update in 2019. Low Urin Tract Symptoms. 2020;12(1):2–7.
46. Giarenis I, Malde S, Harding C, Robinson D, Gajewski J, Rahnamai M, et al. Do we need better information to advise women with stress incontinence on their choice of surgery? Report from the ICI-RS 2018. Neurourol Urodyn. 2019;38(Suppl 5):S98–S103.
47. McGuire EJ, Lytton B. Pubovaginal sling procedure for stress incontinence. J Urol. 1978;119:82–4.
48. Parker WP, Gomelsky A, Padmanabhan P. Autologous fascia pubovaginal slings after prior synthetic anti-incontinence procedures for recurrent incontinence: a multi-institutional prospective comparative analysis to de novo autologous slings assessing objective and subjective cure. Neurourol Urodyn. 2016;35(5):604–8.
49. Milose JC, Sharp KM, He C, Stoffel J, Clemens JQ, Cameron AP. Success of autologous pubovaginal sling after failed synthetic mid urethral sling. J Urol. 2015;193(3):916–20.
50. Petrou SP, Davidiuk AJ, Rawal B, Arnold M, Thiel DD. Salvage autologous fascial sling after failed synthetic midurethral sling: greater than 3-year outcomes. Int J Urol. 2016;23(2):178–81.
51. Albo ME, Richter HE, Brubaker L, Norton P, Kraus SR, Zimmern PE, et al. Burch colposuspension versus fascial sling to reduce urinary stress incontinence. N Engl J Med. 2007;356:2143–55.
52. Aberger M, Gomelsky A, Padmanabhan P. Comparison of retropubic synthetic mid-urethral slings to fascia pubovaginal slings following failed sling surgery. Neurourol Urodyn. 2016;35(7):851–4.
53. Walsh CA. Recurrent stress urinary incontinence after synthetic mid-urethral sling procedures. Curr Opin Obstet Gynecol. 2011;23(5):355–61.
54. Sanses TV, Brubaker L, Xu Y, Kraus SR, Lowder JL, Lemack GE, et al. Preoperative hesitating urinary stream is associated with postoperative voiding dysfunction and surgical failure following Burch colposuspension or pubovaginal rectus fascial sling surgery. Int Urogynecol J. 2011;22(6):713–9.
55. Malde S, Moore JA. Autologous mid-urethral sling for stress urinary incontinence: preliminary results and description of a contemporary technique. J Clin Urol. 2015;9(1):40–7.
56. Preece PD, Chan G, O'Connell HE, Gani J. Optimising the tension of an autologous fascia pubovaginal sling to minimize retentive complications. Neurourol Urodyn. 2019;38(5):1409–16.
57. Zivanovic I, Rautenberg O, Lobodasch K, von Bunau G, Walser C, Viereck V. Urethral bulking for recurrent stress urinary incontinence after midurethral sling failure. Neurourol Urodyn. 2017;36(3):722–6.
58. Toozs-Hobson P, Al-Singary W, Fynes M, Tegerstedt G, Lose G. Two-year follow-up of an open-label multicenter study of polyacrylamide hydrogel (Bulkamid(R)) for female stress and stress-predominant mixed incontinence. Int Urogynecol J. 2012;23(10):1373–8.
59. Brosche T, Kuhn A, Lobodasch K, Sokol ER. Seven-year efficacy and safety outcomes of Bulkamid for the treatment of stress urinary incontinence. Neurourol Urodyn. 2021;40(1):502–8.
60. Pai A, Al-Singary W. Durability, safety and efficacy of polyacrylamide hydrogel (Bulkamid(®)) in the management of stress and mixed urinary incontinence: three year follow up outcomes. Cent Eur J Urol. 2015;68(4):428–33.
61. Rodriguez D, Jaffer A, Hilmy M, Zimmern P. Bladder neck and urethral erosions after Macroplastique injections. Low Urin Tract Symptoms. 2021;13(1):93–7.

62. Lee HN, Lee YS, Han JY, Jeong JY, Choo MS, Lee KS. Transurethral injection of bulking agent for treatment of failed mid-urethral sling procedures. Int Urogynecol J. 2010; 21(12):1479–83.
63. Rodriguez D, Carroll T, Alhalabi F, Carmel M, Zimmern PE. Outcomes of Macroplastique injections for stress urinary incontinence after suburethral sling removal. Neurourol Urodyn. 2020;39(3):994–1001.
64. Siddiqui ZA, Abboudi H, Crawford R, Shah S. Intraurethral bulking agents for the management of female stress urinary incontinence: a systematic review. Int Urogynecol J. 2017;28(9):1275–84.
65. Kim J, Lee W, Lucioni A, Govier F, Kobashi K. 1360 long-term efficacy and durability of Durashpere® urethral bulking after failed urethral sling for stress urinary incontinence. The J Urol. 2012;187:552.
66. Gaddi A, Guaderrama N, Bassiouni N, Bebchuk J, Whitcomb EL. Repeat midurethral sling compared with urethral bulking for recurrent stress urinary incontinence. Obstet Gynecol. 2014;123(6):1207–12.
67. Schierlitz L, Dwyer PL, Rosamilia A, Murray C, Thomas E, De Souza A, et al. Three-year follow-up of tension-free vaginal tape compared with transobturator tape in women with stress urinary incontinence and intrinsic sphincter deficiency. Obstet Gynecol. 2012;119(2 Pt 1):321–7.
68. Speed JM, Mishra K. What to do after a mid-urethral sling fails. Curr Opin Obstet Gynecol. 2020;32(6):449–55.
69. Kim A, Kim MS, Park YJ, Choi WS, Park HK, Paick SH, et al. Retropubic versus transobturator mid urethral slings in patients at high risk for recurrent stress incontinence: a systematic review and meta-analysis. J Urol. 2019;202(1):132–42.
70. Ford AA, Rogerson L, Cody JD, Aluko P, Ogah JA. Mid-urethral sling operations for stress urinary incontinence in women. Cochrane Database Syst Rev. 2017;7:CD006375.
71. Abdel-Fattah M, Cao G, Mostafa A. Long-term outcomes of transobturator tension-free vaginal tapes as secondary continence procedures. World J Urol. 2017;35(7):1141–8.
72. Ulrich D, Bjelic-Radisic V, Grabner K, Avian A, Trutnovsky G, Tamussino K, et al. Objective outcome and quality-of-life assessment in women with repeat incontinence surgery. Neurourol Urodyn. 2017;36(6):1543–9.
73. Park BH, Kim JC, Kim HW, Kim YH, Choi JB, Lee DH. Midterm efficacy and complications of readjustable midurethral sling (Remeex system) in female stress urinary incontinence with recurrence or intrinsic sphincter deficiency. Urology. 2015;85(1):79–84.
74. Kociszewski J, Majkusiak W, Pomian A, Tomasik P, Horosz E, Kuszka A, et al. The outcome of repeated mid urethral sling in SUI treatment after vaginal excisions of primary failed sling: preliminary study. Biomed Res Int. 2016;2016:1242061.
75. Tincello DG, Armstrong N, Hilton P, Buckley B, Mayne C. Surgery for recurrent stress urinary incontinence: the views of surgeons and women. Int Urogynecol J. 2018;29(1):45–54.
76. De Cuyper EM, Ismail R, Maher CF. Laparoscopic Burch colposuspension after failed suburethral tape procedures: a retrospective audit. Int Urogynecol J Pelvic Floor Dysfunct. 2008;19(5):681–5.
77. Kim S, Son JH, Kim HS, Ko JS, Kim JC. Tape shortening for recurrent stress urinary incontinence after transobturator tape sling: 3-year follow-up results. Int Neurourol J. 2010;14(3):164–9.
78. Schmid C, Bloch E, Amann E, Mueller MD, Kuhn A. An adjustable sling in the management of recurrent urodynamic stress incontinence after previous failed midurethral tape. Neurourol Urodyn. 2010;29(4):573–7.
79. de Landsheere L, Lucot JP, Foidart JM, Cosson M. Management of recurrent or persistent stress urinary incontinence after TVT-O by mesh readjustment. Int Urogynecol J. 2010;21(11):1347–51.
80. Patterson D, Rajan S, Kohli N. Sling plication for recurrent stress urinary incontinence. Female Pelvic Med Reconstr Surg. 2010;16(5):307–9.

81. Maheshwari D, Jones K, Solomon E, Harmanli O. Sling plication for failed midurethral sling procedures: a case series. Female Pelvic Med Reconstr Surg. 2019;25(1):e4–6.
82. Glazener CM, Cooper K, Mashayekhi A. Anterior vaginal repair for urinary incontinence in women. Cochrane Database Syst Rev. 2017;7:CD001755.
83. Dray EV, Cameron AP, Bergman R. Stress urinary incontinence in women with neurogenic lower urinary tract dysfunction. Curr Bladder Dysfunct Rep. 2018;13(2):75–83.
84. Rodriguez AR, Hakky T, Hoffman M, Ordorica R, Lockhart J. Salvage spiral sling techniques: alternatives to manage disabling recurrent urinary incontinence in females. J Urol. 2010;184(6):2429–33.
85. Onol SY, Sevket O, Onol FF, Erdem R, Tepeler A. Minimum 1-year results of mesh spiral-sling procedure in managing refractory and primary disabling stress urinary incontinence. Int Urogynecol J. 2014;25(10):1399–404.
86. Rutman MP, Deng DY, Shah SM, Raz S, Rodríguez LV. Spiral sling salvage anti-incontinence surgery in female patients with a nonfunctional urethra: technique and initial results. J Urol. 2006;175(5):1794–9.
87. Lengmang S, Shephard S, Datta A, Lozo S, Kirschner CV. Pubovesical sling for residual incontinence after successful vesicovaginal fistula closure: a new approach to an old procedure. Int Urogynecol J. 2018;29(10):1551–6.
88. Aboseif SR, Sassani P, Franke EI, Nash SD, Slutsky JN, Baum NH, et al. Treatment of moderate to severe female stress urinary incontinence with the adjustable continence therapy (ACT) device after failed surgical repair. World J Urol. 2011;29(2):249–53.
89. Kocjancic E, Crivellaro S, Ranzoni S, Bonvini D, Grosseti B, Frea B. Adjustable continence therapy for severe intrinsic sphincter deficiency and recurrent female stress urinary incontinence: long-term experience. J Urol. 2010;184(3):1017–21.
90. Phe V, Nguyen K, Roupret M, Cardot V, Parra J, Chartier-Kastler E. A systematic review of the treatment for female stress urinary incontinence by ACT(R) balloon placement (Uromedica, Irvine, CA, USA). World J Urol. 2014;32(2):495–505.
91. Staack A, Rodriguez LV. Stem cells for the treatment of urinary incontinence. Curr Urol Rep. 2011;12(1):41–6.
92. Mitterberger M, Pinggera G-M, Marksteiner R, Margreiter E, Fussenegger M, Frauscher F, et al. Adult stem cell therapy of female stress urinary incontinence. Eur Urol. 2008;53(1):169–75.
93. Tran C, Damaser MS. The potential role of stem cells in the treatment of urinary incontinence. Ther Adv Urol. 2015;7(1):22–40.
94. Gomelsky A, Athanasiou S, Choo MS, Cosson M, Dmochowski RR, Gomes CM, et al. Surgery for urinary incontinence in women: report from the 6th international consultation on incontinence. Neurourol Urodyn. 2019;38(2):825–37.
95. Cour F, Le Normand L, Lapray JF, Hermieu JF, Peyrat L, Yiou R, et al. Intrinsic sphincter deficiency and female urinary incontinence. Prog Urol. 2015;25(8):437–54.
96. Peyronnet B, Greenwell T, Gray G, Khavari R, Thiruchelvam N, Capon G, et al. Current use of the artificial urinary sphincter in adult females. Curr Urol Rep. 2020;21(12):53.
97. Peyronnet B, O'Connor E, Khavari R, Capon G, Manunta A, Allue M, et al. AMS-800 artificial urinary sphincter in female patients with stress urinary incontinence: a systematic review. Neurourol Urodyn. 2019;38(Suppl 4):S28–s41.
98. Phé V, Léon P, Granger B, Denys P, Bitker MO, Mozer P, et al. Stress urinary incontinence in female neurological patients: long-term functional outcomes after artificial urinary sphincter (AMS 800(TM)) implantation. Neurourol Urodyn. 2017;36(3):764–9.
99. Chartier-Kastler E, Van Kerrebroeck P, Olianas R, Cosson M, Mandron E, Delorme E, et al. Artificial urinary sphincter (AMS 800) implantation for women with intrinsic sphincter deficiency: a technique for insiders? BJU Int. 2011;107(10):1618–26.
100. Reus CR, Phe V, Dechartres A, Grilo NR, Chartier-Kastler EJ, Mozer PC. Performance and safety of the artificial urinary sphincter (AMS 800) for non-neurogenic women with urinary incontinence secondary to intrinsic sphincter deficiency: a systematic review. Eur Urol Focus. 2020;6(2):327–38.

101. Vayleux B, Rigaud J, Luyckx F, Karam G, Glémain P, Bouchot O, et al. Female urinary incontinence and artificial urinary sphincter: study of efficacy and risk factors for failure and complications. Eur Urol. 2011;59(6):1048–53.
102. Costa P, Poinas G, Ben Naoum K, Bouzoubaa K, Wagner L, Soustelle L, et al. Long-term results of artificial urinary sphincter for women with type III stress urinary incontinence. Eur Urol. 2013;63(4):753–8.
103. Peyronnet B, Capon G, Belas O, Manunta A, Allenet C, Hascoet J, et al. Robot-assisted AMS-800 artificial urinary sphincter bladder neck implantation in female patients with stress urinary incontinence. Eur Urol. 2019;75(1):169–75.
104. Costa P, Mottet N, Rabut B, Thuret R, Ben Naoum K, Wagner L. The use of an artificial urinary sphincter in women with type III incontinence and a negative Marshall test. J Urol. 2001;165(4):1172–6.
105. Abbassian A. A new operation for insertion of the artificial urinary sphincter. J Urol. 1988;140(3):512–3.
106. Gondran-Tellier B, Boissier R, Baboudjian M, Rouy M, Gaillet S, Lechevallier E, et al. Robot-assisted implantation of an artificial urinary sphincter, the AMS-800, via a posterior approach to the bladder neck in women with intrinsic sphincter deficiency. BJU Int. 2019;124(6):1077–80.

Part V
Other Contributors and Causes of Incontinence

Chapter 20
Prolapse as a Contributing Factor to Stress and Urgency Urinary Incontinence

Whitney Horner and Carolyn W. Swenson

Epidemiology of Prolapse

Definition

Pelvic organ prolapse is a downward displacement of the pelvic organs associated with symptoms [1]. Pelvic organs include the anterior and posterior vaginal walls, uterus, vaginal apex, and neighboring organs such as the bladder, rectum, and bowel. Common prolapse symptoms are vaginal bulge or pressure, incomplete bowel or bladder emptying requiring splinting or digitation, bleeding, discharge, or low backache [1, 2]. Prolapse is most symptomatic when it extends beyond the vaginal opening. Diagnosis is made on clinical exam, and quantification of prolapse can be performed using either the Pelvic Organ Prolapse Quantification (POP-Q) [3] or Baden Walker grading system [4]. Categorization is made by compartment affected: anterior vaginal wall prolapse (cystocele), posterior vaginal wall prolapse (rectocele), uterine/cervical prolapse, vaginal vault prolapse (if status post hysterectomy), and enterocele (posthysterectomy small bowel herniation).

Prevalence

The prevalence of prolapse has been reported to be between 3% and 50% depending on how prolapse is defined. In a population-based study of nearly 2000 U.S. women, 2.9% of respondents self-reported having a symptomatic vaginal bulge [5]. Other

W. Horner · C. W. Swenson (✉)
Female Pelvic Medicine & Reconstructive Surgery, Department of Obstetrics & Gynecology, University of Michigan, Ann Arbor, MI, USA
e-mail: scarolyn@med.umich.edu

© The Author(s), under exclusive license to Springer Nature Switzerland AG 2022
A. P. Cameron (ed.), *Female Urinary Incontinence*,
https://doi.org/10.1007/978-3-030-84352-6_20

371

similar population-based studies have reported a prevalence of self-reported symptomatic prolapse to be 6–8% [6]. When prolapse is defined using physical exam, the prevalence of prolapse is much higher. A study by Swift et al. found that 50.3% of women without prolapse symptoms presenting for routine gynecologic care had POP-Q stage 2 (prolapse within 1 cm of the hymen) or 3 prolapse (prolapse extending >1 cm beyond the hymen) on exam [7].

Of the different types of prolapse, anterior vaginal wall prolapse is the most common affecting more than 1 in 3 women >50 years old, followed by posterior vaginal wall prolapse (approximately 1 in 5) and uterine prolapse (1 in 7) [8]. For U.S. women, the lifetime risk of surgery for prolapse is estimated to be 12.6% [9].

Risk Factors

Prolapse is a multifactorial disorder resulting from a culmination of anatomical factors, childbirth-related structural changes, comorbidities, and genetic risk [10]. Aging is perhaps the biggest risk factor for prolapse with the highest rates of prolapse and surgery for prolapse, among women ≥80 years of age [11]. In a cross-sectional analysis of 16,616 women in the Women's Health Initiative, women aged 70–79 had 36% increased odds of uterine prolapse, 18% increased odds of posterior vaginal wall prolapse, and 35% increased odds of anterior vaginal wall prolapse compared to women 50–59 years of age [9]. The association between aging and prolapse is not yet fully understood; however, age-related skeletal muscle changes, neuromuscular and connective tissue damage, and repetitive pelvic floor loading over time may all play a role.

Vaginal delivery is another significant risk factor for prolapse, and there is a cumulative risk for each additional delivery [12–16]. The levator ani, the skeletal muscles that form the "floor" of the pelvic floor, undergoes significant stretching and deformation with vaginal delivery. Forceps-assisted vaginal delivery is the route associated with the highest risk of levator ani injury carrying an 11- to 26-fold increased odds compared to spontaneous births [17]. Using MRI and ultrasound, major levator ani defects have been observed in 34–55% of women with prolapse [18, 19]. The presence of a major levator ani defect carries a 7-fold increased odds of prolapse [20]. Even in the absence of visible injury, the pelvic floor muscles can sustain neurological impairment related to vaginal delivery. A study of primiparous women undergoing electromyography of the levator ani prior to delivery and again at 6 weeks and 6 months postpartum found that 24.1% of women had levator ani neuropathy with only 64% of recovering by 6 months [21]. In a 3D computer simulation of vaginal delivery, DeLancey et al. found that the inferior rectal nerve and perineal nerve branches to the rectum were both stretched to 35% and 33% of their original lengths, respectively, exceeding the 15% strain threshold known to cause permanent nerve damage [22]. Denervation of the pelvic floor muscles could impair the levator's functional ability to maintain normal pelvic support increasing the risk of prolapse development. In a study assessing levator ani strength using a specially designed instrumented speculum, DeLancey et al. found that vaginal closure force (force generated during maximal pelvic floor muscle contraction) was 40% lower among women with versus without prolapse [18].

While delivery via cesarean section does significantly reduce the risk of pelvic floor disorders, it is not entirely protective. In a longitudinal study of 1528 women 5–10 years following their first delivery, rates of pelvic floor disorders were found to be highest among women with an operative vaginal delivery (forceps or vacuum) and lowest in women who delivered by cesarean with spontaneous vaginal delivery as the reference group. However, the cesarean group still reported pelvic floor symptoms with prolapse present in 5%, stress urinary incontinence in 13%, and overactive bladder in 10.4% [23]. Lukacz et al. performed a number-needed-to-treat analysis and determined that seven women would have to deliver exclusively by cesarean section in order to prevent woman from having a pelvic floor disorder [15]. Therefore, the stress of pregnancy alone, independent of delivery route, may confer a risk of pelvic floor disorders including prolapse.

Genetic predisposition to prolapse is suggested by some studies showing a high concordance of prolapse with twins and increased risk of prolapse among women with connective tissue disorders [20, 24–26]. Women with first-degree family members, such as a sister or mother, with prolapse, have a significant increased risk of prolapse themselves [13]. A recent meta-analysis and systematic review found evidence supporting the association between a collagen gene (COL1A1) and prolapse [27]. HOXa11, a homeobox gene involved in embryonic development of the urogenital tract, has been reported to be significantly reduced in the uterosacral ligaments (USLs), a main support structure of the uterus and upper vagina, in women with prolapse compared to controls. Despite these studies, a "prolapse gene" has yet to be identified, and the genetic risk for prolapse remains unknown.

Finally, repetitive loading on the pelvic floor structures over time can increase the risk of prolapse. Repetitive loading refers to activities or conditions that result in repetitive increases in intraabdominal and pelvic pressure. These include obesity [8, 16], chronic straining with constipation [28], and physical labor requiring heavy lifting such as farm and factory workers [13].

How Could Prolapse Cause Urinary Incontinence?

Common Risk Factors

While not all women with prolapse experience urinary incontinence, the two disorders often coexist due to a shared disease mechanism. Many risk factors for prolapse discussed in the prior section—such as age and vaginal delivery—are also risk factors for urinary incontinence.

Of the different types of prolapse, anterior vaginal wall (AVW) prolapse is most likely to be associated with concomitant urinary incontinence given the anatomical relationship between the bladder, urethra, and anterior vaginal wall. Therefore, this section will focus on the causative association between AVW prolapse and urinary incontinence.

Prolapse and Stress Urinary Incontinence

Up to 80% of women with prolapse also have stress urinary incontinence (SUI) [29, 30]. AVW prolapse (Fig. 20.1) is commonly referred to as a "cystocele" which falsely implies this condition results from a pathology of the bladder. In truth, prolapse of the bladder and urethra is a result, not a cause, of AVW prolapse which can be due to impaired connective tissue support at any of the three levels of pelvic support [31].

As described by DeLancey, the AVW connective tissue and endopelvic fascia form a hammock-like support to the urethra and bladder that is anchored laterally to the arcus tendineus fascia pelvis [32]. With increases in intraabdominal and intra-vesicle pressure, the urethra compresses against this hammock, increasing

Fig. 20.1 Clinical picture of a cystocele showing the upwardly deviated urethral meatus and impaired anterior vaginal wall support

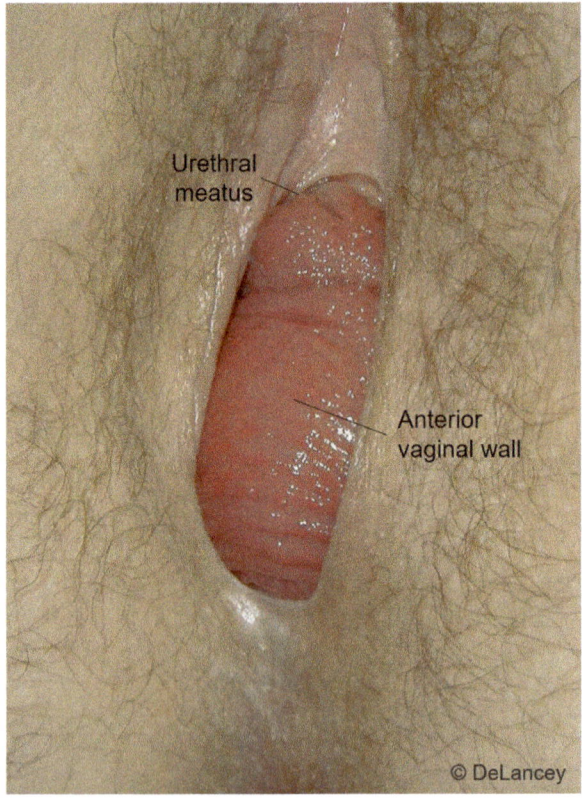

Urethral meatus

Anterior vaginal wall

© DeLancey

Fig. 20.2 Anatomical
drawing showing the
midsagittal relationship
between the bladder,
urethra, and anterior
vaginal wall with a large
anterior vaginal wall
prolapse. "Kinking" of the
urethra can be seen.
Modification of the
original publication from
Halban J, Tandler
J. Anatomie und Aetiologie
der Genital prolapse beim
Weibe. Vienna and
Leipzig, Wilhelm
Braumuller, 1907

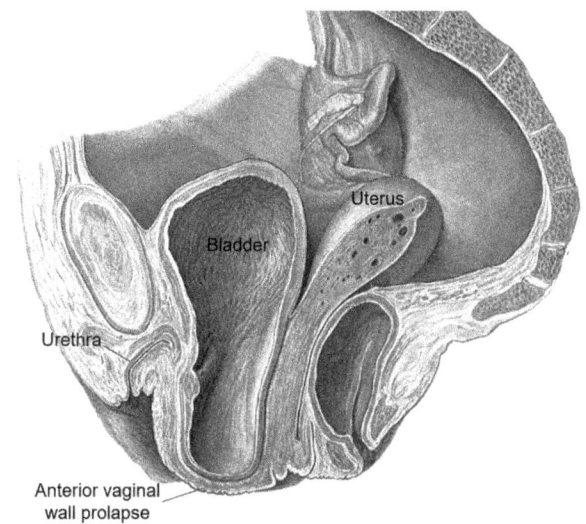

intraluminal urethral pressures and maintaining continence. AVW prolapse is thought to lead to SUI because when the supportive hammock fails, the urethra and urethrovesical junctions have nothing to counteract increases in intraabdominal pressure leading to "urethral hypermobility" and impaired closure of the urethral lumen.

Studies looking at AVW prolapse and SUI have shown that the association is strongest with lower prolapse stages and that once the prolapse becomes large enough to "kink" the urethra and lead to outlet obstruction, rates of SUI actually decrease (Fig. 20.2). Burrows et al. conducted a retrospective study of 330 women to identify the association between prolapse and bladder symptoms and found that maximal AVW prolapse was lower (i.e., more positive on POP-Q) in women without, versus with, SUI (+1.0 vs. 0.0 cm, $p < 0.001$), and apical location was also significantly lower in women without SUI (0.0 vs. −5.0 cm, $p < 0.001$) [33]. Conversely, AVW and apical prolapse were significantly larger among women who had to manually assist bladder emptying (+3.0 vs. 0.0 cm, $p < 0.001$; +1.5 vs. −5.0 cm, $p < 0.001$, respectively). These findings suggest that bladder outlet obstruction is protective of SUI.

The factor most strongly associated with SUI is maximal urethral closure pressure (MUCP) which is 42% lower among women with versus without SUI [34]. As previously mentioned, increasing AVW prolapse size is associated with fewer SUI symptoms, and therefore, one may assume that increased MUCP related to manual obstruction of the urethra is the underlying mechanism for this. Yet, studies looking at the relationship between MUCP and AVW prolapse size show conflicting results. In a study by Bai et al., MUCP was highest among women with stage 4 AVW prolapse (68.7 ± 20.3 (stage 2) vs. 67.0 ± 20.2 (stage 3) vs. 79.0 ± 30.9 (stage 4) mmHg); however, the difference across the three groups did not reach statistical significance ($p = 0.07$) [35]. In contrast, a study by Chang et al. reported that stress urethral closure pressures decreased with increasing stage of prolapse, 69.3 cmH$_2$O, 62.3 cmH$_2$O, and 52.2 cmH$_2$O, respectively, for stages 1, 2, and 3 AVW prolapse (all $p < 0.05$) [36]. However, the significance of these associations was attenuated after controlling for other clinical factors such as age, menopausal status, and vaginal parity. Age is a primary determinant of MUCP with a 15 mmHg decrease seen per decade of life [37] and also a major risk factor for prolapse; therefore, another explanation for the association between SUI and prolapse may simply be the shared risk factor of aging. The seemingly conflicting results of these studies suggest a complex relationship between AVW prolapse and urethral function. The relative contribution of urethral hypermobility and urethral closure pressure to the pathogenesis of SUI may vary depending on each woman's unique risk factors and degree of AVW prolapse. Therefore, a potential area for future research could focus on quantifying the patient-specific contribution of each risk factor to the development of SUI in women with AVW prolapse.

Finally, in women with advanced AVW prolapse, unanticipated SUI can occur with activity or certain position changes due to manual compression of the bladder without preceding urgency and pelvic floor muscle contraction.

Prolapse and Urgency Incontinence

Urgency urinary incontinence (UUI) is present in 22–88% of women with prolapse [38]. The relative risk of UUI with prolapse has been reported to range between 1.1 and 5.8 [39–41]. While treatment of prolapse is associated with improvement in UUI, treatments for UUI do not improve prolapse, suggesting the shared disease mechanism is primarily related to the effects of impaired bladder and urethral support [42].

Several mechanisms for the association between prolapse and UUI have been proposed but none definitively proven in human studies. Advanced AVW prolapse can cause bladder outlet obstruction and incomplete bladder emptying as well as mechanical compression of the displaced bladder. Over time, these factors can lead to irritation and remodeling of the detrusor as well as mechanical trauma to the urothelium. Several animal studies have shown urothelial cells release acetylcholine and ATP in response to chemical or mechanical stimuli, which can trigger detrusor muscle contractions and overactivity [40, 43–45].

How Does Treating Prolapse Improve SUI and UUI?

As discussed in the prior section, prolapse and urinary incontinence commonly coexist due to closely related disease mechanisms. As such, correction of prolapse, by either pessary or surgery, may improve urinary symptoms via resolution of bladder outlet obstruction and/or improved AVW support [38, 46].

Pessary Use

Pessaries have been shown to be effective in both treating prolapse symptoms and improving degree of prolapse [47]. There are also data showing improvement in urinary symptoms including UUI and SUI with pessary use. In one prospective study of 73 women with prolapse, stress incontinence improved in 45%, urge incontinence improved in 46%, and voiding difficulty improved in 53% of women after 2 months of pessary use [48]. Another study reported that out of 97 women successfully fitted with a vaginal pessary, 37% had decrease in urgency and 28% had decrease in UUI after 4 months of use, but no significant improvement in SUI [49]. Conversely, Hanson et al. reported a 58% cure rate for UUI in women using pessary.

In addition to subjective improvement of urinary incontinence symptoms, objective improvement in urinary flow measurements on urodynamic studies with pessary use has been demonstrated. Romanzi et al. found that 72% of women with prolapse had urethral obstruction on urodynamics, and 94% of these women had resolution after pessary insertion [50]. Similarly, another study showed that after 3 months of pessary use, maximum flow rate, mean flow rate, voided volume, and postvoid residual volume significantly improved. In the same study, 76.9% of women reported improvement of UUI and 58.1% of SUI. However, 20% of women developed new SUI with pessary use [51].

Surgery

Surgical repair of prolapse with both reconstructive and obliterative procedures may also improve bothersome urinary symptoms. It is important to note that while correction of prolapse may improve SUI or UUI symptoms, the primary goal of prolapse surgery is to treat prolapse symptoms and not urinary symptoms. Furthermore, correction of prolapse may actually cause new UUI or SUI symptoms making appropriate evaluation and counseling of patients critical prior to prolapse surgery [52].

Baessler et al. in the 6th International Consultation on Incontinence reviewed the effects of prolapse surgery on bladder function. They reported that preoperative overactive bladder (OAB) symptoms may resolve in up to 40% of women undergoing prolapse surgery [53]. Chang et al. showed that lower urinary tract symptoms (LUTS) improved significantly after prolapse repair both subjectively and objectively on bladder diary and urodynamics [32]. In this study, validated questionnaires regarding LUTS and quality of life improved significantly in addition to multiple voiding diary parameters (nocturia episodes, daytime frequency, urgency episodes, and incontinence episodes) despite unchanged fluid intake, total voided volume, and maximum voided volume per micturition. In a review by de Boer et al., OAB symptoms were examined before and after prolapse repair without concomitant incontinence surgery. Postoperative follow-up ranged from 12 to 30 months in the seven studies included. For all studies, detrusor overactivity decreased after surgery, and the proportion of the decrease ranged from 25% to 80% [42]. When comparing reconstructive surgery to obliterative procedures for prolapse, similar improvements in urgency and frequency symptoms are observed [54].

Although several studies show significant improvement in OAB symptoms, there is a risk of new OAB symptoms after prolapse repair. In a Cochrane review on the surgical management of prolapse, new OAB symptoms occurred in 12% of women after undergoing prolapse surgery [55].

In women with existing SUI prior to prolapse surgery, the likelihood that the SUI resolves with prolapse surgery alone without concomitant incontinence procedure is low. The risk of postoperative SUI with prolapse surgery alone was 39%, while the risk with a concomitant midurethral sling was 8–19% [55]. In women with occult SUI, the risk of postoperative SUI with prolapse surgery alone was 34%, while the risk with concomitant midurethral sling was 10–22% [55]. Colombo et al. compared anterior colporrhaphy to Burch colposuspension for treatment of AVW prolapse and SUI. In this study, 52% of the women who underwent anterior repair alone had subjective cure of their SUI [56]. Baessler et al.'s analysis in the 6th International Consultation on Incontinence found that compared to women with a concomitant incontinence procedure at the time of prolapse repair, those without had an 11-fold increased odds of persistent SUI [53]. Similarly, women who were found to have a positive preoperative occult SUI test and did not undergo concomitant incontinence procedure at the time of prolapse repair had a 10-fold increased odds of new or "de novo" SUI after surgery compared to those who had concomitant incontinence procedure. Borstad et al. showed that only 29% of women were cured of SUI after native tissue prolapse surgery alone and did not require continence surgery [57].

The use of vaginal mesh in prolapse repair can also affect risk of de novo SUI. In the Cochrane review on the surgical management of prolapse, anterior vaginal mesh repair was found to slightly increase postoperative de novo SUI when compared to anterior native tissue repair (RR 1.58) [55]. Baessler et al. report a de novo SUI rate of 8% after anterior repair compared to 14% in repairs using anterior armed mesh [53].

When Should an Incontinence Procedure Be Offered with Pelvic Organ Prolapse Repair?

All women who are planning to undergo surgery for prolapse should be screened for urinary symptoms and evaluated for occult SUI to minimize the risk of de novo SUI after prolapse surgery which ranges from 15% to 51% [55, 58–61]. Rates of postoperative SUI are significantly higher in women with occult SUI who undergo prolapse surgery without incontinence procedures as compared to those who have concomitant incontinence procedures (OR 9.8, CI 7.1–13.6) [57, 59, 60, 62]. Liang et al. showed that significantly more patients with preoperative occult SUI with pessary developed de novo SUI after not receiving a midurethral sling compared to those who underwent sling placement at 18–21 months after surgery (53% vs. 0%, $p < 0.001$) [59].

Because preoperative occult SUI significantly increases the risk for de novo SUI after prolapse surgery, routine evaluation should be performed preoperatively in women planning prolapse surgery. Occult SUI can be evaluated using a reduction stress test or urodynamic testing. A reduction stress test evaluates continence with the prolapse "reduced" simulating resolution of prolapse as would occur with a pessary or surgery. There is no consensus on standard protocol for reduction stress test technique; however, the typical procedure is to manually reduce the prolapse and then have the patient cough or Valsalva up to three times with the bladder comfortably full or backfilled to 300 ml. Prolapse reduction can be achieved using a large tip cotton scopette, the examiner's hand, or a pessary. Visco et al. found occult SUI was demonstrated in 27% of otherwise stress-continent women planning sacrocolpopexy for prolapse using reduction stress testing [60]. For women who opt for a pessary trial prior to surgery, this is also an opportunity to assess for occult incontinence.

Unfortunately, the predictive value of reduction stress testing is limited as 39% of women with negative testing will still develop de novo stress incontinence [60]. As there is no way to perfectly predict who will develop de novo SUI, all patients should be counseled on the possibility of de novo SUI despite negative reduction stress test.

Urodynamic studies are commonly performed in women prior to surgery for incontinence to confirm diagnosis or guide treatment decisions. However, Nager et al. showed that for women with uncomplicated, demonstrable stress urinary incontinence, urodynamic testing did not improve treatment success rate when compared to office evaluation alone consisting of provocative stress test, postvoid residual volume, assessment of urethral mobility, and absence of bladder infection (77.2% vs. 76.9%) [63]. When doing urodynamics in women with prolapse, stress maneuvers should be done with the prolapse reduced, especially with advanced prolapse.

When Should a Concomitant Incontinence Procedure Be Offered with Prolapse Surgery?

All women undergoing surgery for prolapse should be counseled about the option for concomitant incontinence procedure. Below, we discuss considerations to help guide counseling and decision making.

Demonstrable SUI

In patients with coexisting SUI and prolapse, a concomitant incontinence procedure is generally recommended at the time of prolapse surgery. Risk of persistent SUI is significantly higher in those who undergo prolapse surgery without incontinence surgery (OR 10.9, 95% CI 7.9–15.0) as compared to those who have concomitant incontinence surgery [55, 53]. However, in a small percentage of women, SUI may improve or resolve after prolapse repair alone [55, 57]. Therefore, a staged approach may be preferred.

Occult SUI

Occult SUI on reduction stress test and history of SUI before prolapse developed or progressed are important factors to consider when counseling patients about risk of postoperative SUI. Similar to demonstrable SUI, women with occult SUI are at risk for de novo SUI after prolapse repair (OR 9.8, 95% CI 7.1–13.6) [53]. Therefore, the option for concomitant or staged incontinence procedure should be offered.

Prophylactic Incontinence Procedure in Continent Women

In continent women undergoing prolapse repair, the risk of de novo SUI and the risks and benefits of a concomitant incontinence procedure should be discussed. Predicting who would benefit from a prophylactic incontinence procedure is clinically challenging. An option to decrease the risk of de novo SUI in previously continent women includes performing an incontinence procedure at time of prolapse repair. Brubaker et al. showed that undergoing concomitant Burch colposuspension at the time of an abdominal sacrocolpopexy significantly reduced the risk of de novo SUI symptoms at two years versus abdominal sacrocolpopexy alone (41.8% vs. 57.9%; $p = 0.020$) [58]. However, number needed to treat with Burch colposuspension to prevent one case of urinary incontinence was 6.2. Wei et al. demonstrated after 12 months that undergoing TVT at the time of vaginal prolapse surgery also significantly decreased the risk of urinary incontinence than prolapse surgery alone (27.3% vs. 43.0%, $p = 0.002$) [61]. Similar to Brubaker's study, number needed to treat with TVT to prevent one case of incontinence was 6.3. Therefore, if all women undergoing prolapse repair received a concomitant incontinence procedure, 57% of women would receive an unnecessary procedure and be subjected to the associated risks.

Presence of Risk Factors and Patient-Centered Outcomes

Shared decision making between the provider and patient is important to determine if a concomitant incontinence procedure at the time of prolapse surgery is appropriate. SUI symptoms prior to prolapse development, current symptoms and quality of life, and results of full bladder reduction stress test and/or urodynamics should help guide counseling. However, it is essential to discuss the patient's preferences and goals prior to surgery as unmet goals are associated with patient dissatisfaction after treatment [64]. For example, if a patient has a strong aversion to mesh, a sling may be declined despite risk factors for de novo SUI. Conversely, if a patient has a strong desire to avoid the risk of de novo SUI, one may perform a concomitant incontinence procedure despite absence of occult SUI or risk factors. Additionally, the decision of whether to add a concomitant incontinence procedure may also depend on the planned surgery. In continent women who have repairs with vaginal mesh, the risk of de novo SUI is higher when compared to native tissue repair; however, these products are no longer on the market (RR 1.58, 95% CI 1.05–2.37) (9% vs. 14%) [55].

Risk Calculator for De Novo SUI

Risk stratification models are often helpful tools in shared decision making. Jelovsek et al. created a model to predict a woman's individual risk of de novo stress incontinence [65]. The nomogram uses risk factors including age at surgery, number of vaginal births, body mass index, preoperative stress test, if incontinence procedure performed, urine leakage associated with a feeling of urgency, and diagnosis of diabetes to predict the risk of de novo SUI for women undergoing prolapse repair. This information can be used to guide the decision to undergo an incontinence procedure at the time of prolapse repair.

Staged Procedure

For those opting for a staged procedure, prolapse repair is performed alone, and urinary symptoms are monitored postoperatively. If bothersome de novo SUI develops, an incontinence procedure can then be performed as a second surgery. There does not seem to be a difference in subjective outcomes when comparing concomitant versus delayed midurethral sling placement (risk of SUI 1–16% vs. 11%) [57].

If prolapse surgery alone does not treat urinary incontinence and intervention is desired, treatment of urinary incontinence should be pursued similarly to someone without a history of prolapse repair.

Conclusion

Pelvic organ prolapse and urinary incontinence are common disorders among women and often coexist due to a shared disease mechanism and shared risk factors. Although urinary symptoms can improve after correction of prolapse, persistent or de novo urinary incontinence is a risk following prolapse repair. Concomitant incontinence procedures can be offered at the time of prolapse repair to either treat preexisting or prevent de novo stress urinary continence.

Risk stratification and patient preferences are important to determine if a concomitant incontinence procedure at the time of prolapse repair is appropriate.

References

1. Haylen BT, Maher CF, Barber MD, Camargo S, Dandolu V, Digesu A, et al. An International Urogynecological Association (IUGA)/International Continence Society (ICS) joint report on the terminology for female pelvic organ prolapse (POP). Int Urogynecol J. 2016;27(4):655–84. https://doi.org/10.1007/s00192-016-3003-y.
2. Rogers RG. Female pelvic medicine and reconstructive surgery: clinical practice and surgical atlas. 1st ed. New York: McGraw-Hill; 2013.
3. Bump RC, Mattiasson A, Bo K, Brubaker LP, DeLancey JO, Klarskov P, et al. The standardization of terminology of female pelvic organ prolapse and pelvic floor dysfunction. Am J Obstet Gynecol. 1996;175(1):10–7.
4. Baden WF, Walker T. Surgical repair of vaginal defects. Philadelphia: Lippincott; 1992.
5. Nygaard I, Barber MD, Burgio KL, Kenton K, Meikle S, Schaffer J, et al. Prevalence of symptomatic pelvic floor disorders in US women. JAMA. 2008;300(11):1311–6. https://doi.org/10.1001/jama.300.11.1311.
6. Barber MD, Maher C. Epidemiology and outcome assessment of pelvic organ prolapse. Int Urogynecol J. 2013;24(11):1783–90. https://doi.org/10.1007/s00192-013-2169-9.
7. Swift SE. The distribution of pelvic organ support in a population of female subjects seen for routine gynecologic health care. Am J Obstet Gynecol. 2000;183(2):277–85. https://doi.org/10.1067/mob.2000.107583.
8. Hendrix SL, Clark A, Nygaard I, Aragaki A, Barnabei V, McTiernan A. Pelvic organ prolapse in the Women's Health Initiative: gravity and gravidity. Am J Obstet Gynecol. 2002;186(6):1160–6.
9. Dieter AA, Wilkins MF, Wu JM. Epidemiological trends and future care needs for pelvic floor disorders. Curr Opin Obstet Gynecol. 2015;27(5):380–4. https://doi.org/10.1097/GCO.0000000000000200.
10. Delancey JO, Kane Low L, Miller JM, Patel DA, Tumbarello JA. Graphic integration of causal factors of pelvic floor disorders: an integrated life span model. Am J Obstet Gynecol. 2008;199(6):610, e1-5. https://doi.org/10.1016/j.ajog.2008.04.001.
11. Wu JM, Vaughan CP, Goode PS, Redden DT, Burgio KL, Richter HE, et al. Prevalence and trends of symptomatic pelvic floor disorders in U.S. women. Obstet Gynecol. 2014;123(1):141–8. https://doi.org/10.1097/AOG.0000000000000057.
12. Akervall S, Al-Mukhtar Othman J, Molin M, Gyhagen M. Symptomatic pelvic organ prolapse in middle-aged women: a national matched cohort study on the influence of childbirth. Am J Obstet Gynecol. 2020;222(4):356, e1-e14. https://doi.org/10.1016/j.ajog.2019.10.007.

13. Chiaffarino F, Chatenoud L, Dindelli M, Meschia M, Buonaguidi A, Amicarelli F, et al. Reproductive factors, family history, occupation and risk of urogenital prolapse. Eur J Obstet Gynecol Reprod Biol. 1999;82(1):63–7. https://doi.org/10.1016/s0301-2115(98)00175-4.
14. Handa VL, Blomquist JL, Roem J, Munoz A. Longitudinal study of quantitative changes in pelvic organ support among parous women. Am J Obstet Gynecol. 2018;218(3):320, e1-e7. https://doi.org/10.1016/j.ajog.2017.12.214.
15. Lukacz ES, Lawrence JM, Contreras R, Nager CW, Luber KM. Parity, mode of delivery, and pelvic floor disorders. Obstet Gynecol. 2006;107(6):1253–60. https://doi.org/10.1097/01. AOG.0000218096.54169.34.
16. Moalli PA, Jones Ivy S, Meyn LA, Zyczynski HM. Risk factors associated with pelvic floor disorders in women undergoing surgical repair. Obstet Gynecol. 2003;101(5 Pt 1):869–74. https://doi.org/10.1016/s0029-7844(03)00078-4.
17. Kearney R, Fitzpatrick M, Brennan S, Behan M, Miller J, Keane D, et al. Levator ani injury in primiparous women with forceps delivery for fetal distress, forceps for second stage arrest, and spontaneous delivery. Int J Gynaecol Obstet. 2010;111(1):19–22. https://doi.org/10.1016/j. ijgo.2010.05.019.
18. DeLancey JO, Morgan DM, Fenner DE, Kearney R, Guire K, Miller JM, et al. Comparison of levator ani muscle defects and function in women with and without pelvic organ prolapse. Obstet Gynecol. 2007;109(2 Pt 1):295–302. https://doi.org/10.1097/01.AOG.0000250901.57095.ba.
19. Dietz HP, Simpson JM. Levator trauma is associated with pelvic organ prolapse. BJOG. 2008;115(8):979–84. https://doi.org/10.1111/j.1471-0528.2008.01751.x.
20. Lammers K, Lince SL, Spath MA, van Kempen LC, Hendriks JC, Vierhout ME, et al. Pelvic organ prolapse and collagen-associated disorders. Int Urogynecol J. 2012;23(3):313–9. https:// doi.org/10.1007/s00192-011-1532-y.
21. Weidner AC, Jamison MG, Branham V, South MM, Borawski KM, Romero AA. Neuropathic injury to the levator ani occurs in 1 in 4 primiparous women. Am J Obstet Gynecol. 2006;195(6):1851–6. https://doi.org/10.1016/j.ajog.2006.06.062.
22. Lien KC, Morgan DM, Delancey JO, Ashton-Miller JA. Pudendal nerve stretch during vaginal birth: a 3D computer simulation. Am J Obstet Gynecol. 2005;192(5):1669–76. https://doi. org/10.1016/j.ajog.2005.01.032.
23. Blomquist JL, Munoz A, Carroll M, Handa VL. Association of delivery mode with pelvic floor disorders after childbirth. JAMA. 2018;320(23):2438–47. https://doi.org/10.1001/ jama.2018.18315.
24. Allen-Brady K, Cannon-Albright L, Farnham JM, Teerlink C, Vierhout ME, van Kempen LCL, et al. Identification of six loci associated with pelvic organ prolapse using genome-wide association analysis. Obstet Gynecol. 2011;118(6):1345–53. https://doi.org/10.1097/ AOG.0b013e318236f4b5.
25. Carley ME, Schaffer J. Urinary incontinence and pelvic organ prolapse in women with Marfan or Ehlers Danlos syndrome. Am J Obstet Gynecol. 2000;182(5):1021–3. https://doi. org/10.1067/mob.2000.105410.
26. Ward RM, Velez Edwards DR, Edwards T, Giri A, Jerome RN, Wu JM. Genetic epidemiology of pelvic organ prolapse: a systematic review. Am J Obstet Gynecol. 2014;211(4):326–35. https://doi.org/10.1016/j.ajog.2014.04.006.
27. Cartwright R, Kirby AC, Tikkinen KA, Mangera A, Thiagamoorthy G, Rajan P, et al. Systematic review and metaanalysis of genetic association studies of urinary symptoms and prolapse in women. Am J Obstet Gynecol. 2015;212(2):199, e1-24. https://doi.org/10.1016/j. ajog.2014.08.005.
28. Snooks SJ, Barnes PR, Swash M, Henry MM. Damage to the innervation of the pelvic floor musculature in chronic constipation. Gastroenterology. 1985;89(5):977–81. https://doi. org/10.1016/0016-5085(85)90196-9.

29. Bai SW, Jeon MJ, Kim JY, Chung KA, Kim SK, Park KH. Relationship between stress urinary incontinence and pelvic organ prolapse. Int Urogynecol J Pelvic Floor Dysfunct. 2002;13(4):256–60.; discussion 60. https://doi.org/10.1007/s001920200053.
30. Muniz KS, Pilkinton M, Winkler HA, Shalom DF. Prevalence of stress urinary incontinence and intrinsic sphincter deficiency in patients with stage IV pelvic organ prolapse. J Obstet Gynaecol Res. 2020;47(2):640–4. https://doi.org/10.1111/jog.14574.
31. Hoyte LPJ, Damaser M. Biomechanics of the female pelvic floor. London/San Diego: Academic Press is an imprint of Elsevier; 2016.
32. DeLancey JO. Structural support of the urethra as it relates to stress urinary incontinence: the hammock hypothesis. Am J Obstet Gynecol. 1994;170(6):1713–20.; discussion 20-3. https://doi.org/10.1016/s0002-9378(94)70346-9.
33. Burrows LJ, Meyn LA, Walters MD, Weber AM. Pelvic symptoms in women with pelvic organ prolapse. Obstet Gynecol. 2004;104(5 Pt 1):982–8. https://doi.org/10.1097/01.AOG.0000142708.61298.be.
34. DeLancey JO, Trowbridge ER, Miller JM, Morgan DM, Guire K, Fenner DE, et al. Stress urinary incontinence: relative importance of urethral support and urethral closure pressure. J Urol. 2008;179(6):2286–90.; discussion 90. https://doi.org/10.1016/j.juro.2008.01.098.
35. Bai SW, Cho JM, Kwon HS, Park JH, Shin JS, Kim SK, et al. The relationship between maximal urethral closure pressure and functional urethral length in anterior vaginal wall prolapse patients according to stage and age. Yonsei Med J. 2005;46(3):408–13. https://doi.org/10.3349/ymj.2005.46.3.408.
36. Chang HW, Ng SC, Chen GD. Correlations between severity of anterior vaginal wall prolapse and parameters of urethral pressure profile. Low Urin Tract Symptoms. 2020;13(2):238–43. https://doi.org/10.1111/luts.12357.
37. Trowbridge ER, Wei JT, Fenner DE, Ashton-Miller JA, Delancey JO. Effects of aging on lower urinary tract and pelvic floor function in nulliparous women. Obstet Gynecol. 2007;109(3):715–20. https://doi.org/10.1097/01.AOG.0000257074.98122.69.
38. Cameron AP. Systematic review of lower urinary tract symptoms occurring with pelvic organ prolapse. Arab J Urol. 2019;17(1):23–9. https://doi.org/10.1080/2090598X.2019.1589929.
39. Bradley CS, Nygaard IE. Vaginal wall descensus and pelvic floor symptoms in older women. Obstet Gynecol. 2005;106(4):759–66. https://doi.org/10.1097/01.AOG.0000180183.03897.72.
40. Fritel X, Varnoux N, Zins M, Breart G, Ringa V. Symptomatic pelvic organ prolapse at midlife, quality of life, and risk factors. Obstet Gynecol. 2009;113(3):609–16. https://doi.org/10.1097/AOG.0b013e3181985312.
41. Tegerstedt G, Maehle-Schmidt M, Nyren O, Hammarstrom M. Prevalence of symptomatic pelvic organ prolapse in a Swedish population. Int Urogynecol J Pelvic Floor Dysfunct. 2005;16(6):497–503. https://doi.org/10.1007/s00192-005-1326-1.
42. de Boer TA, Salvatore S, Cardozo L, Chapple C, Kelleher C, van Kerrebroeck P, et al. Pelvic organ prolapse and overactive bladder. Neurourol Urodyn. 2010;29(1):30–9. https://doi.org/10.1002/nau.20858.
43. Birder LA, de Groat WC. Mechanisms of disease: involvement of the urothelium in bladder dysfunction. Nat Clin Pract Urol. 2007;4(1):46–54. https://doi.org/10.1038/ncpuro0672.
44. Ferguson DR, Kennedy I, Burton TJ. ATP is released from rabbit urinary bladder epithelial cells by hydrostatic pressure changes--a possible sensory mechanism? J Physiol. 1997;505(Pt 2):503–11. https://doi.org/10.1111/j.1469-7793.1997.503bb.x.
45. Keay SK, Birder LA, Chai TC. Evidence for bladder urothelial pathophysiology in functional bladder disorders. Biomed Res Int. 2014;2014:865463. https://doi.org/10.1155/2014/865463.
46. Glazener CM, Cooper K, Mashayekhi A. Anterior vaginal repair for urinary incontinence in women. Cochrane Database Syst Rev. 2017;7:CD001755. https://doi.org/10.1002/14651858.CD001755.pub2.
47. Handa VL, Jones M. Do pessaries prevent the progression of pelvic organ prolapse? Int Urogynecol J Pelvic Floor Dysfunct. 2002;13(6):349–51.; discussion 52. https://doi.org/10.1007/s001920200078.

48. Clemons JL, Aguilar VC, Tillinghast TA, Jackson ND, Myers DL. Patient satisfaction and changes in prolapse and urinary symptoms in women who were fitted successfully with a pessary for pelvic organ prolapse. Am J Obstet Gynecol. 2004;190(4):1025–9. https://doi.org/10.1016/j.ajog.2003.10.711.
49. Fernando RJ, Thakar R, Sultan AH, Shah SM, Jones PW. Effect of vaginal pessaries on symptoms associated with pelvic organ prolapse. Obstet Gynecol. 2006;108(1):93–9. https://doi.org/10.1097/01.AOG.0000222903.38684.cc.
50. Romanzi LJ, Chaikin DC, Blaivas JG. The effect of genital prolapse on voiding. J Urol. 1999;161(2):581–6.
51. Ding J, Chen C, Song XC, Zhang L, Deng M, Zhu L. Changes in prolapse and urinary symptoms after successful fitting of a ring pessary with support in women with advanced pelvic organ prolapse: a prospective study. Urology. 2016;87:70–5. https://doi.org/10.1016/j.urology.2015.07.025.
52. American Urogynecologic Society Guidelines Statements Committee, Carberry CL, Tulikangas PK, Ridgeway BM, Collins SA, Adam RA. American urogynecologic society best practice statement: evaluation and counseling of patients with pelvic organ prolapse. Female Pelvic Med Reconstr Surg. 2017;23(5):281–7. https://doi.org/10.1097/SPV.0000000000000424.
53. Abrams P, Cardozo L, Wagg A, Wein A, editors. Incontinence. 6th ed. Bristol: International Continence Society; 2017.
54. Foster RT Sr, Barber MD, Parasio MF, Walters MD, Weidner AC, Amundsen CL. A prospective assessment of overactive bladder symptoms in a cohort of elderly women who underwent transvaginal surgery for advanced pelvic organ prolapse. Am J Obstet Gynecol. 2007;197(1):82, e1-4. https://doi.org/10.1016/j.ajog.2007.02.049.
55. Maher C, Feiner B, Baessler K, Schmid C. Surgical management of pelvic organ prolapse in women. Cochrane Database Syst Rev. 2013;(4):CD004014. https://doi.org/10.1002/14651858.CD004014.pub5.
56. Colombo M, Vitobello D, Proietti F, Milani R. Randomised comparison of Burch colposuspension versus anterior colporrhaphy in women with stress urinary incontinence and anterior vaginal wall prolapse. BJOG. 2000;107(4):544–51. https://doi.org/10.1111/j.1471-0528.2000.tb13276.x.
57. Borstad E, Abdelnoor M, Staff AC, Kulseng-Hanssen S. Surgical strategies for women with pelvic organ prolapse and urinary stress incontinence. Int Urogynecol J. 2010;21(2):179–86. https://doi.org/10.1007/s00192-009-1007-6.
58. Brubaker L, Cundiff GW, Fine P, Nygaard I, Richter HE, Visco AG, et al. Abdominal sacrocolpopexy with Burch colposuspension to reduce urinary stress incontinence. N Engl J Med. 2006;354(15):1557–66. https://doi.org/10.1056/NEJMoa054208.
59. Liang CC, Chang YL, Chang SD, Lo TS, Soong YK. Pessary test to predict postoperative urinary incontinence in women undergoing hysterectomy for prolapse. Obstet Gynecol. 2004;104(4):795–800. https://doi.org/10.1097/01.AOG.0000140689.90131.01.
60. Visco AG, Brubaker L, Nygaard I, Richter HE, Cundiff G, Fine P, et al. The role of preoperative urodynamic testing in stress-continent women undergoing sacrocolpopexy: the Colpopexy and Urinary Reduction Efforts (CARE) randomized surgical trial. Int Urogynecol J Pelvic Floor Dysfunct. 2008;19(5):607–14. https://doi.org/10.1007/s00192-007-0498-2.
61. Wei JT, Nygaard I, Richter HE, Nager CW, Barber MD, Kenton K, et al. A midurethral sling to reduce incontinence after vaginal prolapse repair. N Engl J Med. 2012;366(25):2358–67. https://doi.org/10.1056/NEJMoa1111967.
62. Ellstrom Engh AM, Ekeryd A, Magnusson A, Olsson I, Otterlind L, Tobiasson G. Can de novo stress incontinence after anterior wall repair be predicted? Acta Obstet Gynecol Scand. 2011;90(5):488–93. https://doi.org/10.1111/j.1600-0412.2011.01087.x.
63. Nager CW, Brubaker L, Litman HJ, Zyczynski HM, Varner RE, Amundsen C, et al. A randomized trial of urodynamic testing before stress-incontinence surgery. N Engl J Med. 2012;366(21):1987–97. https://doi.org/10.1056/NEJMoa1113595.

64. Hullfish KL, Bovbjerg VE, Steers WD. Patient-centered goals for pelvic floor dysfunction surgery: long-term follow-up. Am J Obstet Gynecol. 2004;191(1):201–5. https://doi.org/10.1016/j.ajog.2004.03.086.
65. Jelovsek JE. Predicting urinary incontinence after surgery for pelvic organ prolapse. Curr Opin Obstet Gynecol. 2016;28(5):399–406. https://doi.org/10.1097/GCO.0000000000000308.

Chapter 21
Incontinence After Complex Urinary Reconstruction: Orthotopic Neobladder and Gender-Affirming Surgery

Amanda C. Chi, Nancy Ye, Virginia Li, Krystal DePorto, and Polina Reyblat

Introduction

Urinary incontinence can develop as a consequence or a complication of a variety of urinary reconstructive surgeries. In this chapter, we focus on various types of incontinence after orthotopic neobladder construction and after gender-affirming feminizing and masculinizing surgery. Although the workup should start the same with a thorough history and physical exam, there are important nuances and considerations when treating these patients.

Urinary Incontinence in Women After Orthotopic Urinary Diversion

The gold standard for treatment of muscle-invasive bladder cancer and high-risk noninvasive bladder cancer is radical cystectomy (RC) and urinary diversion [1]. In female patients, this historically referred to total anterior pelvic exenteration, including cystectomy, hysterectomy, bilateral salpingo-oophorectomy, anterior vaginal wall resection, and urethrectomy, with ileal conduit or continent cutaneous reservoir urinary diversion [2]. When orthotopic neobladders were first introduced, there were initial concerns regarding the oncologic and functional outcomes in women, given their shorter urethral length. Studies since have addressed these concerns, suggesting that there is a relatively small percentage of urethral involvement in

A. C. Chi (✉) · N. Ye · V. Li · K. DePorto · P. Reyblat
Department of Urology, Kaiser Permanente Southern California, Los Angeles, CA, USA
e-mail: amanda.c.chi@kp.org; nancy.y.ye@kp.org; virginia.y.li@kp.org; krystal.a.deporto@kp.org; polina.x.reyblat@kp.org

women with bladder cancer, providing a more detailed understanding of the continence mechanism in women, and showing acceptable oncologic and functional outcomes while preserving the urethra for the creation of orthotopic neobladders in selected female patients [3–10].

Principles of Continent Orthotopic Urinary Diversion

While there are many different surgical approaches to orthotopic urinary diversion, the key principles to successful outcomes remain constant: (1) nonobstructed urethra with preservation of an adequate external sphincter mechanism, (2) compliant reservoir that allows for low-pressure storage of urine, and (3) adequate capacity (~300–500 mL) when the reservoir is mature [11]. Various bowel segments may be used to construct a urinary reservoir; however, ileal neobladders have been shown to be more compliant than colonic neobladders [12]. Regardless of the bowel segment used, it is important to have adequate detubularization and creation of a spherical shape. It is thought that detubularizing the bowel segment disrupts the peristaltic contractions, thus allowing for decreased intraluminal pressure and low-pressure storage. The spherical geometry allows for the greatest volume of storage for a given surface area [13].

Continence Mechanism

In order to understand functional outcomes relating to urinary continence after orthotopic urinary diversion in women, one must appreciate female urethral continence mechanisms. The female urethral sphincter is composed of striated and smooth muscles. Historically, it was thought that in women, the bladder neck was required for urinary continence, which accounted for the initial skepticism in creating orthotopic urinary diversions for women; however, studies have shown that the striated rhabdosphincter is most critical for urinary continence. The anatomy of the female rhabdosphincter was carefully evaluated through cadaveric dissections and showed that the striated muscle is most robust at the anterior and lateral aspects of the midurethra deep to the endopelvic fascia [3]. Branches of the pudendal nerve travel deep to the endopelvic fascia and enter the caudal portion of the urethra laterally to innervate the rhabdosphincter [3, 14]. Urodynamic studies have also shown that the primary continence zone in women after cystectomy and orthotopic urinary diversion is the middle third of the urethra [15]. Careful surgical technique should be used to limit urethral dissection superficial to the endopelvic fascia to avoid damaging the rhabdosphincter and its innervation, in an effort to preserve postoperative incontinence.

The smooth muscle component of the urethral sphincter is primarily innervated by autonomic nerves that travel lateral to the vagina. The necessity of preservation of these autonomic nerves is controversial. While some argue that preservation of the autonomic nerves is critical to continence and avoiding retention [6, 9, 16–18], others rely on pudendal innervation of the rhabdosphincter alone [19, 20]. Given lack of randomized controlled trials answering this question, it is prudent to preserve the autonomic plexus when oncologically feasible [21].

Incontinence After Orthotopic Urinary Diversion

It is very challenging to evaluate the true incidence and prevalence of urinary incontinence after orthotopic diversion due to the lack of standardized outcomes reporting. Reservoirs take 6–12 months postoperatively to mature and acquire stable maximum capacity [22]. Some suggest that further evaluation and management should be delayed until 12–18 months to allow for the continence status to plateau [10, 15, 23]. The varied definitions of continence, severity of incontinence, methods of collecting and reporting data, length and timing of follow-up, and infrequent use of validated questionnaires make it difficult to meaningfully compare results between studies. Furthermore, studies reporting continence postorthotopic neobladder tend to categorize continence by timing of continence (daytime vs. nighttime) rather than symptomatology (stress vs. urge vs. overflow).

Reported rates for daytime continence range from 77% to 90%, and nighttime continence from 57% to 86% [5, 23–25]. There appears to be gradual improvement in daytime continence during the first 6–12 months, while nighttime continence is typically slower to improve and can extend into the second year [11]. Studies have shown diabetes and hysterectomy to be risk factors for incontinence [26–28]. Anderson et al. conducted a retrospective study of 49 women who underwent RC and creation of orthotopic neobladder between 1996 and 2011, and determined that the only predictor of daytime incontinence was having a previous or concurrent hysterectomy. In patients with preserved continence, a higher percentage (51.2%) had uterine sparing surgery versus patients with incontinence, and only 13.3% had preserved uterus ($p < 0.01$). In the continent patients, bilateral nerve sparing was attempted in 62.8% and unilateral in 34.9%; in incontinent patients, bilateral nerve sparing was attempted in 36.7% and unilateral in 53.3% ($p = 0.02$) [17]. In 2017, a systematic review of 15 studies evaluated the oncologic and functional outcomes of pelvic organ-preserving radical cystectomy (POPRC) compared to standard RC in women who received orthotopic diversion. POPRC included nerve-sparing, vagina-sparing, or genital-sparing. There was great variability in daytime continence rates of 57.1–100% and nighttime continence rates of 42.9–100% of patients who underwent POPRC [29]. Several limitations exist, including the heterogeneity between studies, narrative synthesis approach, and lack of preoperative continence status; however, this was the first systematic review of POPRC and points to the need for prospective multicenter studies to further assess functional outcomes in women undergoing POPRC.

Careful patient selection is likely to improve outcomes as well. Women with higher preoperative urethral closing pressure at rest and longer functional urethral length were associated with postoperative continence [17]. Preoperative stress urinary incontinence was associated with daytime incontinence severity. Age has also been proposed as a contributing factor; in a study of 41 patients with mean follow-up of 5.7 years, age >65 years at the time of surgery was the only factor associated with daytime incontinence [30]. In a separate study, older age was associated with the presence and severity of nocturnal incontinence [27]. A component of this may be secondary to physiological nocturnal polyuria associated with increasing age [31].

Nighttime incontinence is thought to be due to rhabdosphincter relaxation, physiologic diuresis, and decreased sensation resulting in overdistension of the neobladder with the excess volume overcoming the urethral closure mechanism [28]. Initial management may include fluid reduction in the evening, emptying just prior to sleeping, awakening a few times overnight in order to empty the neobladder, and the use of an alarm clock as needed [28, 32].

Evaluation and Workup

Initial evaluation of urinary incontinence should include review of relevant history and physical exam. Focused physical examination, including sensation and appropriate reflex testing of the abdomen, urethra, vagina, perineum, rectum, anus, and lower extremities, is indicated. Vaginal examination should include the use of a speculum to identify potential neobladder vaginal fistula [33]. Laboratory studies including a basic metabolic panel and urine culture can be helpful to assess renal function and rule out an infectious etiology of incontinence. Outpatient diagnostic testing including uroflowmetry, postvoid residual measurements, voiding diary to assess for polydipsia or nocturnal polyuria, and urodynamic studies can be utilized [28]. Patients with a high postvoid residual may need additional workup for prolapse, which occurs in approximately 6% of this population [34]. The presence of a neobladder vaginal fistula must be ruled out prior to the initiation of any treatment (Fig. 21.1).

Treatment

Physical Therapy

Pelvic floor physical therapy (PFPT) was introduced by Dr. Arnold Kegel in 1948 and is a first-line noninvasive treatment option for stress urinary incontinence [35]. Targeted therapeutic exercises help strengthen the pelvic floor musculature and enhance urethral stability, ultimately improving urinary control. In those

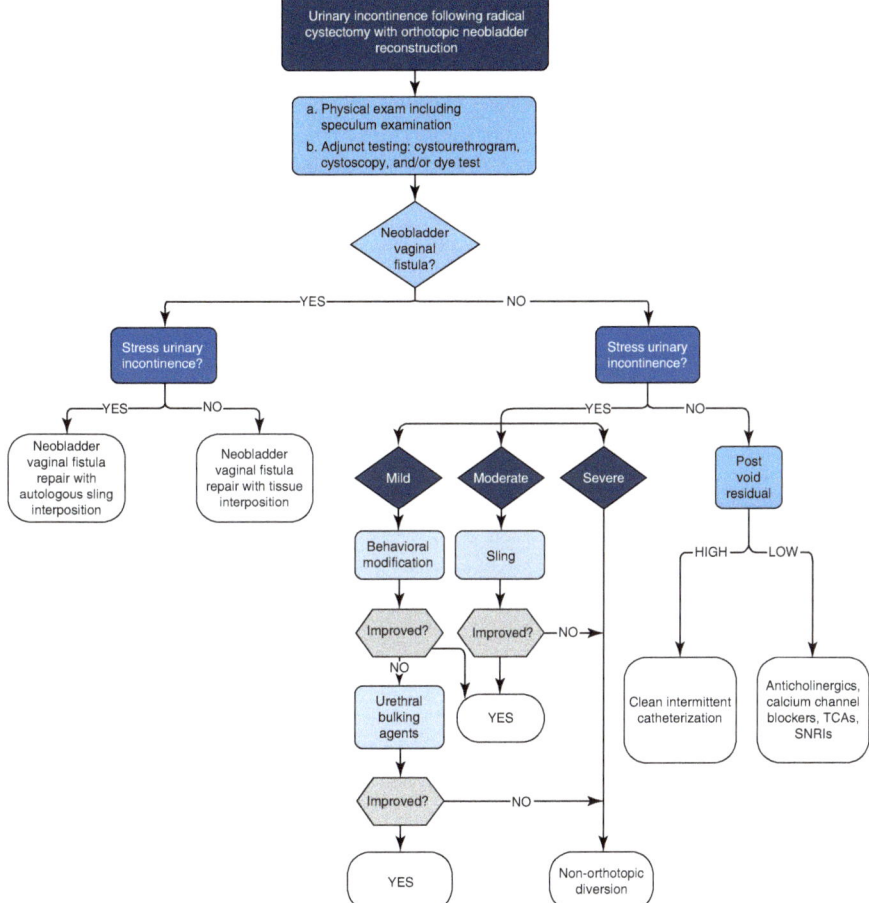

Fig. 21.1 Flowchart detailing workup of patients with neobladder presenting with incontinence

undergoing radical cystectomy with orthotopic neobladder reconstruction, it is recommended that pelvic floor physical therapy starts prior to surgical intervention [36, 37]. This recommendation has been extrapolated from data published by Centemero et al. who studied the return of postprostatectomy continence in patients randomized to pre- and postoperative pelvic floor physical therapy versus postoperative pelvic floor physical therapy alone. Those who completed pre- and postoperative pelvic floor physical therapy reported continence rates 24% higher than their counterparts 1 month after surgery. By initiating pelvic floor physical therapy preoperatively, patients can more expeditiously localize the pelvic floor muscles during the critical stages of neuromuscular reeducation. While there is no gold-standard treatment protocol for women with incontinence after cystectomy and neobladder reconstruction, Johnson et al. proposed a protocol that can be seen in Table 21.1. Visual biofeedbacks via mirrors, cameras, electromyography tracings, or abstract

Table 21.1 Guideline for PFPT protocol [36]

1. Preoperative pelvic floor training (*initiate 4–6 weeks prior to surgery*)	Pelvic floor coordination training and awareness training
	Quick flicks 10 × 4 sets/day
	Endurance training 5–10 s holds 10 × 2 sets/day
2. Postop	Early mobilization: modifying mobility strategies for getting out of bed (log roll), sit to stand with abdominal bracing, avoiding heavy lifting and straining
	Improving daily activity: short 10 min walks at least 3 times/day to improve endurance and assist in GI motility
	Adequate hydration with emphasis on water
3. Post-catheter removal (~3 weeks post-op)	Begin PFM awareness training: learning to isolate the pelvic floor muscles and decrease accessory use of the gluteals, abdominals, and hips to improve sphincter control
	Avoiding valsalva
	Neobladder retraining: timed voiding (improving interval between voids to at least every 1.5 h) with the use of alarms, fluid pacing, and PFM exercises
	Nighttime voiding alarms: every 2 h
4. Neuromuscular reeducation with PFPT (4–6 weeks)	Biofeedback training (either visual or via manual feedback) for PFM awareness training with isolating sphincter closure
	Quick flicks 10 × 4 sets, endurance holds (based on objective findings) 5 s holds 10 × 3 sets/day
	Anticipatory pelvic floor contraction reflex training with coughing to improve coordination
	Initiate gluteal/core strengthening in supine position
	Progress to functional strengthening with mobility (sit to stand) and use of PFM with transverse abdominous coactivation brace prior to movement
	Patient reeducation: liber health and diet, toileting techniques, and PFM coordination for voiding/bowel evacuation
5. Hypertrophy phase (8–12 weeks)	Progress PFM strengthening to upright positions (seated on physioball, standing) with cocontraction of PFM with the transverse abdominous
	Progress endurance holds to 10 s, 15 s, 20 s as tolerated
	Progress motor control to combination quick flick and endurance PFM training in upright positions
	Biofeedback progression with motor control: pyramid, step-up, step-down PFM visual training
	Pelvic floor muscle exercises with cognitive distraction to influence involuntary motor plan development
	Functional mobility training: lifting, bending, gait, return to previous level of activity (sports, hiking, gym exercises)
	Achieve voiding interval of every 4 h during day and night with minimal leakage

graphic representations are important adjuncts to assist patients in the redevelopment of neuromuscular connections [36]. Pelvic floor physical therapy should be considered for 8–12 months postoperatively, even if continence is present [37].

Medications

Anticholinergic agents are indicated for the management of detrusor overactivity. Common side effects include dry eyes, dry mouth, and decreased intestinal motility, which may contribute to improved urinary continence in neobladder patients. The use of either *oxybutynin* or *verapamil*, a calcium channel blocker, alone has shown to improve volume at first desire to void as well as decreased frequency and amplitude of uninhibited neobladder contractions. In the original studies, *oxybutynin* had a subjectively better response with 70% of patients reporting improvement of nocturnal enuresis compared to 55% with the use of *verapamil* [38]. Either medication can be considered in those with intestinal reservoir overactivity. However, given the average age of women undergoing radical cystectomy, anticholinergic agents are advised to be avoided given increased risk of negative side effects and dementia. There has been no evaluation to date of more contemporary anticholinergic agents or novel beta-adrenergic agonists in postcystectomy patients, but since these patients no longer have a detrusor muscle, it is possible that these medications that have no effect on bowel are not effective.

Desmopressin, a synthetic analog of antidiuretic hormone, has shown clinical efficacy in improving urinary incontinence and nocturia in several trials [39–41]. Goldberg et al. studied the use of low-dose *desmopressin* in patients with nocturnal enuresis following orthotopic neobladder reconstruction. By decreasing the volume of urine excreted, 50% of patients experienced longer intervals between voids and reported improved quality of life. Common side effects of *desmopressin* include headaches, dizziness, insomnia, dry mouth, and nausea. Patients should be monitored for electrolyte abnormalities with use of *desmopressin*, given the risk for hyponatremia [42].

While there are no published data available on the use of *imipramine* or *duloxetine* as therapeutic options to improve continence in those with an orthotopic neobladder, the use of these medications has been suggested by various investigators [37, 43]. *Imipramine*, a tricyclic amine (TCA) antidepressant, has been shown to cause detrusor relaxation and contraction of the bladder neck and urethra, making it an effective option for mixed urinary incontinence [44, 45]. *Duloxetine's* effectiveness for stress urinary incontinence stems from its presynaptic reuptake inhibition of serotonin and norepinephrine in Onuf's nucleus. Stimulation of receptors in Onuf's nucleus leads to increased urethral tone through the guarding reflex during bladder filling [46].

The use of intravesical botulinum toxin is well defined in those with idiopathic and neurogenic detrusor overactivity. Its use has also been described for fecal urgency via injection into the rectal submucosa [47]. Michel et al. studied the use of botulinum toxin type A (BTXA) injections in those with augmentation enterocystoplasty for neurogenic detrusor overactivity. Patients received BTXA injections into both the native bladder and augmented intestinal patch with no severe complications [48]. Hoag et al. injected 100–200 units of BTXA into patient's intestinal reservoirs to manage neobladder overactivity. Patients reported varying degrees of subjective improvement at mean follow-up of 8.3 months. The combination of likely sphincter insufficiency and reliance on voiding via Valsalva places these patients at low risk for urinary retention following intravesical botulinum toxin type A injections; therefore, injection of 200 units is recommended, but with limited data on its use [49].

Transurethral Bulking Agents

In carefully selected patients, transurethral injection of bulking agents may provide a minimally invasive treatment option for persistent stress urinary incontinence following orthotopic neobladder reconstruction. Small studies have shown variable and nondurable responses. In a study of 12 patients with a total of 25 injections of collagen or nonabsorbable carbon-coated beads, 17% of patients had complete resolution of urinary leakage, 33% had some improvement, and 50% experienced no change in symptoms at mean follow-up of 22.5 months. When stratified by disease severity, 66% of those with mild-to-moderate disease, defined as use of four pads or less per day, had improvement or cure, while only 33% of those with severe disease derived benefit [50]. Tchetgen et al. reported on three women who underwent transurethral collagen injections; initial outcomes were promising with all women being rendered dry or almost completely dry. However, maintenance injections were required for sustained symptom control, and one patient reverted back to her baseline level of preprocedural incontinence [51].

Presently, collagen is no longer available for transurethral injection. Bailey et al. described their experience treating six women with Deflux, Macroplastique, Coaptite, Contingen, or Durasphere. Seventy-five percent of patients experienced only temporary symptom improvement, with one unfortunately developing a secondary neobladder vaginal fistula [33]. The exact location of transurethral bulking agent injections was not identified in the aforementioned study, but prior work by Pruthi et al. recommended anterior injection of bulking agents, away from the neobladder neck [52]. In summary, transurethral injection of bulking agents is a therapeutic option one can consider with caution and proper counseling and only for those with mild stress urinary incontinence following orthotopic neobladder reconstruction. Patients should be counseled regarding the high likelihood of requiring multiple procedures, uncertain efficacy, the risk of neobladder vaginal fistula formation, and unproven long-term benefit.

Slings

The use of pubovaginal autologous slings and synthetic transobturator slings has been described for the treatment of stress urinary incontinence in patients who fail more conservative treatment options. Similar to data supporting other treatment modalities, studies assessing the outcomes of sling placement are limited, and long-term results show variability with the potential for significant morbidity and mortality.

In a series of four patients who underwent pubovaginal sling placement after orthotopic neobladder reconstruction, two autologous rectus slings and two dermal slings, 50% of patients experienced severe complications related to the retropubic dissection [53]. Passage of trocars through the retropubic space unfortunately led to the development of an entero-neobladder fistula in one patient and an enterotomy in another who subsequently died from sepsis. Those who underwent dermal graft sling placement were hypercontinent postoperatively, requiring clean intermittent catheterization. Given the risk of neobladder and bowel injury, some advocate for the use of infrapubic bone anchors to avoid pelvic entry during sling placement [21, 33, 54].

A small series of four pubovaginal slings placed utilizing a subperiosteal approach and four transobturator slings showed poor results; none of the women were continent secondary to sling placement alone. Transobturator sling placement is advantageous in this population as it avoids pelvic entry, decreasing the risk of neobladder and/or bowel injury [33]. More promising results were seen in a series of six patients who underwent transobturator vaginal tape (inside-out) placement; 66% showed complete day and nighttime dryness, 17% showed relative improvement, and 17% reported no change. Outcomes were durable at mean follow-up of 18 months. The patient who reported no improvement in leakage had severe stress urinary incontinence preoperatively [54].

Although midurethral synthetic sling placement is the gold standard for treatment of stress urinary incontinence in index patients, it has shown only modest success in those with stress urinary incontinence after orthotopic neobladder reconstruction. The extensive pelvic dissection required during radical cystectomy leads to scarring and a relatively ischemic environment, both of which complicate sling placement. Midurethral slings are traditionally placed tension-free; however in this population, the goal is relative urethral obstruction to regain continence. With partial urethral obstruction, there is in turn a high risk of retention and subsequent need for long-term intermittent catheterization. Patients must be counseled preoperatively and be willing and able to perform clean intermittent catheterization. Additionally, placement of a sling under tension in an ischemic environment increases the risk of erosion [55].

In patients with severe stress urinary incontinence postneobladder reconstruction, less-invasive treatment options are likely to be of limited success and carry risks. Frequently patients face a decision to convert the neobladder into an ileal conduit or consider a catheterizable pouch [43]. Given limited treatment options for stress urinary incontinence in this setting, continence status needs to be carefully assessed prior to choosing a urinary diversion type. Counseling and shared decision making regarding the options for urinary diversion should be strongly influenced by the patient's preoperative continence status.

Neobladder Vaginal Fistula

An uncommon, but devastating, complication of orthotopic neobladder reconstruction is the development of a neobladder vaginal fistula, with an incidence of 0–10% [33, 55–57]. Known risk factors for the development of neobladder vaginal fistula include injury to the anterior vaginal wall during dissection, especially at the level of the urethra [58], overlapping suture lines, poorly vascularized tissue due to prior surgery or radiation, cancer recurrence, and the use of transurethral bulking agents [55, 57]. Additionally, the relatively thin wall of the neobladder makes it more prone to fistulization [58]. Neobladder vaginal fistulas can present immediately or months after cystectomy, with most identified in the three- to six-month range [33, 56]. The presence of intermittent versus constant urinary incontinence cannot reliably differentiate a neobladder vaginal fistula from other causes of postoperative urinary incontinence [56]. One must be vigilant in identifying neobladder vaginal fistula formation from other categories of incontinence, as they may present similarly or simultaneously and require different management. The majority of neobladder vaginal fistulas can be identified on exam. Other diagnostic options include voiding cystourethrogram, cystoscopy, and/or a dye test [28, 56, 59]. When a neobladder vaginal fistula is identified, the most likely location is at the urethral neobladder anastomosis, followed by the vaginal stump.

Precise surgical technique is the most important factor in the prevention of neobladder vaginal fistula formation [56]. Meticulous dissection of the vesicovaginal plane is required to prevent inadvertent damage to the vagina [58, 60]. Additional maneuvers to prevent neobladder vaginal fistula formation include closing the vaginal stump and embedding it posteriorly away from the neobladder urethral anastomosis, suture fixation of the peritoneal edge of the anterior rectal wall to the vaginal stump, and securing a pedicalized omental flap between the vaginal stump and neobladder urethral anastomosis [23, 60].

Conservative management of neobladder vaginal fistulas with total parenteral nutrition and bladder decompression has historically proven futile; most patients will require surgical repair [13]. If the clinical exam is suspicious for cancer recurrence, biopsy of the fistula needs to be performed prior to surgical repair. Use of transvaginal estrogen is recommended prior to surgery to optimize vaginal tissue quality. Transvaginal approach of fistula repair is generally recommended over transabdominal approach or conversion to a continent or incontinent diversion.

Transvaginal approach, when feasible, can provide good functional outcomes and does not compromise the external urinary sphincter [57, 61].

The key to repair of a neobladder vaginal fistula is closure in multiple nonoverlapping layers. Tissue options for an interposition layer include Martius flaps, omental flaps, gracilis flaps, peritoneal flaps, autologous fascial grafts, and in rare cases, biologic glue [55–57]. An interposition layer provides additional vascularity, lymphatic drainage, and surface area for epithelization, and prevents suture line overlap. If there is suspicion for simultaneous stress urinary incontinence at initial presentation, an autologous fascial sling can be considered intraoperatively during repair as an interposition layer. Use of infrapubic bone anchors is recommended to prevent dissection into the retropubic space. Synthetic slings should not be used with concomitant fistula repair [33].

Success rates of neobladder vaginal fistula repair vary widely, ranging from 25% to 100% [33, 55, 57, 61]. Those with a fistula at the urethral-neobladder anastomosis tend to fare worse than those with more proximal defects and have a higher rate of conversion to a nonorthotopic neobladder diversion [55]. In those who retain their orthotopic neobladder, many continue to experience urinary incontinence secondary to intrinsic sphincter deficiency and eventually require treatment [56].

Hypercontinence

Although urinary incontinence can be common in women after orthotopic urinary diversion, up to 69% of women also reported some degree of hypercontinence [27, 62]. Hypercontinence after orthotopic neobladder has been defined in the literature as more than 150 mL postvoid residual or inability to void [63]. Factors known to be protective against incontinence after orthotopic neobladder reconstruction can also contribute to the risk of hypercontinence. These include preservation of the uterus, bilateral nerve sparing, and longer functional urethral length [17]. Preservation of the vagina along with colposacropexy was associated with hypercontinence in up to 80% of patients [64]. Patients can also fail to empty due to a large reservoir, dyssynergia of the neobladder and sphincter complex, or formation of pouchocele leading to urethral kinking [18, 63, 65]. Finley et al. found that patients with an average of 18 degrees of urethral kinking after orthotopic neobladder had associated urinary retention, and these were usually due to pouchocele. Patients who are in retention can be managed with clean intermittent catheterization initially. In those with pouchoceles, they can place a finger into the vagina to reduce neobladder prolapse in order to void. Patients whose hypercontinence persist after the initial postoperative period may benefit from correction of the prolapse in order to straighten the urethra and allow for improved emptying [66, 67].

Incontinence After Gender-Affirming Surgery

Feminizing Surgery

In male-to-female genitourinary gender-affirming surgery (MtF GAS), nearly half of patients will have voiding complaints, with the reported rate of incontinence ranging from 5% to 19% [68–70]. Although patients present with external female genitourinary complex, internally, the prostate remains in place. Briefly, full depth vaginoplasty includes bilateral orchiectomy, removal of the corporal bodies, development of the neovaginal canal, lining the canal with skin or peritoneal grafts, urethroplasty with shortening of the urethra, clitoroplasty, and labiaplasty. Patients can also undergo zero-depth vaginoplasty (synonymous with vulvoplasty or shallow-depth vaginoplasty), where a neovaginal canal is not created. Multiple techniques and approaches are currently in practice without clear evidence to support one specific technique. Development of the neovaginal canal relies on careful dissection of the potential space between the posterior aspect of the prostate and anterior aspect of the rectum, along Denonvilliers' Fascia. The foundation to understanding of this anatomy was developed by Hugh Hampton Young in describing techniques for perineal prostatectomy [71].

Patients often have a variety of voiding complaints in the short-term period after vaginoplasty or vulvoplasty. The majority of complaints focus on variation of urinary stream, spraying, postvoid dribbling, and overall increased moisture in the perineal area. These symptoms are common early in the recovery period as incisions heal and postoperative edema improves. Additionally, new voiding dynamics in the sitting position with a shortened urethra will inevitably lead to occasional urine spray on the labia or inner thigh. Once complete emptying is confirmed, patients should be reassured that most urinary stream abnormalities will resolve as their recovery progresses.

When voiding symptoms persist past the acute postsurgical period, a complete evaluation of the patient should include a thorough examination of the urethra in combination with a speculum exam. A thorough exam can identify meatal stricture, urethroneovaginal or vesiconeovaginal fistula, and abnormal kinking/angulation of the urethra. Urethral stricture occurs in 1–6% of postvaginoplasty patients, while urethroneovaginal fistula occurs in 0.9–3.9% of patients [72–74]. Patients with urethral stricture can present with overflow incontinence and obstruction-associated irritative symptoms. Patients with urethrovaginal fistula can experience split stream, vaginal pooling, and continuous wetness depending on the location of the fistula. Additionally, an isolated symptom of vaginal pooling in the absence of a fistula can also be perceived as urinary incontinence. In most cases, vaginal pooling can be explained by the nonphysiologic angulation of the urethra, retracted position of the urethral meatus, or redirection of stream due to redundant tissue near the meatus. In some cases, we have observed patients not opening their legs to straddle the toilet during voiding, which can lead to urine being trapped in the vagina and leakage of trapped urine upon standing. Excessive upward urethral angulation or meatal asymmetry can also cause spraying or upward stream; this can be corrected by surgically revising the location of the urethral meatus.

Workup should start with a thorough history and physical exam, assessment of postvoid residual, and noninvasive flowmetry studies if indicated. It is important to recognize that although most transfeminine patients have been on long-term estrogen supplementation with or without androgen blockade, they may still be at risk for development of benign prostatic hyperplasia (BPH) with lower urinary tract symptoms. The evidence remains unclear regarding the effect of castration on development of BPH, though the literature does show several instances of MtF patients developing prostate cancer despite castration, suggesting that alternative sources of androgen synthesis still influence prostate growth [75–78]. In addition, depending on the age at which patients began their hormone blockade, patients may have already developed BPH-related bladder outlet obstruction symptoms prior to transitioning. On the other end of the spectrum, studies theorize that having a smaller prostate from hormone therapy may lead to easier urine passage and potential stress urinary incontinence [79].

Detailed history can help parse out if a patient is experiencing urge, stress, overflow, continuous, or mixed incontinence. Baseline urinary symptoms prior to GAS are also helpful in identifying the source of incontinence. Lower urinary tract symptoms are likely to remain stable postoperatively, with the exception of patients who are at risk for stress urinary incontinence preoperatively. It is imperative to assess patients' voiding symptoms prior to undergoing a vaginoplasty. At a minimum, we recommend the American Urological Association Symptom Score (AUASS) at the time of the initial consultation. Workup of the identified symptoms should ensue. Additionally, involvement of pelvic floor physical therapy early, before the surgical reconstruction, has shown to improve voiding function and minimize voiding dysfunction in a number of patients. Those patients who have had at least one preoperative pelvic floor physical therapy session were less likely to have pelvic floor dysfunction as compared to patients that did only postoperative therapy (27% vs. 86%). However, patients will still benefit from pelvic floor physical therapy postoperatively even if not diagnosed preoperatively [80].

Patients with a history of prior radical prostatectomy present a special challenge. Conventional approaches to postprostatectomy incontinence, such as placement of an artificial urinary sphincter (AUS) or a male sling, become difficult and potentially risky. During vaginoplasty, corpus spongiosum is typically tapered at the bulbar urethra, leaving very little tissue between the urethra and the overlying sling or sphincter cuff. Furthermore, because the bulbospongiosus muscle is routinely removed, the implanted device may lack adequate coverage. Several approaches have been considered, including simultaneous AUS or male sling placement at the time of vaginoplasty, staged procedures, or robotic approach to position the sphincter cuff at the bladder neck. To date, no data are available to make meaningful conclusions. In postprostatectomy patients who at the time of evaluation do not exhibit urinary incontinence, counseling needs to include the possibility of development of de novo stress urinary incontinence from perineal dissection near the levator complex. Zero-depth vaginoplasty is strongly recommended for patients with prior history of radical prostatectomy. This is mainly due to increased risk of rectal injury and strong potential for de novo development or worsening of existing urinary incontinence. To some extent, this also applies to patients with prior history of transurethral resection of the prostate (TURP), where the functional internal sphincter has been resected as part of the operation [81].

Masculinizing Surgery

Phalloplasty and metoidioplasty can be performed to achieve gender-affirming goals in transmasculine patients. Metoidioplasty includes creation of a neophallus using existing genital tissue. The hormonally enlarged clitoris becomes the neophallus shaft. For those who wish to urinate from the tip of their neophallus, urethral lengthening is completed, whereby the mucosal lining of the vestibule of the introitus is rearranged and tubularized to construct a neourethra spanning from the native meatus to the tip of the neophallus. This segment of the urethra is termed the pars fixa (Fig. 21.2). Typically, vaginectomy is also performed at the timing of urethral lengthening. Phalloplasty involves creation of the neophallus using a tissue flap. Common donor sites include radial forearm, anterolateral thigh, latissimus dorsi, and abdominal flap. Depending on the flap donor site, a neourethra within the penile shaft can either be made at the time of phalloplasty by nestling a fasciocutaneous flap within the penile shaft or it can be made in separate stages. As can be expected, areas of potential urethral complications center mostly around watershed areas,

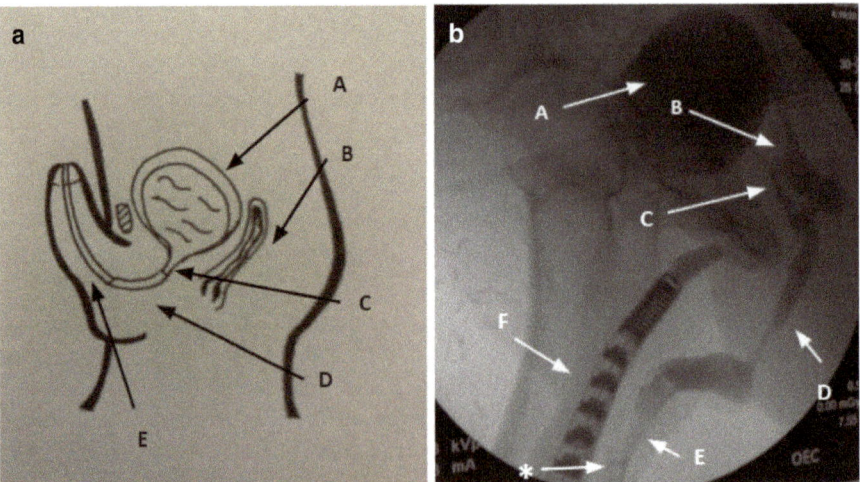

Fig. 21.2 (**a**) Sagittal view of transmasculine neophallus anatomy (**b**) Retrograde urethrogram (RUG) of neophallus. *A:* Bladder, *B:* Vaginal remnant, *C:* Native urethra, *D:* Pars fixa, *E:* Pars pendulans, *F:* Penile implant, *:* filling defect in urethra

typically at the anastomosis between native meatus and pars fixa and the anastomosis between pars fixa and penile urethra (pars pendulous) [82].

Vaginectomy and neourethral reconstruction are components of masculinizing surgery that commonly contribute to voiding dysfunction. The most notable urethral complications are stricture and fistula formation. Incidence of urethral strictures is high and exceeds 50%, while fistulae occur in 10–64% of patients [83–89]. Strictures may lead to urinary retention and symptoms of overflow incontinence, while fistulas may initially appear as incontinence. Strictures at or distal to pars fixa and native meatus anastomosis may lead to reopening of the vaginal remnant and formation of a pseudodiverticulum. These patients can present with weak stream and postvoid dribbling of often foul-smelling urine and/or recurrent urinary tract infections. Evaluation of these patients requires cystoscopy with or without retrograde urethrogram to identify the reconstructed anatomy. At the time of urethral stricture repair, resection of any vaginal remnant and reobliteration of the vaginal cavity are performed. In some instances, a gracilis muscle flap is used to provide additional support to the repair. For patients who present with fistula, up to 66% of these fistulas will resolve with conservative management such as urinary diversion with a catheter [84]. For those with persistent urethrocutaneous fistula, it is important to first evaluate the entire urethra to rule out any distal areas of stricture that may be contributing to fistula formation. Once this has been addressed, the reconstructive repair is similar to patients who have urethrocutaneous fistulas, with excision of the fistula tract and closure in multiple layers with flap coverage as needed. Urethral strictures in postphalloplasty patients typically require surgical repair. In our experience, strictures usually recur after urethral dilation. Excision and primary anastomosis is rarely a viable option due to the lack of urethral mobility and tissue redundancy. Substitution urethroplasty using buccal graft or full thickness skin graft is employed. Short strictures and strictures in pars fixa can usually be repaired with single-stage urethroplasty using buccal mucosal graft, whereas longer strictures and strictures in pars pendulous usually require staged urethroplasty using skin graft.

Phalloplasty patients can experience postvoid dribbling, usually from urine retained in the urethra [90]. Since the neourethra does not have supportive structures such as bulbospongiosus muscle, the neourethra is more likely to contain residual urine when compared to native urethra. These patients learn to manually press from the base of the phallus to the tip to express urine [91].

Conclusion

Urinary incontinence after construction of an orthotopic neobladder and gender-affirming surgery varies in presentation and structural etiology. Initially, women undergoing cystectomy only had the options of an incontinent diversion or a catheterizable pouch. The advancement of surgical techniques and a better understanding of female pelvic floor anatomy have enabled postcystectomy women to void per urethra. This advance did not come without challenges of various types of urinary incontinence. A number of approaches exist to improve the continence of women with orthotopic neobladder; however, if all efforts fail, conversion to an ileal conduit or catheterizable channel construction may be required to achieve socially desirable dryness. In gender-affirming surgery, a thorough understanding of the reconstructed and retained native anatomy is essential in the workup of incontinence. Thorough history and physical examination in combination with a variety of diagnostic investigations from the urological armamentarium are key to determining the cause of incontinence. These cases present technical and intellectual challenges in both identification and treatment.

References

1. Stein JP, Lieskovsky G, Cote R, Groshen S, Feng AC, Boyd S, Skinner E, Bochner B, Thangathurai D, Mikhail M, Raghavan D, Skinner DG. Radical cystectomy in the treatment of invasive bladder cancer: long-term results in 1,054 patients. J Clin Oncol. 2001;19:666–75.
2. Marshall FF, Treiger BFG. Radical cystectomy (anterior exenteration) in the female patient. Urol Clin North Am. 1991;18:765–75.
3. Colleselli K, Stenzl A, Eder R, Strasser H, Poisel S, Bartsch G. The female urethral sphincter: a morphological and topographical study. J Urol. 1998;160:49–54.
4. Stein JP, Penson DF, Wu SD, Skinner DG. Pathological guidelines for orthotopic urinary diversion in women with bladder cancer: a review of the literature. J Urol. 2007;178:756–60.
5. Stein JP, Penson DF, Lee C, Cai J, Miranda G, Skinner DG. Long-term oncological outcomes in women undergoing radical cystectomy and orthotopic diversion for bladder cancer. J Urol. 2009;181:2052–8. discussion 2058–9
6. Stenzl A, Colleselli K, Poisel S, Feichtinger H, Pontasch H, Bartsch G. Rationale and technique of nerve sparing radical cystectomy before an orthotopic neobladder procedure in women. J Urol. 1995;154:2044–9.
7. Stenzl A, Colleselli K, Poisel S, Feichtinger H, Bartsch G. The use of neobladders in women undergoing cystectomy for transitional-cell cancer. World J Urol. 1996;14:15–21.
8. Nesrallah LJ, Almeida FG, Dall'Oglio MF, Nesrallah AJ, Srougi M. Experience with the orthotopic ileal neobladder in women: a mid-term follow-up. J Urol. 2006;175:987–8.
9. Turner WH, Danuser H, Moehrle K, Studer UE. The effect of nerve sparing cystectomy technique on postoperative continence after orthotopic bladder substitution. J Urol. 1997;158:2118–22.
10. Studer UE, Burkhard FC, Schumacher M, Kessler TM, Thoeny H, Fleischmann A, Thalmann GN. Twenty years experience with an ileal orthotopic low pressure bladder substitute- lessons to be learned. J Urol. 2006;176:161–6.
11. Skinner EC, Daneshmand DS. Orthotopic urinary diversion. In: Partin AW, Peters CA, Kavoussi LR, Dmochowski RR, Wein AJ, editors. Campbell-Walsh-Wein urology. 12th ed. Philadelphia: Elsevier; 2020. p. 3233–57.
12. Hinman F. Selection of intestinal segments for bladder substitution: physical and physiological characteristics. J Urol. 1998;139:519–23.
13. Amini E, Djaladat H. Long-term complications of urinary diversion. Curr Opin Urol. 2015;25:50–7.
14. Hinata N, Murakami G, Abe S-I, Honda M, Isoyama T, Sejima T, Takenaka A. Detailed histological investigation of the female urethra: application to radical cystectomy. J Urol. 2012;187:451–6.
15. Grossfeld GD, Stein JP, Bennett CJ, Ginsberg DA, Boyd SD, Lieskovsky G, Skinner DG. Lower urinary tract reconstruction in the female using the kock ileal reservoir with bilat-

eral ureteroileal urethrostomy: update of continence results and fluorourodynamic findings. Urology. 1996;48:383–8.

16. Dhar NB, Kessler TM, Mills RD, Burkhard F, Studer UE. Nerve-sparing radical cystectomy and orthotopic bladder replacement in female patients. Eur Urol. 2007;52:1006–14.

17. Gross T, Meierhans Ruf SD, Meissner C, Ochsner K, Studer UE. Orthotopic ileal bladder substitution in women: factors influencing urinary incontinence and hypercontinence. Eur Urol. 2015;68:664–71.

18. Hautmann RE. The ileal neobladder to the female urethra. Urol Clin North Am. 1997;24:827–35.

19. Ali-El-Dein B. Oncological outcome after radical cystectomy and orthotopic bladder substitution in women. Eur J Surg Oncol. 2009;35:320–5.

20. Stein JP, Dunn MD, Quek ML, Miranda G, Skinner DG. The orthotopic T pouch ileal neobladder: experience with 209 patients. J Urol. 2004;172:584–7.

21. Zlatev DV, Skinner EC. Orthotopic urinary diversion for women. Urol Clin North Am. 2018;45:49–54.

22. Hautmann RE. Urinary diversion: ileal conduit to neobladder. J Urol. 2003;169:834–42.

23. Granberg CF, Boorjian SA, Crispen PL, Tollefson MK, Farmer SA, Frank I, Blute ML. Functional and oncological outcomes after orthotopic neobladder reconstruction in women. BJU Int. 2008;102:1551–5.

24. Stenzl A, Jarolim L, Coloby P, Golia S, Bartsch G, Babjuk M, Kakizoe T, Robertson C. Urethra-sparing cystectomy and orthotopic urinary diversion in women with malignant pelvic tumors. Cancer. 2001;92:1864–71.

25. Lee CT, Hafez KS, Sheffield JH, Joshi DP, Montie JE. Orthotopic bladder substitution in women: nontraditional applications. J Urol. 2004;171:1585–8.

26. Ahmadi H, Skinner EC, Simma-Chiang V, Miranda G, Cai J, Penson DF, Daneshmand S. Urinary functional outcome following radical cystoprostatectomy and ileal neobladder reconstruction in male patients. J Urol. 2013;189:1782–8.

27. Anderson CB, Cookson MS, Chang SS, Clark PE, Smith JA, Kaufman MR. Voiding function in women with orthotopic neobladder urinary diversion. J Urol. 2012;188:200–4.

28. Steers WD. Voiding dysfunction in the orthotopic neobladder. World J Urol. 2000;18:330–7.

29. Veskimäe E, Neuzillet Y, Rouanne M, MacLennan S, Lam TB, Yuan Y, Comperat E, Cowan NC, Gakis G, van der Heijden AG, Ribal MJ, Witjes JA, Lebret T. Systematic review of the oncological and functional outcomes of pelvic organ-preserving radical cystectomy (RC) compared with standard RC in women who undergo curative surgery and orthotopic neobladder substitution for bladder cancer. BJU Int. 2017;120:12–24.

30. Rouanne M, Legrand G, Neuzillet Y, Ghoneim T, Cour F, Letang N, Yonneau L, Hervé J-M, Botto H, Lebret T. Long-term women-reported quality of life after radical cystectomy and orthotopic ileal neobladder reconstruction. Ann Surg Oncol. 2014;21:1398–404.

31. Kim S-O, Kim JS, Kim HS, Hwang EC, Oh KJ, Kwon D, Park K, Ryu SB. Age related change of nocturia in women. Int Neurourol J. 2010;14:245–9.

32. Hoy NY, Cohn JA, Kowalik CG, Kaufman MR, Stuart Reynolds W, Dmochowski RR. Management of voiding dysfunction after female neobladder creation. Curr Urol Rep. 2017;18:33.

33. Bailey GC, Blackburne A, Ziegelmann MJ, Lightner DJ. Outcomes of surgical management in patients with stress urinary incontinence and/or neovesicovaginal fistula after orthotopic neobladder diversion. J Urol. 2016;196:1478–83.

34. Badawy AA, Abolyosr A, Mohamed ER, Abuzeid AM. Orthotopic diversion after cystectomy in women: a single-centre experience with a 10-year follow-up. Arab J Urol. 2011;9:267–71.

35. Marques A, Stothers L, Macnab A. The status of pelvic floor muscle training for women. Can Urol Assoc J. 2010;4:419–24.

36. Johnson EV, Kirages DJ. Pelvic floor rehabilitation for orthotopic diversion. In: Daneshmand S, editor. Urinary diversion. Los Angeles: Springer; 2017. p. 143–52.

37. Zhang Y-G, Song Q-X, Song B, Zhang D-L, Zhang W, Wang J-Y. Diagnosis and treatment of urinary incontinence after orthotopic ileal neobladder in China. Chin Med J. 2017;130:231–5.

38. El-Bahnasawy MS, Shaaban H, Gomha MA, Nabeeh A. Clinical and urodynamic efficacy of oxybutynin and verapamil in the treatment of nocturnal enuresis after formation of orthotopic ileal neobladders. A prospective, randomized, crossover study. Scand J Urol Nephrol. 2008;42:344–51.
39. Hjalmas K, Hanson E, Hellstrom AL, Kruse S, Sillen U. Long-term treatment with desmopressin in children with primary monosymptomatic nocturnal enuresis: an open multicentre study. Swedish enuresis trial (SWEET) group. Br J Urol. 1998;82:704–9.
40. Naghizadeh S, Kefi A, Serkan Dogan H, Burgu B, Akdogan B, Tekgul S. Effectiveness of oral desmopressin therapy in posterior urethral valve patients with polyuria and detection of factors affecting the therapy. Eur Urol. 2005;48:819–25.
41. Eckford SD, Carter PG, Jackson SR, Penney MD, Abrams P. An open, in-patient incremental safety and efficacy study of desmopressin in women with multiple sclerosis and nocturia. Br J Urol. 1995;76:459–63.
42. Goldberg H, Baniel J, Mano R, Gillon G, Kedar D, Yossepowitch O. Low-dose oral desmopressin for treatment of nocturia and nocturnal enuresis in patients after radical cystectomy and orthotopic urinary diversion. BJU Int. 2014;114:727–32.
43. Schneider MP, Burkhard FC. Management of incontinence after orthotopic bladder substitution post-radical cystectomy. Curr Bladder Dysfunct Rep. 2019;14:125–9.
44. Dave S, Grover VP, Agarwala S, Mitra DK, Bhatnagar V. The role of imipramine therapy in bladder exstrophy after bladder neck reconstruction. BJU Int. 2002;89:557–60.
45. Mahony DT, Laferte RO, Mahoney JE. Studies of enuresis. VI. Observations on sphincter-augmenting effect of imipramine in children with urinary incontinence. Urology. 1973;1:317–23.
46. Jost W, Marsalek P. Duloxetine: mechanism of action at the lower urinary tract and Onuf's nucleus. Clin Auton Res. 2004;14:220–7.
47. Bridoux V, Gourcerol G, Kianifard B, Touchais J-Y, Ducrotte P, Leroi A-M, Michot F, Tuech J-J. Botulinum A toxin as a treatment for overactive rectum with associated faecal incontinence. Color Dis. 2012;14:342–8.
48. Michel F, Ciceron C, Bernuz B, Boissier R, Gaillet S, Even A, Chartier-Kastler E, Denys P, Game X, Ruffion A, Le Normand L, Perrouin-Verbe B, Saussine C, Manuta A, Forin V, De Seze M, Grise P, Tournebise H, Schurch B, Karsenty G. Botulinum toxin type A injection after failure of augmentation enterocystoplasty performed for neurogenic detrusor overactivity: preliminary results of a salvage strategy. The ENTEROTOX study. Urology. 2019;129:43–7.
49. Hoag N, Tse V, Wang A, Chung E, Gani J. Intravesical onabotulinumtoxinA injection for overactive orthotopic ileal neobladder: feasibility and efficacy. Int Neurourol J. 2016;20:81–5.
50. Wilson S, Quek ML, Ginsberg DA. Transurethral injection of bulking agents for stress urinary incontinence following orthotopic neobladder reconstruction in women. J Urol. 2004;172:244–6.
51. Tchetgen MB, Sanda MG, Montie JE, Faerber GJ. Collagen injection for the treatment of incontinence after cystectomy and orthotopic neobladder reconstruction in women. J Urol. 2000;163:212–4.
52. Pruthi RS, Petrus CD, Bundrick WS. New onset vesicovaginal fistula after transurethral collagen injection in women who underwent cystectomy and orthotopic neobladder creation: presentation and definitive treatment. J Urol. 2000;164:1638–9.
53. Quek ML, Ginsberg DA, Wilson S, Skinner EC, Stein JP, Skinner DG. Pubovaginal slings for stress urinary incontinence following radical cystectomy and orthotopic neobladder reconstruction in women. J Urol. 2004;172:219–21.
54. Badawy AA, Saleem MD, Abolyosr A, Abuzeid AM. Transobturator vaginal tape (inside-out) for stress urinary incontinence after radical cystectomy and orthotopic reconstruction in women. Arab J Urol. 2012;10:182–5.
55. Rosenberg S, Miranda G, Ginsberg DA. Neobladder-vaginal fistula: the University of Southern California experience. Neurourol Urodyn. 2018;37:1380–5.

56. Kaufman MR. Neobladder-vaginal fistula: surgical management techniques. Curr Urol Rep. 2019;20:67.
57. Carmel ME, Goldman HB, Moore CK, Rackley RR, Vasavada SP. Transvaginal neobladder vaginal fistula repair after radical cystectomy with orthotopic urinary diversion in women. Neurourol Urodyn. 2016;35:90–4.
58. Rapp DE, Corey O'Connor R, Katz EE, Steinberg GD. Neobladder-vaginal fistula after cystectomy and orthotopic neobladder construction. BJU Int. 2004;94:1092–5.
59. Ali-El-Dein B, Shaaban AA, Abu-Eideh RH, El-Azab M, Ashamallah A, Ghoneim MA. Surgical complications following radical cystectomy and orthotopic neobladders in women. J Urol. 2008;180:206–10.
60. Tunuguntla HSGR, Tunuguntla HSG, Manoharan M, Gousse AE. Management of neobladder-vaginal fistula and stress incontinence following radical cystectomy in women: a review. World J Urol. 2005;23:231–5.
61. Ali-El-Dein B, Ashamallah A. Vaginal repair of pouch-vaginal fistula after orthotopic bladder substitution in women. Urology. 2013;81:198–203.
62. Hautmann RE, Paiss T, de Petriconi R. The ileal neobladder in women: 9 years of experience with 18 patients. J Urol. 1996;155:76–81.
63. Ismail MAA, Wishahi MM, Elsherbeeny M, Sewallam TA, Lockhart J. Hypercontinence in women after orthotopic neobladder diversion. UroToday Int J. 2009;2:1.
64. Neymeyer J, Abdul-Wahab W, Beer M. Prevention of hypercontinence and preservation of womanhood in patients undergoing cystectomy and ileum neobladder creation for invasive bladder cancer by preserving the vagina and performing a colposacropexy with titanium coated polypropeleium mesh all in a single session; the berliner neobladder. Eur Urol Suppl. 2008;7:220.
65. Arai Y, Okubo K, Konami T, Kin S, Kanba T, Okabe T, Hamaguchi A, Okada Y. Voiding function of orthotopic ileal neobladder in women. Urology. 1999;54:44–9.
66. Finley DS, Lee U, McDonough D, Raz S, de Kernion J. Urinary retention after orthotopic neobladder substitution in females. J Urol. 2011;186:1364–9.
67. Stearns G, Donahue T, Fathollahi A, Dalbagni G, Sandhu J. Formal sacrocolpopexy reduces hypercontinence rates in female neobladder formation. Neurourol Urodyn. 2018;37:2281–5.
68. Hoebeke P, Selvaggi G, Ceulemans P, De Cuypere G, T'Sjoen G, Weyers S, Decaestecker K, Monstrey S. Impact of sex reassignment surgery on lower urinary tract function. Eur Urol. 2005;47:398–402.
69. Ferrando CA. Vaginoplasty complications. Clin Plast Surg. 2018;45:361–8.
70. Shoureshi P, Dy GW, Dugi D. Neovaginal canal dissection in gender-affirming vaginoplasty. J Urol. 2021;205:1110–8.
71. Jewett HJ. The case for radical perineal prostatectomy. J Urol. 1970;103:195–9.
72. Krege S, Bex A, Lümmen G, Rübben H. Male-to-female transsexualism: a technique, results and long-term follow-up in 66 patients. BJU Int. 2001;88:396–402.
73. Reed HM. Aesthetic and functional male to female genital and perineal surgery: feminizing vaginoplasty. Semin Plast Surg. 2011;25:163–74.
74. Rossi Neto R, Hintz F, Krege S, Rübben H, Vom Dorp F. Gender reassignment surgery – a 13 year review of surgical outcomes. Int Braz J Urol. 2012;38:97–107.
75. van Kesteren P, Meinhardt W, van der Valk P, Geldof A, Megens J, Gooren L. Effects of estrogens only on the prostates of aging men. J Urol. 1996;156(4):1349–53.
76. Roy AK, Lavrovsky Y, Song CS, Chen S, Jung MH, Velu NK, Bi BY, Chatterjee B. Regulation of androgen action. Vitam Horm. 1999;55:309–52.
77. Deebel NA, Morin JP, Autorino R, Vince R, Grob B, Hampton LJ. Prostate cancer in transgender women: incidence, etiopathogenesis, and management challenges. Urology. 2017;110:166–71.
78. Turo R, Jallad S, Prescott S, Cross WR. Metastatic prostate cancer in transsexual diagnosed after three decades of estrogen therapy. Can Urol Assoc J. 2013;7:544–6.

79. Kuhn A, Hiltebrand R, Birkhäuser M. Do transsexuals have micturition disorders? Eur J Obstet Gynecol Reprod Biol. 2007;131:226–30.
80. Jiang DD, Gallagher S, Burchill L, Berli J, Dugi D. Implementation of a pelvic floor physical therapy program for transgender women undergoing gender-affirming vaginoplasty. Obstet Gynecol. 2019;133:1003–11.
81. Chen ML, Reyblat P, Poh MM, Chi AC. Overview of surgical techniques in gender-affirming genital surgery. Transl Androl Urol. 2019;8:191–208.
82. Jun MS, Santucci RA. Urethral stricture after phalloplasty. Transl Androl Urol. 2019;8:266–72.
83. Santucci RA. Urethral complications after transgender phalloplasty: strategies to treat them and minimize their occurrence. Clin Anat. 2018;31:187–90.
84. Ascha M, Massie JP, Morrison SD, Crane CN, Chen ML. Outcomes of single stage phalloplasty by pedicled anterolateral thigh flap versus radial forearm free flap in gender confirming surgery. J Urol. 2018;199:206–14.
85. Matti BA, Matthews RN, Davies DM. Phalloplasty using the free radial forearm flap. Br J Plast Surg. 1988;41:160–4.
86. Fang RH, Kao YS, Ma S, Lin JT. Phalloplasty in female-to-male transsexuals using free radial osteocutaneous flap: a series of 22 cases. Br J Plast Surg. 1999;52:217–22.
87. Leriche A, Timsit M-O, Morel-Journel N, Bouillot A, Dembele D, Ruffion A. Long-term outcome of forearm free-flap phalloplasty in the treatment of transsexualism. BJU Int. 2008;101:1297–300.
88. Kim S-K, Moon J-B, Heo J, Kwon Y-S, Lee K-C. A new method of urethroplasty for prevention of fistula in female-to-male gender reassignment surgery. Ann Plast Surg. 2010;64:759–64.
89. Doornaert M, Hoebeke P, Ceulemans P, T'Sjoen G, Heylens G, Monstrey S. Penile reconstruction with the radial forearm flap: an update. Handchir Mikrochir Plast Chir. 2011;43:208–14.
90. Nassiri N, Maas M, Basin M, Cacciamani GE, Doumanian LR. Urethral complications after gender reassignment surgery: a systematic review. Int J Impot Res. 2020; https://doi.org/10.1038/s41443-020-0304-y.
91. Heston AL, Esmonde NO, Dugi DD III, Berli JU. Phalloplasty: techniques and outcomes. Transl Androl Urol. 2019;8:254–65.

Chapter 22
Rare Conditions Causing Incontinence and Their Treatment

Ariana L. Smith and Andrea C. Yeguez

Vesicovaginal Fistula

Continuous urinary leakage approximately 1 week after benign hysterectomy is the sine qua non of vesicovaginal fistula (VVF). A fistula is defined as an extra-anatomic communication between two or more epithelial- or mesothelial-lined body cavities or the skin surface. The potential exists for fistula formation between any portion of the urinary tract (kidney, ureters, bladder, and urethra) and virtually any other body cavity including the reproductive organs, gastrointestinal tract, chest (pleural cavity), lymphatics, vascular system, genitalia, and skin. Fistulas are named based on the two organ systems that are communicating (Table 22.1). Although most fistulas in the industrialized world are iatrogenic, they may also occur as a result of childbirth (the most common etiology worldwide), congenital anomalies, malignancy, inflammation and infection, radiation therapy, surgical injury, external tissue trauma, foreign bodies, ischemia, and a variety of other processes (Table 22.2) [1–3]. Vesicovaginal fistula (VVF) is the most common acquired fistula of the urinary tract and, as the name suggests, is a communication between the bladder and vagina.

Etiology

In the developing world where routine obstetrical care may be limited, VVFs most commonly occur as a result of prolonged obstructed labor with resulting pressure necrosis and tissue ischemia to the pelvic floor [4, 5]. In sub-Saharan Africa, the

A. L. Smith (✉) · A. C. Yeguez
Division of Urology, Department of Surgery, University of Pennsylvania Health System, Philadelphia, PA, USA
e-mail: ariana.smith@pennmedicine.upenn.edu

A. P. Cameron (ed.), *Female Urinary Incontinence*,
https://doi.org/10.1007/978-3-030-84352-6_22

Table 22.1 Urinary Tract Fistulas: Fistulas are named based on the two organ systems in communication

Name	Organs involved	
Urogynecologic Fistulas		
Vesicovaginal	Bladder	Vagina
Ureterovaginal	Ureter	Vagina
Vesicouterine	Bladder	Uterus
Urethrovaginal	Urethra	Vagina
Uroenteric Fistulas		
Vesicoenteric	Bladder	Intestine
Ureteroenteric	Ureter	Intestine
Pyeloenteric	Renal Pelvis	Intestine
Rectourethral	Rectum	Urethra
Urovascular Fistulas		
Renovascular	Kidney	Vasculature
Pyelovascular	Renal Pelvis	Vasculature
Ureterovascular	Ureter	Vasculature
Other Fistulas		
Nephropleural	Kidney	Lung pleura
Nephrobronchial	Kidney	Bronchia
Vesicocutaneous	Bladder	Skin
Ureterocutaneous	Ureter	Skin
Urethrocutaneous	Urethra	Skin
Pyelocutaneous	Renal pelvis	Skin

incidence rate of obstetric VVF has been estimated at 10.3/100,000 deliveries [6]. The anterior vaginal wall, trigone, and urethra generally experience the greatest direct pressure from the trapped fetus [3]. In some instances, VVF may result from the use of forceps or other instrumentation during operative delivery. Obstetric fistulas tend to be larger, located distally in the vagina, and may involve the proximal urethra. The constellation of problems resulting from obstructed labor is not limited to VVF, has been termed the "obstructed labor injury complex," and includes varying degrees of each of the following: urethral loss, stress incontinence, hydroureteronephrosis, renal failure, rectovaginal fistula, rectal atresia, anal sphincter incompetence, cervical destruction, amenorrhea, pelvic inflammatory disease, secondary infertility, vaginal stenosis, osteitis pubis, and foot drop [7].

In the United States, the most common cause is injury to the bladder at the time of gynecologic surgery—usually hysterectomy for benign conditions (80%) [8]. Obstetric events (10%), surgical intervention for gynecologic malignancy (5%), and pelvic radiotherapy (5%) are less common etiologies of VVF [8, 9]. Fistulas associated with malignancy and prior radiation therapy are generally complex.

Posthysterectomy VVFs are thought to result most commonly from an unrecognized cystotomy near the vaginal cuff (Fig. 22.1). Other potential contributing causes include suture placement into the bladder leading to pressure necrosis and

Table 22.2 Etiology of urinary tract Fistulas

Causes	Examples
Parturition	Prolonged obstructed labor Obstetric trauma/forceps laceration Uterine rupture
Postoperative/iatrogenic	Gynecologic, urologic, or pelvic surgery Cesarean section Synthetic mesh surgery
Congenital anomalies	Cloacal variants
Malignant disease	Gynecologic, urologic, or other pelvic cancer
Inflammation	Endometriosis Pelvic inflammatory disease Urethral diverticulum
Infection	Pelvic abscess Perirectal abscess
Ischemia	Bladder neck/trigone compression leading to ischemia
Radiation therapy	External beam therapy Brachytherapy
Foreign body	Neglected pessaries Intrauterine device Residual surgical material
Trauma	Pelvic facture Sexual violence

Fig. 22.1 A posthysterectomy fistula demonstrating a small vesicovaginal fistula at the level of the posterior bladder wall near the apex of vagina (blue catheter is traversing the fistula tract)

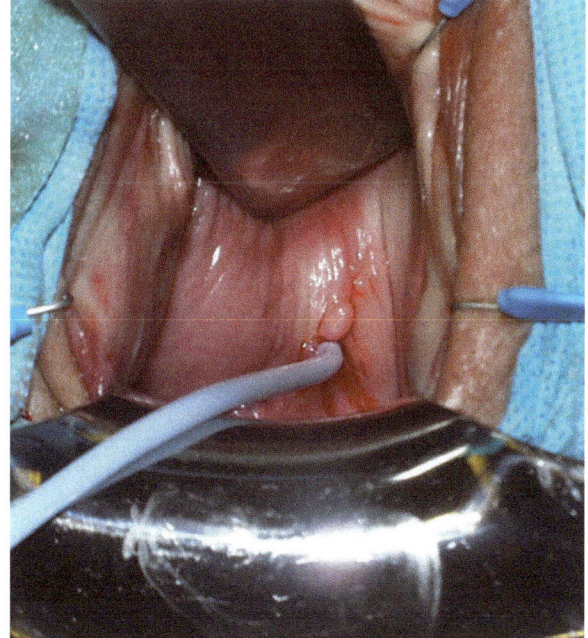

tissue loss, improper placement of clamps or cautery, and infections of the vaginal or perivaginal tissue. The operative approach to hysterectomy is an important factor, as bladder injuries are at least two times more common during laparoscopic hysterectomy compared to total abdominal hysterectomy, and the rate of bladder injury may also be higher during robotic hysterectomy [2, 10]. Subtotal abdominal hysterectomy and vaginal hysterectomy have lower risk of fistula [11]. Patients who develop a VVF are more likely to have a large cystotomy, greater tobacco use, larger uterine size, longer surgery time, and more operative blood loss [12, 13]. Fistulas are more common in women who are over 50 years of age at the time of hysterectomy, presumably due to estrogen deficiency and resultant changes in vaginal tissue quality [11].

Impact

The physical and psychological impact of VVF can be considerable for the affected individual and the medicolegal implications daunting for the provider. Expeditious management to minimize patient discomfort is critical as is an honest, positive doctor–patient relationship. Prevention of iatrogenic injury to the urinary tract through enhanced education, careful execution of pelvic surgery, and precise delivery of radiotherapy may decrease fistula formation.

Diagnosis

The presenting signs and symptoms of urinary tract fistulas are variable and depend to a large degree on the involved organs, the presence of underlying urinary obstruction or infection, the size of the fistula, and associated medical conditions such as malignancy. The most common complaint with VVF is constant urinary drainage per vagina, although small fistulas may present with intermittent wetness that is positional in nature and mistaken for stress incontinence. VVF must be distinguished from urinary incontinence due to other causes including stress (urethral) incontinence, urgency (bladder) incontinence, and overflow incontinence. Patients may also complain of recurrent cystitis, perineal skin irritation due to constant wetness, vaginal fungal infections, or rarely pelvic pain. When a large VVF is present, patients may not void at all and simply have continuous leakage of urine into the vagina. VVF following hysterectomy or other surgical procedures may present on removal of the urethral catheter or may present 1–3 weeks later with urinary drainage per vagina. VVFs resulting from hysterectomy are usually located high in the vagina at or just anterior to the vaginal cuff. VVF resulting from radiation therapy may not present for months to years following completion of radiation. These tend to represent some of the most challenging reconstructive cases in urology due to the size, complexity, and the associated voiding dysfunction due to the radiation effects on the bladder. The tissue ischemia that results from radiation therapy may involve the surrounding tissues, limiting reconstructive options.

A pelvic exam with a speculum should always be performed in an attempt to locate the fistula and assess the size and number of fistulas present. Palpation to assess for masses or other pelvic pathology, which may need to be addressed at the time of fistula repair, should be performed. Additionally, an assessment of inflammation surrounding the fistula is necessary as it may affect timing of the repair. Instilling blue dye into the bladder and observing for discolored vaginal drainage can confirm the presence of a VVF. A double dye test may confirm the diagnosis of urinary fistula as well as suggest the possibility of an associated ureterovaginal or urethrovaginal fistula. To perform this test, a tampon is placed in the vagina, oral phenazopyridine is administered, and blue dye is instilled into the bladder. If the tampon is discolored yellow-orange at the top, it is suggestive of a ureterovaginal fistula. Blue discoloration in the midportion of the tampon suggests VVF, whereas blue staining at the bottom suggests a urethrovaginal fistula. Diagnosis and localization of urinary tract fistulae and evaluation of concomitant injury or pathology generally involve the use of voiding cystourethrography, urography (intravenous, CT, or retrograde pyelography), or other cross-sectional imaging, with or without endoscopic evaluation.

Voiding cystourethrography (VCUG) can be used to assess the size and location of a vesicovaginal or urethrovaginal fistula. Some small fistulas may not be seen radiographically unless the bladder is filled to capacity and a detrusor contraction is provoked. VCUG can also assess for vesicoureteral reflux. Intravenous urography, computed tomography urography (CTU), and/or retrograde pyeloureterography (RPG) can assess for concomitant ureteral injury, stricture, and/or ureterovaginal fistula, which has been reported to occur in up to 12% of patients [14]. Contrast material in the vagina, air in the bladder, and bladder wall thickening are signs suggestive of the presence of a fistula. Cross-sectional pelvic imaging (magnetic resonance imaging [MRI]/computed tomography [CT]) is recommended if malignancy is suspected. CT cystography can be useful when VCUG is nondiagnostic for reasons such as large body habitus or when the fistula tract is very small.

Cystoscopy and possible biopsy of the fistula tract are performed in the setting of prior pelvic malignancy or if a new malignancy is suspected. Cystoscopy allows visualization of the location of fistula relative to ureters since repair of the fistula may require ureteral reimplantation if the fistula involves the ureteral orifice(s). In addition, an assessment of whether the fistula can be reached vaginally is made. The presence of foreign bodies including suture material, mesh, and/or bladder calculi is also assessed.

Treatment

Treatment of urinary fistula depends on several factors including its location, size, etiology (malignant or benign), and surrounding tissue quality.

Nonsurgical Management VVF Effective conservative management of urinary tract fistulae with maximal drainage and diversion of urine (and stool, when involved) may obviate the need for surgical intervention. Foley catheter drainage is the initial treatment in most cases when the VVF is recognized early in the clinical course and an epithelialized tract has not yet had an opportunity to form. Antibiotics, anticholinergics, and topical estrogen creams are adjuvant measures to prevent infection, promote bladder relaxation, and facilitate healing. Fulguration of the fistula tract with electrocautery followed by catheter drainage has been shown to have some efficacy in small (<5 mm), uncomplicated fistulas. Adjuvant measures such as fibrin glue have been reported in small series in conjunction with fulguration and catheter drainage as a "plug" in the fistula as well as "scaffolding" to allow the ingrowth of healthy tissue.

Surgical Management VVF Surgical intervention for urinary tract fistulae involves multilayer, tension-free closure with interposition of well-vascularized tissue. Adherence to basic surgical principles is essential to achieve successful repair of all urinary fistulas. Cystoscopic evaluation of the bladder and ureters at the start of the procedure can aid in identifying the precise location of the fistula tract and intubating it with a catheter or wire. Adequate exposure of the fistula tract is imperative to allow complete dissection and separation of the bladder wall from the vaginal wall regardless of the approach. Adequate hemostasis to prevent ongoing bleeding or postoperative hematoma is necessary without excessive use of monopolar cautery, which can cause delayed necrosis and tissue breakdown overtime. Devitalized and ischemic tissue should be debrided to prevent necrosis and breakdown of the fistula closure, but healthy fistula tract tissue need not be excised. If any residual surgical material or other foreign body is noted, this should be removed to allow a clean, unobstructed, and watertight closure of the bladder wall. A second layer closure of the bladder wall is often performed by imbricating or buttressing the first suture line. Instillation of blue irrigation fluid into the bladder can test the adequacy of the bladder closure and indicate if additional sutures are needed. Interposition of healthy tissue prior to a watertight vaginal wall closure is recommended.

The timing of the repair should take into consideration the degree of inflammation present, presence of infection, general health and nutritional status of the patient, as well as patient comfort [15]. Early intervention is advocated for the vast majority of situations in the developed world. In the setting of significant inflammation, infection, or radiation damage, a 3–6-month waiting period is advised. Success rates approach 90–98% regardless of surgical approach.

Choice of the optimal surgical approach to VVF (transabdominal or transvaginal) is controversial and generally depends on the skill set of the surgeon [16, 17]. No single approach is applicable to all VVFs, but all VVFs should be managed by a well-trained surgeon with adequate expertise in fistula management. The transabdominal (including laparoscopic or robotic) approach is ideally suited for fistulas located near the ureteral orifice when ureteral reimplantation may be necessary and for fistulas located high on the posterior wall in an area difficult to reach through the vagina. The transvaginal approach is ideally suited when the etiologic surgery was performed abdominally.

Transabdominal Approach Through a midline infraumbilical incision, a Pfannenstiel incision, a laparoscopic, or a robotic approach, the bladder is exposed. Cystoscopic placement of a catheter or wire through the fistula track can aid in identifying the area involved. Either an extravesical or transvesical approach can be used to identify the fistulous connection. With an extravesical approach, the bladder is mobilized and reflected off the underlying vaginal cuff, often with the assistance of a sizer or sponge stick in the vagina. With a transvesical approach, the bladder is opened in the sagittal plane down to the level of the fistula. The bladder is separated off the vagina beyond the level of the fistula. The fistulous tract is biopsied if there is any concern for malignancy and debrided back to healthy tissue if necrotic. The bladder and vaginal walls are closed separately, in multiple layers, with incorporation (rather than excision) of the fistula tract in most situations. Often, well-vascularized tissue, such as omentum, is interposed between the vagina and bladder as an additional layer to promote healing and prevent recurrence. When omentum cannot be mobilized, peritoneum is used as an interposition layer.

Transvaginal Approach Many vaginal approaches have been described including those by Sims, Latzko, and Raz [18–23]. Fixed retraction using hooks and a ring retractor as well as a weighted speculum can be a setup for success. A catheter or wire traversing the fistula track allows easy identification of the vaginal opening. Generally, an inverted U incision is made in the vaginal wall and extended around the fistula tract. The vaginal wall is carefully mobilized circumferentially around the fistula tract, and separation of the vagina wall from the underlying bladder is performed. This requires delicate dissection to avoid tearing the bladder and vaginal walls and often requires use of self-retaining and hand-held retractors. Either the fistula tract is excised (if ischemic or necrotic) with edges of the debrided tract forming the first layer of closure, or the tract is left in situ with fistula edges rolled over forming the primary layer of closure. The perivesical fascia on either side of the first layer of closure is then imbricated over the primary suture line forming the second layer. Interposition of healthy tissue from a labial fat pad (Martius flap), peritoneal flap, or gracilis muscle flap may be placed over the suture lines as a well-vascularized flap similar to the omental flap in the transabdominal approach [24]. Alternatively, or in some instances, the modified Latzko technique can be utilized to provide additional coverage. This involves extending the vaginal wall incision to expose the anterior rectal wall at the level of the vaginal apex. The perirectal tissue is then used to cover the closed bladder wall similar to the technique of a partial colpocleisis. While this technique can shorten the vagina a few centimeters and may not be desirable in all sexually active women, it can often be used with little noticeable change in vaginal depth. Finally, a flap of vaginal wall is advanced over the repair forming the final layer of closure.

In properly selected patients, similar success rates can be obtained using transabdominal or transvaginal approach. Adjuvant tissue flaps can be utilized with either approach and can aid in preventing surgical failure in patients with complex or recurrent fistulas, history of pelvic radiation, or those with surrounding extensive tissue loss. Regardless of approach, maximal urinary drainage (with urethral and/or suprapubic catheter) is maintained postoperatively. A cystogram is usually obtained 2–3 weeks following repair to confirm successful closure. Antimuscarinic or beta-3 agonist medications may be prescribed to help promote bladder relaxation and assist the patient in tolerating the catheter(s). When appropriate, topical vaginal estrogen may be added to aid in improving vaginal tissue quality.

Ureterovaginal Fistula

Continuous urinary leakage with preservation of volitional voiding approximately 1–4 weeks after benign hysterectomy or pelvic surgery is the most common presentation of ureterovaginal fistula (UVF).

Etiology

Ureterovaginal fistulas form between the ureter and the vagina. Most ureterovaginal fistulas are secondary to unrecognized distal ureteral injuries sustained during gynecologic procedures including laparoscopic, abdominal or vaginal hysterectomy, caesarean section, prolapse surgery, and anti-incontinence surgery [25]. These injuries may include laceration of the ureter, complete ureteral transection, delayed necrosis secondary to devitalization of blood supply or cautery injury, suture ligation, or blunt avulsion. The incidence of iatrogenic ureteral injury during major gynecologic surgery is estimated at 0.03–1.5% [10]. The injured ureter spills urine into the peritoneal or extraperitoneal space generally resulting in urinoma formation. The increasing size and tension of the urinoma lead to drainage out of the vaginal cuff [18]. Occasionally, ureterovaginal fistulas may be secondary to endoscopic instrumentation, radiation therapy, pelvic malignancy, penetrating pelvic trauma, or other pelvic surgery (vascular, enteric, etc.). Risk factors for ureteral injuries include a prior history of pelvic surgery, pelvic malignancy, obesity, endometriosis, radiation therapy, and pelvic inflammatory disease (PID); however, many ureteral injuries occur without an identifiable risk factor [9, 18, 26]. Up to 12% of vesicovaginal fistulas may have an associated ureterovaginal fistula [14, 27].

Diagnosis

Ureterovaginal fistulas generally present 1–4 weeks after surgery with urinary leakage per vagina or unilateral hydroureteronephrosis and flank pain secondary to partial ureteral obstruction. Flank pain, nausea, and fever that improve with the initiation of urinary leakage following pelvic surgery are very suggestive of ureteral injury. Unlike a VVF, patients a ureterovaginal fistula will continue to have a normal voiding pattern as long as the contralateral kidney is unaffected. A fluid creatinine can confirm that the vaginal leakage is urine, and a double dye test (as noted above) can differentiate a VVF from a ureterovaginal fistula.

Ureterovaginal fistula is generally evaluated with intravenous urography or CT urography. A urogram may demonstrate partial obstruction, hydroureteronephrosis, and drainage into the vagina. Cystoscopy and retrograde pyelography can be performed to evaluate for concomitant bladder injury and to visualize the distal ureteral segment if not well visualized on the urogram. An attempt at retrograde stenting is reasonable if the pyeloureterogram demonstrates ureteral continuity. Prolonged internal diversion (6–8 weeks) with ureteral stenting may result in resolution of the fistula. Cross-sectional imaging with CT or MRI may be useful to evaluate for pelvic malignancy when indicated or to evaluate for a urinoma in patients with persistent fevers. In cases in which a long segment of distal ureter is involved and a Boari flap is being considered for reconstruction, a cystogram or cystometrogram may be useful to evaluate the bladder capacity.

Percutaneous nephrostomy and antegrade nephrostogram can be helpful especially in situations where complete occlusion of the ureter exists. Percutaneous drainage of the involved kidney followed by antegrade instillation of contrast can provide decompression of a partially obstructed kidney as well as anatomic localization and demonstration of the fistula.

Treatment

Ureterovaginal fistulas can be treated conservatively with ureteral stenting as noted above [28]. If high-grade partial obstruction exists in the setting of sepsis, percutaneous drainage and a course of antibiotic therapy are indicated prior to definitive repair. If retrograde stenting is unsuccessful but the pyeloureterogram shows continuity of the ureteral lumen, then an attempt at antegrade stenting may be undertaken. The goal of stenting is to decompress the upper urinary tract and prevent further extravasation of urine and urosepsis.

When stenting is unsuccessful and the fistula is located distally, ureteroneocystostomy (ureteral reimplantation, with or without psoas hitch and Boari flap) is performed. This is approached transabdominally, laparoscopically, or robotically. The psoas hitch maintains the anatomic position of the bladder and maintains stability during filling and emptying of the bladder. It is not necessary to excise the distal ureteral segment or even close the fistula tract to the vagina unless vesicoureteral reflux is present. Fistulas located in the middle third of the ureter may be amenable to ureteroneocystostomy in conjunction with a Boari flap advancement from the bladder or a ureteroureterostomy. A proximal fistula requires proximal and distal mobilization and primary ureteroureterostomy over a stent, ileal interposition for longer lengths of ureteral injury, or even autotransplantation.

Urethrovaginal Fistula

Worsening urinary leakage following anti-incontinence surgery, periurethral mesh removal, urethral diverticulectomy, anterior vaginal wall prolapse repair, or genital reconstruction can indicate the development of a urethrovaginal fistula. The degree of urinary leakage depends on the size and location of the fistula tract along the urethral lumen. Dyspareunia or recurrent urinary tract infections (UTIs) are sometimes found in these patients and can be greatly improved with optimal surgical care.

Etiology

Urethrovaginal fistulas form between the urethra and vagina. Urethrovaginal fistulas are usually iatrogenic and postsurgical in the industrialized world (anti-incontinence surgery, periurethral mesh removal, urethral diverticulectomy, anterior vaginal wall prolapse repair, genital reconstruction, etc.), although they may occur as a result of trauma, instrumentation (prolonged catheterization), radiation, pelvic fracture, vaginal neoplasm, or childbirth (Fig. 22.2) [29, 30]. The incidence of urethrovaginal fistulas is extremely low with the majority due to obstructed labor in the developing world. In the industrialized world, the frequency appears to be increasing secondary to iatrogenic injury of the urethra at the time of sling surgery [31, 32]. It is important to note that approximately 20% of the time a urethrovaginal fistula will be accompanied by a VVF [33].

Diagnosis

Urethrovaginal fistulas may be asymptomatic if located in the distal third of the urethra (beyond the continence mechanism); otherwise, the presentation is similar to VVF. The diagnosis can often be made with careful physical examination of the distal vagina. Cystourethroscopy can also be used to visualize the urethral lumen; however, technical considerations such as using a female cystoscope, flexible cystoscope, or fully distending the urethra and carefully manipulating the standard cystoscope may be needed for visualization. Cystoscopy is also useful to evaluate for concurrent abnormalities of the bladder and urethra, specifically the presence of any foreign body or mesh material from prior sling, residual urethral diverticulum or urethral stricture, and the tissue integrity of the remaining intact urethra. Occasionally, these patients may present with symptoms suggestive of stress or urgency incontinence, and physical examination and cystoscopy do not confirm the diagnosis. In this setting, voiding cystourethrography (VCUG) can be extremely useful in making the diagnosis. Voiding images must be obtained in patients with a competent bladder neck, and proximal sphincter mechanism or the fistula will not be demonstrated.

Fig. 22.2 A urethrovaginal fistula following removal of an eroded mesh sling (yellow catheter is in the urethra)

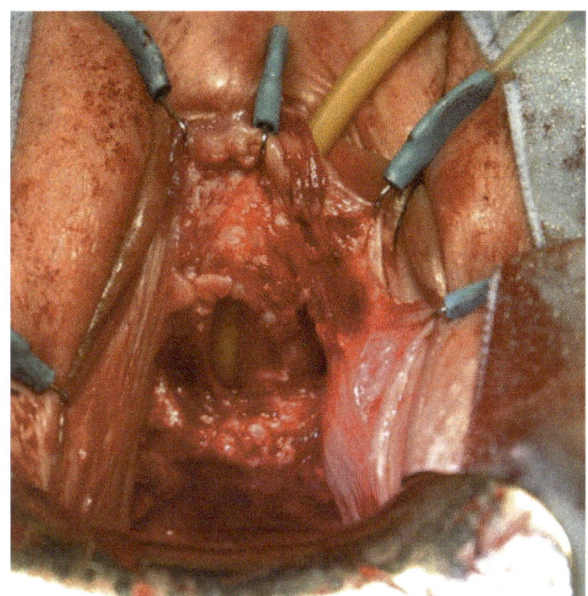

Treatment

Catheter drainage may be useful in a limited number of cases if the urethrovaginal fistula is noted promptly following the causative event. A vaginal approach to repair is most commonly used and allows anatomic restoration of the urethral lumen, the periurethral tissues, and the vagina similar to the principals of VVF surgery. The first step includes identification of the urethrovaginal fistula tract and careful anatomic dissection of the plane between the vagina and urethra. Optimal visualization and retraction can be achieved using a ring retractor with hooks and should facilitate preservation of the periurethral fascia as a distinct layer for interposition between the urethra and vagina. Transvaginal surgical excision of any foreign body material including prior surgical material or mesh is necessary to allow a successful urethral reconstruction. Urethral reconstruction can often be performed primarily over a urethral catheter, but buccal mucosa or vaginal wall may be needed in cases of significant urethral tissue loss. A multiple layer closure is optimal using periurethral fascia, a labial fat pad (Martius flap), and the vaginal wall flap. This multilayered closure technique allows for concomitant or subsequent treatment of SUI should it exist. It should be noted that concomitant stress urinary incontinence treatment with synthetic mesh midurethral sling placement at the time of urethrovaginal fistula repair is not advised according to the recent stress urinary incontinence guideline by the American Urologic Association (AUA)/ Society of Urodynamics, Female Pelvic Medicine & Urogenital Reconstruction (SUFU) [34]. However, use of an autologous pubovaginal sling is considered safe and effective. The optimal timing of treatment of SUI is controversial, and some authors argue that SUI treatment should be deferred until the urethrovaginal fistula is healed and the patient reassessed for the presence of persistent SUI [35].

Vesicouterine Fistula

In the setting of a competent cervix, urinary leakage may not be a part of this condition; rather, cyclic hematuria and watery vaginal discharge can indicate the presence of a vesicouterine fistula. With an incompetent cervix, as in the setting of antecedent vaginal delivery, symptoms may mimic VVF.

Etiology

Vesicouterine fistulas form between the bladder and the uterus. These are rare fistulas that most commonly occur following low-segment caesarean section [36, 37]. Other potential inciting factors include ruptured uterus during obstructed labor, operative vaginal delivery, vaginal birth after prior cesarean section (VBAC), and placenta percreta [38]. Foreign body reaction to intrauterine device (IUD), uterine artery embolization, endometrial ablation, induced abortion, traumatic bladder catheterization, and brachytherapy have been reported causes of vesicouterine fistula. Generally, simultaneous injury to the uterus and the bladder ensues, and if unrecognized or inadequately repaired, fistula formation between the two can occur. It is presumed that some vesicouterine fistulas go unrecognized in the postpartum period, masked by the normal lochia that follows childbirth. Lochiauria (urine mixing with the lochia) may be identified, but may still resolve spontaneously in the postpartum period, potentially assisted by the hormonal suppression and amenorrhea associated with breastfeeding [39]. Spontaneous healing has also been reported in the setting of hormonal suppression with oral contraceptives and luteinizing hormone-releasing hormone (LHRH) agonists.

Diagnosis

The presenting symptoms vary based on the competence of the cervix, and therefore, a high level of suspicion generally accompanies an evaluation for a vesicouterine fistula. Vesicouterine fistulas may present with Youssef syndrome (menouria, cyclic hematuria with apparent amenorrhea, infertility, and urinary continence) or with incontinence similar to a VVF. Diagnosis generally relies on a combination of cystoscopy and imaging. VCUG in the setting of a vesicouterine fistula may demonstrate contrast extravasating from the bladder and filling the uterine cavity. Conversely, hysterosalpingogram may demonstrate contrast extravasating from the uterus and filling of the bladder. Cross-sectional imaging with contrast enhancement of the urine with either CT or MRI can demonstrate the fistula tract and may be able to simultaneously exclude involvement of the ureters.

Treatment

Nonsurgical management of a vesicouterine fistula is possible and, as described for VVF, prolonged catheterization may allow successful healing in patients with small or immature fistulas. Alternatively, or in addition to prolonged catheterization, prevention of menstrual flow through the fistula by administering continuous oral contraceptives or with hormonal induction of uterine involution (amenorrhea) has been reported as successful [39].

Most commonly, these fistulas are treated surgically. The approach to surgery is dictated by the patient's reproductive wishes and should be thoroughly discussed with the patient. If preservation of fertility is desired, dissection of the vesicouterine fistula tract with primary closure of the bladder and uterus and interposition of omentum as described for VVF can be performed. If childbearing is complete, hysterectomy and closure of the bladder with interposition of omentum to prevent a VVF can be performed. Successful delivery has been reported after vesicouterine fistula repair [40].

Radiation Cystitis and Radiation Fistula

Irritative storage symptoms such as urinary frequency, urgency, and urgency incontinence are the most common symptoms associated with radiation cystitis; however, gross hematuria, detrusor hypocontractility, poor bladder emptying, fistulous connection to the vagina, and bladder/urethral pain may all be symptoms of more advanced radiation cystitis.

Etiology

Radiation cystitis can result from pelvic irradiation delivered locally (e.g., brachytherapy) or by external beam to neighboring tissues in the pelvis. Despite significant advances in techniques to deliver radiation to the target organ, effects on surround organs can be profound. An early radiation reaction, approximately 4 weeks after initiation of therapy, has been described in rats demonstrating a change in bladder morphology (e.g., fibrosis, ischemia) as well as function (e.g., compliance, capacity) [41]. Bladder symptoms are common during this period and urodynamic testing often demonstrates early sensations, decreased cystometric capacity, and reduced bladder compliance that can be expected to improve by 6 months. Late radiation effects are less common, but can be progressive and difficult to treat. Rates of deleterious effects on the urinary tract vary between 1% and 12% in the literature with fistula rates of 1–5% [38]. Radiation fistula risk likely depends on the dose of radiation administered and possibly on the type of underlying cancer.

Diagnosis

Diagnosis of radiation cystitis can be made based on clinical history and cystoscopic evaluation of the bladder. Diagnosis of a radiation fistula may be made more difficult by a slow, insidious onset of symptom and lack of a recent surgery to raise suspicion. But it is important to remember that even a remote history of radiation can be responsible. The evaluations needed to make the diagnosis of a fistula in the setting of prior radiation are the same as those describe above for VVF (Sect. 22.1.3). It is imperative that tissue sampling be obtained to assess for cancer recurrence.

Treatment

Symptom-directed therapy with medications to treat the irritative symptoms of frequency, urgency, and urgency incontinence is often employed. Sodium pentosan polysulfate has been used to restore the defective glycosaminoglycans layer of the bladder with some success; however, concerns about vision changes secondary to pigmentary maculopathy limit its utility. Bladder irrigation alone or in combination with intravesical agents such as hyaluronic acid, formalin, aminocaproic acid, or prostaglandins has been used with limited success [42]. Cystoscopic evaluation with bladder fulguration may be effective in stopping most active bleeding. In cases of severe bleeding, selective embolization of the hypogastric arteries may be indicated. Hyperbaric oxygen treatment can greatly improve gross hematuria and irritative bladder symptoms as a result of increased oxygen transfer and restoration of normal cellular composition of the tissue and regeneration of normal urothelium [43]. Resolution of gross hematuria has been seen in upward of 80% of patients.

Treatment of radiation fistula often proves more difficult than nonradiated fistula management. Options to optimize tissue health and integrity prior to surgery include use of topical vaginal estrogen when cancer history allows and hyperbaric oxygen therapy. Surgical repair is the same as that described above for VVF (Sect. 22.1.4). It is imperative to utilize tissue interposition to maximize success in this difficult-to-treat population. When primary closure is not possible, urinary diversion may be needed. Consideration of the radiation field is important in deciding whether to use ileum or transverse colon. If major surgery is not possible, bilateral nephrostomy tubes with or without ureteral coils can be considered as a method of containing the urine.

Urethral Diverticulum

The three Ds, dysuria, dyspareunia, and dribbling, are included in the classic description of a urethral diverticulum; however, it's uncommon for a single patient to experience all of these symptoms. Patients may present with recurrent urinary tract infections, often with persistence of the same organism. Given the elusive nature of urethral diverticula, a high index of suspicion is needed to identify this pathology.

Etiology

A urethral diverticulum/vaginal cyst is an outpouching or sac that forms between the urethra and vaginal wall. This is caused by weakness in the urethra wall, which can be due to repeated urinary tract infections (UTI), a blockage in the glands near the urethra, or trauma to the area during vaginal birth. Women who have had prior vaginal or urethral surgery can develop diverticula or cysts. A diverticulum or cyst may cause no symptoms, but for some they may cause pain, recurrent urinary tract infections, and discomfort with urination or intercourse. When they cause problems, they can be removed with vaginal surgery.

Diagnosis

The astute practitioner may notice persistence of the same offending organism on urine culture and sensitivity raising suspicion for a urinary tract source. All women with recurrent urinary tract infections should undergo careful pelvic examination looking for potential causes including urethral diverticula; although only a small percentage of cases will be found. Vaginal examination may identify a fullness or fluctuance of the midurethra with or without drainage per urethra upon palpation of the anterior vaginal wall. Magnetic resonance imaging (MRI), VCUG, or cystoscopy may aid in diagnosis. T2-weighted sagittal, axial, and coronal MRI views are often the most helpful since fluid-filled structure appears bright white and urethral anatomy can be well defined, often identifying an ostium to the urethra if present. Lateral voiding images on VCUG are generally needed to appreciate the diverticulum and may be limited by body habitus, the indwelling catheter, or the patient's ability to urinate in that position or in front of others. Cystourethroscopy may identify an ostium to the diverticulum. Technique is important when inspecting the female urethra and can be aided by the use of a female cystoscope or a flexible cystoscope as well as hydrodistension of the urethra with irrigant fluid. Careful and thorough visualization of the 5 and 7 o'clock positions of the urethra (which are often in the urethral folds) is important as the ostium can be hidden in the depths of these folds.

Treatment

Monitoring of a urethral diverticulum in asymptomatic patients is appropriate and patients can be reassured that there is a very low risk of cancer found in diverticula. Most commonly, surgery is performed to remove a symptomatic urethral diverticulum. Urethral diverticulectomy is approached through a vaginal incision with dissection of a full-thickness vaginal wall flap off the underlying periurethral fascia. When possible, the periurethral fascia is incised horizontally over the diverticulum and carefully dissected off the underlying urethral diverticulum. If the diverticulum has a horseshoe configuration or extends around to the anterior urethra, urethra dissection and mobilization is needed. Once the whole diverticulum is exposed in the surgical field it is removed from the urethra at the ostium. Many times, an ostium cannot be identified, and removal occurs without a clear opening in the urethra. Not uncommonly, extensive inflammation surrounds the urethral diverticulum and tissue planes become difficult to preserve, limiting the preservation of the periurethral fascia and urethral plane. If the diverticulum is inadvertently entered during dissection, culturing with a tissue swab should be performed and copious irrigation used. After removal of the diverticulum, the urethra should be reconstructed over a Foley catheter using absorbable suture. Irrigation of the urethra with blue dye can confirm a watertight closure. If periurethral tissue is available, a second layer is closed over the urethral closure, generally with nonoverlapping suture lines. A Martius interposition flap may be used if there are any concerns about tissue integrity, if the fascial layer was not preserved, or if subsequent stress incontinence surgery is anticipated. Finally, the vaginal wall incision is closed. The entire surgery is done through the vagina, allowing for minimal discomfort during the recovery period.

Postoperative Care

There are no postoperative pathways that can universally be followed for patients with fistulas and urethral diverticula given their variable characteristics and differences in surgical approaches. However, there are some general principles that are commonly followed postoperatively. A bladder catheter and/or ureteral stent is usually used for several days to weeks after surgical repair to aid in tissue healing. The optimal duration of catheterization is not currently clear, but studies have investigated if shorter catheterization times are sufficient [44, 45]. Prior to catheter and/or stent removal, many surgeons will re-evaluate the fistula or diverticulum using either imaging (e.g., VCUG, CT cystogram) and/or physical exam with the help of dyes (e.g., methylene blue); currently, there is no universally accepted method for evaluating fistula or diverticulum resolution. In terms of pharmacotherapy, several drugs can be used in the postoperative period in addition to pain medications.

Anticholinergics and/or beta-3 agonists may help prevent bladder spasms and irritation due to the Foley catheter. Vaginal estrogen may help improve and maintain vaginal tissue quality and promote healing. An antibiotic or urinary antiseptic (e.g., methenamine) can be used to help prevent bacteriuria when Foley catheters are removed, though the need for ongoing suppressive therapy during the postoperative period is not supported.

Recurrence/Retreatment

Postoperative imaging of the fistula may reveal an ongoing leak. In many cases, prolonged catheter drainage for an additional 3 weeks can allow ample time for the fistula to heal. During this time, every effort is made to maximize healing potential by encouraging a healthy diet, regular ambulation, prevention of infection, use of vaginal estrogen if appropriate, and continued anticholinergic or beta-3 agonist therapy. If a fistula persists despite prolonged catheter drainage a second attempt at repair may be considered. Often a different route of repair is taken for a second surgery (an abdominal approach if the first repair was done vaginal or vaginally if the first repair was done abdominally). For low-volume fistula surgeons, it is appropriate to refer to a center of excellence for repeat surgery. Similarly, if imaging is obtained after urethral diverticulectomy, a small residual diverticulum or a leak from the urethra may be seen. Prolonged catheter drainage for an additional week may allow resolution. In rare circumstances is additional surgery needed if the primary procedure was performed correctly. Recurrent diverticula have been reported and may require subsequent surgery.

Ongoing Symptoms Management

It is not uncommon for patients who have undergone fistula or urethral diverticula surgery to experience irritative bladder symptoms such as urinary, frequency, urgency, nocturia, or urgency urinary incontinence during the postoperative period. These symptoms may extend well beyond the period of indwelling catheterization and may prompt the patient to feel as though their surgery was unsuccessful or complicated. It is important to reassure patients once postoperative evaluation has confirmed their fistula or diverticulum is gone. A combination of pharmacologic therapy, behavioral modification, and pelvic floor muscle exercises can greatly improve bladder symptoms and continence. With time, many patients are able to discontinue pharmacologic therapy. A small percentage of patients may persist with refractory overactive bladder symptoms and may need additional third-line overactive bladder therapy to effectively address their symptoms.

Conclusion

Urinary tract fistulae, radiation cystitis, and urethral diverticula are potentially treatable causes of urinary incontinence. Appropriate diagnosis and treatment of these conditions can greatly improve urine leakage and quality of life. Careful history-taking along with a thorough pelvic examination may be diagnostic or may prompt the clinician to order additional diagnostic studies. Once identified, these reversible causes of urinary incontinence can often be cured surgically, alleviating the burden of incontinence and improving quality of life.

References

1. De Ridder DAP, De Vries C, Elneil S, Emasu A, Esegbono G, Gueye S, Mohammad R, Muleta M, Hilton P, Mourad S, Pickard R, Stanford E, Fistula RE. International Consultation on I. In: Abrams P, Cardozo L, Khoury S, Wein AJ, International Continence S, editors. Incontinence: 5th International Consultation on Incontinence, Paris, February 2012. Paris: ICUD-EAU; 2013. p. 1527–80.
2. Aarts JWM, Nieboer TE, Johnson N, Tavender E, Garry R, Mol BWJ, et al. Surgical approach to hysterectomy for benign gynaecological disease. Cochrane Database Syst Rev. 2015; https://doi.org/10.1002/14651858.CD003677.pub5.
3. Netsch C, Bach T, Gross E, Gross AJ. Rectourethral fistula after high-intensity focused ultrasound therapy for prostate cancer and its surgical management. Urology. 2011;77(4):999–1004. https://doi.org/10.1016/j.urology.2010.10.028.
4. Wall L, Karshima JA, Kirschner C, Arrowsmith SD. The obstetric vesicovaginal fistula: characteristics of 899 patients from Jos, Nigeria. Am J Obstet Gynecol. 2004;190(4):1011–6. https://doi.org/10.1016/j.ajog.2004.02.007.
5. Hillary CJ, Osman NI, Hilton P, Chapple CR. The aetiology, treatment, and outcome of urogenital fistulae managed in well- and low-resourced countries: a systematic review. Eur Urol. 2016;70(3):478–92. https://doi.org/10.1016/j.eururo.2016.02.015.
6. Vangeenderhuysen C, Prual A, et al. Obstetric fistulae: incidence estimates for sub-Saharan Africa. Int J Gynecol Obstet. 2001;73(1):65–6. https://doi.org/10.1016/S0020-7292(00)00374-X.
7. Arrowsmith S, Hamlin EC, Wall LL. Obstructed labor injury complex: obstetric fistula formation and the multifaceted morbidity of maternal birth trauma in the developing world. Obstet Gynecol Surv. 1996;51(9):568–74. https://doi.org/10.1097/00006254-199609000-00024.
8. Chen CW, Mark D, Karram MM. Lower urinary tract fistulas. Urogynecology and reconstructive pelvic surgery. 4th ed. Elselvier Health Sciences; 2015. p. 602–21.
9. Moss RL. Management of enterovesical fistulas. Am J Surg. 1990;159(5):514–7. https://doi.org/10.1016/s0002-9610(05)81259-0.
10. Teeluckdharry B, Gilmour D, Flowerdew G. Urinary tract injury at benign gynecologic surgery and the role of cystoscopy: a systematic review and meta-analysis. Obstet Gynecol. 2015;126(6):1161–9. https://doi.org/10.1097/AOG.0000000000001096.
11. Forsgren C, Lundholm C, Johansson ALV, Cnattingius S, Altman D. Hysterectomy for benign indications and risk of pelvic organ fistula disease. Obstet Gynecol. 2009;114(3):594–9. https://doi.org/10.1097/AOG.0b013e3181b2a1df.
12. Duong TH, Gellasch TL, Adam RA. Risk factors for the development of vesicovaginal fistula after incidental cystotomy at the time of a benign hysterectomy. Am J Obstet Gynecol. 2009;201(5):512, e1-e4. https://doi.org/10.1016/j.ajog.2009.06.046.

13. Duong TH, Taylor DP, Meeks GR. A multicenter study of vesicovaginal fistula following incidental cystotomy during benign hysterectomies. Int Urogynecol J. 2011;22(8):975–9. https://doi.org/10.1007/s00192-011-1375-6.
14. Goodwin WE, Scardino PT. Vesicovaginal and ureterovaginal fistulas: a summary of 25 years of experience. J Urol. 1980;123(3):370–4. https://doi.org/10.1016/S0022-5347(17)55941-8.
15. Ehlert M, Haraway AM, Atiemo HO. Lesson 7: contemporary evaluation and management of vesicovaginal fistula. AUA Update Series. 2013;32:66–75.
16. Lee D, Zimmern P. Vaginal Approach to Vesicovaginal Fistula. Urol Clin North Am. 2019;46(1):123–33. https://doi.org/10.1016/j.ucl.2018.08.010.
17. McKay E, Watts K, Abraham N. Abdominal approach to vesicovaginal fistula. Urol Clin North Am. 2019;46(1):135–46. https://doi.org/10.1016/j.ucl.2018.08.011.
18. Bai SW, Huh EH, Jung DJ, Park JH, Rha KH, Kim SK, et al. Urinary tract injuries during pelvic surgery: incidence rates and predisposing factors. Int Urogynecol J. 2006;17(4):360–4. https://doi.org/10.1007/s00192-005-0015-4.
19. Sims J. On the treatment of vesico-vaginal fistula. Am J Med Sci. 1852;45:59–82. https://doi.org/10.1007/BF01901610.
20. Eilber KS, Kavaler E, Rodrìguez LV, Rosenblum N, Raz S. Ten-year experience with transvaginal vesicovaginal fistula repair using tissue interposition. J Urol. 2003;169(3):1033–6. https://doi.org/10.1097/01.ju.0000049723.57485.e7.
21. Latzko W. Postoperative vesicovaginal fistulas. Am J Surg. 1942;58(2):211–28. https://doi.org/10.1016/S0002-9610(42)90009-6.
22. Raz S, Bregg KJ, Nitti VW, Sussman E. Transvaginal repair of vesicovaginal fistula using a peritoneal flap. J Urol. 1993;150(1):56–9. https://doi.org/10.1016/S0022-5347(17)35396-X.
23. Luo D-Y, Shen H. Transvaginal repair of apical vesicovaginal fistula: a modified latzko techniqueóoutcomes at a high-volume referral center. Eur Urol. 2019;76(1):84–8. https://doi.org/10.1016/j.eururo.2019.04.010.
24. Margules AC, Rovner ES. The use of tissue flaps in the management of urinary tract fistulas. Curr Urol Rep. 2019;20(6):32. https://doi.org/10.1007/s11934-019-0892-6.
25. Shaw J, Tunitsky-Bitton E, Barber MD, Jelovsek JE. Ureterovaginal fistula: a case series. Int Urogynecol J. 2014;25(5):615–21. https://doi.org/10.1007/s00192-013-2272-y.
26. Vakili B, Chesson RR, Kyle BL, Shobeiri SA, Echols KT, Gist R, et al. The incidence of urinary tract injury during hysterectomy: a prospective analysis based on universal cystoscopy. Am J Obstet Gynecol. 2005;192(5):1599–604. https://doi.org/10.1016/j.ajog.2004.11.016.
27. Seth J, Kiosoglous A, Pakzad M, Hamid R, Shah J, Ockrim J, et al. Incidence, type and management of ureteric injury associated with vesicovaginal fistulas: report of a series from a specialized center. Int J Urol. 2019;26(7):717–23. https://doi.org/10.1111/iju.13965.
28. Chen YB, Wolff BJ, Kenton KS, Mueller ER. Approach to ureterovaginal fistula: examining 13 years of experience. Female Pelvic Med Reconstr Surg. 2019;25(2):e7–e11. https://doi.org/10.1097/SPV.0000000000000690.
29. Badlani GDR, Mettu JR, Rovner ES, Wein AJ, Kavoussi LR, Partin AW. Urinary tract fistulae. Campbell-Walsh urology. 11th ed. Elsevier Saunders; 2016. p. 2103–39.
30. Thompson IM, Marx AC. Conservative the of rectourethralfistula: five-year follow-up. Urology. 1990;35(6):533–6. https://doi.org/10.1016/0090-4295(90)80111-Y.
31. Reisenauer C, Wallwiener D, Stenzl A, Solomayer F-E, Sievert K-D. Urethrovaginal fistulaóa rare complication after the placement of a suburethral sling (IVS). Int Urogynecol J. 2007;18(3):343–6. https://doi.org/10.1007/s00192-006-0139-1.
32. Blaivas JG, Mekel G. Management of urinary fistulas due to midurethral sling surgery. J Urol. 2014;192(4):1137–42. https://doi.org/10.1016/j.juro.2014.04.009.
33. Lee RA, Symmonds RE, Williams TJ. Current status of genitourinary fistula. Obstet Gynecol. 1988;72(3 Pt 1):313–9.
34. Kobashi K, Albo M, et al. Surgical treatment of female stress urinary incontinence: AUA/SUFU guideline. J Urol. 2017;198:875.

35. Webster GD, Sihelnik SA, Stone AR. Urethrovaginal fistula: a review of the surgical management. J Urol. 1984;132(3):460–2. https://doi.org/10.1016/s0022-5347(17)49691-1.
36. Porcaro AB, Zicari M, Antoniolli SZ, Pianon R, Monaco C, Migliorini F, et al. Vesicouterine fistulas following cesarean section: report on a case, review and update of the literature. Int Urol Nephrol. 2002;34(3):335–44. https://doi.org/10.1023/A:1024443822378.
37. Rajamaheswari N, Chhikara AB. Vesicouterine fistulae: our experience of 17 cases and literature review. Int Urogynecol J. 2013;24(2):275–9. https://doi.org/10.1007/s00192-012-1798-8.
38. De Ridder DJMK. Urinary tract fistula. In: Partin AW, Kavoussi LR, Dmochowski RR, AJW W, editors. Campbell-Walsh-Wein urology. 12th ed; 2021.
39. Jozwik M. Spontaneous closure of vesicouterine fistula. Account for effective hormonal treatment. Urol Int. 1999;62(3):183–7. https://doi.org/10.1159/000030388.
40. Lotocki WJ, Jozwick M. Prognosis of fertility after surgical closure of vesicouterine fistula. Eur J Obstet Gynecol Reprod Biol. 1996;64(1):87–90. https://doi.org/10.1016/0301-2115(95)02251-1.
41. Vale JA, Bowsher WG, Liu K, Tomlinson A, Whitfield HN, Trott KR. Post-irradiation bladder dysfunction: development of a rat model. Urol Res. 1993;21(6):383–8. https://doi.org/10.1007/BF00300073.
42. Smit SG, Heyns CF. Management of radiation cystitis. Nat Rev Urol. 2010;7(4):206–14. https://doi.org/10.1038/nrurol.2010.23.
43. Degener S, Pohle A, Strelow H, Mathers MJ, Zumbé JR, Roth S, et al. Long-term experience of hyperbaric oxygen therapy for refractory radio- or chemotherapy-induced haemorrhagic cystitis. BMC Urol. 2015;15:38. https://doi.org/10.1186/s12894-015-0035-4.
44. Barone MA, Widmer M, Arrowsmith S, Ruminjo J, Seuc A, Landry E, et al. Breakdown of simple female genital fistula repair after 7 day versus 14 day postoperative bladder catheterisation: a randomised, controlled, open-label, non-inferiority trial. Lancet. 2015;386(9988):56–62. https://doi.org/10.1016/S0140-6736(14)62337-0.
45. Nardos R, Menber B, Browning A. Outcome of obstetric fistula repair after 10-day versus 14-day Foley catheterization. Int J Gynecol Obstet. 2012;118(1):21–3. https://doi.org/10.1016/j.ijgo.2012.01.024.

Part VI
Incontinence in Special Populations

Chapter 23
Incontinence in Older Girls and Adolescents

Esther K. Liu and Kristina D. Suson

Introduction

Female incontinence is widely thought to be a disease process mainly affecting adult women with multiparity or who are perimenopausal or postmenopausal. Urinary incontinence (UI) in the older pediatric or adolescent female is an under-recognized entity. Incontinence can have a negative impact on the quality of life: changing underwear, concern for odor, avoiding fluid intake, avoiding sexual activity, avoiding physical activity, or social isolation during formative years [1–3]. It is also important to note that it may be a harbinger of continued lower urinary tract symptoms (LUTS) into adulthood [4]. This chapter discusses the epidemiology of stress urinary incontinence (SUI) and urgency urinary incontinence (UUI) in this group, along with congenital causes, evaluation, and treatment.

Background and Epidemiology

Prevalence of UI in Older Girls and Adolescents

Limited studies focus on adolescent female UI. One factor that may enable comparison with older females is parity status. Excluding the confounding factor of childbearing distinguishes the UI in this younger population from the more

E. K. Liu
Detroit Medical Center Urology, Detroit, MI, USA
e-mail: eliu@dmc.org

K. D. Suson (✉)
Children's Hospital of Michigan, Pediatric Urology, Detroit, MI, USA

© The Author(s), under exclusive license to Springer Nature   429
Switzerland AG 2022
A. P. Cameron (ed.), *Female Urinary Incontinence*,
https://doi.org/10.1007/978-3-030-84352-6_23

well-recognized adult female incontinence that is often associated with trauma from childbearing, menopause, and comorbidities. As such, we may also extrapolate some of the experience of "young, healthy, nulliparous" female populations that typically include those aged up to 30 years to postpubertal girls.

The prevalence of SUI in adolescent females is reported to range from 6.2% to 79% [1, 5–10]. Most studies found that SUI is more common than UUI, a difference from adult women, with studies quoting rates of UUI between 3.4% and 41.6% [1, 5, 7, 8]. In a systematic review of 18 studies of younger nulliparous females, Almousa et al. quoted SUI rates from 12.5% to as high as 79% (median 49.4%), and rates of UUI ranged from 15.6% to 41.6% (median 31.3%) [10].

A large community study including 15,055 participants from China found a prevalence of UI of 6.6% among 14–21-year-olds. UI was more common in females (7.2% vs 6.0%), and it became more common with increasing age, to a maximum of 12.3% among 19–20-year-olds. Physical and mental health diseases also increased the risk, as did chronic constipation. Increased sexual activity was also a risk factor. In this study, however, UUI occurred more frequently than SUI [11]. Female gender also increased the risk of incontinence in a study from the Netherlands that included patients aged 8–17 years. While 30% of girls reported any daytime or nighttime incontinence, only 14.2% of boys noted UI ($p = 0.003$). They did not find any difference when comparing 8–12-year-olds to 13–17-year-olds (21.5% vs 21.8%, $p = 0.962$). [12].

A US study of 216 patients aged between 14 and 21 years who presented to adolescent gynecology found that 31.5% had any UI. This study also found a higher incidence of UUI (15.7%), followed by mixed incontinence (8.8%), and SUI (6.9%). Nocturnal enuresis (NE) was present in 4.2%. Importantly, most of these patients presented with other chief complaints, commonly seeking contraception or concerned about abnormal periods. Despite the large number who reported any incontinence, only 8% had episodes once or more in a month and less than 1% reported daily/nightly episodes. Generally, their incontinence did not negatively impact their lives; 4.6% of patients reported it as a "very small problem," 0.9% as a small problem, and 0.5% as a medium problem, with no patients perceiving it as a big problem [13].

There is a high incidence of LUTS among pregnant adolescents, with nearly 80% complaining of at least one symptom. UI was reported in 27.2% of 206 pregnant adolescents. More than half of the patients in the study were in their third trimester. Worse symptoms were associated with daily coffee consumption, smoking, chronic cough/constipation, and the history of urinary tract infection (UTI) [14]. As with adult women, adolescent females may develop incontinence after childbirth. Episiotomy increases the risk, as does giving birth to an infant that was large for gestational age and having less frequent prenatal appointments [15].

Urologists have long recognized the connection between the brain and the bladder. Behavioral and psychiatric disorders have been linked to incontinence in children through the age of 18, although these disorders occur less frequently in females than in males [16]. A study that included adolescent boys and girls found a higher incidence of social anxiety among patients with primary NE. Further, social anxiety could lead to a delay in the treatment of enuresis [17]. Children who exhibit internalizing (depression, anxiety, social withdrawal, somatic complaints) and externalizing (aggressive) behaviors and inattention at 10 years of age are more likely to have NE as adolescents [18]. While children and adolescents with any LUTS are more likely to have emotional and behavioral problems, it is even more pronounced that they have concomitant bowel dysfunction [19]. It is difficult to ascertain specifically the psychological findings in female patients, as the studies typically include both genders [17–19]. Developmental and physical delays and sleep disorders are also associated with NE [20].

Stress Urinary Incontinence in the Adolescent Females

SUI is more common in the adolescent female than UUI [10]. Risk factors associated with SUI in this younger population include obesity, strenuous activities or high-intensity training, and pulmonary diseases such as cystic fibrosis (CF) [8]. The pathophysiology behind SUI in the parous woman has been attributed to the trauma from childbirth to the pelvic floor. There are few studies that have explored the pathophysiology in nulliparous or adolescent women. Based on prior studies demonstrating differences in collagen content in women with pelvic organ prolapse, Keane et al. hypothesized similar collagen content differences in nulliparous women with SUI, suggesting an innate risk factor. When comparing nulliparous women with urodynamically proven SUI to a control group of continent young women, they found a significant reduction in collagen content in periurethral biopsies and a reduction in the type I to type III collagen ratio. Type I collagen is more rigid and commonly found in bone, tendon, and dentine, whereas type III collagen is commonly found in more elastic tissues, like the vascular system and intestines. These authors suggested that due to the inherent collagen weakness, pelvic floor training, often the first line of treatment, may be futile and that surgical interventions may be more beneficial [21].

Obesity

Elevated body mass index (BMI) correlates positively with increased intra-abdominal pressures, which, over time, puts stress on the pelvic floor musculature and innervation. Subak et al. demonstrated that each 5-unit increase in BMI can increase the risk of urinary incontinence by 20–70% among adult women [22]. Among girls aged 15–19 years, those who admitted SUI on a questionnaire weighed significantly more than continent adolescents (61 kg vs 56 kg, $p = 0.0188$) [8].

Among a group of 40 obese girls (defined as >95th% BMI) aged 12–17 years, 12.5% reported UI as frequently as once per week compared to none of the 20 non-obese girls. Another 18 girls in the obese group reported UI occurring less than once per month. Differences were found in a metric called the incontinence severity score, leakage frequency multiplied by leakage volume. In the obese group, the score averaged 1.3 compared to 0.3 in the nonobese group ($p = 0.009$) [23]. Finally, an Italian study including 1936 women from 10 universities, with a mean age of 21 years, reported that a BMI >30 kg/m^2 was associated with an increased risk of UI (AOR 3.0, 95% CI 1.4–6.2) [1]. There is still some debate, as there was no association between weight and UI found among 862 boys and girls between the ages of 5 and 18 who presented to an incontinence clinic in Australia [24].

High-Intensity Athletic Training

SUI has been well documented in female athletes. Increases in intra-abdominal pressure cause hypermobility of the bladder neck and urethra, which likely leads to UI with no intrinsic urethral sphincter deficiency. Carls demonstrated that of the 86 female athletes with an average age of 17 years (range 14–21) who spent 3–25 hours/week training or competing in a multitude of sports, 28% reported incidences of SUI during sports activities. Of the 28% who reported SUI, 26% reported associated urgency symptoms. SUI in these athletes also occurred off the playing field, in 11.6% while walking to the bathroom, 11.6% during coughing, and 6.9% during sneezing. Among those with UI, 92% had never told anyone of their symptoms prior to the questionnaire, an unfortunate finding in the study that highlights the stigma [2].

Eliasson et al. had studied urinary incontinence in a very specific group: elite trampolinists [25, 26]. In one study, 35 female trampolinists completed an incontinence questionnaire; 80% admitted involuntary urinary leakage starting an average of 2.5 years after initiating training. All patients over 15 years of age reported urinary leakage. Of note, none of the women admitted leakage outside of trampoline practice [25]. In a second study, former trampolinists were more likely to report incontinence than the nontrampolinists. Additionally, the frequency and duration of training, along with years of training after menarche, were associated with UI [26].

Although the trampolinists did not note UI outside of their sport, a group of female high school athletes, more than 34% of whom experienced UI during sports, also complained of leakage while laughing or during other daily activities. The greater the number of seasons in which a girl competed, the more likely UI was to occur. Although most girls with incontinence reported small volumes, 21% had moderate leakage with urine creating spots on outerwear, and 7% would soak their shorts or pants [27]. SUI in female athletes negatively impacts their quality of life. Those reporting incontinence had statistically significantly lower scores in the total quality of life scores, avoidance and limiting behavior scores, psychosocial impacts scores, and social embarrassment scores [28].

Disordered Eating

Anorexia nervosa has been suggested as a risk factor for UI. A study of 348 patients, 96.3% of whom were female with a mean age of 15.2 ± 1.8 years, found 1.8% had nocturnal enuresis and 1.8% had daytime urinary incontinence, thus concluding they did not have an increased risk [29]. However, a study of elite female athletes with a mean age of 21 ± 5.3 years found that those with disordered eating, as screened with the Eating Disorder Examination Questionnaire, were three times more likely to have urinary incontinence than those without disordered eating [30].

Pulmonary Disease

Chronic lung disease contributes to UI, likely secondary to repetitive increases in abdominal pressure and stress on the pelvic floor from coughing. The connection between the two entities was first described in adults with CF by White et al. They reported a 38% incidence of UI in adult females with CF [31]. Given that CF is a lifelong disease process, Blackwell et al. examined the prevalence of UI in pediatric CF patients. A total of 72 subjects aged 5–18 years at the Pediatric Cystic Fibrosis service in Southampton responded to a questionnaire regarding involuntary urine loss severity and frequency. Eight of the 26 girls (31%) admitted to SUI. Severity of SUI increased with worsening CF as measured by forced expiratory volume [32]. Nixon et al. surveyed adolescent females with CF, finding patients developed UI at a median age of 13 years. The most common precipitators of UI were cough and laugh. Of the 55 patients who responded, 47% reported ever having an incontinence episode, while 22% reported incidences at least twice a month. Concerningly, 42% felt that it interfered with their CF physiotherapy, and only two of the patients with UI had ever mentioned to their physician [33].

Urgency Urinary Incontinence in Female Adolescents

A study of 18–30-year-old "presumably healthy" young female medical students revealed that LUTS, including nocturia, daytime frequency, hesitancy, straining, and intermittency, are more prevalent in this age-group than likely previously assumed. Of the 159 women, 94.3% admitted the presence of any LUTS, and 20% admitted UI. Although overall bother scores were low for the group, the highest bother scores were associated with urgency. None of the subjects had previously sought medical advice, accentuating the likelihood that UI in young women is more prevalent than encountered clinically [7]. It has been suggested that overactive bladder (OAB) in the adult woman may be linked to childhood and adolescent bladder symptoms. Rather than OAB and UUI solely arising in adulthood, consider these on a continuum that could have its origins in childhood [34].

Link Between Childhood and Adult Urinary Incontinence

UUI in adult women may not be a new problem, but rather a newly acknowledged issue. Unresolved or unaddressed urinary issues in childhood can persist into adolescence and adulthood. In 2006, 2109 female participants with the mean age of 56 years were asked to recall their urinary symptoms between the first grade and high school. Childhood diurnal incontinence and NE were associated with a twofold increase with adult UUI (OR 2.6, 95% CI 1.1–5.9 and OR 2.7, 95% CI 1.3–5.5) [35]. Male and female adolescents and adults with a mean age less than 20 treated at an NE clinic completed a questionnaire about their childhood voiding habits and current voiding symptoms. There was a significant correlation between those who reported childhood symptoms of urgency, frequency, UUI, infrequent voiding, or sensation of incomplete emptying and those with current adult symptoms of urgency, UUI, and SUI [36].

A group in Italy mailed surveys, the International Consultation on Incontinence Questionnaire for females with LUTS, to adult women who had been treated as children for UI and LUTS. The questionnaire was returned by 47 former patients and 111 healthy controls. Of the 47 patients, 28 had been treated for diurnal incontinence between the ages of 5 and 20 years (median 11 years), while 19 had been treated for NE between the ages of 5 and 15 years (median 10 years). Women in the patient arm were more likely to currently have UI (34% vs. 7%) [4].

One has to remember that NE resolves spontaneously at a rate of 14% per year as children enter adolescence [37]. The prevalence after age 16 remains constant at 2.3%, suggesting that if NE is still present, the likelihood of spontaneous resolution is low [38]. In a study of 107 Italian male and female adolescents with NE, 74% had primary NE while the remaining 26% admitted to a period of achieving nocturnal dryness for >6 months [39].

Giggle Incontinence

The International Children's Continence Society defines giggle incontinence, also known as giggle micturition or enuresis risoria, as a rare condition in which urine leakage or emptying occurs "during or immediately after laughing." A key distinction about giggle incontinence is that bladder function is otherwise normal in the absence of laughter [40]. There is a little consensus as to the etiology behind giggle incontinence. Logan et al. reviewed the historical discussions of giggle incontinence, first described in 1959, stressing the varying opinions as to the pathophysiology: Is it a neurologic or urologic phenomenon [41]? Although some have emphasized central components of giggle incontinence, it is likely a combination of neurologic factors, abdominal contractions, and detrusor and pelvic floor function and may even carry a familial component. Giggle incontinence seems to share similar pathophysiology as cataplexy, the loss of muscle tone after laughter or after intense feelings such as surprise or fear and associated with narcolepsy [42]. Narcolepsy and cataplexy can be treated with stimulant medications; similarly, methylphenidate has been shown to be effective in treating giggle incontinence [42, 43].

Congenital Causes of Urinary Incontinence

Most congenital causes of UI associated with major birth defects, such as bladder exstrophy or myelomeningocele, will be identified at birth or shortly thereafter. However, there are other more subtle anatomic causes (Table 23.1). Ectopic ureters in females can insert beyond the urethral sphincter and should be considered in patients with persistent, continuous UI. The evaluation begins with renal ultrasound, but frequently magnetic resonance urography is necessary to confirm the diagnosis (Fig. 23.1). Not all patients exhibit the same symptoms; thus, it is important to maintain a high index of suspicion. Viers et al. reported a 12-year-old female who presented with lifelong NE and new onset UI after failing numerous treatments. Computerized tomography revealed an upper pole moiety associated with an ectopic ureteral insertion near the external sphincter. The authors postulated that the NE and new onset leakage occurred at times of decreased sphincteric muscle tone [44].

Complete female epispadias (CFE) is another congenital cause of incontinence. On the exstrophy spectrum, CFE is exceedingly rare, with an incidence of roughly 1/500,000. On the surface, it seems less clinically significant than bladder exstrophy

Table 23.1 Congenital causes of incontinence

Congenital cause	History	Evaluation	Treatment
Ectopic ureter	Continuous incontinence, may have history of febrile UTIs if reflux into lower pole system	Renal ultrasound, MR-urogram, possibly voiding cystourethrography and cystoscopy	Upper-to-lower pole ureteroureterostomy, upper pole heminephrectomy, ureteroneocystostomy
Complete female epispadias	Continuous incontinence	Renal ultrasound, pelvic radiographs, cystoscopy/bladder capacity measurement and cystogram, urodynamics	Epispadias repair, likely will require bladder neck reconstruction, may require ureteral ureteroneocystostomy
Tethered spinal cord	Lower urinary tract symptoms may include UTI, diurnal incontinence, nocturnal enuresis, urgency, frequency. Other symptoms may include back pain, constipation, and gain anomalies	Renal ultrasound, lumbar MRI, urodynamics	Referral to neurosurgery. Depending on urodynamic findings, may require anticholinergics, clean intermittent catheterization, or other bladder therapies

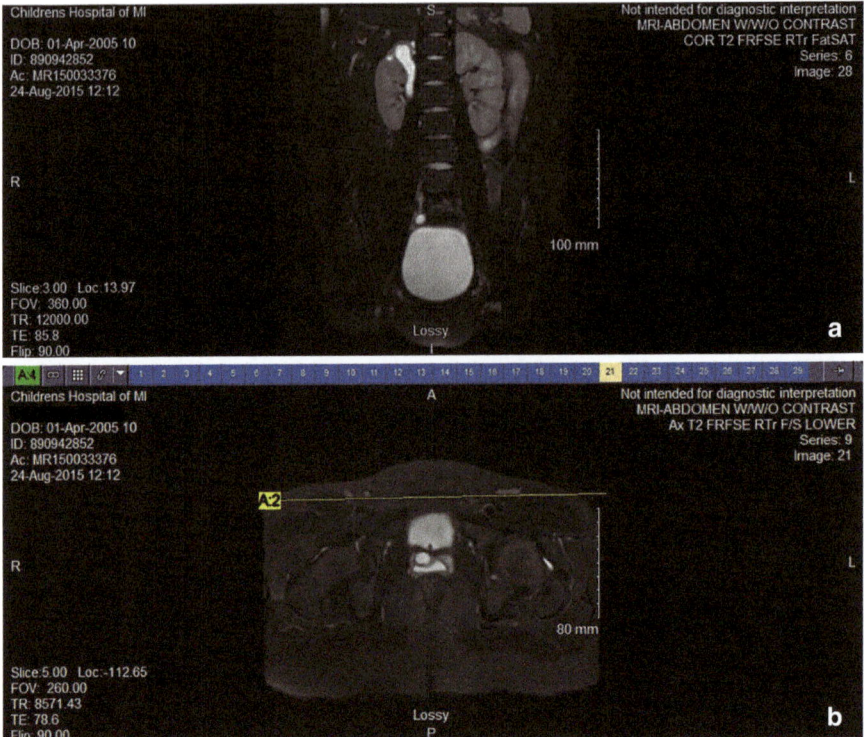

Fig. 23.1 A 14-year-old presented with continuous incontinence since birth. Renal ultrasound demonstrated a right duplicated collecting system with mild dilation of the upper pole, thus magnetic resonance imaging (MRI) was obtained. Coronal T2-weighted MRI (**a**) demonstrated a dilated right upper pole collecting system and the distal ureter inserting into the vagina, also seen on axial imaging (**b**). The patient's incontinence resolved following ureteroureterostomy

in female patients, as the abdominal wall and bladder are closed. However, secondary to the open bladder neck, the continence outcomes are similar [45]. The physical examination findings of CFE may be subtle. While typically picked up earlier in childhood, there are reports of patients who are missed until adolescence, then presenting with continuous incontinence [46, 47].

Other congenital causes of incontinence among adolescent females include spina bifida. Occasionally, even adults may present with primary tethered cord syndrome. Over 90% of adult patients will complain of urologic symptoms, 18.6% of which will have no neurologic complaints. NE may be the only complaint [48]. A retrospective study of girls and adolescents presenting to a pediatric and adolescent gynecology clinic identified 32 for whom there was a clinical suspicion of tethered cord syndrome. The mean age of the 18 eventually diagnosed with tethered cord was 11 ± 4.6 years. Ten of the 18 presented with incontinence. Importantly, 17 of the 18 underwent detethering. Of the 14 patients with follow-up after surgery, 13 experienced a resolution of their symptoms by 6 weeks [49].

Evaluation of the Adolescent with Incontinence

History

Consultation with the incontinent adolescent differs from the younger child or adult (Table 23.2). Adolescents are in a transition period during which they gain independence. Rapid growth and physical changes can often be accompanied by insecurity. This requires a physician who is comfortable interacting with adolescents directly as an individual in a nonjudgmental fashion. Limitations to confidentiality should be set with the adolescent, although sexual history is generally protected [50].

A careful history is the basis for evaluating incontinence. Assess whether the patient has ever been dry or if this has been a lifelong problem. Is the incontinence associated with any particular activities? How frequently does it occur, and what is the volume?

Table 23.2 Evaluation of the older girl and adolescent female with incontinence

History
Does leakage occur during the day, at night, or both?
What is the volume of the leakage?
Have your ever been totally dry?
Do you have a history of urinary tract infections?
Does the leakage occur with activity, cough, laugh, or urgency?
Do you have postvoid dribbling?
How many times a day do you void?
Do you have a history of respiratory issues or snoring?
Is there a family history of nocturnal enuresis or bowel and bladder dysfunction?
On review of symptoms, does the patient have constipation, gait anomalies, back/neck pain, or obesity?
Physical examination
Would the patient like their parent present? (if not, have a chaperone available. Consider having a chaperone even if the parent is present.)
Abdomen: Is the abdomen distended? Is stool palpable?
GU: Is there costovertebral angle tenderness? Is the bladder palpable and/or tender? Are there skin changes near/on the genitalia? Is there urine pooling in the vagina? Is there an ectopic ureteral orifice(s) visualized? Is there a bifid clitoris? Does the urethra appear patulous?
Neurologic: Is the gait normal? Is there an anal wink?
Back: Are there any abnormalities in the area of the sacrum, such as a hairy patch or dimple?
Evaluation
Postvoid residual
Urine analysis
Consider:
Uroflow with EMG if persistent symptoms or elevated postvoid residual
Ultrasound if repeated infections or continuous incontinence
Voiding cystourethrogram if repeated febrile infections or abnormal ultrasound
MR-urogram if concern for ectopic ureter
MRI–lumbar spine if concern for tethered cord syndrome
Urodynamics if persistent symptoms, concerning neurologic findings, or specific concerning findings on ultrasound, voiding cystourethrogram, or spine MRI

Does the leakage occur during the day or at night? What are the patient's voiding habits? A thorough history of bowel habits is also crucial. It is important to note if there is a history of pediatric urologic interventions. Inquiries into the sexual history and potential risk factors for sexually transmitted infections should be performed in this age-group. Additionally, it is important to be sensitive to the possibility of sexual abuse, as there may be an association [51]. Also solicit if the patient could be pregnant.

More objective data can help with counseling. Bladder diaries that include volume and frequency may identify UI triggers and potentially prove therapeutic. The International Consultation on Incontinence Questionnaire Paediatric Lower Urinary Tract Symptoms (ICIQ-CLUTS) is a validated questionnaire that screens for other associated LUTS. The 12-item questionnaire has been shown sensitive and specific in the ages of 5–18 [52]. For the older pediatric patients aged 11–17 years with UI, authors at the University of Michigan developed and performed initial validation of the Incontinence Symptom Index–Pediatric (ISI-P). This 11-item patient-reported questionnaire objectifies UI severity and other scores [53].

A thorough review of symptoms can also provide clues for diagnosis. In girls and adolescents presenting to a pediatric and adolescent gynecology office, in addition to stress urinary incontinence, patients noted constipation and back pain [49]. Especially in patients with NE, it is important to ascertain whether they snore or have other sleep disorders. Consider administering behavioral questionnaires, as these may identify occult behavioral or psychiatric disease [16, 54]. Similarly, patients who present with primary NE may benefit from screening for social anxiety [17].

Physical Examination

Patients should be asked whether they prefer parents/guardians to stay in the room during physical examination [50]. Abdominal examination may demonstrate a large fecal burden, organomegaly, or distended bladder. Carefully examine the genitalia to look for ectopic ureteral orifices. Note any skin changes. Findings of a bifid clitoris and patulous urethra are consistent with CFE [46]. Examination of the lower back may reveal signs of an occult spinal dysraphism. The neurologic examination may demonstrate gait abnormalities. An absent anal wink is suspicious for decreased sensation and possible tethered cord [49].

Adjunct Testing

Urinalysis should be obtained to rule out infection, high or especially low specific gravity, and the presence of glucose. Pyridium pad testing is of value when there is uncertainty about the presence of urine leakage versus physiologic vaginal discharge that may be new for a pubertal girl. A postvoid residual raises the concern for dysfunctional voiding, neurogenic etiology, or pelvic floor dysfunction. Renal bladder ultrasounds may reveal structural abnormalities, upper tract dilation, or bladder wall thickening. Uroflowmetry may demonstrate abnormal flow curves or a decreased Q-max, suggesting obstruction or dysfunctional voiding. A plain film of the Kidneys–Ureters–Bladder (KUB) is helpful in assessing fecal load and may also reveal occult spinal dysraphism. Urodynamic evaluation, although invasive, is used for the diagnosis of detrusor overactivity, dysfunctional voiding, increased bladder capacity, decreased sensation, and intrinsic sphincter deficiency. It should be performed if there is concern for a neurogenic bladder, but may also prompt further neurologic workup.

Treatment

Behavioral Modification and Urotherapy

Urotherapy is often the first-attempted line of therapy and refers to the nonpharmacologic, nonsurgical intervention for LUTS. Urotherapy involves education on regular voiding habits and proper voiding posture to encourage complete emptying. Patients are counseled regarding daily fluid intake, avoiding beverages that may irritate the bladder, and prevention of constipation, along with other voiding suggestions. Table 23.3 lists common steps for improving bladder control, along with escalating therapies.

Table 23.3 Escalating treatment options for incontinence in older girls and adolescent females	
	Urotherapy
	Timed voiding
	Double voiding
	Correct toileting position
	Increased water intake
	Decreased intake of beverages with caffeine, carbonation, artificial colors, and sugars
	Increased fiber and stool softeners
	Referral to weight management clinic as appropriate
	Biofeedback
	Pelvic floor physical therapy
	Medications
	Anticholinergics, including oxybutynin, tolterodine, solifenacin, and fesoterodine
	Mirabegron
	Desmopressin (for nocturnal enuresis)
	Tricyclic antidepressants, including imipramine (for nocturnal enuresis)
	Methylphenidate (for giggle incontinence)
	Transcutaneous electrical nerve stimulation
	Sacral
	Parasacral
	Posterior tibial
	Surgical options
	Sacral neuromodulation
	Intravesical botulinum A toxin

The International Children's Continence Society outlines six specific types of urotherapies in their standardization document: timed voiding, bladder training, pelvic floor muscle training, central inhibition training, neurostimulation, and clean intermittent catheterization. Each urotherapy has specific urologic complaints for which it is best suited. They suggest bladder training for all forms of incontinence. Urgency incontinence may also be treated with timed voiding, central inhibition training, and neurostimulation. Effective bowel management, potentially including laxatives, is a key. Cognitive behavioral therapy is also central to urotherapy, from education and self-monitoring to conditioning and response prevention [55].

In the European Bladder Dysfunction Study, which included both girls and boys (171 girls and 46 boys) between the ages of 7 and 12 years, 44% of children with incontinence secondary to OAB randomized to standard therapy and 6–12 bladder training sessions achieved full continence. This is in comparison with 15% who achieved continence on standard therapy or three sessions of counseling with an urotherapist, alone [56].

For children with NE, both monosymptomatic and nonmonosymptomatic, the bed-wetting alarm has been demonstrated to be the most successful therapy. Patients who had only NE required fewer clinic visits and achieved dryness more quickly than those with other LUTS. The alarm alone was prescribed to patients with a smaller-than-expected bladder capacity, while those with polyuria were prescribed desmopressin, and patients with small bladders and polyuria were prescribed both. They reported continence rates with the alarm of 39.9% with monosymptomatic NE and 36.4% of patients with nonmonosymptomatic NE. Desmopressin worked for 27.8% of monosymptomatic NE and 14.9% of nonmonosymptomatic NE. Combination therapy worked for 13.2% of monosymptomatic NE and 18.2% of nonmonosymptomatic NE [57].

Urotherapy can be successful in treating patients with giggle incontinence, specifically biofeedback. A retrospective review included 10 girls and 2 boys between 6 and 15 years of age who were offered biofeedback after failing anticholinergics and/or pseudoephedrine. Girls who had at least four sessions had a complete response that was durable at 6 months, although some did remain on pharmacologic therapy. They believe that the treatment was successful because of the new ability to recruit the external sphincter muscles to prevent incontinence. Additionally, 40% of the patients had dysfunctional voiding identified on urodynamics, despite only having symptoms of giggle incontinence; biofeedback also helped them learn how to relax the sphincter [58].

For patients with SUI, pelvic floor therapy is a helpful adjunct. In Eliasson's study of 35 elite trampolinists, of whom 80% reported stress urinary incontinence, 21 of the athletes reported leakage "at the end of the exercise session," suggesting fatigue of the pelvic floor muscles [25]. Similarly, Ree et al. found a decrease of maximum voluntary contraction pressure by 17% after 90 minutes of strenuous activity in young women (mean age 24 ± 1.7 years) [59]. In a study by Da Roza et al., 16 women had high levels of physical activity classified according to the International Physical Activity Questionnaire–Short Form (IPAQ-SF), 3000 metabolic equivalent minutes/week or 4 hours/week of intense physical activity. Seven of those women suffered from UI. They each underwent an 8-week pelvic floor rehabilitation program. After completion, there was a significant increase in both vaginal resting and maximum voluntary contraction pressures from baseline. The UI frequency and volume improved significantly, resolving completely in six of the patients [60].

In the European Bladder Dysfunction Study, 49% of the children with incontinence secondary to dysfunctional voiding randomized to standard therapy plus pelvic floor training achieved continence; 25% achieved continence from standard therapy or three counseling sessions with an urotherapist. As a control for the pelvic floor training, patients were also randomized to a cognitive therapy arm, where 52% of patients achieved continence. Researchers hypothesized that social stress may be an important mediator of symptoms [56]. This justifies a multidisciplinary approach to these complicated patients.

Given that weight loss is an effective treatment for overweight and obese women with UI [22], the same recommendation has been studied in adolescents. A prospective study included 242 obese adolescents, 33 females (18%) with a mean age of 17.1 years and an BMI of 50.5 kg/m^2 reported urinary incontinence prior to bariatric surgery. They were followed up postoperatively, with UI decreasing to 7% at 6-month and 3-year follow-ups [61].

Medical Therapy

In pediatric patients, anticholinergics, such as oral oxybutynin, have been considered the "gold standard" for symptoms of OAB; however, as in adults, the side effects and potential need for multiple daily doses are problematic [62]. Anticholinergics are also a recommended treatment option for NE in patients who have failed desmopressin and the bed-wetting alarm. It is important to monitor these patients for increasing postvoid residuals and to avoid developing or worsening constipation [54].

Gleason et al. investigated the efficacy and side effect profile of the oxybutynin patch in patients between 4 and 16 years old. This eliminated the need for multiple daily doses, as it is changed every 3–4 days. They found that the only significant side effect was skin irritation at the patch site in 35% of patients. Within the study group, 69% had discontinued oral oxybutynin therapy because of dry mouth, constipation, or behavior changes, none of which were experienced with the patch. The patch was highly effective, with 97% of patients reporting improved symptoms; 57% reported complete resolution [62].

Solifenacin has been proposed for therapy-resistant OAB, after failing oxybutynin and tolterodine [63, 64]. One study included 138 boys and girls who had some degree of diurnal or nocturnal incontinence, most of whom had been on other anticholinergics. After 3 months of therapy, 99 patients were evaluated, of whom 45 gained complete continence. An additional 39 patients had partial responses, 17 of whom became dry during the day. Side effects were noted in 6.5% of patients, including hyperactivity, drowsiness, constipation, abdominal pain, and fecal impaction [63]. Another study reported a solifenacin success rate of 94% for incontinence secondary to OAB. Although it was effective, 38% of patients did experience side effects, most commonly dry mouth and constipation. When considering urodynamic data, bladder capacity increased from 128 mL to 340 mL, and uninhibited detrusor contractions decreased in magnitude from 70 cm H_2O to 18 cm H_2O. The number of incontinence episodes per day significantly decreased, and patient and parent perception of continence also improved [64].

Fesoterodine has also been utilized to treat incontinence in pediatric and adolescent patients with OAB. A study comparing fesoterodine 4–8 mg to extended-release oxybutynin demonstrated equal efficacy between the two. There was no difference in side effects such as constipation and dry mouth; however, those randomized to fesoterodine experience an increase in their heart rate. Median voided volume and the number of incontinence episodes improved for both medications, as did the quality of life. The authors extended treatment by 12 months for 23 children. For the 34 children who were not enrolled in the extension, 68% had gained continence at a mean follow-up of 18 months. Of those enrolled in the extension, 78% gained continence [65].

Although mirabegron, a β3-adrenoreceptor agonist used to treat OAB in adults, has not been approved as a treatment option for children, studies have reported good outcomes. Of the 58 patients at a median age of 10.1 years with OAB who failed anticholinergic therapy or had unacceptable side effects, 52 reported improved continence. No severe side effects were noted [66].

Tricyclic antidepressants have historically been used to treat NE in children. A Cochran review found that tricyclics reduced the number of wet nights when compared to placebo. Further, a greater proportion of patients were able to achieve a dry 14-day stretch. The medications for which they found a benefit over placebo included imipramine, amitriptyline, and desipramine. They noted a recurrence of NE upon cessation of therapy. The studies did not include enough data to compare tricyclics to each other. They did compare their efficacy to desmopressin and found it similar to monotherapy, although one study found that desmopressin/oxybutynin combination therapy was superior to imipramine monotherapy. While tricyclics were more effective than behavioral modification, the bed-wetting alarm was more effective in the short term and upon stopping therapy [67]. The International Children's Continence Society only recommends tricyclics if patients have failed desmopressin, the bed-wetting alarm, and anticholinergics because of the risk of cardiotoxicity [54].

Double anticholinergic therapy may be an option when patients have persistent incontinence with a partial response on one well-tolerated agent. In a study that included six females with nonneurogenic bladder dysfunction at a mean age of 10.5 ± 2 years, a second anticholinergic was offered, with combinations that included oxybutynin and tolterodine, oxybutynin and solifenacin, and tolterodine and solifenacin. The most common side effect was dry mouth, but no patients stopped therapy because of it. All patients had improved continence [68].

Rather than adding a second anticholinergic, Morin et al. reported their experience of adding mirabegron. Their prospective study included 35 patients (median age 10.3 years), mostly males, who had persistent incontinence and a partial response to an extended-release anticholinergic. Ultimately, 29 patients received solifenacin and mirabegron, three patients received extended-release oxybutynin and mirabegron, and three patients received fesoterodine and mirabegron. All patients reported an improvement in symptoms, with 34% reporting total continence and 66% reporting a 50–99% reduction in incontinence episodes. The voided urine volumes increased with treatment. Side effects were reported by 20% of patients, with moderate side effects reported by 3% [69].

Similarly, dual therapy with desmopressin and oxybutynin improves response rates in patients with NE. A retrospective review of 61 patients (mean age 11.6 ± 2.6 years) with either monosymptomatic NE or NE with controlled daytime symptoms found a 69% response rate to a maximum of 0.6 mg desmopressin. They would then add oxybutynin 5 mg nightly and increase by 2.5 mg to a maximum of 10 mg nightly for patients who failed desmopressin monotherapy. Of the 25 patients who started combination therapy, 68% became dry on 5 mg of oxybutynin. Of the eight that went on to high-dose oxybutynin, 75% became dry, for an ultimate success rate of 97% on either desmopressin monotherapy or combination therapy. Male and female patients had similar responses to monotherapy, but female patients seemed to respond better than males to combination therapy, with 100% achieving dryness. Among the patients, there were no reported side effects with desmopressin monotherapy, nor were any children on combination therapy treated for dry mouth or constipation [70].

Giggle incontinence is its own subset of UI and, as such, has a unique medical therapy. A group of 20 patients with pure giggle incontinence at a mean age of 12.4 years were first treated with standard behavioral modifications, along with anticipatory voiding before activities that may increase laughter. Thirteen of these patients reported no improvement in symptoms. All patients were offered a trial of methylphenidate, and 15 accepted. UI resolved in 12 of the 15 patients during school hours. At 2 months, the medication was stopped, and 9 of the 12 previously dry patients had recurrence of symptoms [43].

More Intensive Therapies

Urinary incontinence can have a significant impact on quality of life. A group in Canada surveyed patients and caregivers, reporting that 71% of patients and 89% of caregivers appreciated a moderate-to-severe impact on their quality of life. Further, they were willing to try either transcutaneous neurostimulation (54%) or implanted sacral neuromodulation (42%) [3]. Modifications to the sacral neuromodulation technique may allow for it to be even less invasive, with decreased radiation exposure and improved cosmesis [71].

Transcutaneous Neuromodulation

Less invasive than an implanted device, transcutaneous electrical nerve stimulation (TENS) has been proposed as a better option for pediatric patients. Various electrode locations have been described, including sacral, parasacral, and posterior tibial. A placebo-controlled trial of sacral TENS that included children up to the age of 14 found that 61% of the patients in the active arm had a decrease in daytime incontinence severity compared to 17% in the sham group ($p < 0.01$). They also experienced fewer daytime accidents. The investigators also evaluated urodynamic parameters, in an attempt to elucidate why it worked, but they could not identify differences in bladder volumes [72].

A prospective study of 83 patients treated with parasacral TENS, most of whom were female but only 25% were older than 10 years, identified a lower success rate when NE was present. A significant improvement was reported by 96.4% of patients, with complete resolution in 56.6% of cases. When specifically comparing patients with or without NE, only 45.5% of those with NE had a complete response, as compared to 78.6% of those without NE. There was no statistically significant difference in age 10 or greater when compared to those aged nine or younger (66.7% complete response vs. 55.9%, $p = 0.97$) [73]. Parasacral TENS also improves constipation, but the effect seems to be independent of curing UI [74].

Posterior tibial TENS has also been shown to be effective in curing daytime incontinence and NE in boys and girls with OAB and dysfunctional voiding. Those with dysfunctional voiding had an even better response than those with OAB, with 85% achieving daytime continence. Most children with dysfunctional voiding maintained their response at 2 years. Many of those who were not cured had excellent responses to chronic monthly stimulation [75].

One study compared biofeedback and parasacral TENS in a prospective fashion as treatment modalities for OAB, dysfunctional voiding, or both OAB and dysfunctional voiding. They found that both options result in improved daytime incontinence, with no difference in their success. They did note, however, that biofeedback was successful after fewer sessions [76]. Another study compared parasacral TENS to oxybutynin. They randomized patients to either parasacral TENS and placebo or sham scapular electrical therapy and oxybutynin. They found that all patients in the parasacral TENS group had improved constipation, and no patients had the anticholinergic side effects noted in the oxybutynin group. They found no difference in treatment success when evaluating improvement in dysfunctional voiding severity scores. Both the groups demonstrated improved maximum and mean voided volumes and the number of voids per day [77].

Surgical Treatments

Sacral neuromodulation can be used successfully to treat UI in select adolescent patients. Most studies require conservative and/or medical treatment failure. In a study including three boys and 15 girls with varied lower urinary tract dysfunction at a mean age of 15 years, 15 had at least a 50% improvement in their symptoms after the test phase and had the pulse generator implanted. Of those with a device, 50% experienced a full response, and 28% experienced a partial response in the short term. This dropped slightly to 73% of patients reporting a full or partial response at a mean follow-up of 28.8 ± 43.8 months. When looking specifically at the 10 patients whose primary indication was incontinence, six patients had a full response and three had a partial response [78]. Over a moderate length of follow-up, with a median of 3.9 years, 74% of children who had sacral neuromodulation performed after failing conservative management endorsed improvement in their symptoms, with improvement persisting after device removal for some [79].

As with TENS, implanted sacral neuromodulation seems more successful for diurnal UI. In a study of patients with diurnal or nocturnal incontinence, 75% of the 16 patients with diurnal incontinence had resolution of their symptoms, with an additional 13% having improvement, while of the 16 patients with NE, 38% had resolution and an additional 25% had improvement [80].

In addition to improving continence, sacral neuromodulation also positively impacts psychosocial quality of life scores, without a difference in physical quality of life scores [81]. Patients with longer follow-up seem to have persistently improved urinary symptom and quality of life scores. Patients with uninhibited contractions in particular may respond better to sacral neuromodulation [82].

While, in most studies, it is difficult to ascertain the ages of the patients, one study did stratify response to sacral neuromodulation in children with refractory dysfunctional elimination syndrome/bowel and bladder dysfunction. They found that of the 52 patients, 9 years of age or older, 87% experienced improvement in their daytime incontinence, with it resolving in 44%. Of the 44 patients in that age-group with NE, 73% had improvement, with 23% reporting resolution [83].

One downside to implanted sacral neuromodulation is the need for additional surgeries. Even when the procedure is a success, the device will ultimately be explanted. Of the 61 patients, 32.4% had their devices removed within 4 years of placement for cure, where the device had been turned off for 6 months or greater without a recurrence of symptoms [84]. Patients may also require revision/replacement or removal because of complications. The removal rate for complications varies from 8% to 25%, for reasons such as infection or treatment failure [79, 84, 85]. The reoperation rate, most commonly for lead migration or breakage, or device malfunction, ranges between 19.7% and 54% [79, 83–85]. Patients with low body mass index may be at an increased risk of leads breaking with minimal trauma [82], although others have not found age, gender, or body mass index to predict complications [85].

Intravesical botulinum A toxin injection has also been used for older children and adolescents with UI. As with sacral neuromodulation, patients should first exhaust conservative options. Success rates vary, with a complete response in 32–55% and additional patients reporting a partial response [86–88]. In addition to improved UI, patients may also have decreased symptoms of frequency, urgency, and nocturia [87]. Quality of life scores also improve [89]. In a study that included pre- and postinjection urodynamics, 75% of the patients had resolution of uninhibited contractions, while the remaining 25% had contractions of decreased magnitude [90]. The complication rates vary, from no complications

[86, 90] to postoperative urinary retention and urinary tract infection [87, 88, 90]. Patient and parent satisfaction is high, with only one of the 43 patients who underwent intravesical botulinum A toxin injection finding it poor/disappointing [91].

Burch colposuspensions, both open and laparoscopic, have been reported in girls with refractory urinary incontinence and video-urodynamically proven bladder neck insufficiency. A study of 18 consecutive laparoscopic and 18 consecutive open colposuspensions included girls who first failed ambulatory urotherapy and then an intensive 10-day inpatient training. Ultimately, all girls had been resistant to therapy for at least 2 years. The mean age of girls undergoing the laparoscopic procedure was 13.5 years and those undergoing open surgery was 11.5 years. Complete dryness was achieved in 44% of the patients undergoing the laparoscopic procedure and 38% of the open group, while partial dryness, where the patients reported fewer episodes of stress incontinence, was achieved for 28% of the laparoscopic group and 17% of the open group. They reported no complications [92]. A PubMed search revealed no reports of sling procedures or artificial urinary sphincters for pediatric or adolescent nonneurogenic bladder dysfunction in the absence of other congenital anomalies, such as bladder exstrophy or epispadias.

Conclusion

In conclusion, UI is an under-recognized, yet potentially life-affecting diagnosis in older girls and adolescent females, with athletes and those with chronic health conditions such as obesity or lung disease at particular risk. Although rare, the cause may be anatomic; thus, congenital causes should be excluded during evaluation. Treatment begins with behavior modification and urotherapy, but may escalate to transcutaneous or implanted neuromodulation or intravesical botulinum A toxin injection. Unfortunately, those who suffer in their youth are at risk of continued LUTS as adults, but their quality of life can be improved with intervention.

References

1. Bardino M, Di Martino M, Ricci E, Parazzini F. Frequency and determinants of urinary incontinence in adolescent and young nulliparous women. J Pediatr Adolesc Gynecol. 2015;28(6):462–70.
2. Carls C. The prevalence of stress urinary incontinence in high school and college-age female athletes in the Midwest: implications for education and prevention. Urol Nurs. 2007;27(1):21–4, 39
3. Dos Santos J, Marcon E, Pokarowski M, Vali R, Raveendran L, O'Kelly F, Amirabadi A, Elterman D, Foty R, Lorenzo A, Koyle M. Assessment of needs in children suffering from refractory non-neurogenic urinary and fecal incontinence and their caregivers' needs and attitudes toward alternative therapies (SNM, TENS). Front Pediatr. 2020;8:558.

4. Petrangeli F, Capitanucci ML, Marciano A, Mosiello G, Alvaro R, Zaccara A, Finazzi-Agro E, De Gennaro M. A 20-year study of persistence of lower urinary tract symptoms and urinary incontinence in young women treated in childhood. J Pediatr Urol. 2014;10(3):441–5.
5. O'Halloran T, Bell RJ, Robinson PJ, Davis SR. Urinary incontinence in young nulligravid women: a cross-sectional analysis. Ann Intern Med. 2012;157(2):87–93.
6. Hägglund D, Olsson H, Leppert J. Urinary incontinence: an unexpected large problem among young females. Results from a population-based study. Fam Pract. 1999;16(5):506–9.
7. van Breda HM, Bosch JL, de Kort LM. Hidden prevalence of lower urinary tract symptoms in healthy nulligravid young women. Int Urogynecol J. 2015 ov;26(11):1637–43.
8. Alnaif B, Drutz HP. The prevalence of urinary and fecal incontinence in Canadian secondary school teenage girls: questionnaire study and review of the literature. Int Urogynecol J Pelvic Floor Dysfunct. 2001;12(2):134–7.
9. Parden AM, Griffin RL, Hoover K, Ellington DR, Gleason JL, Burgio KL, Richter HE. Prevalence, awareness, and understanding of pelvic floor disorders in adolescent and young women. Female Pelvic Med Reconstr Surg. 2016;22(5):346–54.
10. Almousa S, Bandin van Loon A. The prevalence of urinary incontinence in nulliparous adolescent and middle-aged women and the associated risk factors: a systematic review. Maturitas. 2018;107:78–83.
11. Luo Y, Zou P, Wang K, Cui Z, Li X, Wang J. Prevalence and associated factors of urinary incontinence among Chinese Adolescents in Henan Province: a cross-sectional survey. Int J Environ Res Public Health. 2020;17(17):6106.
12. Linde JM, Nijman RJM, Trzpis M, Broens PMA. Prevalence of urinary incontinence and other lower urinary tract symptoms in children in the Netherlands. J Pediatr Urol. 2019;15(2):164.e1–7.
13. Arbuckle JL, Parden AM, Hoover K, Griffin RL, Richter HE. Prevalence and awareness of pelvic floor disorders in female adolescents seeking gynecologic care. J Pediatr Adolesc Gynecol. 2019;32(3):288–92.
14. Aydın A, Kocaöz S, Kara P. Prevalence of lower urinary tract symptoms in pregnant adolescents and the influencing factors. J Pediatr Adolesc Gynecol. 2020;33(2):160–6.
15. Babini D, Lemos A. Risk factors for urinary incontinence in primiparous adolescents after vaginal delivery: a cohort study. J Pediatr Adolesc Gynecol. 2020;33(5):500–5.
16. von Gontard A, Mattheus H, Anagnostakou A, Sambach H, Breuer M, Kiefer K, Holländer T, Hussong J. Behavioral comorbidity, overweight, and obesity in children with incontinence: an analysis of 1638 cases. Neurourol Urodyn. 2020;39(7):1985–93.
17. Eray Ş, Tekcan D, Baran Y. More anxious or more shy? Examining the social anxiety levels of adolescents with primary enuresis nocturna: a controlled study. J Pediatr Urol. 2019;15(4):343.e1–5.
18. Vasconcelos MMA, East P, Blanco E, Lukacz ES, Caballero G, Lozoff B, Gahagan S. Early behavioral risks of childhood and adolescent daytime urinary incontinence and nocturnal enuresis. J Dev Behav Pediatr. 2017;38(9):736–42.
19. Dourado ER, de Abreu GE, Santana JC, Macedo RR, da Silva CM, Rapozo PMB, Netto JMB, Barroso U. Emotional and behavioral problems in children and adolescents with lower urinary tract dysfunction: a population-based study. J Pediatr Urol. 2019;15(4):376.e1–7.
20. Shah S, Jafri RZ, Mobin K, Mirza R, Nanji K, Jahangir F, Patel SJ, Ejaz MS, Qaiser I, Iftikhar H, Aziz K, Khan W, Maqbool HS, Ahmed H. Frequency and features of nocturnal enuresis in Pakistani children aged 5 to 16 years based on ICCS criteria: a multi-center cross-sectional study from Karachi, Pakistan. BMC Fam Pract. 2018;19(1):198.
21. Keane DP, Sims TJ, Abrams P, Bailey AJ. Analysis of collagen status in premenopausal nulliparous women with genuine stress incontinence. Br J Obstet Gynaecol. 1997;104(9):994–8.
22. Subak LL, Whitcomb E, Shen H, Saxton J, Vittinghoff E, Brown JS. Weight loss: a novel and effective treatment for urinary incontinence. J Urol. 2005;174(1):190–5.
23. Schwartz B, Wyman JF, Thomas W, Schwarzenberg SJ. Urinary incontinence in obese adolescent girls. J Pediatr Urol. 2009;5(6):445–50.

24. Monkhouse K, Caldwell PH, Barnes EH. The relationship between urinary incontinence and obesity in childhood. J Paediatr Child Health. 2019;55(6):625–31.
25. Eliasson K, Larsson T, Mattsson E. Prevalence of stress incontinence in nulliparous elite trampolinists. Scand J Med Sci Sports. 2002;12(2):106–10.
26. Eliasson K, Edner A, Mattsson E. Urinary incontinence in very young and mostly nulliparous women with a history of regular organised high-impact trampoline training: occurrence and risk factors. Int Urogynecol J Pelvic Floor Dysfunct. 2008;19(5):687–96.
27. Logan BL, Foster-Johnson L, Zotos E. Urinary incontinence among adolescent female athletes. J Pediatr Urol. 2018;14(3):241.e1–9.
28. Hagovska M, Svihra J, Bukova A, Horbacz A, Svihrova V. The impact of physical activity measured by the International Physical Activity questionnaire on the prevalence of stress urinary incontinence in young women. Eur J Obstet Gynecol Reprod Biol. 2018;228:308–12.
29. Mattheus HK, Wagner C, Becker K, Bühren K, Correll CU, Egberts KM, Ehrlich S, Fleischhaker C, Föcker M, Hahn F, Hebebrand J, Herpertz-Dahlmann B, Jaite C, Jenetzky E, Kaess M, Legenbauer T, Pfeiffer JP, Renner TJ, Roessner V, Schulze U, Sinzig J, Wessing I, von Gontard A. Incontinence and constipation in adolescent patients with anorexia nervosa-Results of a multicenter study from a German web-based registry for children and adolescents with anorexia nervosa. Int J Eat Disord. 2020;53(2):219–28.
30. Carvalhais A, Araújo J, Natal Jorge R, Bø K. Urinary incontinence and disordered eating in female elite athletes. J Sci Med Sport. 2019;22(2):140–4.
31. White D, Stiller K, Roney F. The prevalence and severity of symptoms of incontinence in adult cystic fibrosis patients. Physiother Theory Pract. 2000;16:35–42.
32. Blackwell K, Malone PS, Denny A, Connett G, Maddison J. The prevalence of stress urinary incontinence in patients with cystic fibrosis: an under-recognized problem. J Pediatr Urol. 2005;1(1):5–9.
33. Nixon GM, Glazner JA, Martin JM, Sawyer SM. Urinary incontinence in female adolescents with cystic fibrosis. Pediatrics. 2002;110(2 Pt 1):e22.
34. Salvatore S, Serati M, Origoni M, Candiani M. Is overactive bladder in children and adults the same condition? ICI-RS 2011. Neurourol Urodyn. 2012;31(3):349–51.
35. Fitzgerald MP, Thom DH, Wassel-Fyr C, Subak L, Brubaker L, Van Den Eeden SK, Brown JS, Reproductive Risks for Incontinence Study at Kaiser Research Group. Childhood urinary symptoms predict adult overactive bladder symptoms. J Urol. 2006;175(3 Pt 1):989–93.
36. Bower WF, Sit FK, Yeung CK. Nocturnal enuresis in adolescents and adults is associated with childhood elimination symptoms. J Urol. 2006;176(4 Pt 2):1771–5.
37. Forsythe WI, Redmond A. Enuresis and spontaneous cure rate. Study of 1129 enuretis. Arch Dis Child. 1974;49(4):259–63.
38. Yeung CK, Sihoe JD, Sit FK, Bower W, Sreedhar B, Lau J. Characteristics of primary nocturnal enuresis in adults: an epidemiological study. BJU Int. 2004;93(3):341–5.
39. Nappo S, Del Gado R, Chiozza ML, Biraghi M, Ferrara P, Caione P. Nocturnal enuresis in the adolescent: a neglected problem. BJU Int. 2002;90(9):912–7.
40. Austin PF, Bauer SB, Bower W, Chase J, Franco I, Hoebeke P, Rittig S, Vande Walle J, von Gontard A, Wright A, Yang SS, Nevéus T. The standardization of terminology of lower urinary tract function in children and adolescents: update report from the Standardization Committee of the International Children's Continence Society. J Urol. 2014;191(6):1863–1865.e13.
41. Logan BL, Blais S. Giggle incontinence: evolution of concept and treatment. J Pediatr Urol. 2017;13(5):430–5. https://doi.org/10.1016/j.jpurol.2017.04.021.
42. Sher PK, Reinberg Y. Successful treatment of giggle incontinence with methylphenidate. J Urol. 1996;156(2 Pt 2):656–8.
43. Berry AK, Zderic S, Carr M. Methylphenidate for giggle incontinence. J Urol. 2009;182(4 Suppl):2028–32.
44. Viers BR, Trost LW, Kramer SA. Ectopic ureter in an adolescent female presenting with primary nocturnal enuresis and new onset urinary incontinence. J Urol. 2011;185(2):689.

45. Suson KD, Preece J, Baradaran N, Di Carlo HN, Gearhart JP. The fate of the complete female epispadias and exstrophy bladder--is there a difference? J Urol. 2013;190(4 Suppl):1583–8.
46. Tantibhedhyangkul J, Copland SD, Haqq AM, Price TM. A case of female epispadias. Fertil Steril. 2008;90(5):2017.e1–3.
47. Atilgan D, Uluocak N, Erdemir F, Parlaktas BS. Female epispadias: a case report and review of the literature. Kaohsiung J Med Sci. 2009;25(11):613–6.
48. Son HS, Kim JH. Urological presentations of adult primary tethered cord syndrome. Neurourol Urodyn. 2020;39(2):633–41.
49. Granada C, Loveless M, Justice T, Moriarty T, Mutchnick I, Dietrich JE, LaJoie AS, Hertweck P. Tethered cord syndrome in the pediatric-adolescent gynecologic patient. J Pediatr Adolesc Gynecol. 2015;28(5):309–12.
50. Barnes HV. The adolescent patient. In: Walker HK, Hall WD, Hurst JW, editors. Clinical methods: the history, physical, and laboratory examinations. 3rd ed. Boston: Butterworths; 1990. Chapter 223.
51. Yildirim A, Uluocak N, Atilgan D, Ozcetin M, Erdemir F, Boztepe O. Evaluation of lower urinary tract symptoms in children exposed to sexual abuse. Urol J. 2011;8(1):38–42.
52. De Gennaro M, Niero M, Capitanucci ML, von Gontard A, Woodward M, Tubaro A, Abrams P. Validity of the international consultation on incontinence questionnaire-pediatric lower urinary tract symptoms: a screening questionnaire for children. J Urol. 2010;184(4 Suppl):1662–7.
53. Nelson CP, Park JM, Bloom DA, Wan J, Dunn RL, Wei JT. Incontinence Symptom Index-Pediatric: development and initial validation of a urinary incontinence instrument for the older pediatric population. J Urol. 2007;178(4 Pt 2):1763–7.
54. Nevéus T, Fonseca E, Franco I, Kawauchi A, Kovacevic L, Nieuwhof-Leppink A, Raes A, Tekgül S, Yang SS, Rittig S. Management and treatment of nocturnal enuresis-an updated standardization document from the international Children's continence society. J Pediatr Urol. 2020 Feb;16(1):10–9.
55. Nieuwhof-Leppink AJ, Hussong J, Chase J, Larsson J, Renson C, Hoebeke P, Yang S, von Gontard A. Definitions, indications and practice of urotherapy in children and adolescents: - A standardization document of the International Children's Continence Society (ICCS). J Pediatr Urol. 2020:S1477-5131(20)30630-6.
56. van Gool JD, de Jong TP, Winkler-Seinstra P, Tamminen-Möbius T, Lax H, Hirche H, Nijman RJ, Hjälmås K, Jodal U, Bachmann H, Hoebeke P, Walle JV, Misselwitz J, John U, Bael A, European Bladder Dysfunction Study (EU BMH1-CT94-1006). Multi-center randomized controlled trial of cognitive treatment, placebo, oxybutynin, bladder training, and pelvic floor training in children with functional urinary incontinence. Neurourol Urodyn. 2014;33(5):482–7.
57. Rittig N, Hagstroem S, Mahler B, Kamperis K, Siggaard C, Mikkelsen MM, Bower WF, Djurhuus JC, Rittig S. Outcome of a standardized approach to childhood urinary symptoms-long-term follow-up of 720 patients. Neurourol Urodyn. 2014;33(5):475–81.
58. Richardson I, Palmer LS. Successful treatment for giggle incontinence with biofeedback. J Urol. 2009;182(4 Suppl):2062–6.
59. Ree ML, Nygaard I, Bø K. Muscular fatigue in the pelvic floor muscles after strenuous physical activity. Acta Obstet Gynecol Scand. 2007;86(7):870–6.
60. Da Roza T, Poli de Araujo M, Viana R, Viana S, Jorge RN, Bo K, Mascarenhas T. Pelvic floor muscle training to improve urinary incontinence in young, nulliparous sport students: a pilot study. Int Urogynecol J. 2012;23:1069–73.
61. DeFoor WR Jr, Inge TH, Jenkins TM, Jackson E, Courcoulas A, Michalsky M, Brandt M, Kollar L, Xie C. Prospective evaluation of urinary incontinence in severely obese adolescents presenting for weight loss surgery. Surg Obes Relat Dis. 2018;14(2):214–8.
62. Gleason JM, Daniels C, Williams K, Varghese A, Koyle MA, Bägli DJ, Pippi Salle JL, Lorenzo AJ. Single center experience with oxybutynin transdermal system (patch) for management of symptoms related to non-neuropathic overactive bladder in children: an attractive, well tolerated alternative form of administration. J Pediatr Urol. 2014;10(4):753–7.

63. Hoebeke P, De Pooter J, De Caestecker K, Raes A, Dehoorne J, Van Laecke E, Vande WJ. Solifenacin for therapy resistant overactive bladder. J Urol. 2009;182(4 Suppl):2040–4.
64. Nadeau G, Schröder A, Moore K, Genois L, Lamontagne P, Hamel M, Pellerin E, Bolduc S. Long-term use of solifenacin in pediatric patients with overactive bladder: extension of a prospective open-label study. Can Urol Assoc J. 2014;8(3–4):118–23.
65. Ramsay S, Naud É, Simonyan D, Moore K, Bolduc S. A randomized, crossover trial comparing the efficacy and safety of fesoterodine and extended-release oxybutynin in children with overactive bladder with 12-month extension on fesoterodine: the FOXY study. Can Urol Assoc J. 2020;14(6):192–8.
66. Blais AS, Nadeau G, Moore K, Genois L, Bolduc S. Prospective pilot study of mirabegron in pediatric patients with overactive bladder. Eur Urol. 2016;70(1):9–13.
67. Caldwell PH, Sureshkumar P, Wong WC. Tricyclic and related drugs for nocturnal enuresis in children. Cochrane Database Syst Rev. 2016;1:CD002117.
68. Bolduc S, Moore K, Lebel S, Lamontagne P, Hamel M. Double anticholinergic therapy for refractory overactive bladder. J Urol. 2009;182(4 Suppl):2033–8.
69. Morin F, Blais AS, Nadeau G, Moore K, Genois L, Bolduc S. Dual therapy for refractory overactive bladder in children: a prospective open-label study. J Urol. 2017;197(4):1158–63.
70. Berkenwald A, Pires J, Ellsworth P. Evaluating use of higher dose oxybutynin in combination with desmopressin for refractory nocturnal enuresis. J Pediatr Urol. 2016;12(4):220.e1–6.
71. McGee SM, Routh JC, Granberg CF, Roth TJ, Hollatz P, Vandersteen DR, Reinberg Y. Sacral neuromodulation in children with dysfunctional elimination syndrome: description of incisionless first stage and second stage without fluoroscopy. Urology. 2009;73(3):641–4.
72. Hagstroem S, Mahler B, Madsen B, Djurhuus JC, Rittig S. Transcutaneous electrical nerve stimulation for refractory daytime urinary urge incontinence. J Urol. 2009;182(4 Suppl):2072–8.
73. Hoffmann A, Sampaio C, Nascimento AA, Veiga ML, Barroso U. Predictors of outcome in children and adolescents with overactive bladder treated with parasacral transcutaneous electrical nerve stimulation. J Pediatr Urol. 2018;14(1):54.e1–6.
74. Veiga ML, Costa EV, Portella I, Nacif A, Martinelli Braga AA, Barroso U Jr. Parasacral transcutaneous electrical nerve stimulation for overactive bladder in constipated children: The role of constipation. J Pediatr Urol. 2016;12(6):396.e1–6.
75. Capitanucci ML, Camanni D, Demelas F, Mosiello G, Zaccara A, De Gennaro M. Long-term efficacy of percutaneous tibial nerve stimulation for different types of lower urinary tract dysfunction in children. J Urol. 2009;182(4 Suppl):2056–61.
76. Dos Reis JN, Mello MF, Cabral BH, Mello LF, Saiovici S, Rocha FET. EMG biofeedback or parasacral transcutaneous electrical nerve stimulation in children with lower urinary tract dysfunction: a prospective and randomized trial. Neurourol Urodyn. 2019;38(6):1588–94.
77. Quintiliano F, Veiga ML, Moraes M, Cunha C, de Oliveira LF, Lordelo P, Bastos Netto JM, Barroso JU. Transcutaneous parasacral electrical stimulation vs oxybutynin for the treatment of overactive bladder in children: a randomized clinical trial. J Urol. 2015;193(5 Suppl):1749–53.
78. Groen LA, Hoebeke P, Loret N, Van Praet C, Van Laecke E, Ann R, Vande Walle J, Everaert K. Sacral neuromodulation with an implantable pulse generator in children with lower urinary tract symptoms: 15-year experience. J Urol. 2012;188(4):1313–7.
79. Boswell TC, Hollatz P, Hutcheson JC, Vandersteen DR, Reinberg YE. Device outcomes in pediatric sacral neuromodulation: a single center series of 187 patients. J Pediatr Urol. 2020:S1477-5131(20)30568-4.
80. Roth TJ, Vandersteen DR, Hollatz P, Inman BA, Reinberg YE. Sacral neuromodulation for the dysfunctional elimination syndrome: a single center experience with 20 children. J Urol. 2008;180(1):306–11.
81. Stephany HA, Juliano TM, Clayton DB, Tanaka ST, Thomas JC, Adams MC, Brock JW 3rd, Pope JC 4th. Prospective evaluation of sacral nerve modulation in children with validated questionnaires. J Urol. 2013;190(4 Suppl):1516–22.

82. Mason MD, Stephany HA, Casella DP, Clayton DB, Tanaka ST, Thomas JC, Adams MC, Brock JW 3rd, Pope JC 4th. Prospective evaluation of sacral neuromodulation in children: outcomes and urodynamic predictors of success. J Urol. 2016;195(4 Pt 2):1239–44.
83. Dwyer ME, Vandersteen DR, Hollatz P, Reinberg YE. Sacral neuromodulation for the dysfunctional elimination syndrome: a 10-year single-center experience with 105 consecutive children. Urology. 2014;84(4):911–7.
84. Rensing AJ, Szymanski KM, Dunn S, King S, Cain MP, Whittam BM. Pediatric sacral nerve stimulator explanation due to complications or cure: a survival analysis. J Pediatr Urol. 2019;15(1):39.e1–6.
85. Fuchs ME, Lu PL, Vyrostek SJ, Teich S, Alpert SA. Factors predicting complications after sacral neuromodulation in children. Urology. 2017;107:214–7.
86. McDowell DT, Noone D, Tareen F, Waldron M, Quinn F. Urinary incontinence in children: botulinum toxin is a safe and effective treatment option. Pediatr Surg Int. 2012;28(3):315–20.
87. Blackburn SC, Jones C, Bedoya S, Steinbrecher HA, Malone PS, Griffin SJ. Intravesical botulinum type-A toxin (Dysport®) in the treatment of idiopathic detrusor overactivity in children. J Pediatr Urol. 2013;9(6 Pt A):750–3.
88. Uçar M, Akgül AK, Parlak A, Yücel C, Kılıç N, Balkan E. Non-invasive evaluation of botulinum-A toxin treatment efficacy in children with refractory overactive bladder. Int Urol Nephrol. 2018;50(8):1367–73.
89. Al Edwan GM, Mansi HH, Atta ONM, Shaath MM, Al Adwan R, Mahafza W, Afram KM, Ababneh O, Al Adwan D, Muheilan MM. Objective and subjective improvement in children with idiopathic detrusor overactivity after intravesical botulinum toxin injection: a preliminary report. J Pediatr Surg. 2019;54(3):595–9.
90. Léon P, Jolly C, Binet A, Fiquet C, Vilette C, Lefebvre F, Bouché-Pillon-Persyn MA, Poli-Mérol ML. Botulinum toxin injections in the management of non-neurogenic overactive bladders in children. J Pediatr Surg. 2014;49(9):1424–8.
91. El-Dakhakhny AS, El-Karamany TM, El-Atrebi M, Gharib T. Efficacy and safety of intradetrusor onabotulinumtoxinA injection for managing paediatric non-neurogenic overactive bladder: a prospective case-series study. Arab J Urol. 2019;17(2):143–9.
92. Dobrowolska-Glazar BA, Groen LA, Nieuwhof-Leppink AJ, Klijn AJ, de Jong TPVM, Chrzan R. Open and laparoscopic colposuspension in girls with refractory urinary incontinence. Front Pediatr. 2017;5:284.

Chapter 24
Female Neurogenic Incontinence

Jenny N. Nguyen and Doreen E. Chung

Introduction

It is well known that urinary incontinence can have a serious negative impact on quality of life. However, in women with neurogenic lower urinary tract dysfunction (NLUTD), who often have limited mobility, urinary incontinence can have an even greater negative impact on their quality of life [1–4]. Women with NLUTD can suffer from the same types of incontinence as women without NLUTD. However, some additional disease processes may be superimposed. Depending on the neurologic insult, the resultant bladder manifestations can vary. Neurogenic incontinence in women can sometimes be protective against upper tract dysfunction and can serve as a warning that the lower urinary tract poses danger for the upper tracts. Furthermore, in these women, urinary incontinence can also be a risk factor for skin breakdown, decubitus ulcers, and wound complications. This chapter describes the causes, different presentations including urodynamic studies, workup, and treatment of neurogenic incontinence in women.

Etiology of Neurogenic Urinary Incontinence

The etiology of neurogenic urinary incontinence in females can be broken down based on the location of the neurologic lesion. The normal micturition reflex involves multiple locations throughout the central nervous system. These include the pontine micturition center (brainstem), the parasympathetic and somatic

J. N. Nguyen (✉) · D. E. Chung
Department of Urology, Columbia University Irving Medical Center, New York, NY, USA
e-mail: dec2154@cumc.columbia.edu

© The Author(s), under exclusive license to Springer Nature
Switzerland AG 2022
A. P. Cameron (ed.), *Female Urinary Incontinence*,
https://doi.org/10.1007/978-3-030-84352-6_24

components of the sacral micturition center as well as the thoracolumbar sympathetics [5, 6].

Lesions above the brainstem affect the brain's inhibitory effect on micturition reflex. This leads to detrusor overactivity (DO) and subsequent urinary urgency, frequency, and nocturia [7]. Additionally, some patients may have urinary incontinence from voiding involuntarily, as they are able to sense their involuntary detrusor contraction and voluntarily contract their striated sphincter muscle, but are unable to actually stop their detrusor contraction [8].

Lesions below the level of the pons and above the sacral spinal cord have interrupted the pathway that previously allowed for simultaneous detrusor muscle contraction and urethral sphincter relaxation. This interruption thereby results in detrusor sphincter dyssynergia and an uncoordinated relationship between detrusor muscle contraction and relaxation with urethral sphincter contraction [9, 10]. In other words, neurogenic detrusor overactivity and uninhibited bladder contractions occur alongside a discordant contraction of the external sphincter. The involuntary detrusor contractions lead to urinary incontinence, while the discordant sphincter contractions cause bladder outlet obstruction and urinary retention and potentially high storage pressures [11].

Sacral neurologic insults can vary in presentation depending on injury to the parasympathetic, sympathetic, or somatic portions of the neurologic tract. For injuries causing complete parasympathetic disruption, this results in detrusor areflexia and urinary retention. With urinary retention, there may also be resultant overflow incontinence. Injuries causing sympathetic nerve injury can manifest as sphincteric urinary incontinence due to a nonfunctioning proximal urethra. Finally, somatic neurologic injuries affecting the pudendal nerves result in loss of perineal and perianal sensation as well as loss of the bulbocavernosus reflex which then alters voluntary contraction of the urethral and anal sphincters. The latter may manifest as urinary and fecal incontinence and contribute to intrinsic sphincter deficiency (ISD).

Common causes of somatic neurologic insults include herniated disks, diabetes, multiple sclerosis, and sacral tumors. Additionally, extensive pelvic surgery such as abdominoperineal resection of the rectum and radical hysterectomy are both common surgical causes of sacral as well as somatic nerve injury [8]. For example, one such study examining patients requiring urologic intervention for urinary retention after radical hysterectomy after stage IB1-IIB cervical cancer showed nearly 54% of patients developing postvoid residuals of >100 cc [12].

It is important not to forget that the chronic indwelling urethral catheters encountered in neurogenic female patients can overtime cause erosion and patulous urethras with no functional sphincteric mechanism, leading to overt urinary incontinence (Fig. 24.1) [13]. Additionally, in patients with a history of pelvic radiation, pelvic surgery, or recent traumatic vaginal birth history, it is also important to keep in mind that urinary fistulae can develop and be a cause for urinary incontinence even in the setting of the neurogenic female patient.

Fig. 24.1 Urethral erosion occurring gradually over time after progressive upsizing of Foley catheter from 14 F to 24 F and upsizing of retention balloon from 10 cc to 30 cc in a woman with T6 spinal cord injury (SCI). Erosion is so profound; the trigone is visible on pelvic examination. Patient failed vaginal approach at urethral closure with Martius flap and ultimately required a urinary diversion. (Image courtesy Anne Cameron MD)

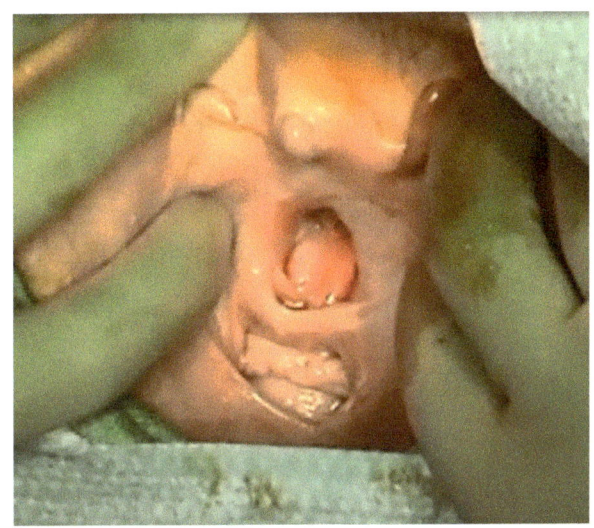

Different Clinical Presentations

When urinary incontinence occurs in patients with an NLUTD, it can be attributed to one of three dysfunctions, alone or in combination. These are detrusor overactivity, poor bladder compliance, and urethral sphincter/bladder neck incompetence [11].

A. Urinary Incontinence due to Detrusor Overactivity with Complete Bladder Emptying (Balanced Voiding)

    Patients with neurologic conditions above the sacral spinal cord will have detrusor overactivity and resultant urgency incontinence. This can often be compounded by limited mobility. Although these patients are able to completely empty, occasionally these patients only void by involuntary detrusor contractions and cannot void by volition, and in this case, they may need to be treated with clean intermittent catheterization (CIC) to give the patient continence. This is in addition to therapies to treat bladder storage.

B. Urinary Incontinence due to Detrusor Overactivity (DO) and/or Poor Compliance with Incomplete Bladder Emptying

    Patients with lesions below the pontine micturition center usually have detrusor overactivity with DESD. These patients will often have poor emptying (due to bladder outlet obstruction from DESD) in addition to incontinence from detrusor overactivity. Their functional capacity is much lower as well due to reflex DO that can occur at low volume or high bladder storage pressures from poor compliance.

C. Overflow Incontinence due to Atonic Bladder with Sphincteric Incompetence or Infrequent Bladder Emptying with CIC

Patients with sacral or peripheral nerve injury typically have an atonic bladder resulting in urinary retention, which is a low storage pressure; however, these women may still leak if they have an incompetent sphincter or reach terminal capacity. Having them catheterize more frequently is often a good solution.

D. Stress Urinary Incontinence

Some patients have neurologic injury to one or more urinary sphincters. These patients will have stress incontinence of varying degrees with sometimes total incontinence or stress urinary incontinence with changing position or increased intra-abdominal pressure. Some patients will also have stress incontinence due to urethral hypermobility from prior pregnancy and delivery. These women may have a milder stress urinary incontinence that only occurs with any increase in intra-abdominal pressure, similar to the stress urinary incontinence that occurs in nonneurogenic women.

Urodynamic Investigation

Urodynamics are a key in the evaluation of NLUTD patients due to the potentially silent risk of renal injury and ultimately renal failure. This type of renal failure is usually due to high intravesical pressure, poor bladder compliance, vesicoureteral reflux, infection, and/or hydronephrosis [11, 14]. In addition to assessing for potential upper tract damage, urodynamics can also be used to evaluate the etiology of symptoms and direct treatment. (See Chap. 4 for in-depth description of urodynamics.)

Storage Issues

Low bladder pressures during filling are a key to preventing upper tract injury. Detrusor leak-point pressures and storage pressures greater than 40 cm H_2O have been found to put the upper tracts at risk [15]. Additionally, during filling, uninhibited detrusor contractions can also be seen and can contribute to urinary incontinence.

In patients with sacral or peripheral nerve injuries, a fixed open urinary sphincter may be seen which can result in urinary incontinence. Sphincteric damage may also ensue due to chronic indwelling catheterization, also leading to an incompetent outlet and stress incontinence. A Valsalva leak-point pressure less than 60 cm H_2O in the absence of a detrusor contraction can also be found in neurogenic patients and can identify intrinsic sphincter deficiency [16].

Finally, bladder compliance can be calculated as the change in volume over change in detrusor pressure with abnormal bladder compliance generally perceived as less than 20 ml/cm H_2O [16]. Bladder compliance is an important urodynamic parameter as abnormal compliance is a risk factor for urologic complications.

Emptying Issues

Urodynamic evaluation showing poor detrusor contractility, detrusor atony, or sphincteric dyssynergia can also provide information on the neurogenic patient and help direct management. With these findings, incomplete emptying and urinary retention are typically found. Additionally, for women, it is important to evaluate for pelvic organ prolapse as a contributor for incomplete emptying due to urethral kinking, even as a neurogenic patient [16].

Timing of Urodynamics

It is imperative to obtain a baseline urodynamic study in all newly diagnosed NLUTD patients after the period of spinal shock is resolved, at approximately 90 days or when spinal reflexes can be elicited on examination [17]. Typically, periodic urodynamics are performed along with upper tract imaging; however, this is tailored to the patient's symptoms and/or changes in the upper tract or renal function [14, 18].

Safety Workup

Prior to regular urologic care for NLUTD patients, renal failure was the most common cause of mortality [19]. The safety workup for neurogenic urinary incontinence in females relies solely on the principles of NLUTD management. While there is no consensus on the exact time frame of follow-up and surveillance, published data recommend routine urologic care of NLUTD patients at least every 2 years and at most every 3–6 months [14, 18, 20]. Follow-up should include a history, physical examination, and serum creatinine. However, in NLUTD patients with little muscle mass, serum creatinine can be inaccurate, and substantial renal function loss can occur prior to any noticeable rise in serum creatinine. In such cases where renal dysfunction is suspected, a functional renal scan can be obtained as it is the most sensitive test for decreased renal function or obstruction. Cystatin C, while costly, can also serve as an alternate and more accurate representation of renal function and GFR as it is not affected by mass, age, or gender [21].

In terms of regular upper urinary tract imaging, most urologists consider a renal ultrasound as sufficient imaging to rule out hydronephrosis as well as to evaluate renal stone disease. Other tests useful in detecting stone disease include an intravenous pyelogram or a noncontrast CT scan, but these expose the patient to ionizing radiation [14, 20].

As mentioned previously, urodynamic evaluation should be performed at the time of initial evaluation (after any such spinal shock period has resolved) and at subsequent intervals at the discretion of the clinician. Important urodynamic parameters for neurogenic patients include assessing bladder compliance and detrusor leak-point pressure. Low bladder filling pressures are imperative to upper tract protection, and bladder storage pressures greater than 40 cm H_2O put the patient at risk for upper tract impairment. Additionally, a detrusor leak-point pressure higher than40 mm Hg has also been shown to be a risk factor for upper tract deterioration [15].

Routine urine cytology is generally not recommended due to lack of quality data showing utility. While asymptomatic bacteriuria is common in NLUTD patients, it should not be treated except in the context of a urologic procedure [22].

While historical data showed a higher incidence of bladder cancer in chronic indwelling catheter spinal cord injury (SCI) patients [22], more updated studies have shown a significant decrease in the risk of bladder cancer in spinal cord injury patients, especially with the advent of intermittent catheterization. Due to a higher risk of bladder stones and increased duration of catheterization being risk factors for bladder cancer, some urologists do incorporate screening cystoscopy as part of routine urologic surveillance. However, there is insufficient evidence to support screening cystoscopy for bladder cancer in asymptomatic spinal cord injury patients. These same principles can be applied to all NLUTD patients [14, 20].

Should there be any change in urinary incontinence, recurrent urinary tract infection (UTI), gross hematuria, or new signs or symptoms, follow-up and further urinary tract imaging, cystoscopy, or urodynamic evaluation should be performed sooner [14].

Treatment of the Bladder

Patients with detrusor overactivity (with or without urinary incontinence) and/or poor bladder compliance can first be trialed on antimuscarinic medications [23]. Common antimuscarinic drugs such as oxybutynin, solifenacin, and tolterodine work by blocking the muscarinic M3 receptors located in the bladder smooth muscle. However, given data on cognitive impairment related to these anticholinergic medications, newer anticholinergic medications targeting the β3 adrenergic receptors of the bladder are more favored, but have not been FDA approved or formally trialed in NLUTD patients [24]. These include mirabegron and the newest FDA-approved drug vibegron [25, 26]. Especially in NLUTD patients who may also have concurrent cognitive impairment issues, such as multiple sclerosis or Parkinson's disease, the newer β3 adrenergic receptor–targeting medications are increasingly being used as first-line oral agents over anticholinergics on this population. For example, a combination of mirabegron and desmopressin in one study of multiple sclerosis patients has been shown to improve detrusor overactivity than in solifenacin alone [27].

NLUTD patients refractory to oral medication can be trialed on intradetrusor botulinum toxin injections. The most commonly used serotype produced by

Clostridium botulinum bacteria is onabotulinum toxin A. Onabotulinum toxin A works by inhibiting the release of presynaptic acetylcholine from nerve terminals and thereby decreasing muscarinic receptor activation [28]. This leads to improved bladder capacity and decreased detrusor overactivity and clinically improves incontinence episodes. The commercially available form of onabotulinum toxin A in the United States is Botox™, and studies have used both 200 unit injections and 300 unit injections for NLUTD patients [28]. Patients who do voluntarily void must be counseled on the risk of urinary retention. For patients who catheterize, 200U is the best starting dose since retention is not a concerns, whereas for voiding patients 100U is more appropriate and less likely to result in retention. An increase in the frequency of injections up to every 3 months can be undertaken in the case of weaning efficacy followed by either augmentation cystoplasty or dose increase (Fig. 24.2).

Specifically to multiple sclerosis patients and other NLUTD patients where voiding is preserved, sacral nerve neuromodulation has also been studied for both urinary retention and detrusor overactivity [23, 29]. Newer generation of sacral nerve stimulators are now MRI-compatible since MRI is critical in neurologic follow-up for many of these conditions.

Augmentation cystoplasty for low bladder capacity/compliance in NLUTD patients entails using a small portion of detubularized small intestine or colon sewn to a widely opened bladder to increase overall urinary storage. This in turn mitigates any high detrusor filling pressures and can help prevent leakage as well as increases

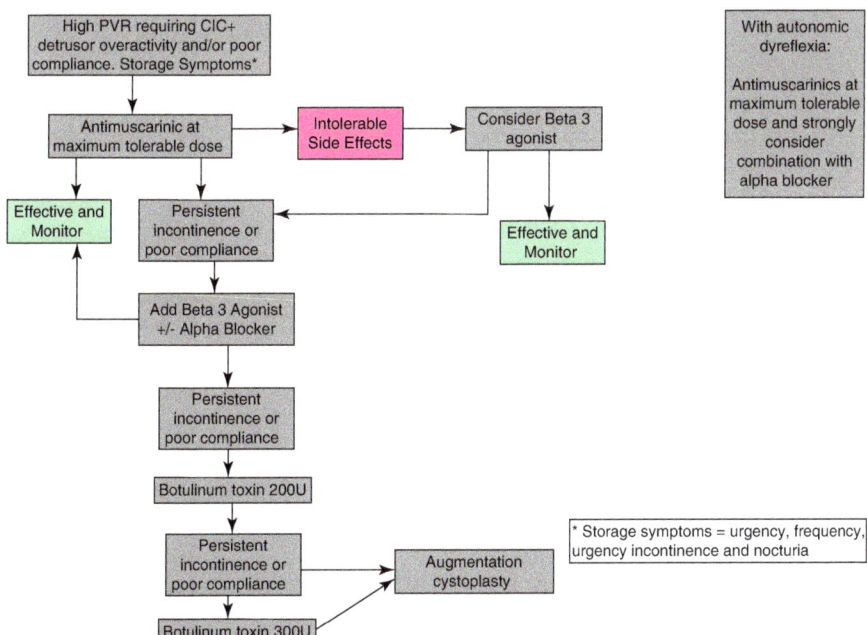

Fig. 24.2 Flowchart for the treatment of poor bladder compliance or neurogenic detrusor overactivity in NLUTD patients

overall bladder capacity. In the appropriately worked-up NLUTD patient, this can be another option to help manage incontinence and the overall bladder and may be an early option in younger patients where countless botulinum toxin injections are anticipated, and they may desire a more definitive option or have difficulty with catheterizing and need construction of a catheterizable channel [23]. Complete description of this procedure is discussed in Chap. 12.

Treatment of the Outlet

In female NLUTD patients with urinary incontinence, treatment of the outlet is often required and a range of options exist. Options include pubovaginal sling, bladder neck reconstruction, urethral bulking agents, artificial urinary sphincter (AUS), and urinary diversion.

For female NLUTD patients with patulous urethras or intrinsic sphincter deficiency, an autologous fascial pubovaginal sling is one of the best surgical options with high efficacy and low morbidity. Patients can easily perform clean intermittent catheterization (CIC) through a pubovaginal sling without concerns about mesh erosion that exists with midurethral slings. Neurogenic women with ISD appear to have comparable outcomes to nonneurogenic women [30]. One study of 33 female patients with myelomeningocele or spinal cord injury and ISD showed a 91% satisfaction rate after the placement of pubovaginal sling with 25 patients completely dry and five patients markedly improved [31]. While synthetic mesh options do exist, autologous fascial pubovaginal slings may be the more suitable option in NLUTD patients who require daily lifelong intermittent catheterization.

Bladder neck reconstruction is another option for female NLUTD patients with ISD. Several techniques exist with the main objective of increasing bladder outlet resistance [30]. In female NLUTD patients with devastating patulous urethras from chronic indwelling urethral catheters, bladder neck closure may be necessary due to inadequate residual urethral tissue to reconstruct or permit a pubovaginal sling. A continent catheterizable stoma, typically using appendix or ileum, is concurrently created to allow for bladder drainage if the patient desires continence and has good manual dexterity. Otherwise, a suprapubic tube is placed concurrently [32, 33]. The approach to bladder neck closure can be transvaginal versus retropubic. One study of 64 women who underwent bladder neck closure and suprapubic catheter placement showed no significant difference in achieving urethral continence between either approach; however, the transvaginal group had a significantly shorter mean operative time, hospital stay, and fewer short-term complications [34]. See Chap. 13 for details of this procedure.

Injecting urethral bulking agents can be performed in an outpatient clinic setting without general anesthesia and involve minimal morbidity. However, they are not efficacious in patients with severe stress urinary incontinence. The bulking agent is injected periurethrally or intraurethrally through a cystoscope. Due to its minimal invasiveness, intraurethral bulking agents are a good option for patients who are poor surgical candidates. The following are the four FDA-approved agents currently on the market: silicon microparticles (Macroplastique®), pyrolytic carbon-coated zirconium oxide bead (Durasphere®), calcium hydroxyapatite (Coaptite®), and polyacrylamide hydrogel (Bulkamid®) [16]. The majority of the bulking agent literature as it pertains to intrinsic sphincter deficiency population is within the pediatric NLUTD population. However, in one adult study, it has been used as an adjuvant procedure for persistent low pressure incontinence after pubovaginal sling. Long-term follow-up of 8 years showed that only two of 27 patients were continent, despite repeat injections. Despite there being low success, bulking agents can serve as a useful option due to low complication rate after other failed outlet procedures [30].

While placing an artificial urinary sphincter (AUS) in females is not FDA-approved in the United States, European countries such as France recommend AUS placement in females with intrinsic sphincter deficiency. In the female NLUTD patient population, AUS placement would only be viable in select candidates with good manual dexterity and who would not normally require catheterization. One such study has suggested satisfactory outcomes in female neurogenic stress urinary incontinence with low rates of infection and erosion [35].

Salvage Treatment with Urinary Diversion

In select patients with small poorly compliant bladders and/or persistent urinary incontinence refractory to conservative measures or serious complications such as urethral erosion or unreconstructable fistulae, salvage treatment with urinary diversion may be required. For patients with limited upper extremity function, cognitive impairment, or poor renal function, an ileal conduit is the best option. For patients with good renal function and good manual dexterity, a continent diversion, such as an Indiana pouch, is an excellent option. The Indiana pouch is a particularly good option for patients with a devastated bladder outlet.

At the time of surgery, a simple cystectomy or Spence–Allen procedure (iatrogenic vesicovaginal fistula) can be performed to prevent pyocystis.

Conclusion

While most of the management of NLUTD is irrespective of gender, the management of neurogenic incontinence in females can differ from that in males. Treatment options such as pubovaginal slings are often more appropriate for female NLUTD patients given anatomy. Additionally, it is vital to assess for other nonneurogenic causes for voiding dysfunction in these females such as pelvic organ prolapse or urinary fistula. Understanding the unique workup and management for NLUTD patients, especially that for female NLUTD patients, is essential for providing excellent urologic care in this population.

References

1. Clanet B. Management of multiple sclerosis patients. Curr Opin Neurol. 2000;13:263–70.
2. Hicken BL, Putzke JD, et al. Bladder management and quality of life after spinal cord injury. Am J Phys Med Rehabil. 2001;80:916–22.
3. Westgren N, Levi R. Quality of life and traumatic spinal cord injury. Arch Phys Med Rehabil. 1998;79:1433–9.
4. Tang DH, Colayco D, Piercy J, et al. Impact of urinary incontinence on health-related quality of life, daily activities, and healthcare resource utilization in patients with neurogenic detrusor overactivity. BMC Neurol. 2014;14:74. https://doi.org/10.1186/1471-2377-14-74.
5. Blaivas JG. The neurophyisiology of micturition: a clinical study of 550 patients. J Urol. 1982;127:958.
6. Unger CA, Tunitsky-Bitton E, Muffly T, et al. Neuroanatomy, neurophysiology and dysfunction of the female lower urinary tract: a review. Female Pelvic Med Reconstr Surg. 2014;20(2):65–75. https://doi.org/10.1097/spv.0000000000000058.
7. Abrams P, Cardozo L, Fall M, et al. The standardization of terminology of lower urinary tract function: report from the standardization subcommittee of the international continence society. Neurol Urodyn. 2002;21:167–78.
8. Blaivas JG, Chancellor M, Weiss J, Verhaaren M. Atlas of Urodynamics. 2nd ed. Blackwell Publishing; 2007.
9. Wein A. Lower urinary tract dysfunction in neurologic injury and disease. In: Wein A, Kavoussi L, Novick A, et al., editors. Campbell-Walsh urology. New York: Saunders; 2007. p. 2011–45.
10. Chancellor M, Blaivas J. Spinal cord injury. In: Chancellor M, Blaivas J, editors. Practical neurourology. Boston: Butterworth-Heinemann; 1995. p. 99–118.
11. Nitti VW. Evaluation of the female with neurogenic voiding dysfunction. Int Urogynecol J. 1999;10:119–29. https://doi.org/10.1007/s001920050031.
12. Komatsu H, et al. Long-term evaluation of renal function and neurogenic bladder following radical hysterectomy in patients with uterine cervical cancer. J Obstet Gynaecol Res. 2020;46(10):2108–14. https://doi.org/10.1111/jog/14394.
13. Chancellor MB, Erhard MJ, Kiiholma PJ, et al. Functional urethral closure with pubovaginal sling for destroyed female urethra after long-term urethral catheterization. Urology. 1994;43:499–505. https://doi.org/10.1016/0090-4295(94)90241-0.
14. Kreydin E, Welk B, Chung D, et al. Surveillance and management of urologic complications after spinal cord injury. World J Urol. 2018;36:1545–53.
15. McGuire EJ, Woodside JR, Borden TA. Prognostic value of urodynamic testing in myelodysplasia patients. J Urol. 1981;126:205–9.
16. Cameron AP, Gupta P. Surgery for female stress urinary incontinence. AUA Core Curriculum; 2021.
17. Danfort TL, Ginsberg DA. Neurogenic lower urinary tract dysfunction: how, when and with which patients do we use urodynamics? Urol Clin North Am. 2014;41(3):445–52.
18. Consortium for Spinal Cord Medicine. Bladder management for adults with spinal cord injury: a clinical practice guideline. Washington, DC: Paralyzed Veterans of America; 2016. Urologic evaluation. p. 16–7.
19. Greenwell MW, et al. Kidney disease as a predictor of mortality in chronic spinal cord injury. Am J Kidney Dis. 2007;49(3):383–93.
20. Cameron AP, Rodriguez GM, Schomer KG. Systematic review of urological followup after spinal cord injury. J Urol. 2012;187(2):391–7.
21. Dharnidharka VR, Kwon C, Stevens G. Serum cystatin C is superior to serum creatinine as a marker of kidney function: a meta-analysis. Am J Kidney Dis. 2002;40(2):221–6.
22. Broecker BH, Klein FA, Hackler RA. Cancer of the bladder in spinal cord injury patients. J Urol. 1981;125(2):196–7.
23. Barboglio Romo PG, Cameron AP. Neurogenic lower urinary tract dysfunction. AUA Core Curriculum; 2021.

24. Welk B, McArther E. Increased risk of dementia among patients with overactive bladder treated with an anticholinergic medication compared to a beta-3 agonist: a population-based cohort study. BJU Int. 2020;126(10):183–90. https://doi.org/10.1111/bju.15040.
25. Nitti VW, et al. Results of a randomized phase III trial of mirabegraon in patients with overactive bladder. J Urol. 2013;189:1388–95.
26. Staskin D, Frankel J, Varano S, et al. International phase III, randomized, double-blind, placebo and active controlled study to evaluate the safety and efficacy of Vibegron in patients with symptoms of overactive bladder: EMPOWUR. J Urol. 2020;204(2):316–24.
27. Zachariou A, Filiponi M, Baltogiannis D, et al. Effective treatment of neurogenic detrusor overactivity in multiple sclerosis patients using desmopressin and mirabegron. Can J Urol. 2017;24:9107–13.
28. Ginsberg D, Gousse A, Keppenne V, Sievert KD, et al. Phase 3 efficacy and tolerability study of onobotulinumtoxin a for urinary incontinence from neurogenic detrusor overactivity. J Urol. 2021;187(6):2131–9.
29. Engeler DS, Meyer D, Abt D, Muller S, et al. Sacral neuromodulation for the treatment of neurogenic lower urinary tract dysfunction caused by multiple sclerosis: a single-centre prospective series. BMC Urol. 2015;15:105. https://doi.org/10.1186/s12894-015-0102-x.
30. Myers JB, Mayer EN, Lenherr S, et al. Management options for sphincteric deficiency in adults with neurogenic bladder. Transl Androl Urol. 2016;5(1):145–57. https://doi.org/10.3978/j.issn.2223-4683.2015.12.11.
31. Athanasopoulos A, Gyftopoulos K, McGuire EJ. Treating stress urinary incontinence in female patients with neuropathic bladder: the value of autologous fascia rectus sling. Int Urol Nephrol. 2012;44:1363–7.
32. Chancellor MB, et al. Functional urethral closure with pubovaginal sling for destroyed female urethra after long-term urethral catheterization. Urology. 1994;43(4):499–505.
33. Zimmern PE, et al. Transvaginal closure of the bladder neck and placement of a suprapubic catheter for destroyed urethra after long-term indwelling catheterization. J Urol. 1985;134(3):554–7.
34. Willis H, Safiano N, Lloyd LK. Comparison of transvaginal and retropubic bladder neck closure with suprapubic catheter in women. J Urol. 2015;193(1):196–02. https://doi.org/10.1016/j.juro.2014.07.091.
35. Peyronnet B, Greenwell T, Gray G, et al. Current use of the artificial urinary sphincter in adult females. Curr Urol Rep. 2020;21:53. https://doi.org/10.1007/s11934-020-01001-1.

Chapter 25
Urinary Incontinence in the Elderly

Casey G. Kowalik and Lara S. MacLachlan

Introduction

The prevalence of urinary incontinence increases with age and affects up to 30% of women over the age of 60 [1]. As the population ages, the number of women with urinary incontinence will increase. In addition to the standard evaluation reviewed in Chap. 3, it is critical to understand the particular factors that need to be addressed in an elderly population. The morbidity associated with urinary incontinence in the elderly can be significant and has been independently associated with nursing home admission [2]. It is essential to not only understand the patient's condition, but also incorporate any comorbidities, degree of bother, goals of care, and the involvement of any caregivers into the decision algorithm. Additionally, age itself may not be as important, versus the degree of frailty, which has been associated with adverse outcomes. While frailty does increase with age, the concept of frailty as it relates to the care of patients is becoming increasingly important. For example, a robust 75-year-old woman will have different considerations than a frail 65-year-old. It is also important to emphasize that urinary incontinence is a chronic condition and the goal of treatment is to provide improvement in symptoms and quality of life, not necessarily the cure of the incontinence.

C. G. Kowalik (✉)
Department of Urology, University of Kansas Health System, Kansas City, KS, USA
e-mail: ckowalik@kumc.edu

L. S. MacLachlan
Institute of Urology, Lahey Hospital & Medical Center, Burlington, MA, USA
e-mail: lara.maclachlan@lahey.org

A. P. Cameron (ed.), *Female Urinary Incontinence*,
https://doi.org/10.1007/978-3-030-84352-6_25

Table 25.1 Effects of aging on the lower urinary tract

Bladder contractility decreases [3, 6]
Bladder capacity decreases [5]
Decreased maximum urethral closure pressure [3, 4]
Slower flow rate [5]
Increased postvoid residual [5]

Conditions Contributing to Urinary Incontinence in Elderly Women

The development of urinary incontinence in women is largely multifactorial, but many of these factors are more common in the elderly. First, aging itself is a risk factor for lower urinary tract dysfunction (Table 25.1). There are numerous anatomic, physiologic, metabolic, and hormonal changes that occur with aging, along with the effects of other coexistent disease processes. In studies of healthy women, without a history of neurologic disease, pelvic surgery, or diabetes, there was a decline in detrusor contractility, bladder sensation with filling, and maximum urethral closure pressure (MUCP) with each decade of aging [3, 4]. Another study of age-related urodynamic changes found an association of age with slower flow rates, reduced bladder capacity, and increased postvoid residual [5]. Investigation of muscarinic receptors in the detrusor of patients with normal bladder function found an age-related decrease in mRNA expression for M3 receptors, which could explain the decreased detrusor contractility with aging [6]. Reduced bladder contractility can result in elevated residual urine, leading to overflow incontinence. Also, incomplete emptying coupled with lower MUCP may increase stress urinary incontinence (SUI) symptoms.

Beyond lower urinary tract pathology, there may be other influences increasing the likelihood of urinary incontinence in the elderly [7]. Some comorbid conditions can exacerbate urinary incontinence. For example, any condition with chronic coughing, such as emphysema, can increase stress urinary incontinence symptoms. Medical conditions that result in polyuria such as diabetes mellitus, diabetes insipidus, diuretic use, or primary polydipsia will contribute to polyuria and can exacerbate urinary incontinence. Conditions such as congestive heart failure, venous insufficiency, and nephrotic syndrome can cause peripheral edema. When recumbent during sleep, this fluid mobilizes and may result in increased nocturnal urine production. Disorders that result in cognitive impairment, such as Alzheimer's disease or delirium, can lead to increased urinary incontinence due to a lack of awareness or motivation for toileting. Additionally, in patients with cognitive impairment, the use of validated questionnaires is unlikely to be useful. Severe constipation is more common in elderly women and can lead to urinary dysfunction. Urogenital atrophy is most likely to result in symptoms of vaginal dryness and burning, but urinary symptoms can also be present, comprising the genitourinary syndrome of menopause, and vaginal estrogen treatment can help [8].

Polypharmacy is another major issue affecting the elderly as many medications can modify lower urinary tract function and, thus, may have some effects on continence. For example, α-blockers have been linked to a reversible cause of stress urinary incontinence [9]. Other medications, such as diuretics, may increase urine production. It is not only the medication itself that can influence urinary symptoms, but the side effects from the medication may influence them. Angiotensin-converting enzyme inhibitors may cause a cough and increase urinary incontinence. Many medications cause dry mouth, which may result in increased fluid intake or can worsen constipation, both side effects contributing to the propensity for urinary incontinence. Compounding the effects of polypharmacy can be the addition of medical treatment for urinary incontinence, leading to a complex situation where the treatment of the incontinence causes secondary effects (i.e., constipation) that actually worsen the incontinence.

It is important to assess mobility and manual dexterity in elderly women as both can affect the likelihood of functional incontinence or urinary leakage that occurs due to reasons unrelated to the bladder. It is understandable that women with urinary urgency and urgency incontinence will more likely have an incontinence episode if it takes a prolonged amount of time to reach the toilet. In some cases, assistance may be required to transfer to the toilet, thus making the patient dependent on others to avoid incontinence episodes. Evaluation of mobility can be done formally with assessments such as Timed Up and Go (TUG) test that involves measuring in seconds the time to stand up from a chair, walk 3 m, and return to sit in the chair and is a validated measure of frailty [10]. An informal measure may be observation of the patient's ability to move from their chair to the exam table. Mobility-related issues may be improved by ensuring a direct route to the toilet or acquiring a portal commode. Poor manual dexterity may result in longer time needed to undress and could be ameliorated by clothing without buttons.

Figure 25.1 is a schematic that highlights the interwoven complexity of these issues.

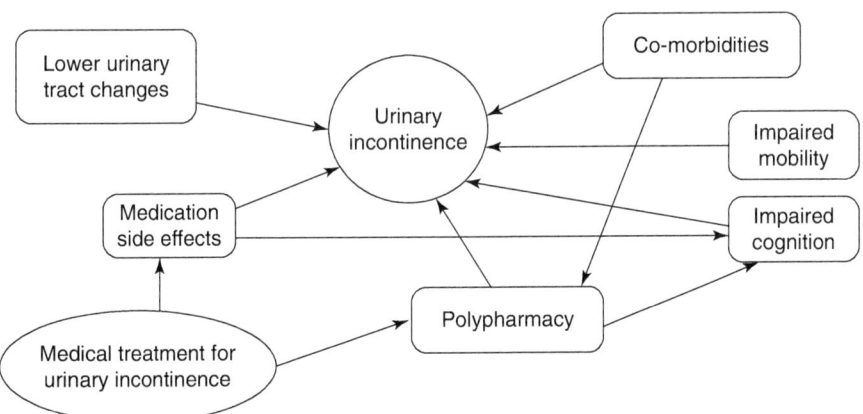

Fig. 25.1 Schematic highlighting the complex interactions of effects associated with aging and urinary incontinence

General Treatment Considerations in Elderly Women

In elderly women, the same treatment options are available for both SUI and urge urinary incontinence (UUI) as in younger women, but there are additional considerations to account for, which are highlighted in Table 25.2.

Elderly women with urinary incontinence have an increased risk of concomitant pelvic floor disorders, such as pelvic organ prolapse or fecal incontinence [11]. It is generally agreed that the pathophysiology of these conditions shares a common origin, with intrinsic predisposing factors such as genetics, age, race, menopause, and extrinsic risk factors affecting the pelvic floor, such as obstetric history, pelvic floor surgery, comorbidities, and obesity [12, 13]. It is essential to evaluate for these because their presence may alter your treatment recommendations. For example, a woman with urinary and fecal incontinence may have more potential benefits from sacral neuromodulation (SNS) that could potentially treat both. The relationship between pelvic organ prolapse and bladder dysfunction is complex, and there is likely an association between the degree of prolapse and urinary incontinence [14]. In these patients, correcting prolapse, either nonoperatively or surgically, may improve incontinence symptoms.

Frailty is a defined syndrome characterized by an increased vulnerability. Frailty has been associated with increased risk of surgical complications, increased length of hospital stay, and probability of discharge to a nursing facility [15]. Currently, there is no standard method for screening and measuring frailty, but several assessment tools exist, such as the Fried frailty index, gait speed (measured by TUG), or grip strength [16, 17]. The importance of frailty as it relates to urinary incontinence is twofold in that pelvic floor disorders are associated with frailty and the presence of frailty influences treatment options and outcomes.

Table 25.2 Special considerations for elderly patients with urinary incontinence

	Assessment options
Mobility	"Is the bathroom on the same floor or do you have to go upstairs/downstairs?" Timed Up and Go test, observation of transfer to exam table
Frailty	Fried frailty index, Timed Up and Go test
Involvement of caregivers	"Who helps with self-care?" "How often are your caregivers available?"
Cognition	Mini-Mental Status Exam
Falls prevention	"Are there any obstacles in the path to the bathroom?" (e.g., rugs, stairs)
Polypharmacy	Review list of medications
Comorbid conditions	Assess how each may contribute to urinary incontinence
Primary sleep disorders	Referral for formal sleep assessment
Concomitant pelvic floor disorders	Physical examination for pelvic organ prolapse, ask about fecal incontinence: "Do you ever have accidental leakage of stool?"

If medication treatment is going to be recommended, then keep in mind that the interactions of overactive bladder medications with their current medication list are crucial. For example, starting an antimuscarinic can increase the anticholinergic burden on patients who may already be on other anticholinergic medications, which could theoretically increase the risk of dementia [18]. Furthermore, anticholinergics have been associated with an increased risk of falls.

Urinary incontinence can lead to skin breakdown and dermatitis, which may be compounded by decreased mobility with prolonged sitting or lying. Minimizing skin damage caused by incontinence can be achieved by successfully improving urinary incontinence, keeping the skin dry, and applying an emollient as a barrier between the urine and skin. In significant cases, catheterization may be warranted for diversion of urine away from the wounds.

Treatment of Urge Urinary Incontinence

First-Line Treatments: Behavioral Modifications

Behavioral modifications have generally been the mainstay for the treatment of urge urinary incontinence (UUI) in the elderly and can be individualized for people with varying levels of cognitive and physical impairments who may need assistance with self-care activities.

In an attempt to reduce urinary incontinence episodes, many elderly patients will report that they restrict their fluid intake. Although counter-intuitive, a small randomized control trial suggests that adequate hydration is more useful in the management of urinary incontinence [19] Older women were randomized to one of three groups: increase fluid intake to 500 cc, maintain fluid intake at baseline level, or decrease fluid intake by 300 cc. Although compliance to the fluid intake protocols was poor, follow-up interviews revealed that women who had reported a decrease in UI episodes felt that increasing their fluid intake was the most significant learning point.

In addition to fluid management, toileting therapy programs that include prompted voiding techniques and habit retraining can be utilized to improve UUI. Prompting the individual to toilet is designed to increase the patient's requests for toileting and self-initiated toileting, which will in turn decrease the number of UUI episodes. This is an effective short-term treatment of daytime UUI in nursing home residents and home care clients when caregivers comply with the protocol [20]. Habit retraining first requires identification of the individual's baseline toileting pattern with incontinence episodes. Once a baseline toileting pattern is established, a new toileting schedule can be created to preempt the UUI episodes.

Pelvic floor muscle training (PFMT) is an exercise program that involves intentional contraction of the pelvic floor muscles which can suppress detrusor overactivity and strengthen urethral support. Studies on the use of PFMT to treat UUI in the elderly have demonstrated a reduction in the number of UUI episodes as well as an increase in patient satisfaction [21]. Behavioral modification therapy can often take a combined approach that includes elements of all of the above techniques. In fact, studies in community-dwelling older women have shown that a combined approach to behavioral modification that includes PFMT, habit retraining, and lifestyle modifications can improve UUI [22].

Although behavioral modifications can be an effective treatment option for UUI in the elderly, the approach needs to be tailored to the individual's abilities and disabilities. Elderly patients with cognitive impairment may require active involvement of their caregivers for prompted voiding or assistance with fluid management. Elderly patients with functional limitations may have difficulty with toileting programs if they are not able to safely transfer to the toilet. In an effort to achieve success with behavioral therapy, one must keep in mind that a one-size-fits-all approach will not accommodate the diverse needs of older patients.

Second-Line Treatments: Pharmacologic Treatment

Medication therapy is considered a second-line treatment for UUI treatment but can present challenges in the elderly population due to the risk of medication noncompliance, polypharmacy, and increased side effects (Fig. 25.1). Following a comprehensive evaluation and a trial of appropriate behavioral therapy, pharmacologic treatment can be considered in the elderly population. In fact, it has been suggested that pharmacologic treatment in the elderly who are eligible for medication therapy is underutilized. A study of nursing home residents in the United States found that only 7% of eligible residents received medication therapy for their incontinence [23].

Medication therapy for UUI includes antimuscarinics and $\beta3$-adrenoreceptor agonists. Oxybutynin has been well studied and is available in several preparations. Oxybutynin's efficacy to decrease episodes of UUI in the elderly has also been well established; however, its known risk of acute cognitive impairment is why it is not used readily in the elderly population [24, 25]. The use of the transdermal formulation of oxybutynin may be more favorable in the elderly due to the avoidance of first pass metabolism, which would reduce its side effect profile [26]. Fesoterodine has also been well studied in the older population with good efficacy results and similar side effect profiles when compared to a younger population [27, 28]. Trospium is the only antimuscarinic with a quaternary amine structure, while the others are tertiary amines, giving it hydrophilic properties so that it is less likely to cross the blood-brain barrier and contribute to central nervous system effects, such as cognitive impairment [26]. A randomized controlled trial demonstrated no changes in cognitive function in women older than 50 years who were given trospium when compared to placebo [29]. Of all the antimuscarinic choices, trospium may be preferred in older patients with UUI given its unique chemical structure. Mirabegron is the only approved $\beta3$-adrenoreceptor agonist on the market, but there is a paucity of published data on its use in the elderly population; however, given its low side effect profile, overall it may be a better first choice in those patients without contraindications (uncontrolled HTN or drug interactions).

Although medication therapy may be successful in improving UUI in the elderly, this has to be weighed against the potential side effects in this vulnerable population. Mitigating these side effects is essential. For example, constipation as a side effect of antimuscarinics may ultimately worsen urinary incontinence, resulting in no significant improvement in symptoms. Studies have demonstrated an association between higher cumulative antimuscarinic use and increased risk of dementia [18, 30]. The AUA/SUFU guidelines for overactive bladder recommend using caution when prescribing medications in the frail older patient, given the risk of cognitive impairment. A baseline assessment of patient cognition using the Mini-Mental State Examination is recommended in those patients who are at risk of cognitive impairment prior to receiving antimuscarinic therapy to assess the risk of further cognitive decline [31]. Additional considerations prior to prescribing medications to the elderly are the age-related changes that could affect the pharmacokinetics and metabolism of medications. Slow gastric emptying can be seen in increasing age, which may reduce drug absorption. In addition, older patients can have decreased serum albumin that can lead to increased plasma levels of free drug [32]. Given the risk profile of medication therapy for UUI, a proactive approach with close monitoring is recommended when using medication therapy in the elderly.

Third-Line Treatments: Intradetrusor Onabotulinum Toxin A and Neuromodulation

In patients who are refractory to first- and second-line therapies, the AUA/SUFU guidelines recommend consideration of third-line therapies such as intradetrusor onabotulinum toxin A (BoNT-A), posterior tibial nerve stimulation (PTNS), or sacral neuromodulation.

Intradetrusor onabotulinum toxin A (BoNT-A) injections can be considered in carefully selected and thoroughly counseled elderly patients who are refractory to first- and second-line therapies. Studies have demonstrated no difference in reduction of mean daily UUI episodes between older and younger patients receiving BoNT-A injections; however, older patients did have a higher rate of urinary tract infections [33]. Another study investigated BoNT-A injections in three groups: frail elderly patients, elderly patients without frailty, and younger patients. They found that all three groups had similar success rates following BoNT-A injections at 3 and 6 months; however, the frail elderly group had significantly lower long-term success rates at 12 months. In addition, the frail elderly group had increased postvoid residuals and slower return to spontaneous voiding for those in urinary retention [34].

In drug-naive patients who prefer to avoid medications due to potential side effects or cost, the guidelines suggest consideration of PTNS as it is minimally invasive and reversible in nature [31]. A retrospective study on the effectiveness of

PTNS on an elderly population demonstrated a subjective success rate of 70% that is comparable to published success rates for PTNS in a younger population [35]. One of the potential barriers to the elderly receiving PTNS treatment is related to the need for weekly 30-min treatments for 12 weeks followed by monthly maintenance sessions. This commitment could pose an issue for those elderly patients who require transportation assistance to appointments.

Sacral neuromodulation (SNS) can be considered for the treatment of refractory UUI in the carefully selected elderly patient who is a candidate for a surgical procedure. Previous studies have reported lower success rates in older patients following SNS when compared to younger patients [36, 37]. However, a more recent study looking at the impact of age on SNS outcomes challenges the existing literature. This particular study demonstrated no difference in response to SNS test stimulation trials or in the implantation rate in older patients when compared to younger patients [38]. When considering SNS as a treatment for UUI in the elderly population, an important factor to consider is the patient's cognitive status and ability to operate the neurostimulator device, since poor understanding of the device is a contraindication for the therapy as it will not be efficacious if misused.

Treatment of Stress Urinary Incontinence

Nonsurgical Treatment Options

Pelvic floor muscle training (PFMT) improves pelvic floor muscle strength, endurance, and power, which is a commonly used treatment for women with stress urinary incontinence (SUI). PFMT has been well studied and has been shown to cure or improve SUI in all age groups [39]. In the elderly population specifically, PFMT has been studied and shown to significantly improve SUI symptoms [40, 41].

Incontinence pessaries are a nonsurgical option for the treatment of SUI for the elderly who prefer a nonsurgical intervention. Vaginal pessaries are one of the oldest medical devices and have been used for centuries as a treatment for pelvic organ prolapse. More recently, vaginal pessaries have been redesigned into incontinence pessaries for the treatment of SUI. They are designed to support the urethra and bladder wall, increasing urethral length, and provide gentle compression of the urethra against the pubic bone [42]. A retrospective review of women treated with an incontinence pessary for their SUI demonstrated complete resolution or a decrease in their incontinence in 59% of the women, and advanced age did not affect the success of the treatment [43]. Common complications of incontinence pessary use include an increase in vaginal discharge with or without odor, new onset difficulty in voiding, and spontaneous expulsion. A rare complication is vaginal erosion that can often be treated with topical estrogen cream with concomitant removal and subsequent refitting of the pessary. Pessaries do require regular removal and inspection of the vaginal epithelium, so they would not be a viable option for those patients who would be unlikely to follow up.

Surgical Treatment Options

Injection of a urethral bulking agent is a minimally invasive treatment of SUI, which is an option for elderly patients who are not considered surgical candidates. Injection of a bulking agent into the submucosa of the urethra elevates the urethral mucosa restoring coaptation, which then will increase urethral resistance and improve continence. A meta-analysis evaluating the efficacy and effectiveness of bulking agents in all age groups demonstrated a pooled objective treatment success rate of 46% in women with a follow-up of >12 months [44]. However, studies of older patients treated with urethral bulking agent injection have reported objective success rates between 73.2% and 77% [45, 46]. Potential complications include urinary retention, urinary tract infection, and worsening urinary incontinence. Complication rates are low and have been reported between 0% and 5.7% [44, 45]. Given the high success rates and low adverse event rates seen in the elderly, the injection of a urethral bulking agent can be considered a valid alternative to surgery in older patients and does not require anesthesia or halting of any medications prior to procedure.

Surgical procedures for the treatment of SUI are being more commonly performed in the elderly with a significant increase in SUI surgery in older women recently when compared to younger women [47]. Over the last two decades, there has been a shift from colposuspension and pubovaginal (autologous fascia) sling surgery to the more minimally invasive surgery of midurethral sling procedures. In an older population, colposuspension and pubovaginal sling surgery may not be as successful when compared to a younger population. The Stress Incontinence Surgical Treatment Efficacy Trial (SISTEr) that compared Burch colposuspension to pubovaginal slings revealed that older women were more likely to have a positive stress test and less subjective improvement of SUI at follow-up when compared to younger patients [48]. There was no difference in postoperative adverse events, but older women were more likely to require repeat surgery.

The minimally invasive nature of the midurethral sling procedure has increased the number of women, especially older women, who may be considered candidates for a surgical procedure to treat their SUI. The efficacy of midurethral sling surgery in the elderly has been investigated and demonstrated no significant difference in subjective cure between older and younger groups [49]. However, multiple studies have demonstrated an increase in perioperative complications such as longer hospitalization time, higher incidence of short-term voiding difficulties, increase in hospital readmissions, increase in recurrent urinary tract infections, and higher rates of de novo overactive bladder symptoms [49–51]. In summary, elderly women have similar outcomes from midurethral sling surgery but incur a higher associated morbidity when compared to younger women. The risks would need to be carefully weighed against the potential benefits on an individual basis prior to proceeding with midurethral sling surgery.

Conclusion

There is a need to continually personalize clinical care pathways for elderly patients with urinary incontinence in order to capture all the additional diagnostic and therapeutic considerations that go into decision-making in this population. There are still a lot of unanswered questions regarding the ideal treatment of elderly women with urinary incontinence and the impacts of different treatment options on factors specific to this population (i.e., cognition, role of caregivers). For this reason, further research in this arena is imperative to reduce the burden of urinary incontinence on this vulnerable population.

References

1. Hunskaar S, Lose G, Sykes D, Voss S. The prevalence of urinary incontinence in women in four European countries. BJU Int. 2004;93(3):324–30.
2. Andel R, Hyer K, Slack A. Risk factors for nursing home placement in older adults with and without dementia. J Aging Health. 2007;19(2):213–28.
3. Pfisterer MH-D, Griffiths DJ, PhD WS, Resnick NM. The effect of age on lower urinary tract function: a study in women. J Am Geriatr Soc. 2006;54(3):405–12.
4. Trowbridge ER, Wei JT, Fenner DE, Ashton-Miller JA, DeLancey JOL. Effects of aging on lower urinary tract and pelvic floor function in nulliparous women. Obstet Gynecol. 2007;109(3):715–20.
5. Madersbacher S, Pycha A, Schatzl G, Mian C, Klingler CH, Marberger M. The aging lower urinary tract: a comparative urodynamic study of men and women. Urology. 1998;51(2):206–12.
6. Mansfield KJ, Liu L, Mitchelson FJ, Moore KH, Millard RJ, Burcher E. Muscarinic receptor subtypes in human bladder detrusor and mucosa, studied by radioligand binding and quantitative competitive RT–PCR: changes in ageing. Br J Pharmacol. 2005;144(8):1089–99.
7. Wu JM, Vaughan CP, Goode PS, Redden DT, Burgio KL, Richter HE, et al. Prevalence and trends of symptomatic pelvic floor disorders in U.S. women. Obstet Gynecol. 2014;123(1):141–8.
8. Gandhi J, Chen A, Dagur G, Suh Y, Smith N, Cali B, et al. Genitourinary syndrome of menopause: an overview of clinical manifestations, pathophysiology, etiology, evaluation, and management. Am J Obstet Gynecol. 2016;215(6):704–11.
9. Marshall HJ, Beevers DG. α-Adrenoceptor blocking drugs and female urinary incontinence: prevalence and reversibility. Br J Clin Pharmacol. 1996;42(4):507–9.
10. Ansai JH, Farche ACS, Rossi PG, de Andrade LP, Nakagawa TH, Takahashi AC de M. Performance of different timed up and go subtasks in frailty syndrome. J Geriatr Phys Ther. 2019;42(4):287–93.
11. Nygaard I, Barber MD, Burgio KL, Kenton K, Meikle S, Schaffer J, et al. Prevalence of symptomatic pelvic floor disorders in US women. JAMA. 2008;300(11):1311–6.
12. Heilbrun ME, Nygaard IE, Lockhart ME, Richter HE, Brown MB, Kenton KS, et al. Correlation between levator ani muscle injuries on MRI and fecal incontinence, pelvic organ prolapse, and urinary incontinence in primiparous women. Am J Obstet Gynecol. 2010;202(5):488.e1–6.
13. Rodríguez-Mias Núria L, Martínez-Franco E, Aguado J, Sánchez E, Amat-Tardiu L. Pelvic organ prolapse and stress urinary incontinence, do they share the same risk factors? Eur J Obstet Gynecol Reprod Biol. 2015;190:52–7.
14. Cetinkaya SE, Dokmeci F, Dai O. Correlation of pelvic organ prolapse staging with lower urinary tract symptoms, sexual dysfunction, and quality of life. Int Urogynecol J. 2013;24(10):1645–50.

15. Makary MA, Segev DL, Pronovost PJ, Syin D, Bandeen-Roche K, Patel P, et al. Frailty as a predictor of surgical outcomes in older patients. J Am Coll Surg. 2010;210(6):901–8.
16. Savva GM, Donoghue OA, Horgan F, O'Regan C, Cronin H, Kenny RA. Using timed up-and-go to identify frail members of the older population. J Gerontol A Biol Sci Med Sci. 2013;68(4):441–6.
17. Abellan van Kan G, Rolland Y, Houles M, Gillette-Guyonnet S, Soto M, Vellas B. The assessment of frailty in older adults. Clin Geriatr Med. 2010;26(2):275–86.
18. Gray SL, Anderson ML, Dublin S, Hanlon JT, Hubbard R, Walker R, et al. Cumulative use of strong anticholinergics and incident dementia: a prospective cohort study. JAMA Intern Med. 2015;175(3):401–7.
19. Dowd TT, Campbell JM, Jones JA. Fluid intake and urinary incontinence in older community-dwelling women. J Community Health Nurs. 1996;13(3):179–86.
20. Wagg A, Gibson W, Ostaszkiewicz J, Johnson T, Markland A, Palmer MH, et al. Urinary incontinence in frail elderly persons: report from the 5th international consultation on incontinence. Neurourol Urodyn. 2015;34(5):398–406.
21. Burgio KL, Goode PS, Locher JL, Umlauf MG, Roth DL, Richter HE, et al. Behavioral training with and without biofeedback in the treatment of urge incontinence in older women: a randomized controlled trial. JAMA. 2002;288(18):2293–9.
22. Diokno AC, Sampselle CM, Herzog AR, Raghunathan TE, Hines S, Messer KL, et al. Prevention of urinary incontinence by behavioral modification program: a randomized, controlled trial among older women in the community. J Urol. 2004;171(3):1165–71.
23. Narayanan S, Cerulli A, Kahler KH, Ouslander JG. Is drug therapy for urinary incontinence used optimally in long-term care facilities? J Am Med Dir Assoc. 2007;8(2):98–104.
24. Aaron LE, Morris TJ, Jahshan P, Reiz JL. An evaluation of patient and physician satisfaction with controlled-release oxybutynin 15 mg as a one-step daily dose in elderly and non-elderly patients with overactive bladder: results of the STOP study. Curr Med Res Opin. 2012;28(8):1369–79.
25. Katz IR, Sands LP, Bilker W, DiFilippo S, Boyce A, D'Angelo K. Identification of medications that cause cognitive impairment in older people: the case of oxybutynin chloride. J Am Geriatr Soc. 1998;46(1):8–13.
26. McFerren SC, Gomelsky A. Treatment of overactive bladder in the elderly female: the case for trospium, oxybutynin, fesoterodine and darifenacin. Drugs Aging. 2015;32(10):809–19.
27. Dubeau CE, Kraus SR, Griebling TL, Newman DK, Wyman JF, Johnson TM, et al. Effect of fesoterodine in vulnerable elderly subjects with urgency incontinence: a double-blind, placebo controlled trial. J Urol. 2014;191(2):395–404.
28. Wagg A, Khullar V, Marschall-Kehrel D, Michel MC, Oelke M, Darekar A, et al. Flexible-dose fesoterodine in elderly adults with overactive bladder: results of the randomized, double-blind, placebo-controlled study of fesoterodine in an aging population trial. J Am Geriatr Soc. 2013;61(2):185–93.
29. Geller EJ, Dumond JB, Bowling JM, Khandelwal CM, Wu JM, Busby-Whitehead J, et al. Effect of trospium chloride on cognitive function in women aged 50 and older: a randomized trial. Female Pelvic Med Reconstr Surg. 2017;23(2):118–23.
30. Richardson K, Fox C, Maidment I, Steel N, Loke YK, Arthur A, et al. Anticholinergic drugs and risk of dementia: case-control study. BMJ. 2018;361:k1315.
31. Gormley EA, Lightner DJ, Burgio KL, Chai TC, Clemens JQ, Culkin DJ, et al. Diagnosis and treatment of overactive bladder (non-neurogenic) in adults: AUA/SUFU guideline. J Urol. 2012;188(6 Suppl):2455–63.
32. Wagg AS. Antimuscarinic treatment in overactive bladder: special considerations in elderly patients. Drugs Aging. 2012;29(7):539–48.
33. Komesu YM, Amundsen CL, Richter HE, Erickson SW, Ackenbom MF, Andy UU, et al. Refractory urgency urinary incontinence treatment in women: impact of age on outcomes and complications. Am J Obstet Gynecol. 2018;218(1):111.e1–9.

34. Liao C-H, Kuo H-C. Increased risk of large post-void residual urine and decreased long-term success rate after intravesical onabotulinumtoxinA injection for refractory idiopathic detrusor overactivity. J Urol. 2013;189(5):1804–10.
35. Palmer C, Nguyen N, Ghoniem G. Clinical experience with percutaneous tibial nerve stimulation in the elderly; do outcomes differ by gender? Arab J Urol. 2019;17(1):10–3.
36. Levin PJ, Wu JM, Siddiqui NY, Amundsen CL. Does obesity impact the success of an InterStim test phase for the treatment of refractory urge urinary incontinence in female patients? Female Pelvic Med Reconstr Surg. 2012;18(4):243–6.
37. Amundsen CL, Webster GD. Sacral neuromodulation in an older, urge-incontinent population. Am J Obstet Gynecol. 2002;187(6):1462–5; discussion 1465
38. Faris AER, Gill BC, Pizarro-Berdichevsky J, Dielubanza E, Clifton MM, Okafor H, et al. Impact of age and comorbidities on use of sacral neuromodulation. J Urol. 2017;198(1):161–6.
39. Dumoulin C, Cacciari LP, Hay-Smith EJC. Pelvic floor muscle training versus no treatment, or inactive control treatments, for urinary incontinence in women. Cochrane Database Syst Rev. 2018;04(10):CD005654.
40. Leong BS, Mok NW. Effectiveness of a new standardised urinary continence physiotherapy programme for community-dwelling older women in Hong Kong. Hong Kong Med J Xianggang Yi Xue Za Zhi. 2015;21(1):30–7.
41. Dumoulin C, Morin M, Danieli C, Cacciari L, Mayrand M-H, Tousignant M, et al. Group-based vs individual pelvic floor muscle training to treat urinary incontinence in older women: a randomized clinical trial. JAMA Intern Med. 2020;180(10):1284–93.
42. Al-Shaikh G, Syed S, Osman S, Bogis A, Al-Badr A. Pessary use in stress urinary incontinence: a review of advantages, complications, patient satisfaction, and quality of life. Int J Women's Health. 2018;10:195–201.
43. Farrell SA, Singh B, Aldakhil L. Continence pessaries in the management of urinary incontinence in women. J Obstet Gynaecol Can JOGC. 2004;26(2):113–7.
44. Capobianco G, Saderi L, Dessole F, Petrillo M, Dessole M, Piana A, et al. Efficacy and effectiveness of bulking agents in the treatment of stress and mixed urinary incontinence: a systematic review and meta-analysis. Maturitas. 2020;133:13–31.
45. Mohr S, Siegenthaler M, Mueller MD, Kuhn A. Bulking agents: an analysis of 500 cases and review of the literature. Int Urogynecol J. 2013;24(2):241–7.
46. Zullo MA, Ruggiero A, Montera R, Plotti F, Muzii L, Angioli R, et al. An ultra-miniinvasive treatment for stress urinary incontinence in complicated older patients. Maturitas. 2010;65(3):292–5.
47. Lee J, Dwyer PL. Age-related trends in female stress urinary incontinence surgery in Australia – Medicare data for 1994-2009. Aust N Z J Obstet Gynaecol. 2010;50(6):543–9.
48. Richter HE, Goode PS, Brubaker L, Zyczynski H, Stoddard AM, Dandreo KJ, et al. Two-year outcomes after surgery for stress urinary incontinence in older compared with younger women. Obstet Gynecol. 2008;112(3):621–9.
49. Stav K, Dwyer PL, Rosamilia A, Schierlitz L, Lim YN, Lee J. Midurethral sling procedures for stress urinary incontinence in women over 80 years. Neurourol Urodyn. 2010;29(7):1262–6.
50. Groutz A, Cohen A, Gold R, Pauzner D, Lessing JB, Gordon D. The safety and efficacy of the "inside-out" trans-obturator TVT in elderly versus younger stress-incontinent women: a prospective study of 353 consecutive patients. Neurourol Urodyn. 2011;30(3):380–3.
51. Cohen AJ, Packiam VT, Nottingham CU, Alberts BD, Faris SF, Bales GT. 30-day morbidity and reoperation following midurethral sling: analysis of 8772 cases using a national prospective database. Urology. 2016;95:72–9.

Chapter 26
Maximizing Intraoperative Performance and Safety During Incontinence Surgery

Kristin Chrouser and Keow Mei Goh

Patient Safety in the Operating Room

The last several decades have seen widespread institutional adoption of patient safety practices such as huddles, preoperative briefings, and preprocedural "time-outs." These team-based tools are intended to maximize communication and improve outcomes by preventing adverse events such as wrong site surgery, surgical site infections, and intraoperative errors. Best practices to protect patient safety are available in many guidelines and white papers from various surgical societies [1, 2]. Here, we will focus on selected patient and safety considerations that are particularly relevant to incontinence surgery.

Safe Patient Positioning

Correct positioning of the patient is crucial in preventing injury in the operating room (OR). Once under anesthesia, the patient will be unable to communicate discomfort or adjust their position. Many risk factors influence positioning including the type and length of surgical procedure, need for access to the operative site, patient's height, weight, age, nutritional status, level of mobility, and comorbidities [3]. General guidelines for patient positioning should be followed [4]. The OR staff need to be well versed in the use of advance positioning devices and supplies. All equipment (e.g., stirrups, padding, and arm boards) required for positioning should

K. Chrouser (✉) · K. M. Goh
University of Michigan Department of Urology, VA Ann Arbor Healthcare System,
Ann Arbor, MI, USA
e-mail: chrouser@med.umich.edu; mgoh@med.umich.edu

A. P. Cameron (ed.), *Female Urinary Incontinence*,
https://doi.org/10.1007/978-3-030-84352-6_26

be in the room before the patient's arrival. The OR bed should be able to support the patient's weight and be of sufficient width.

Supine Positioning

Ulnar neuropathy is the most common injury associated with supine positioning. The goal is to minimize pressure on the ulnar grove and avoid both arm hyperextension and flexion >90° [5]. In addition, hyperabduction of the shoulder, external rotation and dorsal extension of the arm, and flexion of the head to the contralateral side will increase the risk of brachial plexus injury. In order to avoid this, the head should be in midline and straight. Arms should be in a neutral position, rotated medially and tucked under the draw sheet. Alternatively, the arms can be placed laterally on an arm board and abducted <90° to prevent dorsal hyperextension [6]. Radial nerve injury can occur if the supinated arm is inadvertently hanging off the table or from a distally misplaced blood pressure cuff. The median nerve can be injured if the arm is pronated and hanging off the table. Hyperextension of the elbow also places the median nerve at risk. Even when taking safety precautions, idiopathic nerve injuries have been documented [6].

Trendelenburg Positioning

The Trendelenburg position is a common position with vaginal as well as laparoscopic/robotic pelvic surgery that can lead to increases in central venous, intracranial, pulmonary venous, and intraocular pressures [7]. In addition to decreases in functional residual capacity and pulmonary compliance, the practice of taping the patient's chest to secure them into place for this position has resulted in compromised lung function [8]. Severe head and neck edema has resulted in laryngeal edema requiring reintubation and posterior ischemic optic neuropathy resulting in loss of vision following robotic prostatectomy [9, 10]. In the past, shoulder braces have been used to prevent cephalad migration of the patient on the table. However, the use of shoulder braces has resulted in documented brachial plexus injuries [6].

Nerve injuries related to incorrect positioning have been estimated at 0.02% and 0.16% for the upper extremities and 1.5–1.8% for the lower extremities during laparoscopic gynecologic surgery and 1% in robotic-assisted surgeries. Note that the exact incidence may be higher due to underreporting and the fact that many of these injuries are self-limited [11]. Patient factors that increase the risk of nerve injury include the following: very high or very low body mass index (BMI), age >60 years, a history of smoking or alcohol intake, hypovolemia, hypotension, electrolyte imbalance or malnutrition at the time of surgery, and higher ASA scores [12, 13]. Historically, operative time was felt to play a major role in nerve injury after lithotomy positioning, but recent data are less convincing [11]. In order to avoid nerve injuries, patient positioning is crucial. When positioning the patient's legs in stirrups or tucking the arms against the OR table, attention should be paid to extra padding to cushion nerves where they are at risk for compression. Excessive hip flexion

(>80°–90°), extreme abduction and external rotation while in lithotomy, and pressure on the patient's inner thigh all place the femoral nerve at risk for a compression injury [14].

Avoiding the cephalad movement of the patient while in steep Trendelenburg has been the subject of much debate; however, there is not clear evidence which technique is best given few direct comparisons [15]. In addition to shoulder braces, other techniques for stabilizing patient position on the table include bean bags, egg crate or foam mattress pads, or the Pink Pad® system [15, 16]. Continuous intraoperative neuromonitoring using upper extremity somatosensory evoked potentials was recommended as a novel way to monitor for intraoperative neuropathic injury in real time [17]. When focusing on proper positioning, the team should take care to pad all pressure points and avoid hyperflexion, overrotation, or excess abduction of the limbs. In addition, the minimum amount of Trendelenburg needed to achieve visualization should be used [11].

Lithotomy Positioning

Lithotomy position is commonly utilized for incontinence procedures. There are multiple levels of lithotomy position which vary in the degree of hip angulation and leg height, from low lithotomy (legs at approximately 35° relative to the axis of the bed) up to exaggerated lithotomy (legs at >90°) [18]. In standard lithotomy position, legs are abducted 30–45° from the midline, hips flexed at 80–100°, and lower legs parallel to the torso [5]. Care should be taken to limit the leg elevation and abduction to provide adequate surgical exposure without compromising lower extremity circulation or impacting patient hemodynamics [19]. Lower extremity injuries from lithotomy position are well documented. The peroneal nerve is at risk of compression between head of fibula and the stirrup. In a similar fashion, the saphenous vein can be compressed at the medial tibial condyle. Hyperflexion of the hips and extension of the knees risk injury to the sciatic nerve [5]. In a retrospective study of patients undergoing surgery in the lithotomy position at the Mayo Clinic, Warner et al. found a one in 3608 incidence of motor neuropathy lasting >3 months with the common peroneal nerve involved in 78% of these cases [20]. Risk factors for injury include extremes of body size and surgery >2 hours. Compartment syndrome requiring fasciotomy and rhabdomyolysis has also been reported in cases lasting >4.5 hours [5, 19]. In a study of 177 patients placed into exaggerated lithotomy position, 28 patients experienced peroneal nerve injury with 27 of the cases resolving [21].

While in lithotomy, legs can be supported in candy cane stirrups, knee crutch stirrups, or boot-type stirrups (Fig. 26.1). When using candy cane stirrups, the patient's legs should not be allowed to rest on the vertical bar. Padding can be placed between the bar and the patient's leg, but this does not guarantee safety. Care should be taken to avoid overrotation of the patient's hips with rotation of the candy canes. Gel boots and wide straps can help with reducing pressure to the ankle and the foot [22]. The knee crutch–type stirrups place the weight of the lower extremity on the popliteal space in the posterior knee, increasing the risk of injury to the posterior

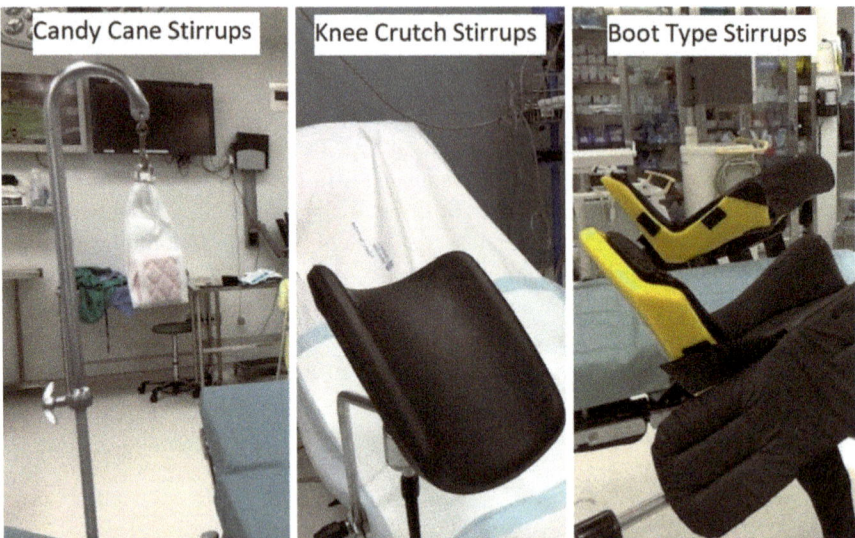

Fig. 26.1 Stirrup options for lithotomy position

and common peroneal nerves and the popliteal artery [23]. Alternatively, the boot-type stirrup allows for the weight of the leg to be distributed over the leg and the foot, while allowing for intraoperative adjustment of hip flexion and leg abduction [22]. If exaggerated lithotomy position is required, the perineum will be almost parallel to the floor and a bolster should be used to support the low back [5]. In order to ensure correct lithotomy positioning in boot-type stirrups, the patient should be positioned so the sacrum is well-supported once the foot of the table is removed and the table rail clamp should be aligned with the patient's hip. The heel should rest in the base of the boot. The knee angle should remain <90° as to avoid hyperflexion (for reference, straight leg is 0°). The long axis of the boot should be directed toward the contralateral shoulder [5]. Upper extremities should be tucked or extended laterally, keeping in mind the same concerns as above in supine positioning. In addition, ensure that the fingers are not injured when removing or replacing the foot of the bed.

Positioning in Challenging Situations

Obese Patients

The prevalence and degree of obesity in Americans continue to increase every year. In 2020, the CDC estimated that 9.8% of the US population was considered severely obese (BMI >40) and this number will continue to rise [24]. These patients create unique challenges in the OR. In addition to addressing all the positioning concerns above, care must be taken to ensure that the patient is not positioned on wrinkled bed linen and that equipment such as compression stockings, blood pressure cuffs, and the OR bed are adequately sized. In moving the patient to the OR table, the use of transfer device such as the HoverMatt® is a useful adjunct to reduce the risk of patient skin shear and musculoskeletal injury to the staff. For severely obese patients, lifting and lowering the patient's legs from stirrups should be done slowly to prevent lumbosacral strain and to avoid rapid changes in circulatory system [4]. There are bariatric boot-type stirrups that have higher weight limits, wider boots, and lift assist. The off-label use of pneumatic Hoyer lifts to support patient's legs has also been reported [22].

Patients with Contractures or Amputations

When positioning a patient with limited flexibility due to joint contractions, consider placing the patient in the position required for surgery prior to the delivery of anesthesia to confirm that the patient is able to comfortably lie in that position. Sometimes contractures can make some surgical approaches (e.g., prone and lithotomy) physically impossible. Placing patients with amputations into lithotomy requires special consideration to support the single amputated limb. For low amputations, boot-type stirrups with extra padding are often adequate. If leg elevation is unnecessary, one strategy is to use a split leg table with shoulder support to brace the stump site [25] (Fig. 26.2).

Fig. 26.2 Positioning amputee using split leg table and shoulder supports. (With permission from Keow Goh (top) and James Williamson (bottom))

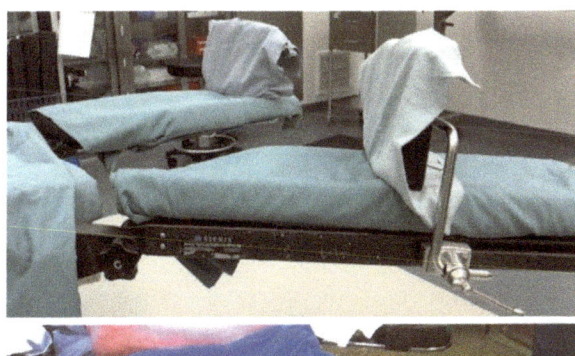
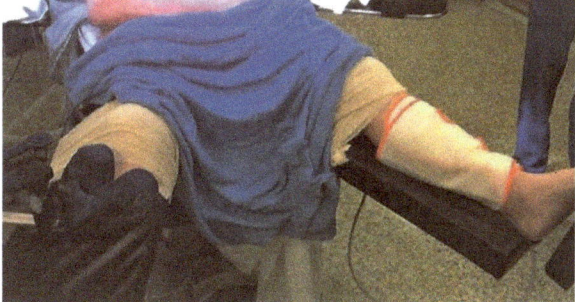

Safe Use of Intraoperative Radiation

Sacral neuromodulation is commonly used for the treatment of refractory urge incontinence. Although the procedure itself is of very low risk, it requires fluoroscopy that exposes both the patient and surgical team to ionizing radiation. Accurate lead placement can be accomplished while minimizing radiation exposure to both patients and surgical staff. Many studies confirm a lack of awareness of the risks (e.g., cancer, infertility, and cataracts) of radiation exposure [26, 27]. Every effort should be made to reduce both dose and exposure time while maximizing shielding (Table 26.1) [1]. Surgeons should optimize fluoroscopy settings by using pulsed radiation, reduced pulse rates and doses, image holding/fluoroscopy store, and image collimation [28].

Patient Protection

The patient should be positioned closest to the image intensifier and farther from the side of the X-ray tube. A designated member of the operative team (nurses or radiology technicians) should monitor the dose and report when the maximal dose has been reached [29]. Institutions should have a policy to screen female patients for possible pregnancies. If a pregnant female must be exposed to ionizing radiation, appropriate shielding should be placed over the abdomen and pelvis to protect the fetus [30].

Table 26.1 Strategies for minimizing radiation exposure of patients and surgical team [1]

Reduce dose and exposure time
Limit fluoroscopy time
Low dose setting (set as default)
Pulsed fluoroscopy on lowest setting (e.g., 1 pulse per second)
Use spot fluoro images, not continuous fluoroscopy
Use "last image hold" and "save and swap" technology
Collimate to narrow area if entire image does not need to be seen
Maximize distance from energy source, minimize distance from image intensifier (reduce scatter)
Minimize the use of image magnification (magnification increases dose)
Use physician foot pedal control (avoids confusion of when fluoroscopy is needed, and whether it needs to be continuous)
Use dedicated surgical radiation technologist who is familiar with case anatomy
Shielding
Use personal protective equipment (lead aprons, thyroid shields, lead glasses, and lead gloves)
Shield patient (e.g., radiosensitive areas like thyroid, pelvis in pregnant patients)

Staff Protection

Perioperative team members should limit exposure time and maximize distance from the source of radiation. The amount of radiation exposure is inversely proportional to the square of the distance to the source. Additionally, the person activating the radiology equipment should provide those in the room an opportunity to don protective equipment [31]. Personnel can use fixed shielding, mobile shields, equipment-mounted shields, or personal protective devices such as aprons and thyroid shields. Care should be taken to provide coverage on the back of the personnel if X-ray exposure is likely. If the hands of the personnel are likely to be in path of the radiation beam, protective gloves and finger dosimeters should be available [31]. The OR staff needs to be consistent in wearing protective lead aprons and thyroid shields while using dosimeters to monitor exposure. In one study, only 50–56% of personnel at academic training centers used dosimeters, and this percentage was even less in private institutions [32]. Notably, the team leaders' adoption of radiation protection practices influences staff compliance [33]. Pregnant personnel need to comply with precautions set by local, state, and federal regulatory bodies. The pregnant team member should wear a radiation monitor under her waist shield, and the monitor should be read monthly. Use of maternity or double-thickness lead apron should be encouraged [30]. If possible, she should minimize her participation in procedures requiring radiation.

Surgeon Safety and Occupational Health

Surgical culture encourages surgeons to sacrifice in service of their patients, including rigorous training, long work hours, and a disregard of personal physical needs. Intraoperatively surgeons do not typically take breaks to eat or empty their bladders. Surgeons are willing to use operative techniques that require poor ergonomic positioning (and cause musculoskeletal discomfort) if they consider it to be in the patient's best interest. In addition, many providers spend long hours in the electronic medical record on computer workstations that have not been ergonomically optimized. Unfortunately, over the course of a long career, long hours filled with repetitive work-related musculoskeletal injury can lead to chronic disability, leading them to shift case modalities/volumes or consider early retirement [34, 35]. Although interest is growing, few residency programs provide instruction in ergonomic principles that can assist young surgeons in minimizing the negative physical impact of their occupational activities [36].

In a recent review, 68% of surgeons reported musculoskeletal pain, 61% noted their pain was exacerbated by operating, while less than a third sought medical attention for their symptoms. Rates of pain vary somewhat based on surgical subspecialty and surgical modality (e.g., open, lap, robotic, and endoscopic). Approximately 41–80% of urologists and 54%–87% of vaginal surgeons report work-related musculoskeletal pain. [35, 37, 38] Surgeons admit to modifying hours spent operating, case mix, and operative technique in order to manage pain [35, 37]. In a study combining surgeons from all subspecialties, wearable technology was used to monitor intraoperative surgeon body position and found that 65% of operative time was spent in high-risk neck positions [39]. Not surprisingly, high-risk positions, loupes, and headlight were all associated with increased subjective pain ratings.

Although surgeons in general report high rates of work-related musculoskeletal disorders, there are concerns that female surgeons may be disproportionally affected. The American Urological Association 2017 census, which is less likely to suffer from response bias than ergonomic-specific surveys, found that female surgeons reported work-related pain more commonly than their male counterparts [35]. Differences were greater in younger surgeons under 45 years of age, where 65% of women had discomfort compared to 42% of men. On average, female surgeons are shorter and have smaller hands than their male counterparts. The da Vinci robotic console is not ergonomically optimized for surgeons shorter than 5′4″ [40]. Small hand size is correlated with difficulty firing staplers [41]. Medical devices are not currently designed to accommodate the range of hand sizes and grip strengths found in the current population of surgeons, especially as more women have entered the profession [42]. Lack of rigorous usability testing of instruments unfortunately leads to increased ergonomic stress and risk of injury in female surgeons. Many companies rely on outdated end-user anthropometric measurement ranges dating from an era when surgery was a male-dominated profession [43]. Surgeons should encourage companies to design devices and equipment that will accommodate a large range of hand sizes and strengths, as this can help ensure equitable access to a safe workplace for all. It is important to note that not all differences in pain rates can be attributed to height and hand size. Objective measures of more serious injury, such as the need for treatment, have been noted at higher rates in female surgeons even when controlling for glove size [44]. Similarly, even after controlling for case length and surgeon height, EMG measurements of muscle activation during laparoscopic surgery were higher among female than those among male surgeons [45]. Additional research is required to assess whether open vaginal or robotic surgery also requires more physical exertion from female surgeons to complete the same procedure.

Since most surgical interventions for incontinence are performed vaginally, we will focus on the particular challenges of operating on patients in the lithotomy position, although many of these principles can also be applied to open, laparoscopic, and robotic approaches. The main risk factors for musculoskeletal pain include awkward postures, high exertion activities, static positions, and long surgeries without breaks [46, 47]. The cramped working space inherent in the lithotomy position makes it almost impossible to maintain a neutral posture. Inappropriate table height can lead to excessive trunk and head flexion [48]. 67% of vaginal surgeries in one observational series caused neck, shoulder back, or hip pain [49]. This correlates with objective assessments of surgeon postures where high-risk shoulder, trunk, and neck postures were identified during vaginal surgery [50]. Additionally, for surgeons in teaching institutions, the attending surgeon often stands beside the resident surgeon in the "assistant" position during vaginal surgery, resulting in postures with excessive lateral rotation and flexion of the trunk and prolonged upper extremity static strain from retracting [38].

Strategies to Maximize Intraoperative Ergonomics and Prevent Injury

A multipronged approach to reduce occupational musculoskeletal injury in surgeons includes adjustments in the physical environment (bed and equipment arrangement), surgeon-specific strategies/activities, as well as prevention strategies outside the operating room.

Strategies to Optimize the Physical Environment

Maintaining proper posture is paramount to optimal surgical ergonomics, and detailed resources are available for guidance [51, 52]. The table height should be adjusted to accommodate the tallest surgeon (patient at elbow height), and others should use steps or platforms if required [48]. The neck, shoulders, back, and hips should be aligned with minimal trunk rotation, weight evenly distributed without locking knees [53]. Limit axial neck rotation to <15° [51]. Vaginal surgeons should sit when possible and adjust table/stool in order to look straight ahead while working [48]. Adjust lights so that they do not require constant repositioning that often requires awkward postures, and tuck the patient's arms when possible as to not inhibit surgeon/assistant freedom of movement [53]. Rotating assistants or using self-retaining retractors can decrease ergonomic stress on assistants [48]. Foot pedals should be placed directly in front of the working foot, which should remain in neutral alignment [52]. Monitors should be positioned 3–4 feet away with the center of the screen approximately 10–20° below the eye level [52]. Placing the top of the screen at the eye level is usually a reasonable approximation. Cushioned floor mats have been found to improve subjective measures of surgeon discomfort in some studies and are commercially available for surgical use [54]. A table-mounted vaginal retractor in conjunction with a mounted camera has been proposed as a potential method to improve both visualization and ergonomics during vaginal surgery [55]. Chairs with chest and limb supports as well as exoskeleton suits are both innovative strategies that have shown promise in improving intraoperative surgeon pain and fatigue but are not widely disseminated to date [56, 57].

Surgeon-Specific Strategies to Improve Ergonomics and Decrease Pain

For surgeons accustomed to risky intraoperative postures, changing habits can be difficult. Postural resets are intermittent postural "check-ins" allowing opportunity for readjustment [53]. Wearing shoes with arch support and pressure support hose can be helpful during long cases, especially in surgeons with chronic lower extremity or back discomfort [48].

Intraoperative Breaks/Stretches

Intraoperative microbreaks involve pausing the procedure at a noncritical juncture (every 20–40 min) and engaging in a short 90-s series of targeted stretches/exercise. These microbreaks are accomplished without breaking scrub and have been shown to decrease surgeon discomfort and improve mental focus without increasing operative time [58]. Surgeons engrossed in surgery are unlikely to remember to take their breaks, so Abdelall et al. operationalized them into an app with automatic reminders and effectively implemented this into the workflow of a small group of surgeons [59]. Information on accessing this resource can be found at ORstretch.mayoclinic.org.

Prevention Strategies Beyond the Operating Room

Workstation Optimization

Outside the operating room, surgeons spend a significant time at computer workstation, which can also contribute to musculoskeletal pain, as most desks are too high. Use an adjustable chair in which the lower back fits snugly against the chair or a pillow, feet on the floor (or a footrest), knees at 90°, and back slightly reclined. Elbows should be open at an angle of 90°–100°, and wrists should remain straight, not resting on the desk. Do not tilt the keyboard toward the user. The top of the monitor should be at or a little below the eye level, so the center of the computer screen is ~20° below the eye level—with the screen at least 20 inches away (about a full arm's length). Bifocal wearers should drop the monitor another 1–2 inches. When doing computer work, reduce eye strain by taking a break every 20 min for 20 s and focusing 20 feet away. Proper ergonomic positioning is almost impossible when using a laptop without a separate monitor and/or keyboard.

Exercise, Physical Therapy, Massage

A survey study suggests that exercise outside the OR appears to have a protective effect against work-related pain in urologists in a dose-dependent fashion [60]. Targeted exercises have been shown to improve work-related neck and shoulder pain in nonsurgeons, although prospective exercise interventions have not yet been reported in surgeons [61]. For surgeons with work-related musculoskeletal pain, physical therapy and/or regular massage can also be helpful to improve pain (therapeutic) and maintain flexibility (preventive).

Ergonomic Education

Many studies assessing the increasing prevalence of work-related musculoskeletal pain in surgeons have also noted the lack of ergonomic instruction during surgical training or continuing medical education offerings. There is a growing consensus that surgical ergonomics instruction should be offered during residency, lest we fail to prepare the next generation to do their job safely [36].

Maximizing Intraoperative Surgeon and Team Performance

Surgical outcomes are influenced by multiple aspects of surgeon performance, including psychomotor/technical performance as well as a diverse collection of other cognitive activities and interpersonal team exchanges that are often referred to as "nontechnical performance" [62, 63]. Nontechnical skills encompass communication, decision-making, situation awareness, teamwork, and leadership [64]. Communication requires receiving and conveying information in a way others can understand. Situational awareness is the surgeon's perception of the team's activity as well as ongoing awareness of physical cues from the surgical field. Decision-making takes place when a surgeon is faced with a challenge and then chooses and implements a course of action. Teamwork involves engaging in a collaborative effort with others toward a goal. Leadership skills include modeling positive behaviors coupled with the ability to engage and motivate others [65]. Although it is tempting to focus narrowly on surgeon technical error as the cause of complications, many patient safety events can be traced back to deficits in nontechnical performance [66, 67]. As a result, individual performance improvement efforts must move beyond a narrow focus on improving just individual technical speed and accuracy and also address a broader range of skills.

Strategies to Optimize Individual Surgeon Performance

Surgical Coaching or Didactic Training

Expert and peer surgical coaching using various modalities (in person, video, simulation) has been found to subjectively improve performance [68]. Most coaching studies and QI projects have focused on technical performance, but some also address nontechnical skills [69]. One author noted that, although surgeons' self-assessment of their technical performance is concordant with expert option, surgeons do a poor job of assessing the quality of their own nontechnical skills, suggesting a potential blind spot [70]. There are didactic and simulation programs, in addition to coaching options, that focus on the acquisition of these critical skills [65]. Some residency programs have developed comprehensive programs that address a wide range of these skills, including communication and professionalism [71].

Encourage Psychological Safety

Surgeons should use their leadership role to improve team performance by nurturing a psychologically safe environment in the operating room. Historically, the operating room has not been an environment that rewards interpersonally risky behaviors such as speaking up with concerns or asking for help. However, psychological safety encourages learning and maximizes team performance [72]. Such an environment is particularly critical in a crisis situation where a high functioning team can prevent a surgeon error from spiraling into a full-blown adverse event.

Mental Practice

Training in mental imagery/mental practice has been used for the past century as a way to improve athletic performance [73]. Mental practice has been shown to have a positive impact on surgical performance in trainees [74]. It can also be useful in experienced surgeons to delay skill decay and accelerate the learning curve when adopting a new technique or in preparation for complex or unfamiliar procedures [75].

Stress, Emotion, Conflict Management

Acute stress is unavoidable in the operating room, yet when poorly managed it puts the patient, surgeon, and team at risk. Lack of emotional management and disruptive behavior can distress staff, disrupt team dynamics, increase tension, and decrease psychological safety [76, 77]. Chronic surgeon stress can lead to burnout and attrition, which also negatively impacts patients and providers. Surgeon stress management intervention trials have included instruction in coping strategies, mental rehearsal, and relaxation techniques [78]. Preoperative mental practice has also been shown to reduce stress in novice surgeons [79]. Mental toughness, a measure of individual resilience and confidence associated with excellence in athletic and military performance literature, has only recently been described in surgeons [80]. Techniques used by soldiers to improve/maintain mental toughness include visualization, self-talk, affirmations, concentration skills, and breathing [81]. These help control the arousal associated with stressful situations and improve physical and psychological performance. Surgeons will also find that honing their skills in conflict management in the operating room can improve both individual and team performance [82].

Optimize Physiology

Optimizing surgeon physiology involves preventing hypoglycemia, dehydration, fatigue, and musculoskeletal pain.

The fast pace and unpredictable nature of surgery lends itself to poor fluid intake and missed meals. Blood glucose levels are associated with both reductions in cognitive performance and increased irritability/anger [83, 84]. Induction of frustration in an experimental setting leads to more negative responses when subjects are fasting [85]. Irritability and negative emotions impact nontechnical skills and influence a team's willingness to work together [86]. This evidence from the nonsurgical literature suggests potential vulnerabilities in technical and nontechnical performance when surgeons are hypoglycemic. Dehydration depresses mood and cognitive function in on-call physicians and nurses although this relationship hasn't been assessed in surgeons [87]. The nonsurgical literature demonstrates that sleep deprivation has the most profound impact on mood, then cognition, followed by psychomotor performance [88]. Studies in surgeons have focused on psychomotor performance, and results are mixed but suggest a negative impact [89]. In contrast, the majority of surgeons and nurses feel their performance during the critical portion of the case is not affected by fatigue [90]. Even if technical performance is maintained, degradation of surgeon's nontechnical performance can adversely affect the surgical team.

Surgeon's musculoskeletal pain can impact performance in several ways. Pain can restrict range of motion, strength, and motor control, thus negatively influencing psychomotor/technical performance [91, 92]. Pain can decrease mental focus and adversely impact intraoperative decision-making and cognition [93]. Pain can also increase irritability toward others and negatively affect psychological safety and team dynamics [94, 95]. Poor nontechnical performance of surgeon can lead to a reduction in team communication and collaboration resulting in adverse events. It should be evident that the ergonomic strategies listed earlier are not only important for surgeon occupational health, but when they prevent or reduce work-related pain, this helps optimize surgeon/team performance and improve patient outcomes.

Strategies to Optimize Surgical Team Performance

Team Training

Strategies to improve surgical team performance overlap to some degree with those already addressed for surgeons, especially regarding nontechnical skill acquisition, training, and practice. Didactic training is helpful but likely insufficient as so many of these skills require practice in order to become habit, particularly when teams are under stress. Team training and coaching using simulation can help build and reinforce the use of these skills [96]. Team simulation is particularly effective to help members better understand the roles and responsibilities of others, and an after-action review provides opportunity to reflect and learn that is rare in the real world.

Crisis Preparation

Some institutions have developed topical (e.g., surgical fire), equipment-specific (e.g., robotic undocking), or specialty-specific crisis management simulations (e.g., code during bypass) [97, 98]. Team simulation is particularly useful for crisis training situations that involve performing procedures or using equipment that is unfamiliar. Crises magnify the importance of nontechnical skills, as crises require a clear understanding of team member roles, enhanced situational awareness, and much higher levels of communication and coordination among team members. Such training can reduce stress and may improve performance in a surgical emergency [99].

Institutional Culture and Policies

Institutions' culture and policies influence day-to-day activities within the operating room. Departmental/union policies affect the timing of intraoperative breaks for team members (ideally not allowed at critical points in the procedure), adherence to safety protocols, provision of regular staff education, and procedures for acquiring and safely rolling out new technology. Institutional resources are required to establish dedicated teams for complex procedures, increase team case familiarity, run crisis drills or simulations (OR fire, rapid robotic takedown, intraoperative code), coach/discipline individuals exhibiting disruptive behaviors, and streamline coordination with "invisible team members" (biomedical engineering/sterile supply/company reps/surgical scheduling) who profoundly impact routine OR functioning.

In summary, excellent patient outcomes are not just the product of a technically talented surgeon, but rely on a team functioning within a high-reliability organization dedicated to patient safety and learning. This chapter provided a variety of practical strategies to maximize intraoperative patient and surgeon safety and optimize surgeon and team performance.

References

1. Chrouser K, Foley F, Goldenberg M, Hyder J, Maranchie JK, Moore JM, et al. Optimizing outcomes in urological surgery: intraoperative patient safety and physiological considerations. Urol Pract. 2020;7(4):309–18.
2. Chrouser K, Kim FJ, Smith A, Stoffel JT, Goldenberg M. Optimizing outcomes in urologic surgery: intraoperative environmental, behavioral, and performance considerations. Urol Pract. 2020;7(5):405–12.
3. Davis SS. The key to safety: proactive prevention. Wiley Online Library; 2018.
4. Guideline for positioning the patient. In: Guidelines for perioperative practice. Association of periOperative Registered Nurses; 2018. p. 673–744.
5. Akhavan A, Gainsburg DM, Stock JA. Complications associated with patient positioning in urologic surgery. Urology. 2010;76(6):1309–16.
6. Winfree CJ, Kline DG. Intraoperative positioning nerve injuries. Surg Neurol. 2005;63(1):5–18.
7. Wilcox S, Vandam LD. Alas, poor Trendelenburg and his position! A critique of its uses and effectiveness. Anesth Analg. 1988;67(6):574–8.
8. Gainsburg DM, Wax D, Reich DL, Carlucci JR, Samadi DB. Intraoperative management of robotic-assisted versus open radical prostatectomy. JSLS: J Soc Laparoendosc Surg. 2010;14(1):1.
9. Phong S, Koh L. Anaesthesia for robotic-assisted radical prostatectomy: considerations for laparoscopy in the Trendelenburg position. Anaesth Intensive Care. 2007;35(2):281–5.
10. Weber ED, Colyer MH, Lesser RL, Subramanian PS. Posterior ischemic optic neuropathy after minimally invasive prostatectomy. J Neuroophthalmol. 2007;27(4):285–7.
11. Han ES, Advincula AP. Safety in minimally invasive surgery. Obstet Gynecol Clin N Am. 2019;46(2):389–98.
12. Abdalmageed OS, Bedaiwy MA, Falcone T. Nerve injuries in gynecologic laparoscopy. J Minim Invasive Gynecol. 2017;24(1):16–27.
13. Bjøro B, Mykkeltveit I, Rustøen T, Candas Altinbas B, Røise O, Bentsen SB. Intraoperative peripheral nerve injury related to lithotomy positioning with steep Trendelenburg in patients undergoing robotic-assisted laparoscopic surgery–a systematic review. J Adv Nurs. 2020;76(2):490–503.
14. Bradshaw AD, Advincula AP. Postoperative neuropathy in gynecologic surgery. Obstet Gynecol Clin N Am. 2010;37(3):451–9.
15. Das D, Propst K, Wechter ME, Kho RM. Evaluation of positioning devices for optimization of outcomes in laparoscopic and robotic-assisted gynecologic surgery. J Minim Invasive Gynecol. 2019;26(2):244–52.e1.
16. Steck-Bayat KP, Henderson S, Aguirre AG, Smith RB, Mahnert NM, Gerkin RD, et al. Prospective randomized controlled trial comparing cephalad migration in robotic gynecologic surgery using egg-crate foam versus the Pink Pad®. J Robot Surg. 2019;1–5.
17. Watson MJ, Koch B, Tonzi M, Xu R, Heath G, Lute B, et al. Decreasing the prospect of upper extremity neuropraxia during robotic assisted laparoscopic prostatectomy: a novel technique. J Robot Surg. 2020;14(5):733–8.
18. AORN bariatric surgery guideline. Perioperative standards and recommended practices. Association of periOperative Registered Nurses; 2010. p. 481–499.
19. Warner ME, LaMaster LM, Thoeming AK, Shirk Marienau ME, Warner MA. Compartment syndrome in surgical patients. J Am Soc Anesthesiol. 2001;94(4):705–8.
20. Warner MA, Martin JT, Schroeder DR, Offord KP, Chute CG. Lower-extremity motor neuropathy associated with surgery performed on patients in a lithotomy position. J Am Soc Anesthesiol. 1994;81(1):6–12.
21. Angermeier K, Jordan G. Complications of the exaggerated lithotomy position: a review of 177 cases. J Urol. 1994;151(4):866–8.
22. Bennicoff G. Perioperative care of the morbidly obese patient in the lithotomy position. AORN J. 2010;92(3):297–312.

23. Graling PR, Colvin DB. The lithotomy position in colon surgery. Postoperative complications. AORN J. 1992;55(4):1029–39.
24. Hales CM, Carroll MD, Fryar C, Ogden CL. Prevalence of obesity and severe obesity among adults. United States, 2017–2018. NCHS Data Brief. 2020;288:1–8.
25. Williamson J, Mahon D. Shouldering responsibility for intraoperative bariatric amputees. Ann R Coll Surg Engl. 2016;98(1):71.
26. Dauer L, Miller D, Schueler B, Silberzweig J, Balter S, Bartal G, et al. Society of Interventional Radiology Safety and Health Committee. Cardiovascular and Interventional Radiological Society of Europe Standards of Practice Committee Occupational radiation protection of pregnant or potentially pregnant workers in IR: a joint guideline of the Society of Interventional Radiology and the Cardiovascular and Interventional Radiological Society of Europe. J Vasc Interv Radiol. 2015;26(2):171–81.
27. Buisson-Valles I, Ollivier S, Gabinski P, Basse-Cathalinat B, Verdun-Esquer C, AQUITAINS MDT. Etat des lieux de la radioprotection dans les blocs opératoires des établissements privés et publics d'Aquitaine. Arch Mal Prof Environ. 2004;65(2–3):263.
28. Galonnier F, Traxer O, Rosec M, Terrasa J-B, Gouezel P, Celier D, et al. Surgical staff radiation protection during fluoroscopy-guided urologic interventions. J Endourol. 2016;30(6):638–43.
29. Spruce L. Back to basics: radiation safety. AORN J. 2017;106(1):42–9.
30. ACR-SPR practice parameter for imaging pregnant or potentially pregnant adolescents and women with ionizing radiation. 2018. https://www.acr.org/-/media/ACR/Files/Practice-Parameters/Pregnant-Pts.pdf. Accessed 4/11/2021.
31. Guidelines for radiation safety. Guidelines for perioperative practice. Denver: Association of PeriOperative Registered Nurses; 2017. p. 339–74.
32. Tok A, Akbas A, Aytan N, Aliskan T, Cicekbilek I, Kaba M, et al. Are the urology operating room personnel aware about the ionizing radiation? Int Braz J Urol. 2015;41(5):982–9.
33. Kuon E, Weitmann K, Hoffmann W, Dörr M, Hummel A, Busch M, et al. Role of experience, leadership and individual protection in the cath lab–a multicenter questionnaire and workshop on radiation safety. RöFo-Fortschritte auf dem Gebiet der Röntgenstrahlen und der bildgebenden Verfahren: © Georg Thieme Verlag KG; 2015. p. 899–905.
34. Tjiam IM, Goossens RH, Schout BM, Koldewijn EL, Hendrikx AJ, Muijtjens AM, et al. Ergonomics in endourology and laparoscopy: an overview of musculoskeletal problems in urology. J Endourol. 2014;28(5):605–11.
35. The State of Urology Workforce and Practice in the United States 2017. Linthicum. Maryland: American Urological Association; 2018.
36. Epstein S, Tran BN, Capone AC, Ruan QZ, Fukudome EY, Ricci JA, et al. The current state of surgical ergonomics education in US surgical training: a survey study. Ann Surg. 2019;269(4):778–84.
37. Kim-Fine S, Woolley SM, Weaver AL, Killian JM, Gebhart JB. Work-related musculoskeletal disorders among vaginal surgeons. Int Urogynecol J. 2013;24(7):1191–200.
38. Dolan L, Martin D. Backache in gynaecologists. Occup Med. 2001;51(7):433–8.
39. Meltzer AJ, Hallbeck MS, Morrow MM, Lowndes BR, Davila VJ, Stone WM, et al. Measuring ergonomic risk in operating surgeons by using wearable technology. JAMA Surg. 2020;155(5):444–6.
40. Lux MM, Marshall M, Erturk E, Joseph JV. Ergonomic evaluation and guidelines for use of the daVinci Robot system. J Endourol. 2010;24(3):371–5. https://doi.org/10.1089/end.2009.0197.
41. Berguer R, Hreljac A. The relationship between hand size and difficulty using surgical instruments: a survey of 726 laparoscopic surgeons. Surg Endosc. 2004;18(3):508–12. https://doi.org/10.1007/s00464-003-8824-3.
42. Stellon M, Seils D, Mauro C. Assessing the importance of surgeon hand anthropometry on the design of medical devices. J Med Devices. 2017;11(4).
43. Meredyth N. Cute little hands. Ann Surg. 2019;270(6):964–5.
44. Sutton E, Irvin M, Zeigler C, Lee G, Park A. The ergonomics of women in surgery. Surg Endosc. 2014;28(4):1051–5. https://doi.org/10.1007/s00464-013-3281-0.

45. Armijo PR, Flores L, Pokala B, Huang C-K, Siu K-C, Oleynikov D. Gender equity in ergonomics: does muscle effort in laparoscopic surgery differ between men and women? Surg Endosc. 2021:1–6.
46. Punnett L, Wegman DH. Work-related musculoskeletal disorders: the epidemiologic evidence and the debate. J Electromyogr Kinesiol. 2004;14(1):13–23.
47. Reyes D, Tang B, Cuschieri A. Minimal access surgery (MAS)-related surgeon morbidity syndromes. Surg Endosc Other Interv Tech. 2006;20(1):1–13.
48. Hullfish KL, Trowbridge ER, Bodine G. Ergonomics and gynecologic surgery: "surgeon protect thyself". Female Pelvic Med Reconstr Surg. 2009;15(6):435–9.
49. Singh R, Leon DAC, Morrow MM, Vos-Draper TL, Mc Gree ME, Weaver AL, et al. Effect of chair types on work-related musculoskeletal discomfort during vaginal surgery. Am J Obstet Gynecol. 2016;215(5):648.e1–9.
50. Zhu X, Yurteri-Kaplan LA, Gutman RE, Sokol AI, Iglesia CB, Park AJ, et al. Postural stress experienced by vaginal surgeons. Proceedings of the Human Factors and Ergonomics Society annual meeting. SAGE Publications Sage CA: Los Angeles; 2014. p. 763–7.
51. Catanzarite T, Tan-Kim J, Whitcomb EL, Menefee S. Ergonomics in surgery: a review. Female Pelvic Med Reconstr Surg. 2018;24(1):1–12.
52. Ronstrom C, Hallbeck S, Lowndes B, Chrouser KL. Surgical ergonomics. In: Surgeons as educators. Cham: Springer; 2018. p. 387–417.
53. Rosenblatt PL, McKinney J, Adams SR. Ergonomics in the operating room: protecting the surgeon. J Minim Invasive Gynecol. 2013;20(6):744.
54. Haramis G, Rosales JC, Palacios JM, Okhunov Z, Mues AC, Lee D, et al. Prospective randomized evaluation of FOOT gel pads for operating room staff COMFORT during laparoscopic renal surgery. Urology. 2010;76(6):1405–8.
55. Woodburn KL, Kho RM. Vaginal surgery: don't get bent out of shape. Am J Obstet Gynecol. 2020;223(5):762–3.
56. Gözen AS, Tokas T, Tschada A, Jalal A, Klein J, Rassweiler J. Direct comparison of the different conventional laparoscopic positions with the ethos surgical platform in a laparoscopic pelvic surgery simulation setting. J Endourol. 2015;29(1):95–9.
57. Liu S, Hemming D, Luo RB, Reynolds J, Delong JC, Sandler BJ, et al. Solving the surgeon ergonomic crisis with surgical exosuit. Surg Endosc. 2018;32(1):236–44.
58. Hallbeck MS, Lowndes BR, Bingener J, Abdelrahman AM, Yu D, Bartley A, et al. The impact of intraoperative microbreaks with exercises on surgeons: a multi-center cohort study. Appl Ergon. 2017;60:334–41. https://doi.org/10.1016/j.apergo.2016.12.006.
59. Abdelall ES, Lowndes BR, Abdelrahman AM, Hawthorne HJ, Hallbeck MS. Mini breaks, many benefits: development and pilot testing of an intraoperative microbreak stretch web-application for surgeons. Proceedings of the Human Factors and Ergonomics Society annual meeting. SAGE Publications Sage CA: Los Angeles; 2018. p. 1042–6.
60. Lloyd GL, Chung AS, Steinberg S, Sawyer M, Williams DH, Overbey D. Is your career hurting you? The ergonomic consequences of surgery in 701 urologists worldwide. J Endourol. 2019;33(12):1037–42.
61. Zebis MK, Andersen LL, Pedersen MT, Mortensen P, Andersen CH, Pedersen MM, et al. Implementation of neck/shoulder exercises for pain relief among industrial workers: a randomized controlled trial. BMC Musculoskelet Disord. 2011;12(1):1–9.
62. Fecso AB, Szasz P, Kerezov G, Grantcharov TP. The effect of technical performance on patient outcomes in surgery. Ann Surg. 2017;265(3):492–501.
63. Agha RA, Fowler AJ, Sevdalis N. The role of non-technical skills in surgery. Ann Med Surg. 2015;4(4):422–7.
64. Yule S, Flin R, Paterson-Brown S, Maran N. Non-technical skills for surgeons in the operating room: a review of the literature. Surgery. 2006;139(2):140–9.
65. Wood TC, Raison N, Haldar S, Brunckhorst O, McIlhenny C, Dasgupta P, et al. Training tools for nontechnical skills for surgeons—a systematic review. J Surg Educ. 2017;74(4):548–78.

66. Gawande AA, Thomas EJ, Zinner MJ, Brennan TA. The incidence and nature of surgical adverse events in Colorado and Utah in 1992. Surgery. 1999;126(1):66–75.
67. Christian CK, Gustafson ML, Roth EM, Sheridan TB, Gandhi TK, Dwyer K, et al. A prospective study of patient safety in the operating room. Surgery. 2006;139(2):159–73.
68. Valanci-Aroesty S, Alhassan N, Feldman LS, Landry T, Mastropietro V, Fiore J Jr, et al. Implementation and effectiveness of coaching for surgeons in practice–a mixed studies systematic review. J Surg Educ. 2020;77(4):837–53.
69. El-Gabri D, McDow AD, Quamme SP, Hooper-Lane C, Greenberg CC, Long KL. Surgical coaching for advancement of global surgical skills and capacity: a systematic review. J Surg Res. 2020;246:499–505.
70. Arora S, Miskovic D, Hull L, Moorthy K, Aggarwal R, Johannsson H, et al. Self vs expert assessment of technical and non-technical skills in high fidelity simulation. Am J Surg. 2011;202(4):500–6.
71. Larkin AC, Cahan MA, Whalen G, Hatem D, Starr S, Haley H-L, et al. Human Emotion and Response in Surgery (HEARS): a simulation-based curriculum for communication skills, systems-based practice, and professionalism in surgical residency training. J Am Coll Surg. 2010;211(2):285–92.
72. Edmondson AC, Higgins M, Singer S, Weiner J. Understanding psychological safety in health care and education organizations: a comparative perspective. Res Hum Dev. 2016;13(1):65–83.
73. Driskell JE, Copper C, Moran A. Does mental practice enhance performance? J Appl Psychol. 1994;79(4):481.
74. Sevdalis N, Moran A, Arora S. Mental imagery and mental practice applications in surgery: state of the art and future directions. Multisens Imagery. 2013:343–63.
75. Hall JC. Imagery practice and the development of surgical skills. Am J Surg. 2002;184(5):465–70.
76. Chrouser KL, Partin MR. Intraoperative disruptive behavior: the medical student's perspective. J Surg Educ. 2019;76(5):1231–40.
77. Villafranca A, Hamlin C, Enns S, Jacobsohn E. Disruptive behaviour in the perioperative setting: a contemporary review. Can J Anesth. 2017;64(2):128–40.
78. Wetzel CM, George A, Hanna GB, Athanasiou T, Black SA, Kneebone RL, et al. Stress management training for surgeons—a randomized, controlled, intervention study. Ann Surg. 2011;253(3):488–94.
79. Arora S, Aggarwal R, Sirimanna P, Moran A, Grantcharov T, Kneebone R, et al. Mental practice enhances surgical technical skills: a randomized controlled study. Ann Surg. 2011;253(2):265–70.
80. Percy DB, Streith L, Wong H, Ball CG, Widder S, Hameed M. Mental toughness in surgeons: is there room for improvement? Can J Surg. 2019;62(6):482.
81. Asken M, Christensen LW, Grossman D. Warrior mindset. 1st ed. Human Factors Research Group. US: warrior science publications. 2010.
82. Rogers D, Lingard L, Boehler ML, Espin S, Klingensmith M, Mellinger JD, et al. Teaching operating room conflict management to surgeons: clarifying the optimal approach. Med Educ. 2011;45(9):939–45.
83. Feldman J, Barshi I. The effects of blood glucose levels on cognitive performance: a review of the literature. NASA Ames Research Center: Moffett Field; 2007.
84. McCrimmon RJ, Ewing FM, Frier BM, Deary IJ. Anger state during acute insulin-induced hypoglycaemia. Physiol Behav. 1999;67(1):35–9.
85. Benton D, Owens D. Is raised blood glucose associated with the relief of tension? J Psychosom Res. 1993;37(7):723–35.
86. Chrouser KL, Xu J, Hallbeck S, Weinger MB, Partin MR. The influence of stress responses on surgical performance and outcomes: literature review and the development of the surgical stress effects (SSE) framework. Am J Surg. 2018;216(3):573–84.

87. El-Sharkawy AM, Bragg D, Watson P, Neal K, Sahota O, Maughan RJ, et al. Hydration amongst nurses and doctors on-call (the HANDS on prospective cohort study). Clin Nutr. 2016;35(4):935–42.
88. Pilcher JJ, Huffcutt AI. Effects of sleep deprivation on performance: a meta-analysis. Sleep. 1996;19(4):318–26.
89. Hull L, Arora S, Aggarwal R, Darzi A, Vincent C, Sevdalis N. The impact of nontechnical skills on technical performance in surgery: a systematic review. J Am Coll Surg. 2012;214(2):214–30.
90. Flin R, Yule S, McKenzie L, Paterson-Brown S, Maran N. Attitudes to teamwork and safety in the operating theatre. Surgeon. 2006;4(3):145–51.
91. Sittikraipong K, Silsupadol P, Uthaikhup S. Slower reaction and response times and impaired hand-eye coordination in individuals with neck pain. Musculoskelet Sci Pract. 2020;50:102273.
92. Huysmans MA, Hoozemans MJ, van der Beek AJ, de Looze MP, van Dieën JH. Position sense acuity of the upper extremity and tracking performance in subjects with non-specific neck and upper extremity pain and healthy controls. J Rehabil Med. 2010;42(9):876–83.
93. Moriarty O, Finn DP. Cognition and pain. Curr Opin Support Palliat Care. 2014;8(2):130–6.
94. Riskin A, Erez A, Foulk TA, Kugelman A, Gover A, Shoris I, et al. The impact of rudeness on medical team performance: a randomized trial. Pediatrics. 2015;136(3):487–95.
95. Rosenstein AH, O'Daniel M. Impact and implications of disruptive behavior in the perioperative arena. J Am Coll Surg. 2006;203(1):96–105.
96. Gordon M, Darbyshire D, Baker P. Non-technical skills training to enhance patient safety: a systematic review. Med Educ. 2012;46(11):1042–54.
97. Huser A-S, Müller D, Brunkhorst V, Kannisto P, Musch M, Kröpfl D, et al. Simulated life-threatening emergency during robot-assisted surgery. J Endourol. 2014;28(6):717–21.
98. Stevens L-M, Cooper JB, Raemer DB, Schneider RC, Frankel AS, Berry WR, et al. Educational program in crisis management for cardiac surgery teams including high realism simulation. J Thorac Cardiovasc Surg. 2012;144(1):17–24.
99. Arora S, Sevdalis N, Nestel D, Tierney T, Woloshynowych M, Kneebone R. Managing intraoperative stress: what do surgeons want from a crisis training program? Am J Surg. 2009;197(4):537–43.

Chapter 27
Experimental Therapies and Research Needs for Urinary Incontinence in Women

Casey G. Kowalik and Rena D. Malik

Abbreviations

ADSC	Adipose-derived stem cells
AMDCs	Autologous muscle-derived cells
OAB	Overactive bladder
P4HB	Poly-4-hydroxybutryate
PGI	Patient global impression
PRP	Platelet-rich plasma
SUI	Stress urinary incontinence
TTT	Tunable-tension transobturator tape
UMB	Urinary bladder matrix
UUI	Urgency urinary incontinence

Introduction

Currently available treatment options for urgency urinary incontinence (UUI) and stress urinary incontinence (SUI) have good outcomes with high patient satisfaction; however, the search for innovative options or modifications to existing therapies is ongoing with the goal of obtaining superior outcomes and fewer side effects.

C. G. Kowalik (✉)
Department of Urology, University of Kansas Health System, Kansas City, KS, USA
e-mail: ckowalik@kumc.edu

R. D. Malik
Department of Surgery, Division of Urology, University of Maryland School of Medicine, Baltimore, MD, USA
e-mail: rmalik@som.umaryland.edu

© The Author(s), under exclusive license to Springer Nature Switzerland AG 2022
A. P. Cameron (ed.), *Female Urinary Incontinence*,
https://doi.org/10.1007/978-3-030-84352-6_27

As a chronic condition, urinary incontinence has a financial impact, which reaches multiple billions of dollars annually [1]. These costs include, but are not limited to, the material costs of incontinence products, loss of income due to missed work, health-care costs related to treatment, and indirect costs such as depression, sexual dysfunction, and poor self-esteem related to urinary incontinence. The current management options for UUI include behavioral modifications, medical therapy with anticholinergics or β3 agonists, onabotulinum toxin injection into the bladder, and tibial or sacral neuromodulation. A new highly selective β3 agonist was recently approved for use in the United States and has demonstrated clinically significant reductions in UUI episodes and few adverse effects in clinical trials [2]. Advancements in neuromodulation technology, including the development of implantable tibial nerve stimulators and MRI-compatible sacral nerve stimulators, may offer additional treatment options to be available to a wider population of women desiring office-based procedures or requiring the use of MRI for other health-care conditions. Gene therapy utilizing a plasmid vector is currently under investigation, and emerging research in the arena of the urinary microbiome shows promise for individualized treatment of UUI. Mesh slings for the treatment of SUI have been in use since the mid-1990s, and modifications to improve outcomes and decrease adverse events continue to be made. For example, nonpermanent materials or drug-eluting mesh has been studied in animal models. Adjustable slings and tunable-tension slings are currently under clinical investigation. Radiofrequency and CO_2 laser therapy delivered via a transvaginal probe are commercially available, but data on improvements on SUI are still accumulating. Novel concepts including an intravesical device to reduce SUI by attenuating sudden increases in intra-abdominal pressures are also being explored in clinical studies. Researchers have been looking at regenerative therapy targeting the urethral sphincter with stem cells in animal models for several years, but recent clinical studies using autologous muscle-derived stem cells had promising results [3].

In this chapter, we review the latest medical therapy and technological advancements for the treatment of UUI and SUI. We conclude by identifying current limitations to research and proposing areas of the future study.

Novel Medical Therapies for Urgency Urinary Incontinence

Vibegron

Vibegron, a highly selective β3 agonist, is a recent addition to treatment options for UUI. Similar to its predecessor mirabegron, it attaches to the β3 adrenergic receptor and encourages relaxation of the bladder wall. Vibegron is unique in its >9000-fold selectivity for the β3 receptor over other β subtypes [4]. β3 selectivity may be attributed to vibegron's structural configuration with a pyrrolidine ring and resultant configuration of its arms for the activation of the β3 receptor [4]. Notably, the pharmaceutical has a mean half-life of 25–38 hours allowing for daily dosing and does not inhibit the CYP2D6 enzyme reducing the risk of drug–drug interactions.

Vibegron's efficacy was analyzed in a four-arm, double-blind, placebo-controlled randomized controlled trial in Japan [5]. Patients with the presence of overactive bladder (OAB) symptoms for at least 6 months were included in the trial and underwent a placebo run-in phase for 2 weeks. Subsequently, they were randomized to one of four treatment groups: vibegron (50 mg or 100 mg once daily), placebo, or anticholinergic therapy with imidafenacin (0.1 mg twice daily) for a total of 12 weeks. The primary outcome evaluated was a change in the mean number of micturitions per day from baseline to study end. In the 50-mg and 100-mg vibegron group, the change in least squares mean of daily micturition episodes from baseline was −2.08 and −2.03 in the 100-mg vibegron group, respectively, compared to −1.21 in the placebo group ($p < 0.001$). In regard to UUI, the 100-mg and 50-mg vibegron groups demonstrated a reduction in daily UUI episodes with a least squares mean change of −1.47 and −1.35, respectively. The study also identified significant improvements for both doses of vibegron in daily urgency, nocturia episodes, and scores on the validated King's Health Questionnaire domains and satisfaction on the Patient Global Impression (PGI). Adverse events were low (5.6–7.6%) with most common including nasopharyngitis and cystitis. In the severe UUI subgroup (≥ 3 episodes daily), significant improvements were noted in the reduction of UUI (−2.95 and −3.28 UUI episodes/day for 50-mg and 100-mg dose, respectively), voided volume, and PGI with both 50 mg and 100 mg. Improvements in urgency were only noted in the 100-mg dose group with increased diary dry rates significant only for the 50-mg dose (37.5% vs 17.9%, $p = 0.020$) [6].

In the international phase III trial, EMPOWUR, 1518 OAB patients, of which 75% had UUI, were randomized to receive 75 mg vibegron daily, 4 mg tolterodine ER daily, or placebo with a coprimary endpoint of change in UUI episodes from baseline to 12 weeks. The vibegron group had a statistically significant decrease in daily UUI episodes at 12 weeks compared with placebo. Adverse events in the vibegron group compared with placebo included headache (4.0% vs 2.4%), nasopharyngitis (2.8% vs 1.7%), diarrhea (2.2% vs 1.1%), and nausea (2.2% vs 1.1%). Hypertension was not noted to be significantly higher than rates of placebo [2]. In extension trials up to 52 weeks, further reduction in UUI was noted with 61% of patients having a ≥75% reduction in UUI, and 41% were dry at week 52, as well as reporting sustained improvements in their quality of life [7, 8].

In a systematic review and pooled analysis of three randomized controlled trials, including a total of 2120 patients with OAB, it was again concluded that vibegron significantly reduced the number of UUI, urinary urgency, and increased volume voided per micturition, with improvements in quality of life over 12 weeks. In addition to nasopharyngitis and cystitis, dry mouth and constipation were also listed as adverse effects [9]. Vibegron (under the trade name of Gemtesa®) was approved by the US Food and Drug Administration in December 2020.

Gene Therapy

Gene therapy utilizing a plasmid vector is currently under investigation for the treatment of UUI. *Uro-902* is a plasmid vector expressing the big potassium channel alpha subunit, which is normally highly expressed on the bladder smooth muscle cells, and activation reduces smooth cell excitability and hence detrusor overactivity [10]. Phase I, double-blind, placebo-controlled, sequential active dose trials have been completed comparing intravesical instillation (ION-02) versus direct injection (ION-03) of the plasmid vector in females with urodynamic detrusor overactivity and symptoms of OAB. In the intravesical instillation arm, seven patients received the 5000 μg dose, six received the 10,000 μg dose, and five received placebo. In the direct injection arm, six patients received the 16,000 μg dose, three received the 24,000 μg dose, and four received placebo. In terms of safety, in the ION-02 arm, one patient had a Mobitz type II second-degree AV block and one had fatigue, headache, shaking chills, and insomnia. In the ION-03 arm, most OAB parameters and quality of life had significant improvements compared with placebo; however, UUI did not. UUI did improve from baseline significantly up to 24 weeks after treatment. There were no increases in postvoid residual compared with placebo in either group. While trials are still in early phases, data seem promising for a therapeutic option that has longer treatment duration without the risk of urinary retention.

Technological Advancements in Neuromodulation

Implantable Tibial Nerve Stimulation

Percutaneous tibial nerve stimulation is a treatment option for UUI; however, it requires weekly office visits for 12 weeks followed by maintenance visits every 4–6 weeks. Due to the inconvenience of requiring several office visits, implantable devices are being explored (Table 27.1). BlueWind RENOVA™ (BlueWind Medical, Herzliya, Israel) is a cylindrical (3.4 mm in diameter, 25 mm in length) battery-less unit that is implanted in close proximity to the tibial nerve and used with an external stimulator shaped as a cuff that goes around the ankle (Fig. 27.1). It is suggested to use 30 min daily with available modifications for pulse width (50–800 μs), amplitude (0–9 mA), and frequency (5–40 Hz). Six-month follow-up of 34 patients implanted with the device revealed 71% achieving a >50% improvement in UUI and a 27.8% dry rate [11, 12]. However, adverse events included implant site pain in 14%, suspected infection in 22%, and wound complications in 8.3% of participants.

eCoin™ (Valencia, California, the USA) is the only fully-implanted tibial nerve stimulator with a leadless design and a primary battery with the size and shape of a US nickel (23.3 mm in diameter and 2.3 mm thick) (Fig. 27.2). It is implanted subcutaneously above the fascia in the outpatient setting using local anesthesia. The

Table 27.1 Summary of implantable tibial nerve stimulation design, use, and clinical trials

Device	Design	Use	Patient-wearable	Clinical programmer	Patient remote control	Author, year	N	Follow-up (months)	≥50% UUI improvement	≥50% severe UUI improvement	Dry rate
BlueWind RENOVA™ (BlueWind Medical, Herzliya, Israel)	Leadless, battery-less, implant (0.3 cm³ volume, diameter 3.4 mm)	Daily, 30 min self-administered	✓	✓	✓	Van Breda, 2017 [70]	11	3	36.4%	71%[a]	18.2%
						Heesakkers, 2018 [11]	29	6	51.7%	NR	27.6%
						Dorsthorst, 2020 [71]	16[b]	36	50%	75–80%[b]	NR
						Dmochowski, 2019 [72]	20	36	75%[c]	NR	NR
eCoin™ (Valencia, CA, USA)	Fully implanted, primary battery, leadless (23.3 mm diameter, 2.3 mm thick), 3-year battery life	Automatic stimulation delivered 30 min twice weekly				MacDiarmid, 2019 [73]	46	6	67.4%	NR	23.9%
						MacDiarmid, 2019 [74]	46	12	65%	NR	26.1%
						Rogers, 2020 [13]	122	8.3	73.0%	NR	30.3%
StimGuard® now Protect PNS (Micron Medical Boca Raton, FL, USA)	Wireless tined lead, rechargeable external power source	Daily stimulation for 6+ hours	✓			Sirls, 2019 [18]	7	12	–	–	–
Bioness StimRouter™	Tined lead, integrated receiver, external pulse transmitter worn externally	30-min sessions for 3–7 days per week	✓		✓	Giusto, 2019 [16]	–	–	–	–	–

NR not reported

[a]Severe UUI = baseline large amount of UI episodes on voiding diary

[b]Extension trial of Heesakkers et al., 75% in per protocol treatment group and 80% in intention to treat, treatment group

[c]Success defined as ≥50% reduction in urgent voids or leaks or normalization of voids

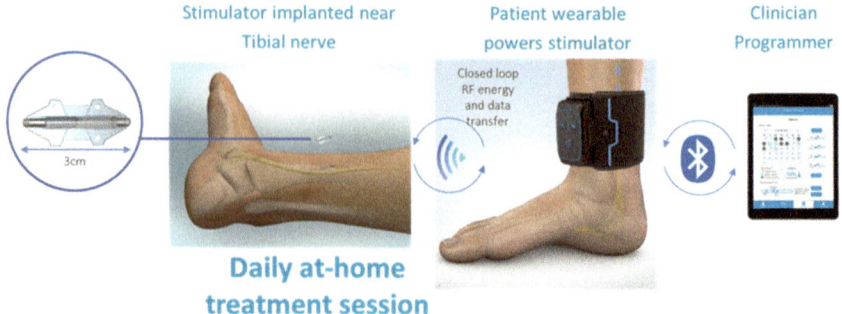

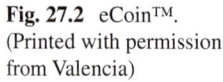

Fig. 27.1 BlueWind RENOVA™. (Printed with permission from BlueWind Medical)

Fig. 27.2 eCoin™.
(Printed with permission
from Valencia)

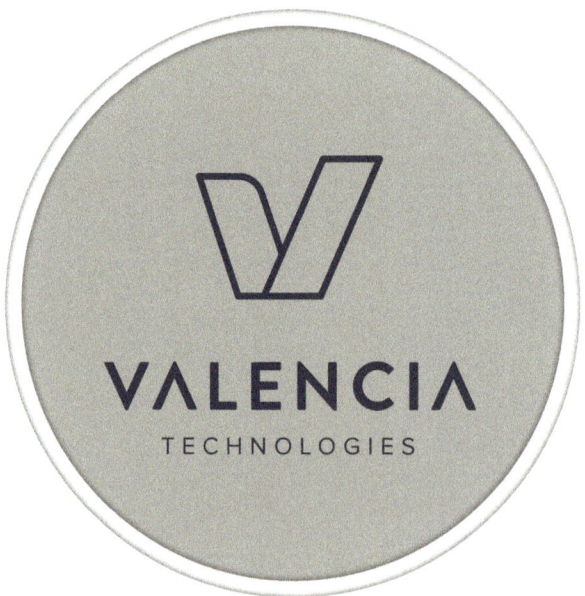

device delivers automatic stimulation for 30 min twice weekly from the center cathode to the anode electrode at the outermost edge. It does not require constant stimulation, recharging, remote use, or repeat office visits. The battery life averages 3 years. It has been trialed in 46 patients with OAB, of which 73% of patients reduced their UUI by 50% or more, with 30% being dry at up to 36-week follow-up. Infection rate was low at 2.3% [13].

Initial data for both BlueWind RENOVA™ and eCoin™ seem promising with improvements in UUI similar to current third-line therapies. Recruitment is ongoing, and long-term follow-up data are being collected [14, 15]. Other implants with limited data available currently include StimGuard® and Bioness [16, 17]. StimGuard® (now Protect PNS) is a wireless implantable tibial tined lead completed in the outpatient setting associated with a rechargeable external power source (Fig. 27.3). Initial data on seven implantations suggested improvement in UUI

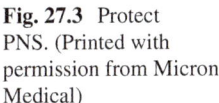

Fig. 27.3 Protect PNS. (Printed with permission from Micron Medical)

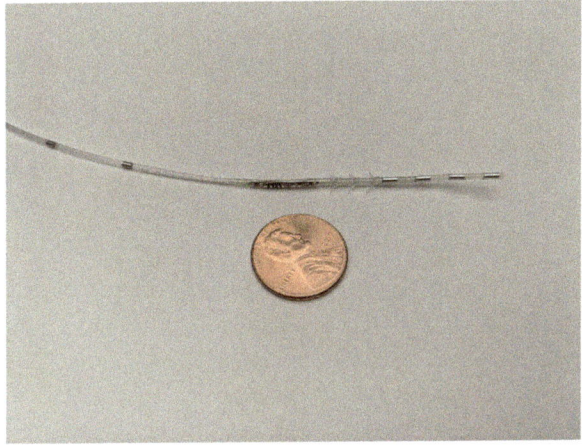

within 6 months of implantation with UUI episodes decreasing from 3.05 to 1.24. Data on three patients at 12 months suggested further improvement to 0.66 UUI episodes per day [18]. Five minor adverse events were reported including lead tenting, suture erosion, and loss of stimulation [19]. Currently, a prospective, randomized, controlled, multicenter study comparing wireless tibial neuromodulation (Chronic Afferent Nerve Stimulation [CAN-Stim]) to standard sacral neuromodulation is actively recruiting with a goal of 150 participants with a primary endpoint of ≥50% reduction in UUI episodes at 3 months [20].

Bioness StimRouter™ is an implanted lead design with an integrated receiver, an anchor, and three electrode contacts (Fig. 27.4). Wireless energy is delivered using an external pulse transmitter attached to an electrode patch to be worn externally. A patient programmer is used to change programs and monitor usage. The device is implanted in the outpatient setting under ultrasound guidance. Suggested treatments are 30-min sessions for 3–7 days per week. Recruitment is currently ongoing for a prospective, multicenter, randomized, double-blind, clinical trial of 180 patients comparing the StimRouter to sham treatment [21]. The external component of the tibial nerve systems is not MRI-compatible and must be removed prior to MRI, but the implanted lead can remain. Implantable tibial nerve devices offer the benefit of implantation in an office-based setting with local anesthesia using anatomic landmarks without the need for fluoroscopy compared with currently available sacral neuromodulation stimulators.

Sacral Neuromodulation

Constant current, rechargeable, and MRI-compatible neuromodulation systems have emerged as treatment options for UUI. The constant current technology automatically adjusts current based on changes in impedance to deliver consistent levels

Fig. 27.4 Bioness StimRouter™. (Printed with permission from Bioness)

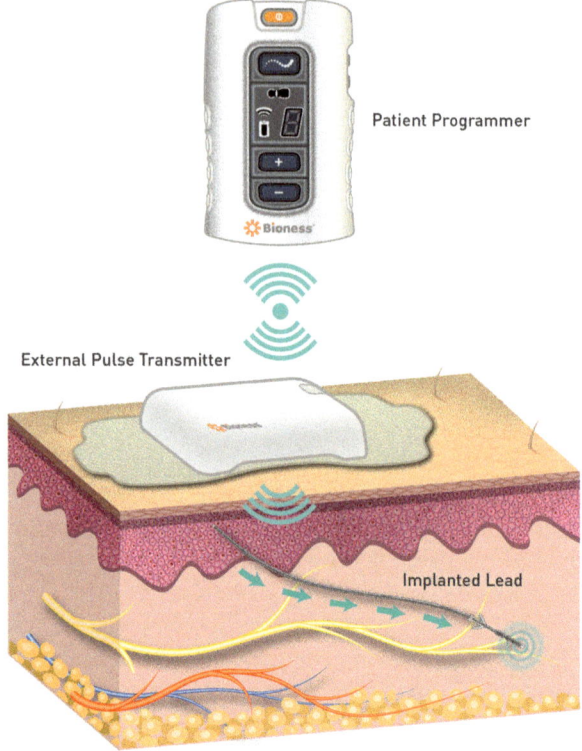

Patient Programmer

External Pulse Transmitter

Implanted Lead

of stimulation. Initial data suggest that this may be beneficial particularly in the first 6 months after implantation at which time impedance increases most significantly [22]. Rechargeable batteries offer a number of benefits including smaller size (Axonics 5.5 cm^3 volume & InterStim Micro 2.8 cm^3 volume) compared with standard implantable pulse generators (14 cm^3 volume) and an extended lifetime of an estimated 15 years. It is anticipated that further modifications will continue to be made in current sacral neuromodulation systems to continue to optimize and standardize lead placement and allow ease of use for the patient.

Targeted Therapy for Urgency Urinary Incontinence

Microbiome

The role of the microbiome in maintaining bladder health is still being uncovered, and some researchers are evaluating the influence of the microbiome on urinary incontinence. In a comparison of catheterized urine samples from women with and without UUI, there were notable differences in the microbiomes of each cohort suggesting that the urinary microbiome is involved in the complex understanding of lower urinary tract symptoms [23]. Furthering the concept that the urinary microbiome has a role in UUI and may help guide individualized treatment was a study by Thomas-White et al. This group examined the urine of women with UUI and found that those women with fewer bacteria and less diversity in their microbiota were more likely to have a clinical response to solifenacin medical therapy [24].

Nonsurgical Options for Stress Urinary Incontinence

Pelvic floor muscle training through physical therapy and biofeedback has been shown in multiple studies not only to improve urinary incontinence, but also to help with prevention. Pulsed magnetic stimulation and electrical stimulation are two technologies aimed at improving pelvic floor muscle contractions. Whether these therapies will gain more widespread acceptance in the United States is likely dependent on insurance coverage, because otherwise the treatments can be costly.

Pulsed Magnetic Stimulation

Pulsed magnetic stimulation is a nonsurgical treatment with varying reported success rates for the treatment of SUI. The proposed mechanism is that pelvic floor muscles are stimulated with resultant contraction by magnetic coils that generate electromagnetic fields. Treatment is generally twice weekly 20-min sessions done in office on a device that resembles a chair. Short-term (2-month) results in a blinded, sham-controlled study of 120 women who underwent twice weekly sessions showed an improvement in subjective urinary incontinence symptoms [25].

Electrical Stimulation

The advantage of electrical stimulation is that treatment can be done at home. A Cochrane review of electrical stimulation concluded that there is a benefit compared to placebo, but it was not possible to make adequate comparisons with traditional pelvic floor physical therapy [26]. External and intravaginal delivery of electrical stimulation has been compared in a randomized trial and shown that external delivery was noninferior to intravaginal electrical stimulation and there were fewer urinary tract infections with external delivery [27].

Slings for Stress Urinary Incontinence

Mid-urethral mesh slings for the treatment of SUI have long been the gold standard for surgical care due to their minimally invasive nature, fast convalescence, and high rates of efficacy. However, synthetic materials are known to generate foreign body reaction and have a risk of postoperative mesh complications. To minimize these complications and increase viscoelasticity, a search for alternative sling materials or nonpermanent materials has been ongoing. Types of biomaterials utilized include the following: (1) synthetic materials enhanced with platelet-rich plasma (PRP) or seeded with human fibroblasts, which may offer improved biocompatibility or decreased inflammatory cell reaction, and (2) extracellular matrix (ECM) alone, cell-seeded or enhanced, which offers the additional benefit of being biodegradable and activating host cell remodeling and collagen deposition. ECM-based materials include cadaveric human dermis, small intestinal submucosa, and urinary bladder matrix (UBM). Also, electrospun materials, technique whereby scaffold is developed by voltage-driven process of a polymer solution, have potentially improved tensile strength and closely mimic physiologic microarchitecture [28]. Enhanced or cell-seeded synthetic materials have been limited to evaluation in prolapse repair in animal models. In these models, implantation of PRP enhanced polypropylene mesh, and collagen-coated polypropylene mesh resulted in reduced inflammatory cell infiltrate and increased collagen production showing improved biocompatibility [29, 30].

Small studies have utilized ECMs for the repair of pelvic organ prolapse with encouraging results; however, due to heterogeneity in manufacturing, processing, materials, small sample sizes, and limitations in the clinical study design, the value of ECMs remains unclear [31]. There is limited contemporary evaluation of ECM for sling material in clinical trials. Currently, cell-seeded ECMs have been under further investigation. UBM and anti-Sca-1 and basic fibroblast growth factor have been cross-linked to recruit host stem cells and result in smooth muscle differentiation. Preclinical studies indicate this unique combination resulted in a biocompatible scaffold with potential for use in pelvic floor reconstruction [32].

Electrospinning is a process of using electric charge to randomly deposit polymer nanoparticles in a random pattern to mimic human physiologic architecture and subsequently facilitate cell attachment and growth [33]. Rabbit models of electrospun polypropylene for SUI have shown increased tensile strength and reduced inflammatory response in comparison with conventional polypropylene mid-urethral sling materials [34]. In vitro studies of adipose-derived stem cells (ADSCs) impregnated with biodegradable materials including electrospun poly-lactic acid with trimethylene carbonate and poly(L-lactide)–trimethylene carbonate–glycolide have been evaluated and have found to result in increased tensile strength, ECM deposition, and angiogenesis [35, 36]. Additionally electrospun synthetic polyurethane with the inclusion of 17-β-estradiol have also been evaluated on human ADSCs and revealed angiogenic potential with suitable tensile strength and ECM production [37].

Nonpermanent Sling Materials

An implant using a single-layer monofilament utilizing biodegradable poly-4-hydroxybutyrate (P4HB), TephaFLEX™, is considered a possible alternative to permanent mesh materials currently utilized for SUI. It is estimated that P4HB undergoes a gradual loss of strength after 3 months with full resorption between 18 and 24 months. In rabbit models comparison of P4HB crochet weave, net weave, and permanent polypropylene mesh, implantation resulted in a similar histologic response with P4HB having higher tensile strength and lowest inflammatory reaction [38]. The TephaFLEX™ sling is currently under investigation in a prospective 24-month single-center observational trial of estimated 25 patients with SUI with a primary outcome of device safety and measurement of treatment-emergent adverse events [39].

Drug-Eluting and Coated Mesh

Local delivery of drugs around the surgical site by mesh has been studied in pelvic organ prolapse. The use of a drug-eluting system that delivers antibiotics resulted in decreased short-term postoperative infection rates while maintaining structural integrity of the mesh [40]. While not specifically studied in mid-urethral slings, the concept is something that could be translated.

Steroid-coated mesh has been studied in animal models with the theory that the steroids will reduce local foreign body reaction. One study found decreased granuloma size, reduced number of inflammatory cells, and decreased collagen formation with the use of mesh coated with steroids [41].

Adjustable Slings

Additional optimization of current mid-urethral slings with adjustable tension is also under investigation. The Altis® sling is a mini, adjustable sling with an integrated tensioning system. Initial prospective industry-sponsored multicenter trials recruited 113 women, and 90% achieved a ≥50% reduction in pad weight with an 81% dry rate (pad weight ≤4 gm). There were also significant improvements in symptom bother and quality of life questionnaires up to 24 months [42]. In an unsponsored, prospective, single-center trial, 110 women were recruited with 83% objective (negative cough stress test) and 88% subjective cure (ICIQ-SF = 0) rates. Complications included 7% with acute urinary retention, 8% with voiding dysfunction, and 7% with pain [43]. A prospective, observational cohort study comparing the Altis® sling to traditional transobturator and retropubic slings has recently completed accrual with 416 participants and results pending. Primary outcomes included reduction in pad weight of ≥50% at 6-month follow-up and device- and/or procedure-related adverse events through 36 months. Adverse events were notable for a 3.5% mesh exposure rate similar to that of traditional mid-urethral slings [44]. Additionally, ongoing, prospective, postmarket, single-arm, multicenter studies are recruiting in Europe [45] (Clinicaltrials.gov Identifier: NCT02049840).

Tunable-tension transobturator tape (TTT), Urosling-T (Lintex, LLC), is a transobturator mid-urethral sling with the ability to modulate tension in the early postoperative periods. A randomized controlled trial enrolling 388 participants to receive the TTT or standard transobturator mid-urethral sling is currently under investigation with a primary outcome of absence of urinary leakage during the International Continence Society–uniform cough stress test [46] (Clinicaltrials.gov Identifier: NCT03958695).

Regenerative Treatments for Stress Urinary Incontinence

Stem Cell Therapy

Research on the use of stem cells in the treatment of SUI has been ongoing, starting with animal models going back several years. More recently, human trials have been underway with the injection of cells into the urethral sphincter. The science behind the effectiveness of stem cells is not well defined, but proposed etiologies include the following: (1) incorporation of injected cells into host cells, (2) release of local factors from the stem cells which can help repair injured host cells, and (3) actual cell differentiation of the stem cells into other cell types. In the case of SUI, there may also be some bulking effects on the urethral sphincter that improves symptoms [47].

Multiple cell types have been looked at including skeletal muscle cells (myoblasts, progenitor cells), bone marrow stem cells, adipose-derived stem cells (ADSCs), and human umbilical cells, with the most promising being autologous muscle-derived cells (AMDCs) (Table 27.2) [3, 48–53]. In a pilot study, Carr et al. injected AMDCs, harvested from thigh muscle, into eight women with SUI and noted a sustained improvement in pad weight at 10 months [48]. Further dose finding and safety trials have found that intrasphincteric injection of AMDC is safe, with biopsy site pain and bruising being reported in three of 38 women. There was also a statistically significant reduction in pad weight [3]. In phase I and II studies, no adverse events attributed to the cells were reported, and procedure-related complications were minor (bruising/pain) [53]. An ongoing phase III randomized, placebo-controlled trial is recruiting women with SUI (ClinicalTrials.gov Identifier: NCT03104517).

Table 27.2 Clinical trials in women with stress urinary incontinence using mesenchymal stem cells

Mesenchymal stem cell type	Study	Site of cell harvest	Study design	Clinical results
Autologous muscle-derived cells	Carr et al. [48]	Thigh	Pilot, $n = 8$	Five completed study, one with cure and four with decreased pad weight at 10 months
	Carr et al. [3]	Quadriceps femoris	Prospective cohort, $n = 38$	33 completed study
	Mitterberger et al. [49]	Biceps	Prospective cohort, $n = 123$	40% improvement in MUCP, 79% subjective cure rate
	Gras et al. [50]	Vastus lateralis	Prospective cohort, $n = 35$	Subjective and objective cure in 14%, improvement in another 37%
	Sebe et al. [51]	Deltoid	Prospective cohort, $n = 12$	25% subjectively dry, 58% improved on pad testing at 12 months
	Blaganje et al. [52]	Biceps	Prospective cohort, $n = 38$, electrical stimulation of cells postinjection	23% cured and 52% improved at 6 months
	Peters et al. [53]	Quadriceps femoris	Pooled data from phase I/II trials, $n = 80$	Subjective improvements at 12 months, higher dose (200×10^6 AMDC-USR) had reduction in pad weight
Adipose-derived stem cells	Kuismanen et al. [54]	Abdominal wall	Prospective cohort, $n = 5$	Improvement in patient-reported outcomes, no difference in urodynamic parameters at 1 year
Human cord blood stem cells	Lee et al. [55]	Umbilical cord vein	Prospective cohort, $n = 39$	80% subjective improvement at 3 months, improved MUCP in 10/10 women

Adipose-derived stem cells (ADSCs) have also been shown to undergo cell differentiation and have been injected into the urethral sphincter in five women [54]. Another research group has studied periurethral injection of human cord stem cells into 30 women with SUI. At 3 months postinjection, 80% reported improved subjective outcomes, and of the 10 women with low preprocedure maximum urethral closure pressures (MUCP), there were significant increases [55]. No trials in humans have been done using bone marrow stem cells, to date, largely due to the inability to harvest large numbers of cells needed and pain associated with bone marrow biopsy.

Low-Intensity Extracorporeal Shockwave Therapy

Animal models have demonstrated that applying low-intensity extracorporeal shockwave therapy (LiSWT) to the lower pelvis activates myotube formation and enhances cell regeneration [56, 57]. The hypothesis is that LiSWT can mobilize stem cells to the site of injury and thereby decrease inflammation, increase pelvic floor blood supply, and enhance bladder stem cell activation, which may lead to decreased detrusor overactivity and improved function of urethral sphincter. In theory, this technique could decrease both UUI and SUI symptoms in women. There is an ongoing randomized (experimental arm with LiSWT vs. sham treatment) clinical trial in Taiwan utilizing LiSWT for the treatment of urinary incontinence (ClinicalTrials.gov Identifier: NCT04059133). In recent years, this therapy has been used for the treatment of erectile dysfunction with variable success. If successful at improving clinical outcomes, LiSWT could become a novel, noninvasive, and widely available approach for female urinary incontinence treatment.

Other Technological Advancements for Stress Urinary Incontinence

Radiofrequency

Cryogen-cooling monopolar radiofrequency (CMRF) devices have been trialed for the treatment of SUI. Initially utilized to treat female sexual dysfunction and vaginal laxity, these devices work by using a vaginal probe that delivers simultaneous monopolar radiofrequency energy to the lamina propria and cryogen cooling to the superficial mucosal layer of the vaginal epithelium. This results in fibroblast activation and collagen production and increased pelvic floor support [58]. In a randomized unblinded trial at a single center of women with mild–moderate SUI (up to 50-gm leakage on a 1-hour pad weight test), 35 patients were randomized to receive either one or two CMRF treatments delivered 6 weeks apart in an office-based setting. The treatment consisted of 220 pulses of 90 J/cm^2 with 25 pulses delivered to four quadrants at the vaginal introitus sparing the area directly underneath the urethra. In both groups, 50–54% of women achieved $\geq 50\%$ reduction in 1-hour pad weight test and 75% achieved cure, or ≤ 1-gm leakage, on 1-hour pad weight in the single CMRF treatment arm at 12 months. No adverse events to the procedure were noted with the exception of one patient having two urinary tract infections during the trial period [59]. While data in this small single-center study are promising, further large-scale randomized controlled trials are needed to confirm results. A randomized single-blind controlled trial comparing CMRF to cryogen-only treatment and sham for patients with mild–moderate SUI has recently been completed pending publication of results [60].

Laser Therapies

Thermoablative fractional CO_2 laser works by inducing collagen denaturation, remodeling, and neogenesis resulting in subsequent increase in elasticity of tissues. Its use transvaginally has been studied for the treatment of SUI in women with symptoms of the genitourinary syndrome of menopause (GSM) [61]. GSM is characterized by thinning of the vaginal epithelium, loss of rugae, alterations in pH, and bacterial flora. In this investigation, 161 postmenopausal women, aged 45–65 years, received one 30- to 45-min laser treatment with the SmartXide[2] V[2]LR fractional microablative CO_2 laser system at the urethrovesical junction followed by yearly sessions as 12, 24, and 36 months. Patients demonstrated significant improvements in 1-hour pad weight tests and SUI based on the validated ICIQ-UI-SF, and histological changes confirmed thickened vaginal epithelium and improved organization of the lamina propria.

In a systematic review of both CO2 and erbium laser treatments for female SUI including 13 studies and 764 patients, significant improvements in ICIQ-SF and 1-hour pad weight were noted at 6 months after a single treatment and out to 24 months with repeated treatments. However, further high-quality investigations are needed to determine the laser type and duration of treatment for optimal results in women with SUI [62].

Vesair® Intravesical Balloon

The Vesair® intravesical balloon is an intravesical polyurethane balloon that is free-floating at the bladder dome meant to attenuate intravesical pressure generated by abdominal pressure increases. This novel device is inflated with 30 mL of air, floats at the bladder dome, and absorbs the pressure generated during transient increases in intravesical pressure during stressful activities that typically result in SUI [63]. The device has completed phase III trials in the United States with 12-month follow-up with promising safety and efficacy data. In the multicenter, randomized, sham-controlled trial, 221 women with SUI and >5 gm pad weight on provocative stress test were randomized to receive the device or a sham procedure. The device is inserted using a proprietary urethral access sheath using cystoscopic guidance and inflated with 30 mL of air and 0.7 mL of liquid perfluorocarbon. At 12 months, 54.7% of treated patients with the balloon achieved the composite endpoint of >75% decrease in pad weight and a 10-point increase in the Incontinence Quality of Life Scale. However, less than half of the patients in the treatment arm remained in the study at 12 months with 84% of those exiting the study due to intolerability of the device or adverse events including irritation, suprapubic discomfort, urgency, or urinary tract infection. While the data are encouraging in the select patients who tolerated the therapy, further investigation in defining the optimal patient population and potential revisions to the balloon to reduce discomfort are needed.

Current Limitations to Research for Urinary Incontinence

Despite all the great advancements in urinary incontinence research, there are still some factors that currently limit widespread comparisons between studies. In the assessment of SUI, leak point pressure (LPP) has a defined threshold for defining intrinsic sphincter deficiency (<60 cmH$_2$O), but the determination of LPP is not standardized between research groups making comparisons between studies difficult. Differences in the methods used to provoke SUI, between pressure recording sites (bladder or urethra), and/or the type of pressure transducer used are not uniform. The International Continence Society has published guidelines on the performance of urodynamics, but also acknowledges that diverse techniques prevail [64].

The development of an animal model for urinary incontinence remains challenging. Most often this is done utilizing an acute insult, resulting in pelvic floor weakness rather than a chronic process, which is how these conditions typically evolve in women.

While the economic burden of urinary incontinence is substantial, so are the costs associated with clinical research. Cost data were analyzed on new market therapeutic agents between 2009 and 2018 and their associated spending on research and development. The median investments to bring a drug to market was $985 million [65]. Furthermore, decreases in NIH grant funding further compound the financial difficulties of conducting high-quality research needed to ensure safe delivery of new treatments to patients [66].

Strategies for Future Research

Novel therapeutics aimed at preventive approaches to urinary incontinence would be a welcome addition to current paradigms that often focus on treatment rather than on prevention. The increasing availability of Internet access combined with familiarity using social media has allowed educational content about urinary incontinence to reach broader audiences [67]. As a result, younger audiences can be targeted with content aimed at prevention. Furthermore, the development of mobile applications and other Internet-based interventions is in progress, and these avenues can be used to distribute information and potentially recruit participants for research trials.

We know urinary incontinence can result from multiple etiologies, and individual subtyping of urinary incontinence may play a major role in the future as we understand more about the underlying causes. Personalized treatment of urinary incontinence based on etiology, anatomy, and genetic factors may result in improved patient outcomes. With more widespread availability of 3D printing technology, tailoring surgical technique to an individual patient's anatomy may become a reality. For example, device-manufacturing companies may be able to commercially produce mesh that is patient-specific for the degree of urethral hypermobility or other variables, such as tensile strength. Paul et al. have combined stem cell and 3D printing technology to bioprint endometrial mesenchymal stromal cells from endometrial lining onto a mesh for potential therapy of pelvic organ prolapse [68]. This concept of tissue engineering may also have a role in the use of mesh slings for SUI.

Further work in the identification of biomarkers important in UUI and SUI may help to guide individualized treatments for women based on the biochemical makeup of their urine. While this has been studied in the past without significant revelations, it may be worth additional investigation as an understanding of different OAB phenotypes emerges [69].

Conclusion

While the current treatment options are effective, there is always a desire for improvements, and the evolving research in pharmacology, gene therapy, and neuromodulation for UUI and regenerative medicine for SUI is promising. For treatments to advance, new technologies must undergo rigorous evaluation from preclinical studies to postmarket analyses. These evaluations should be standardized and reproducible with quantifiable outcome measures in order to allow for multiple studies for confirmatory data. We hope there will continue to be an increase in new medical therapy and technology to improve the quality of lives of women suffering from urinary incontinence.

References

1. Ward-Smith P. The cost of urinary incontinence. Urol Nurs. 2009;29(3):188–94.
2. Staskin D, Frankel J, Varano S, Shortino D, Jankowich R, Mudd PN. International phase III, randomized, double-blind, placebo and active controlled study to evaluate the safety and efficacy of vibegron in patients with symptoms of overactive bladder: EMPOWUR. J Urol. 2020;204(2):316–24.
3. Carr LK, Robert M, Kultgen PL, Herschorn S, Birch C, Murphy M, et al. Autologous muscle derived cell therapy for stress urinary incontinence: a prospective, dose ranging study. J Urol. 2013;189(2):595–601.
4. Di Salvo J, Nagabukuro H, Wickham LA, Abbadie C, DeMartino JA, Fitzmaurice A, et al. Pharmacological characterization of a novel beta 3 adrenergic agonist, vibegron: evaluation of antimuscarinic receptor selectivity for combination therapy for overactive bladder. J Pharmacol Exp Ther. 2017;360(2):346–55.
5. Yoshida M, Takeda M, Gotoh M, Nagai S, Kurose T. Vibegron, a novel potent and selective β3-adrenoreceptor a8, 16gonist, for the treatment of patients with overactive bladder: a randomized, double-blind, placebo-controlled phase 3 study. Eur Urol. 2018;73(5):783–90.
6. Yoshida M, Takeda M, Gotoh M, Yokoyama O, Kakizaki H, Takahashi S, et al. Efficacy of vibegron, a novel β3-adrenoreceptor agonist, on severe urgency urinary incontinence related to overactive bladder: post hoc analysis of a randomized, placebo-controlled, double-blind, comparative phase 3 study. BJU Int. 2020;125(5):709–17.

7. Staskin D, Frankel J, Varano S, Shortino D, Jankowich R, Mudd Jr PN. Once-daily vibegron 75 mg improves quality-of-life and incontinence efficacy endpoints in patients with overactive bladder: double-blind 52-week results from an extension study of the EMPOWUR international phase 3 trial. Neurourol Urodyn [Internet]. 2020 [cited 2020 Dec 20]. Available from: https://www.ics.org/2020/abstract/440.

8. Staskin D, Frankel J, Varano S, Shortino D, Jankowich R, Mudd P. Pd21-01 once-daily vibegron 75 mg for overactive bladder (oab): double-blind 52-week results from an extension study of the international phase 3 trial (EMPOWUR). J Urol. 2020;203(Supplement 4):e453.

9. Shi H, Chen H, Zhang Y, Cui Y. The efficacy and safety of Vibegron in treating overactive bladder: a systematic review and pooled analysis of randomized controlled trials. Neurourol Urodyn. 2020;39(5):1255–63.

10. Rovner E, Chai TC, Jacobs S, Christ G, Andersson K-E, Efros M, et al. Evaluating the safety and potential activity of URO-902 (hMaxi-K) gene transfer by intravesical instillation or direct injection into the bladder wall in female participants with idiopathic (non-neurogenic) overactive bladder syndrome and detrusor overactivity from two double-blind, imbalanced, placebo-controlled randomized phase 1 trials. Neurourol Urodyn. 2020;39(2):744–53.

11. Heesakkers JPFA, Digesu GA, van Breda J, Van Kerrebroeck P, Elneil S. A novel leadless, miniature implantable Tibial Nerve Neuromodulation System for the management of overactive bladder complaints. Neurourol Urodyn. 2018;37(3):1060–7.

12. Yamashiro J, de Riese W, de Riese C. New implantable tibial nerve stimulation devices: review of published clinical results in comparison to established neuromodulation devices. Res Rep Urol. 2019;11:351–7.

13. Rogers A, McCrery R, MacDiarmid S, Lukban J, Kaaki B, Shapiro A, et al. Pivotal study of subcutaneous tibial nerve stimulation with coin-sized implantable tibial neurostimulator (eCoin device) for urgency urinary incontinence. Neurourol Urodyn [Internet]. 2020 [cited 2020 Dec 21]. Available from: https://www.ics.org/2020/abstract/3.

14. Valencia Technologies Corporation. Pivotal study of subcutaneous tibial nerve stimulation with eCoin for overactive bladder (OAB) with urgency urinary incontinence (UUI) [Internet]. clinicaltrials.gov. 2020 [cited 2021 Jan 5]. Report No.: NCT03556891. Available from: https://clinicaltrials.gov/ct2/show/NCT03556891.

15. BlueWind Medical. A prospective study to assess the efficacy and safety of the BlueWind RENOVA iStim™ system in the treatment of patients diagnosed with overactive bladder (OASIS – OverActive Bladder StImulation System Study) [Internet]. clinicaltrials.gov. 2020 [cited 2021 Jan 5]. Report No.: NCT03596671. Available from: https://clinicaltrials.gov/ct2/show/NCT03596671.

16. Giusto L, Zahner P, Goldman H. V12-04 placement of an implantable tibial nerve stimulator under local anesthesia: step by step instructions. J Urol. 2019;201(Supplement 4):e1205.

17. Tipton WA, de Riese WT, de Riese CS. Review of new implantable tibial nerve stimulators in comparison to established third line treatment modalities for nonneurogenic overactive bladder. Urol Pract. 2020;7(6):530–7.

18. Sirls LT, Peters KM, Schonhoff A, Waldvogel A, Hasenau D. Early evaluation of an implanted chronic tibial nerve stimulation device versus percutaneous nerve stimulation for the treatment of urinary urge incontinence. ics.org [Internet]. 2019 [cited 2021 Jan 21]. Available from: https://www.ics.org/2019/abstract/156.

19. Vollstedt A, Gilleran J. Update on implantable PTNS devices. Curr Urol Rep. 2020;21(7):28.

20. Micron Medical Corporation. Multi-center, prospective, randomized, controlled, non-inferiority, clinical trial of chronic afferent nerve stimulation (CAN-Stim) of the tibial nerve versus sacral nerve stimulation (SNS) in the treatment of urinary urgency incontinence resulting from refractory overactive bladder (OAB) [Internet]. clinicaltrials.gov. 2020 [cited 2021 Jan 7]. Report No.: NCT02577302. Available from: https://clinicaltrials.gov/ct2/show/NCT02577302.

21. Bioness Inc. Prospective, multi-center, randomized, double-blinded trial of percutaneous tibial nerve stimulation with the Bioness StimRouter neuromodulation system versus Sham

in the treatment of overactive bladder (OAB) [Internet]. clinicaltrials.gov. 2020 [cited 2021 Jan 7]. Report No.: NCT02873312. Available from:. https://clinicaltrials.gov/ct2/show/ NCT02873312.

22. de Wachter S, McCrery R, Lane F, Benson K, Taylor C, Padron O, et al. Stimulation output and tissue impedance over 6-months of sacral neuromodulation therapy with a constant current system. Neurourol Urodyn [Internet]. 2020 [cited 2020 Dec 21]. Available from: https://www. ics.org/2020/abstract/47.

23. Pearce MM, Hilt EE, Rosenfeld AB, Zilliox MJ, Thomas-White K, Fok C, et al. The female urinary microbiome: a comparison of women with and without urgency urinary incontinence. mBio. 2014;5(4):e01283–14.

24. Thomas-White KJ, Hilt EE, Fok C, Pearce MM, Mueller ER, Kliethermes S, et al. Incontinence medication response relates to the female urinary microbiota. Int Urogynecol J. 2016;27(5):723–33.

25. Lim R, Liong ML, Leong WS, Karim Khan NA, Yuen KH. Pulsed magnetic stimulation for stress urinary incontinence: 1-year Followup results. J Urol. 2017;197(5):1302–8.

26. Stewart F, Berghmans B, Bø K, Glazener CM. Electrical stimulation with non-implanted devices for stress urinary incontinence in women. Cochrane Database Syst Rev [Internet]. 2017 [cited 2021 Jan 24];2017(12). Available from: https://www.ncbi.nlm.nih.gov/pmc/ articles/PMC6486295/.

27. Dmochowski R, Lynch CM, Efros M, Cardozo L. External electrical stimulation compared with intravaginal electrical stimulation for the treatment of stress urinary incontinence in women: a randomized controlled noninferiority trial. Neurourol Urodyn. 2019;38(7):1834–43.

28. Whooley J, Cunnane EM, Do Amaral R, Joyce M, MacCraith E, Flood HD, et al. Stress urinary incontinence and pelvic organ prolapse: biologic graft materials revisited. Tissue Eng Part B Rev. 2020;26(5):475–83.

29. Darzi S, Urbankova I, Su K, White J, Lo C, Alexander D, et al. Tissue response to collagen containing polypropylene meshes in an ovine vaginal repair model. Acta Biomater. 2016;39:114–23.

30. Parizzi NG, Rubini OÁ, de Almeida SHM, Ireno LC, Tashiro RM, de Carvalho VHT. Effect of platelet-rich plasma on polypropylene meshes implanted in the rabbit vagina: histological analysis. Int Braz J Urol. 2017;43(4):746–52.

31. D'Angelo W, Dziki J, Badylak SF. The challenge of stress incontinence and pelvic organ prolapse: revisiting biologic mesh materials. Curr Opin Urol. 2019;29(4):437–42.

32. Li J, Chen X, Ling K, Liang Z, Xu H. Evaluation of the bioactivity about anti-sca-1/basic fibroblast growth factor-urinary bladder matrix scaffold for pelvic reconstruction. J Biomater Appl. 2019;33(6):808–18.

33. Vashaghian M, Zaat SJ, Smit TH, Roovers J-P. Biomimetic implants for pelvic floor repair. Neurourol Urodyn. 2018;37(2):566–80.

34. Lai K, Zhang J, Wang G, Luo X, Liu M, Zhang X, et al. A biomimetic mesh for treating female stress urinary incontinence. Biofabrication. 2017;9(1):015008.

35. Wang X, Chen Y, Fan Z, Hua K. Comparing different tissue-engineered repair materials for the treatment of pelvic organ prolapse and urinary incontinence: which material is better? Int Urogynecol J. 2018;29(1):131–8.

36. Mangır N, Hillary CJ, Chapple CR, MacNeil S. Oestradiol-releasing biodegradable mesh stimulates collagen production and angiogenesis: an approach to improving biomaterial integration in pelvic floor repair. Eur Urol Focus. 2019;5(2):280–9.

37. Shafaat S, Mangir N, Regureos SR, Chapple CR, MacNeil S. Demonstration of improved tissue integration and angiogenesis with an elastic, estradiol releasing polyurethane material designed for use in pelvic floor repair. Neurourol Urodyn. 2018;37(2):716–25.

38. El-Neemany D, O'Shaughnessy D, Grande D, Sajjan S, Jin C, Kohn N, et al. 24: histological and biomechanical characteristics of permanent and absorbable sling mesh in a rabbit model: 3-month time point. Am J Obstet Gynecol. 2019;220(3):S722.

39. Pelvic Floor Research Foundation of South Africa. Prospective study to evaluate use of TephaFLEX™ sling implanted via a retropubic mid-urethral sling procedure for treatment of women with stress urinary incontinence [Internet]. clinicaltrials.gov. 2018 [cited 2021 Jan 7]. Report No.: NCT03673488. Available from: https://clinicaltrials.gov/ct2/show/NCT03673488.
40. Guillaume O, Lavigne J-P, Lefranc O, Nottelet B, Coudane J, Garric X. New antibiotic-eluting mesh used for soft tissue reinforcement. Acta Biomater. 2011;7(9):3390–7.
41. Brandt CJ, Kammer D, Fiebeler A, Klinge U. Beneficial effects of hydrocortisone or spironolactone coating on foreign body response to mesh biomaterial in a mouse model. J Biomed Mater Res A. 2011;99A(3):335–43.
42. Kocjancic E, Erickson T, Tu L-M, Gheiler E, Drie DV. Two-year outcomes for the Altis® adjustable single incision sling system for treatment of stress urinary incontinence. Neurourol Urodyn. 2017;36(6):1582–7.
43. Morán E, Pérez-Ardavín J, Sánchez JV, Bonillo MA, Martínez-Cuenca E, Arlandis S, et al. Mid-term safety and efficacy of the ALTIS® single-incision sling for female stress urinary incontinence: less mesh, same results. BJU Int. 2019;123(5A):E51–6.
44. Coloplast A/S. A post-market evaluation of the Altis® single incision sling system versus transobturator or retropubic mesh sling in the treatment of female stress urinary incontinence [Internet]. clinicaltrials.gov. 2020 [cited 2021 Jan 7]. Report No.: NCT02348112. Available from: https://clinicaltrials.gov/ct2/show/NCT02348112.
45. Coloplast A/S. The European Study of Altis single incision sling system for female stress urinary incontinence [Internet]. clinicaltrials.gov; 2018 Jan [cited 2021 Jan 7]. Report No.: NCT02049840. Available from: https://clinicaltrials.gov/ct2/show/NCT02049840.
46. Dmitry S. A randomized clinical trial comparing a tunable-tension transobturator tape (TTT) versus standard transobturator midurethral tape (TOT) for the surgical treatment of stress urinary incontinence in women [Internet]. clinicaltrials.gov. 2019 [cited 2021 Jan 11]. Report No.: NCT03958695. Available from:. https://clinicaltrials.gov/ct2/show/NCT03958695.
47. Gill BC, Sun DZ, Damaser MS. Stem cells for urinary incontinence: functional differentiation or cytokine effects? Urology. 2018;117:9–17.
48. Carr LK, Steele D, Steele S, Wagner D, Pruchnic R, Jankowski R, et al. 1-year follow-up of autologous muscle-derived stem cell injection pilot study to treat stress urinary incontinence. Int Urogynecol J Pelvic Floor Dysfunct. 2008;19(6):881–3.
49. Mitterberger M, Marksteiner R, Margreiter E, Pinggera GM, Colleselli D, Frauscher F, et al. Autologous myoblasts and fibroblasts for female stress incontinence: a 1-year follow-up in 123 patients. BJU Int. 2007;100(5):1081–5.
50. Gräs S, Klarskov N, Lose G. Intraurethral injection of autologous minced skeletal muscle: a simple surgical treatment for stress urinary incontinence. J Urol. 2014;192(3):850–5.
51. Sèbe P, Doucet C, Cornu J-N, Ciofu C, Costa P, de Medina SGD, et al. Intrasphincteric injections of autologous muscular cells in women with refractory stress urinary incontinence: a prospective study. Int Urogynecol J. 2011;22(2):183–9.
52. Blaganje M, Lukanović A. Ultrasound-guided autologous myoblast injections into the extrinsic urethral sphincter: tissue engineering for the treatment of stress urinary incontinence. Int Urogynecol J. 2013;24(4):533–5.
53. Peters KM, Dmochowski RR, Carr LK, Robert M, Kaufman MR, Sirls LT, et al. Autologous muscle derived cells for treatment of stress urinary incontinence in women. J Urol. 2014;192(2):469–76.
54. Kuismanen K, Sartoneva R, Haimi S, Mannerström B, Tomás E, Miettinen S, et al. Autologous adipose stem cells in treatment of female stress urinary incontinence: results of a pilot study. Stem Cells Transl Med. 2014;3(8):936–41.
55. Lee CN, Jang JB, Kim JY, Koh C, Baek JY, Lee KJ. Human cord blood stem cell therapy for treatment of stress urinary incontinence. J Korean Med Sci. 2010;25(6):813–6.
56. Wang B, Zhou J, Banie L, Reed-Maldonado AB, Ning H, Lu Z, et al. Low-intensity extracorporeal shock wave therapy promotes myogenesis through PERK/ATF4 pathway. Neurourol Urodyn. 2018;37(2):699–707.

57. Zhang X, Ruan Y, Wu AK, Zaid U, Villalta JD, Wang G, et al. Delayed treatment with low-intensity extracorporeal shock wave therapy in an irreversible rat model of stress urinary incontinence. Urology. 2020;141:187.e1–7.
58. Krychman M, Rowan CG, Allan BB, Durbin S, Yacoubian A, Wilkerson D. Effect of single-session, cryogen-cooled monopolar radiofrequency therapy on sexual function in women with vaginal laxity: the VIVEVE I trial. J Women's Health. 2018;27(3):297–304.
59. Allan BB, Bell S, Husarek K. A 12-month feasibility study to investigate the effectiveness of cryogen-cooled monopolar radiofrequency treatment for female stress urinary incontinence. Can Urol Assoc J. 2020;14(7):E313–8.
60. Viveve Inc. Comparison of the Viveve treatment and cryogen-only treatment versus Sham treatment for stress urinary incontinence [Internet]. clinicaltrials.gov. 2020 [cited 2021 Jan 7]. Report No.: NCT04206085. Available from:. https://clinicaltrials.gov/ct2/show/NCT04206085.
61. González Isaza P, Jaguszewska K, Cardona JL, Lukaszuk M. Long-term effect of thermoablative fractional CO2 laser treatment as a novel approach to urinary incontinence management in women with genitourinary syndrome of menopause. Int Urogynecol J. 2018;29(2):211–5.
62. Ni J, Gu B. Up-to-date evidences of laser therapy for female stress urinary incontinence: a systematic review and meta-analysis. ics.org [Internet]. 2020 [cited 2020 Dec 21]. Available from: https://www.ics.org/2020/abstract/98.
63. Winkler H, Jacoby K, Kalota S, Snyder J, Cline K, Robertson K, et al. Twelve-month efficacy and safety data for the "stress incontinence control, efficacy and safety study": a phase III, multicenter, prospective, randomized, controlled study treating female stress urinary incontinence using the vesair intravesical balloon. Female Pelvic Med Reconstr Surg. 2018;24(3):222–31.
64. Rosier PFWM, Schaefer W, Lose G, Goldman HB, Guralnick M, Eustice S, et al. International continence society good urodynamic practices and terms 2016: urodynamics, uroflowmetry, cystometry, and pressure-flow study. Neurourol Urodyn. 2017;36(5):1243–60.
65. Wouters OJ, McKee M, Luyten J. Estimated Research and Development investment needed to bring a new medicine to market, 2009–2018. JAMA. 2020;323(9):844.
66. 2017Factsheet_Restore NIH Funding.pdf [Internet]. [cited 2021 Jan 23]. Available from: https://faseb.org/Portals/2/PDFs/opa/2017/2017Factsheet_Restore%20NIH%20Funding.pdf.
67. Malik RD, Kowalik CG. Patient education for overactive bladder in the digital era. Curr Bladder Dysfunct Rep. 2019;3(14):186–90.
68. Paul K, Darzi S, McPhee G, Del Borgo MP, Werkmeister JA, Gargett CE, et al. 3D bioprinted endometrial stem cells on melt electrospun poly ε-caprolactone mesh for pelvic floor application promote anti-inflammatory responses in mice. Acta Biomater. 2019;97:162–76.
69. Antunes-Lopes T, Cruz F. Urinary biomarkers in overactive bladder: revisiting the evidence in 2019. Eur Urol Focus. 2019;5(3):329–36.
70. van Breda HMK, Martens FMJ, Tromp J, Heesakkers JPFA. A new implanted posterior tibial nerve stimulator for the treatment of overactive bladder syndrome: 3-month results of a novel therapy at a single center. J Urol. 2017;198(1):205–10.
71. te Dorsthorst MJ, Digesu GA, Tailor V, Gore M, van Kerrebroeck PE, van Breda HMK, et al. 3-year followup of a new implantable tibial nerve stimulator for the treatment of overactive bladder syndrome. J Urol. 2020;204(3):545–50.
72. Dmochowski RR, Kerrebroeck PV, Digesu GA, Elneil S, Heesakkers JP. Pd31 02 long-term results of safety, efficacy, quality of life and satisfaction of patients treated for refractory oab using an implantable tibial neurostimulation system: renova istim™ system. J Urol. 2019;201(Supplement 4):e565–6.
73. MacDiarmid S, Staskin DR, Lucente V, Kaaki B, English S, Gilling P, et al. Feasibility of a fully implanted, nickel sized and shaped tibial nerve stimulator for the treatment of overactive bladder syndrome with urgency urinary incontinence. J Urol. 2019;201(5):967–72.
74. MacDiarmid S, Staskin DR, Lucente V, Kaaki B, English S, Gilling P, Meffan P, et al. Lba-06 12 month feasibility data of a fully-implanted, nickel-sized and shaped tibial nerve stimulator for the treatment of overactive bladder syndrome with urgency urinary incontinence. J Urol. 2019;201(Supplement 4):e994.

Index

A

Abdominal leak point pressure (ALPP), 70
Abobotulinum toxin A, 195
Acute stress, 488
Adipose-derived stem cells (ADSCs), 509
Adjustable continence (ACT's), 357–358
Adjustable slings, 507–508
Adrenergic receptors, 148
AMS 800 model, 360, 362
Angiotensin-converting enzyme inhibitors, 467
Anorexia nervosa, 433
Anterior colporrhaphy, 86, 378
Anterior vaginal wall (AVW) prolapse, 372, 373
Anticholinergic agents, 393
Anticholinergics, 441
Anti-incontinence procedures, 85, 248, 249
Antimuscarinics, 148–151, 414, 471
    comparative effectiveness, 152, 153
    effectiveness, 148, 151, 152
    ß3-agonist, efficacy compared to, 156, 157
    transdermal use of, 153
Anus, 41, 42, 44, 49
Aquamid™, 246, 247
Arcus tendineus fascia pelvis (ATFP), 260
Arterial blood supply, 44
Arteries, 43
Artificial urinary sphincter (AUS), 358–362,
        399, 461
    iIndications, 359
    optimal timing, 359
    outcomes, 359–360
    pre-operative considerations, 360–361
Atonic bladder, 73–75
Augmentation cystoplasty for low bladder
        capacity/compliance in NLUTD, 459

Augmentation cystoplasty in non-neurogenic
        bladder patient
    AC laparoscopic/robotic technique,
        215, 216
    AC with/without catheterizable channel,
        211, 213, 214
    decreased bladder capacity, 209
    follow-up, 216, 217
    interstitial cystitis/bladder pain
        syndrome, 208
    overactive bladder, 207, 208
    partial cystectomy, 208, 209
    pregnancy after bladder augmentation, 217
    surgical approach, 210
Auto-augmentation, *see* Detrusor myectomy
Autologous fascia pubovaginal sling, 295
    anaerobic coverage, 298
    cure/improvement rates, 305–307
    de novo urge incontinence, 307
    general/spinal anesthesia, 298
    indications, 296
    labial retraction, 299
    outcomes and complications, 305–309
    patient positioning, 299
    physical examination, 298, 308
    postoperative care, 305
    post-operative voiding dysfunction, 308
    postvoid residual, 298, 308
    pre-operative evaluation, 298
    surgical management of obstruction after
        fascial sling, 308
    synthetic mid-urethral slings, 309
    tensioning of the sling, 308
    urine culture, 298
    urodynamic studies, 298

Autologous fascia use for transobturator
        slings, 312
Autologous fascial sling (AFS),
        309–310, 349–351
Autologous fat, 241
Autologous graft compared to allograft
        materials, 311–312
Autologous tissue retropubic slings, 87–89
Autotransplantation, 415
Axonics® sacral neuromodulation system, 186

B
Beers criteria, 159
Behavioral modification and
        urotherapy, 439–441
Behavioral therapy and lifestyle modifications
    absorbent products, 108, 119, 120
    alcohol consumption, 113, 114
    alcohol reduction, 108
    anticholinergic medications, 113
    bladder training, 108, 115, 116
    bowel management, 108
    caffeine, 112
    caffeine reduction, 108
    dietary components, 110, 111
    dietary modification, 108, 110
    estrogen receptors, 110
    exercise, 108, 117
    fluid and caffeine management, 111–113
    fluid intake, 111
    fluid management, 108
    management/regulation of bowel
        function, 116
    obesity, 118
    patient educational handout, 109
    pelvic floor muscle exercises, 117
    skin protection, 119, 120
    skin protectants, 108
    smoking cessation, 114
    timed/prompted voiding, 108, 114, 115
    tobacco cessation, 108
    tobacco use, 113
    vitamin C and calcium, 110
    weight loss, 108, 118, 119
Benign prostatic hyperplasia (BPH) with
        lower urinary tract symptoms, 399
Bioness StimRouter™, 503, 504
Bladder compliance, 456
Bladder denervation, 97, 98
Bladder diaries, 438
Bladder injury rate from improper retropubic
        needle passage, 309

Bladder neck closure, 460
    indications and methods, 223, 224
    transabdominal approach, 226
    transurethral approach, 226
    transvaginal approach, 224, 225
Bladder neck dissection, 361–362
Bladder neck reconstruction, 460
Bladder neck suspension (BNS), 355
Bladder outflow obstruction (BOO),
        75–77, 344
Bladder outlet obstruction, 75, 319, 321–324
Bladder outlet obstructive index
        (BOOI), 343–344
Bladder pain syndrome (BPS), 208
Bladder training, 115, 116
BlueWind RENOVA™, 174, 500, 502
Body mass index (BMI), 431
Botox injection techniques, 196, 197
Botulinum toxin for overactive bladder, 194
    complications and other
        considerations, 200
    contraindications, 202
    delivery techniques under investigation,
        197, 198
    distant spread, 201
    efficacy, 198, 199
    immunogenicity, 200, 201
    mechanism of action, 194
    neurotoxins
        Abobotulinum toxin A, 195
        Dysport, 195
        incobotulinum toxin A, 195, 196
        Xeomin, 195, 196
    techniques, 196, 197
Bowel management, 116–117, 440
Brink scale, 133
Bulbospongiosus muscles, 32
Bulkamid™, 238, 246, 247
Bulking agents, 351–352
Burch colposuspension, 91, 257, 258, 281,
        378, 446
    complications and adverse events, 265, 269
    mechanism of action, 258–260
    surgical techniques
        abdominal incision, 263
        anatomy, 260
        bladder drainage, 264
        bladder neck and pectineal ligament,
            adequate exposure of, 262
        outcomes, 264, 265
        retroperitoneal space, access to, 261
        suture placement, 262, 263
Burch procedure, 90

C

Calcium hydroxylapatite, 244
Carbon-coated zirconium, 245
Cardinal (transverse cervical) ligaments, 31
Cervix, 36
Children with dysfunctional voiding, 444
Children with refractory dysfunctional
    elimination syndrome, 445
Chronic irritative symptoms, 324–325
Chronic ketamine, 209
Chronic lung disease (CLD), 11, 433
Coaptite™, 244
Coccygeal plexus, 46
Cognitive behavioral therapy, 440
Cognitive impairment, 158, 159
Colon segment, 210
Colposuspension techniques for salvage, 353
Combination therapy, 157
Complete female epispadias (CFE), 435
Compliance calculation, 78
Computed tomography urography (CTU), 411
Congenital causes of incontinence, 435
Constipation, 10
Contigen™, 241
Cooper's ligament, 262
Cough leak point pressure (CLPP), 70
Cough stress test (CST), 53
Counterbracing, 137
Crisis preparation, 490
Cross-linked polydimethylsiloxane elastomer
    particles, 245, 246
Cryogen-cooling monopolar radiofrequency
    (CMRF) devices, 510
Cystic fibrosis (CF), 431
Cystometry, 68
Cystoscopy, 308, 347, 411
Cystourethropexy, 90, 91
Cystourethroscopy, 421

D

Darifenacin, 153, 158
De novo overactive bladder, 346, 347
Decreased bladder capacity, 209
Deep perineal pouch (DPP), 21, 33
Deep transverse perineal muscles, 32
Deflux™, 242
Denervation injury to urethral sphincter
    mechanism, 276
Desmopressin, 393, 442
Detrusor leak point pressure (DLPP), 77
Detrusor myectomy, 99
Detrusor overactivity (DO), 57, 62, 72, 73, 458

Detrusor underactivity (DU), 62, 73–75
Device-guided injection, 238
Dextranomer with hyaluronic acid, 242
Diabetes mellitus (DM), 11
Diagnostic Aspects of Incontinence Study
    (DAISy), 12
Dietary and fluid modifications, 110
Disordered eating, 433
Diurnal incontinence, 434
Double anticholinergic therapy, 442
Double dye test, 411
Drug-eluting and coated mesh, 507
Dual therapy with desmopressin and
    oxybutynin, 443
Duloxetine, 348, 393
Durasphere™, 245, 352
Dye testing, 56
Dysport, 195

E

Eating Disorder Examination
    Questionnaire, 433
eCoin™, 500, 502
Elderly women, urinary incontinence
    age-related urodynamic changes, 466
    behavioral modifications, 469
    behavioral therapy, 470
    catheterization, 469
    comorbid conditions, 466
    development of, 466
    fluid management, 470
    functional incontinence, 467
    intra-detrusor onabotulinum toxin A
        injections, 471
    medication treatment, 469, 470
    morbidity associated, 465
    PFMT, 470
    prevalence, 465
    PTNS, 471
    reduced bladder contractility, 466
    skin breakdown and dermatitis, 469
    slow gastric emptying, 471
    SNS, 472
    toileting programs, 470
    toileting therapy programs, 469
    transdermal formulation of
        oxybutynin, 470
    treatment options, 468
Electrical stimulation, 505
Electrospinning, 506
Electrospun synthetic polyurethane with the
    inclusion of 17-β-estradiol, 506

End stage renal disease (ESRD), 209
Endoscopic management, 331
Endoscopic suprapubic cystotomy, 222
Epidemiology of lower urinary tract symptoms
        (EpiLUTS), 5
Ergonomics, 486, 487
Establishing the Prevalence of Incontinence
        (EPI) study, 7
Ethylene vinyl alcohol (EVA), 242
European Bladder Dysfunction study, 440, 441
Exercise, 487
Extended-SISTEr study, 307
External and intra-vaginal delivery of
        electrical stimulation, 505
Extravesical/transvesical approach, 413

F
Failed sling with recurrent SUI
    conservative and medical therapy, 347–348
    surgical decision making, 348
    surgical management of recurrent
        SUI, 348–362
Fallopian tubes, 36
Fascia lata considerations, 303–305
Fascial pubovaginal sling, 276
Female external genitalia, 34, 35
Female pelvic floor disorders, social
        disparities in, 13, 14
Female pelvic organs
    lower urinary tract organs
        ureters, 41
        urethra, 38, 40
        urinary bladder, 37, 38
    rectum and anus, 41, 42
    reproductive organs
        fallopian tubes, 36
        ovaries, 37
        uterus and cervix, 36
Female urinary incontinence, 20
    lower urinary tract organs
        ureters, 41
        urethra, 38, 40
        urinary bladder, 37, 38
    lymphatics of female pelvis, 48
        reproductive organs, 48, 49
        urinary tract, 48
    pelvic blood supply
        arterial blood supply, 44
        arteries, 43
        internal iliac artery, 43
        rectum and anus, 44

urethra, 44
        vagina, 44
    pelvic bones, 23, 24
    pelvic foramina, 26, 27
    pelvic ligaments, 24–26
    pelvic plexuses and nerve supply of pelvis
        and perineum, 46, 47
    pelvic side wall
        muscles of, 27, 28
        pelvic diaphragm, 29, 30
        pelvic floor, 28
    perineum, 32–35
    rectum and anus, 41, 42
    reproductive organs
        fallopian tubes, 36
        ovaries, 37
        uterus and cervix, 36 (*see also* Urinary
            incontinence)
    uterine supports, 30, 31
    venous, 44, 45
    voiding, physiology of, 22, 23
FemSoft, 131
Fesoterodine, 153, 158, 442, 470
First-stage lead placement (FSLP), 178,
        179, 183
Fistulas, 21, 410
Fluoroscopy, 181
    anatomic diagnoses seen on, 78–80
Food and Drug Administration Public
        Health Notification in 2001
        and 2008, 295
Frailty, 468
Freeze and squeeze, 137
Functional obstruction, 73

G
Gene therapy, 498, 500
Genetic predisposition to prolapse, 373
Genitourinary syndrome of menopause
        (GSM), 511
Geriatrics, *see* Elderly women, urinary
        incontinence
Giggle incontinence, 443
Giggle micturition/enuresis risoria, 434, 435
Gittes needle suspension procedure, 95
Gittes procedure, 95
Glutaraldehyde cross-linked (GAX) collagen
        (Contigen™), 241
Goebell-Frangenheim-Stoeckel operation, 88
Greater sciatic notch, 26
Group Health Cooperative, 5

H
Hammock effect, 259
Harvest of fascial lata, 303
Healthcare costs, 498
High-intensity athletic training, 432
Hovermatt®, 481
Hydrodissection of anterior vaginal wall, 300
Hypercontinence, 397
Hysterectomy, 25, 410

I
Ileal-bladder anastomosis, 216
Ileocystoplasty, 212
Ileum, 210
Imipramine, 393
Immunogenicity, 200, 201
Implantable pulse generator (IPG), 183
Implantable tibial nerve
        stimulation, 500–503
Implanted sacral neuromodulation, 445
Impressa, 131
Incobotulinum toxin A, 195, 196
Incontinence after gender affirming
        surgery, 398–401
Incontinence after orthotopic urinary
        diversion, 389, 390
Incontinence-associated dermatitis, 120
Incontinence Impact Questionnaire short form
        (IIQ-7), 53
Incontinence Quality of Life Scale, 511
Incontinence Symptom Index-Pediatric
        (ISI-Pediatric), 438
Incontinent adolescents
    history, 437
    neurologic work-up, 439
    physical exam, 438
    post-void residual, 438
Individualized programs creation, 137–139
Infection, 190
Ingelman-Sundberg pubococcygeal
        repair, 87, 88
Inguinal ligaments, 25
Institutional culture and policies, 490
Integral theory, 277
Internal iliac artery, 43
Internal pudendal artery, 43
International Children's Continence Society,
        434, 440
International Consultation on Incontinence
        Questionnaire for Females with
        LUTS, 434

International Consultation on Incontinence
        Questionnaire Urinary
        Incontinence short form
        (ICIQ-SF), 53
International Continence Society-Uniform
        Cough Stress test, 508
International Physical Activity
        Questionnaire–Short Form
        (IPAQ-SF), 440
International Urogynecological Association
        (IUGA), 286, 287
Interstim® Medtronic device, 186
Interstitial cystitis (IC), 208
Intraoperative ergonomics, 485
Intraoperative radiation, 482–483
Intraoperative surgeon and team
        performance, 487–490
Intraurethral bulking agents, 460
Intravenous urography, 411
Intravesical botulinum A toxin injection, 445
Intravesical botulinum toxin, 394
Intravesical thermosensitive polymer
        hydrogel, 198
Intrinsic sphincter deficiency (ISD), 72, 235,
        296, 344
Irritative storage symptoms, 419
Ischioanal fossae, 35
Ischiocavernosus muscles, 33

K
Kaiser Permanente Continence Associated
        Risks Epidemiologic Study (KP
        CARES), 5
Kelly plication, 86, 276
Kidneys–ureters–bladder (KUB), 439
King's Health Questionnaire
        [KHQ], 53, 499
Knack maneuver, 137

L
Lacunar ligaments, 25
Laparoscopic hysterectomy, 410
Laser therapies, 511
Lead migration, 189
Lesser sciatic notch, 26
Liposomal formulations, 198
Lithotomy, 479, 480
Low bladder pressures during filling, 456
Low intensity extracorporeal shockwave
        therapy (LiSWT), 510

Lower urinary tract organs
  ureters, 41
  urethra, 38, 40
  urinary bladder, 37, 38
Lower urinary tract symptoms (LUTS), 152,
      377, 430
Lower urinary tract, innervation of, 46, 47
Lowsley retractor, 222
Lymphatics of female pelvis, 48
  reproductive organs, 48
  urinary tract, 48

M
Macroplastique™, 238, 245, 246, 351
Male to female genitourinary gender
      affirming surgery (MtF
      GAS), 398–400
Marshall-Marchetti-Krantz cystourethropexy
      (MMK), 90
Masculinizing surgery, 400–401
Maximal urethral closure pressure
      (MUCP), 375
Medication pharmacology, 148
Mental toughness, 489
Mesh complications, 283–285
Metoidioplasty, 400
Michigan Incontinence Symptoms Index
      (M-ISI), 53
Microbiome, bladder health, 504
Micturition reflex, 453
Middle rectal artery, 43
Mid-stream interruption technique, 135
Mid-urethral mesh slings for the treatment of
      SUI, 506
Midurethral sling, 278–283, 395, 473
Mini Mental State Exam (MMSE),
      158, 471
Minimally invasive mid-urethral sling
      (MUS), 257–258
Minimally invasive sling procedures, 264
Mirabegron, 154, 155
Mixed urinary incontinence
      (MUI), 52, 240
Modified Martius labial fat pad flap
      (MMLFPF), 21
Modified oxford scale (MOS), 132–133
Mother's Outcome after Delivery (MOAD)
      study, 8
Multichannel urodynamics (UDS), 57
Muscle-invasive bladder cancer, 387
Musculoelastic theory, 277
Musculoskeletal pain, 483, 486, 487

N
National Health and Nutrition Examination
      Survey (NHANES), 5, 112
Native tissue plication, 86, 87
Needle suspension procedures, 91–97
Neobladder vaginal fistula, 390,
      394, 396–397
Nerve injuries, 478
Neurogenic lower urinary tract dysfunction
      (NLUTD), 62, 453, 459
Neurogenic urinary incontinence
  biomarkers, 513
  causes of, 454
  chronic indwelling urethral catheters, 454
  clean intermittent catheterization, 460
  clinical presentations, 455–456
  development of animal model, 512
  development of mobile applications, 512
  economic burden, 512
  etiologies, 453–455, 512
  internet-based interventions, 512
  lesions above the brainstem, 454
  limitations to research, 512
  OAB phenotypes, 513
  oral medication, 458
  preventive approaches, 512
  renal failure, 457
  sacral neurologic insults, 454
  subtyping of, 512
  urethral erosion, 455
  urine cytology, 458
  urodynamic evaluation, 457
  using mesenchymal stem cells, 509
Neuromodulation, 166
Nighttime incontinence, 390
Nocturnal enuresis (NE), 430
Non-invasive tests, 54, 56
Non-neurogenic bladder patient, augmentation
      cystoplasty in, see Augmentation
      cystoplasty in non-neurogenic
      bladder patient
Non-permanent sling materials, 507
Nonsurgical management VVF, 412
Nurses' Health Study, 5, 112

O
Obesity, 10, 431–432
Obliterated umbilical artery, 43
Obturator artery, 43
Obturator ligaments, 25
Obturator nerve, 27, 47
Occult SUI on reduction stress test, 380

Onabotulinum Toxin A (BTXA),
  194, 199–202
Oral oxybutynin, 441
Oral pharmacotherapy, 148
Orthotopic neobladders, 387
Orthotopic urinary diversion
  anticholinergic agents, 393
  bowel segments, 388
  detubularization, 388
  evaluation of, 390
  neobladder presenting with
    incontinence, 391
  surgical approaches, 388
Ovaries, 37
Overactive bladder (OAB), 147, 149–151, 177,
    207, 208
  botulinum toxin for, 194
    Abobotulinum toxin A, 195
    complications and other
      considerations, 200
    contraindications, 202
    delivery techniques under investigation,
      197, 198
    distant spread, 201
    Dysport, 195
    efficacy, 198, 199
    immunogenicity, 200, 201
    incobotulinum toxin A, 195, 196
    mechanism of action, 194
    techniques, 196, 197
    Xeomin, 195, 196
  treatment and cognitive impairment,
    158, 159
Overactive Bladder Symptom Score (OABSS)
  subscales, 153
Oxybutynin, 152
Oxybutynin chloride topical gel (OTG), 154
Oxybutynin immediate release (IR), 148

P
Pad tests, 64
Parasympathetic nerves, 46
Partial cystectomy, 208, 209
Patient Global Impression (PGI), 499
Patient Global Impression of Severity Scale
  (PGI-S), 53
Patient safety in operating room, 477–483
Pelvic abscesses, 326
Pelvic blood supply
  arterial blood supply, 44
  arteries, 43
  internal iliac artery, 43

rectum and anus, 44
urethra, 44
vagina, 44
Pelvic bones, 23, 24
Pelvic diaphragm, 29, 30
Pelvic floor, 21, 28
Pelvic floor contraction, 132
  assessment of, 132–134
  education on, 134, 135
Pelvic floor disorders, 373
Pelvic floor muscle pain (PFMP), 11
Pelvic floor muscle therapy (PFMT), 127, 132,
  135, 137, 469, 472
Pelvic floor physical therapy (PFPT), 390
Pelvic floor reconstruction, 506
Pelvic floor therapy, 440
Pelvic foramina, 26, 27
Pelvic ligaments, 24–26
Pelvic organ prolapse (POP), 53, 129, 468
  aging, 372
  anatomical factors, 372
  and stress urinary incontinence, 374–376
  and urgency incontinence, 376
  AVW prolapse and urethral function, 376
  clinical factors, 376
  concomitant incontinence procedure,
    380, 382
  concomitant versus delayed midurethral
    sling placement, 381
  de novo SUI after prolapse surgery, 378
  de novo SUI for women undergoing
    prolapse repair, 381
  definition, 371
  disease mechanism, 382
  epidemiology, 371–373
  major levator ani defect, 372
  OAB symptoms, 377
  outlet obstruction, 375
  patient dissatisfaction, 381
  patient-specific contribution, 376
  pessaries, 377
  population based studies, 372
  preoperative occult SUI, 379
  prevalence of, 371
  risk factors, 373–374, 381, 382
  risk stratification and patient
    preferences, 382
  staged procedure, 381
  surgical repair of prolapse with both
    reconstructive and obliterative
    procedures, 377
  tissue repair, 381
  types of, 372

Pelvic Organ Prolapse Quantification
      (POP-Q), 54, 371
Pelvic pain, 11
Pelvic plexuses and nerve supply of pelvis and
      perineum, 46, 47
Pelvic side wall
   muscles of, 27, 28
   pelvic diaphragm, 29, 30
   pelvic floor, 28
Pelvic surgery, 9
Pelvis, 21
Percutaneous nephrostomy and antegrade
      nephrostogram, 415
Percutaneous nerve evaluation (PNE),
      178, 179
Percutaneous posterior tibial nerve
      stimulation, 169–171
Percutaneous tibial nerve stimulation
      (PTNS), 13, 500
Perineal body, 33
Perineal membrane, 33
Perineometery, 134
Perineum, 21, 32–35, 44
Peritoneal/omental flap, 226
Periurethral injection, 237
Permacol™, 244
Permeability-glycoprotein (P-gp) system, 158
Pessaries, 131
Peyrera needle suspension, 92
Phalloplasty, 400, 401
Physical therapy, 487
Pink Pad®system, 479
Pisces quad foramen electrode, 177
Polyacrylamide hydrogel, 246, 247
Polydimethylsiloxane, 247, 248
Polypharmacy, 159, 466
Polytetrafluoroethylene, 241
Polyuria, 466
Porcine collagen, 244
Post void residual (PVR), 63
Posterior tibial nerve stimulation (PTNS), 165
   mechanism of action, 165, 166
   new technology in, 174
   pathophysiology and treatment, 173, 174
   percutaneous posterior tibial nerve
         stimulation, 169–171
   side effects/complications, 172
   techniques, 167–169
   transcutaneous posterior tibial nerve
         stimulation, 171, 172
Posterior tibial TENS, 444
Posthysterectomy fistula, 409
Post-hysterectomy VVFs, 408

Postoperative bladder outlet obstruction, 322
Postoperative care, 422–423
Post-operative imaging of fistula, 423
Postoperative pain and neuropathy, 327, 328
Post-operative retention, 308
Post-operative voiding dysfunction, 307
Postvoid residual (PVR), 54
Pre-operative mental practice, 489
Pressure flow urodynamics (UDS), 61, 346
Prolapse reduction, 379
Prophylactic incontinence procedure in
      continent women, 380
Psychological safety, 488
Pubic symphysis, 23
Pubocervical ligaments, 31
Pubovaginal autologous slings, 395
Pubovaginal slings, 281
Pudendal nerve, 26, 27, 47
Pudendal neuromodulation (PNM)
   adverse events (AEs)/complications,
         189, 190
   mechanism of action, 177, 178
   operative techniques, 183, 186
   outcomes of, 188, 189
   recent technological advances, 186, 187
Pulmonary disease, 433
Pulsed magnetic stimulation, 505

Q
Q-tip test, 54

R
Radiation cystitis, 419, 420, 424
Radical cystectomy (RC), 387
Radiofrequency and CO_2 laser therapy, 498
Raz needle suspension procedure, 93, 94
Rectum, 41, 42, 44, 49
Rectus fascia graft harvest, 299–300
Rectus fascia versus fascia lata, 310–311
Recurrent diverticula, 423
Reduction stress test, 379
Regenerative medicine for SUI, 513
Relaxation techniques, 489
Repeat mid urethral synthetic sling, 352–353
Repetitive loading, 373
Reproductive organs, 48
   fallopian tubes, 36
   ovaries, 37
   uterus and cervix, 36
Reproductive Risks for Incontinence Study at
      Kaiser (RRISK), 5

Retrograde pyeloureterography (RPG), 411
Retropubic slings using autologous
        tissue, 87–89
Retropubic urethrolysis, 323
Rhabdosphincter, 388
Risk stratification models, 381
Robot-assisted AMS 800 Bladder Neck
        Implantation, 361–362

S

Sacral neuromodulation (SNM), 194, 444,
        445, 459, 472, 482, 498
    adverse events (AEs)/complications,
        189, 190
    failed, 189
    mechanism of action, 177, 178
    operative techniques, 178, 179, 181–183
    outcomes of, 187, 188
    recent technological advances, 186, 187
    stimulators, 503, 504
Sacral plexus, 46
Sacroiliac ligaments, 25
Sacrospinous ligaments, 24
Sacrotuberous ligaments, 24
Sclerosing agent, 241
Sensory nerves, 47
Sequential compression devices (SCDs), 299
Sexual dysfunction, 332
Side-to-side anastomosis, 228
Simple cystometric test, 65
Single-incision sling (SIS), 279
SISTeR trial, 344
Sling incision, 323
Sling mobilization success and continence
        rates, 322
Sling placement and fixation, 301–303
Sling plication and manipulation, 355
Slings failure, SUI treatment, 343
    causes, 344
    management of, 345, 346
    pathophysiology, 345
Smooth muscle component of urethral
        sphincter, 388
Sodium morrhuate, 241
Solifenacin, 153, 157, 441, 442
Somatic nerves, 46, 47
Spence-Allen procedure, 461
Sphincter urethrae, 33
Spiral and obstructing slings, 355–357
Spontaneous perforation, 216
Staff protection, 483
Stamey needle suspension procedure, 93, 94

Stem cell therapy, 358, 508–509
Stimrouter® peripheral nerve stimulation
        system, 174
Stoma, 229
Stress incontinence, 12, 13
Stress Incontinence Surgical Treatment
        Efficacy Trial (SISTEr), 12, 305
Stress urinary incontinence, 21, 52, 87, 456
    in adolescent female, 431–433
    clinical care pathways, 474
    complex interactions of effects
        associated, 467
    definition of, 70
    effects of, 466
    midurethral sling procedure, 473
    nonsurgical treatment, 472
    post-neobladder reconstruction, 395
    surgical procedures, 473
    surgical treatment, 473
    UBA (*see* Urethral bulking agents (UBAs))
    urethral bulking agent, 473
    urodynamics, 71, 72
Study of Women's Health Across the Nation
        (SWAN) study, 14
Subtotal abdominal hysterectomy, 410
Superficial perineal pouch, 21, 33, 34
Superficial transverse perineal muscles, 32
Superior vesical artery, 43
Suprameatal urethrolysis, 324
Suprapubic (SP) catheter
    endoscopic placement of, 222
    indications and methods, 221
    percutaneous procedure, 221, 222
    surgical placement of, 223
Surgeon safety and occupational
        health, 483–487
Surgical coaching or didactic training, 488
Surgical culture, 483
Surgical team performance optimization
        strategies, 490
Surgical techniques, urethral sphincter, 274
Surgical treatment complications, stress
        urinary incontinence
    diagnosis of obstruction, 318
    diagnostic procedures, 318
    evaluation, 318
    preoperative post void residual, 318
    urinalysis and post-void residual, 318
Surgical treatment, stress urinary incontinence,
        success rate, 281
Sustained therapeutics effects of percutaneous
        tibial nerve stimulation (STEP), 170
Sympathetic nerves, 46

Symptom-directed therapy with
        medications, 420
Synthetic mesh midurethral slings, 295, 328
Synthetic transobturator slings, 395

T
Team training, 490
Teflon™, 241
Tegress™, 242
Tension-free vaginal tape procedure
        (TVT), 278
TephaFLEX™ sling, 507
Thermoablative fractional CO_2 laser, 511
3-D printing technology, 512, 513
Timed Up and Go (TUG) test, 467
Tissue engineering, 513
TOMUS trial, 344
Topical vaginal estrogen, 356
Total abdominal hysterectomy, 410
Training in mental imagery/mental
        practice, 488
Transabdominal approach, 226, 413
Transcutaneous electrical nerve stimulators
        (TENS), 167, 444
Transcutaneous neuromodulation, 444
Transcutaneous posterior tibial nerve
        stimulation (T-PTNS), 167,
        171, 172
Transdermal oxybutynin (OXY-TDS), 153
Transmasculine neophallus anatomy, 400
Transobturator based sling, 345
Transobturator midurethral sling, 320
Transurethral approach, 224, 226
Transurethral injection, 237, 394
Transurethral resection of the prostate
        (TURP), 400
Transvaginal approach, 224, 225, 360, 413
Trendelenburg position, 478
Tricyclic antidepressants, 442
Trospium, 152, 153, 158, 470
Tunable-tension transobturator tape
        (TTT), 508

U
Ultrasound, 134
Unilateral hydroureteronephrosis, 414
Ureterovaginal fistulas
        etiology, 414
        intravenous urography or CT
                urography, 415
        risk factors, 414
        treatment, 415

Ureters, 41
Urethra, 38, 40, 44
Urethral bulking, 97
Urethral bulking agents (UBAs), 235, 285,
        348, 460
        anti-incontinence procedures, 248, 249
        autologous fat, 241
        calcium hydroxylapatite, 244
        carbon-coated zirconium, 245
        cross-linked polydimethylsiloxane
                elastomer particles, 245, 246
        dextranomer with hyaluronic acid, 242
        ethylene vinyl alcohol (EVA), 242
        glutaraldehyde cross-linked (GAX)
                collagen (Contigen™), 241
        mode of action, 235, 236
        patient selection and indications, 236
        polyacrylamide hydrogel, 246, 247
        polydimethylsiloxane, 247, 248
        polytetrafluoroethylene, 241
        porcine collagen, 244
        procedural aspects and injection
                techniques, 236
                comparison of injection methods,
                        239, 240
                device-guided injection, 238
                periurethral injection, 237
                post-operative recommendations and
                        findings, 238
                transurethral injection, 237
        as salvage procedure after failed MUS,
                249, 250
        sclerosing agent, 241
Urethral closure pressure, 40
Urethral continence mechanisms, 388
Urethral diverticula, 424
Urethral diverticula surgery, 423
Urethral diverticulum/vaginal cyst, 421, 422
Urethral erosion and vaginal extrusion, 309
Urethral hypermobility and ISD, 296
Urethral mechanics, 296–298
Urethrocutaneous fistula, 401
Urethrolysis, 309, 324
Urethrovaginal fistulas, 416, 417
Urge suppression, 137
Urgency urinary incontinence (UUI), 13,
        147, 165
        bladder neck closure
                indications and methods, 223, 224
                transabdominal approach, 226
                transurethral approach, 226
                transvaginal approach, 224
                transvaginal approach, 224, 225
        in female adolescents, 433

SP catheter placement, 221
  endoscopic placement of, 222
  percutaneous procedure, 221, 222
  surgical placement of, 223
  urinary diversion, simple cystectomy with
    conduit, 227–229
Urinalysis, 438
Urinary bladder, 37, 38
Urinary diversion, 387
  salvage treatment, 461
  simple cystectomy with conduit, 227–229
Urinary fistula, treatment of, 411
Urinary incontinence (UI), 51, 455
  by age, rates of, 6
  cost of, 11–13
  definition of, 3, 4
  diagnosis
    advance testing, 56–58
    non-invasive tests, 54, 56
  differential diagnosis, 51, 52
  epidemiological studies in, 5
  history and physical examination, 52–54
  in older pediatric/adolescent female
    congenital causes, 435, 436
    escalating treatment, 439
    evaluation of, 437
    prevalence, 430
    prevalence of, 429–431
    under-recognized entity, 429
  prevention
    during pregnancy and postpartum,
      128, 129
    in older women, 128
  primary prevention, 128
  by race/ethnicity, rates of, 6, 7
  rates of, 4
  risk factors for, 7
    age, 8
    CLD, 11
    constipation, 10
    diabetes mellitus, 11
    family history, 8
    obesity, 10
    parity and mode of delivery, 8
    pelvic pain, 11
    pelvic surgery, 9
    physical activity, 9
    smoking, 9
  social disparities in female pelvic floor
    disorders, 13, 14
Urinary microbiome, 498
Urinary retention, 310
Urinary tract, 48
Urinary tract erosion, 331–332

Urinary tract fistulas, 408, 424
  etiology of, 409
Urinary tract infection (UTI), 326
Urodynamic evaluation, 457
Urodynamic studies (UDS), 129, 379
Urodynamic testing, 379
Urodynamics, 347, 456, 457
  anatomic diagnoses seen on
    fluoroscopy, 78–80
  antibiotics and patient preparation
    for, 66–68
  bladder outflow obstruction
    (BOO), 75–77
  detrusor overactivity, 72, 73
  detrusor underactivity, 73–75
  diagnosis, 70
  NGB safety/poor compliance, 77, 78
  pad tests, 64
  post void residual (PVR), 63
  principles of, 61, 62
  simple cystometric test, 65
  SUI, 71, 72
  systematic interpretation of, 68–70
  testing and interpretation, 65, 66
  uroflowmetry, 63, 64
  voiding diaries, 63
Uroflowmetry, 63, 64, 439
Urolastic™, 238, 247, 248
Urotherapy, 439–441
Uryx™, 242
Uterine artery, 43
Uterine supports, 30, 31
Uterosacral ligaments, 31
Uterus, 36

V
Vagina, 44
Vaginal and urethral devices, 129–132
Vaginal artery, 43
Vaginal delivery, 372
Vaginal digital palpation, 132
Vaginal dissection, 300–301
Vaginal hysterectomy, 410
Vaginal mesh exposure and
  extrusion, 328–330
Vaginal mesh in prolapse repair, 378
Vaginectomy and neourethral
  reconstruction, 401
Valsalva leak point pressure (VLPP), 70
Venous, 44, 45
Vesair intravesical balloon, 511
Vesicoureteric reflux (VUR), 37
Vesicouterine fistulas, 418, 419

Vesicovaginal fistula (VVF), 407
   diagnosis and localization, 411
   physical and psychological impact, 410
   pressure necrosis and tissue loss, 408–410
   prolonged obstructed labor, 407
   radiation therapy, 410
   signs and symptoms, 410
   vaginal or perivaginal tissue, 410
Vibegron, 156, 498, 499
Videourodynamics, 308, 345
Voiding, definition of, 22
Voiding cystourethrography (VCUG), 411
Voiding diaries, 63
Voiding dysfunction, 307, 344

W
Women's Health Initiative, 5
Work-related musculoskeletal
   pain, 487
Workstation optimization, 486
Wound infections, 326

X
Xeomin, 195, 196

Z
Zuidex, 242